Relearning to See

Relearning to See

Thomas R. Quackenbush

North Atlantic Books
Berkeley, California

This book is solely educational and informational in nature. The reader of this book agrees that the reader, author, and publisher have not formed a professional, or any other, relationship. The reader assumes full responsibility for any changes or lack of changes experienced due to the reading of this book. The reader also assumes full responsibility for choosing to do any of the activities mentioned in this book. The author and publisher are not liable for any use or misuse of the information contained herein.

The educational information in this book is not intended for diagnosis, prescription, determination of function, or treatment of any eye conditions or diseases or any health disorder whatsoever. Readers and students of the Bates method are advised to have an eye doctor monitor their eyesight. The information in this book should not be used as a replacement for proper medical or optometric care.

Any person with disease, pathologies, or accidents of the eyes should be under the care of an eye doctor, and consult with the eye doctor before doing any activity in this book.

Relearning to See

Published by Frog, Ltd.

Frog, Ltd. books are distributed by
North Atlantic Books
P.O. Box 12327
Berkeley, California 94712

Cover photo licensed from PhotoDisc
Cover and book design by Catherine Campaigne

Printed in the United States of America

Library of Congress Cataloging-in-Publication Data

Quackenbush, Thomas R. 1952–
Relearning to see / Thomas R. Quackenbush.
p. cm.
Includes bibliographical references and index.
ISBN 1-55643-205-4
1. Orthoptics. 2. Eye—Care and hygiene.
I. Title.
RE992.07Q33 1997
817.7—dc21 96-54600
CIP

1 2 3 4 5 6 7 8 9 / 01 00 99 98 97

PERMISSIONS

The following individuals and organizations kindly granted permission to use their works in this book:

- "Vision," from the artist Gail E. Hargrove, Edu-Kinesthetics, Inc., Ventura, CA.
- "Scientific Assumptions of the Empirical and Rational Schools of Health and Healing" from "The Health Care Contract: A Model For Sharing Responsibility" from Jerry Green, Mill Valley, CA.
- "Spectral Power Distribution Curves" from GE Lighting, a division of General Electric Company, Cleveland, OH.
- Quotations from *The New Species* from Chérie Carter-Scott of The MMS Institute, Santa Barbara, CA.
- Quotations from *Inside Mac Games* from Tuncer Deniz, Glenview, IL.
- The author's [TQ] photographs of model Lynn Kahn beginning with the "The Sway" from Lynn Kahn.
- "BodyShots"™ Business Images ©1994 from Digital Wisdom Inc., Tappahannock, VA.
- The author's [TQ] photographs of *M.S. Dixie II* boat from Travel Systems, Zephyr Cove, NV.
- Text and images from *Perfect Sight Without Glasses*, ©1920 by William H. Bates, from Henry Holt and Company, Inc., New York.
- "Out of the Night" poem from Adam Schwartz.
- Graph from *The Science of Homeopathy* from Grove Press, Inc., New York.
- "Chart to Iridology" from Bernard Jensen, D.C., Ph.D., Escondido, CA.
- "Health Returns in Cycles" from Share International, Inc., Fort Worth, TX.
- "ClickArt" images from T/Maker® Co., Mountain View, CA.
- "Evolution," from Nevin Berger (Eli) of Laughing Trout, Albany, CA.
- Quotes from the "General Chuck Yeager Air Combat" manual ©1993 from Electronic Arts, Mountain View, CA.
- "Dancer" from Terry Schmidbauer Illustration, Lake Zurich, IL.
- "Georgia's View of Health" from Georgia Dow.
- Artwork "Relaxation," "Movement," "The Three B's," "A Buoy," and "The Three Seeing Mice" from Annie Buttons.
- "Suzie Q's Red Eyes" from Suzie, Bill, and Laura Quackenbush.
- Images from LifeART Super Anatomy 1–4, and Imaging 1, ©1991–95, from TechPool Studios Inc., Cleveland, OH.
- Image of "Ott-Lite" from Environmental Lighting Concepts, Inc., Tampa, FL.
- Images from Photo Pro™, Vol. 1–3, from Wayzata Technologies, Inc., Grand Rapids, MN.
- Images from "©1994 PhotoLab®" from Creative Data, Inc., Scottsdale, AZ.
- Images from PhotoDisc ©1994, Seattle, WA.
- Images from "Art Explosion 40,000 Images" from Nova Development Corp., Calabasas, CA.
- "Cosmosis" Art Stone images from Jim Quackenbush.
- Images from "PowerPhotos™, Series I" from Metatools™, Inc., Carpinteria, CA.
- Images from "Color Digital Photos, Paramount" from Seattle Support Group, Kent, WA.
- Images from "MediaClips™," ©Aris Multimedia Entertainment, Inc. 1994, Marina del Rey, CA.

DEDICATION

William H. Bates, M.D. (1860–1931)

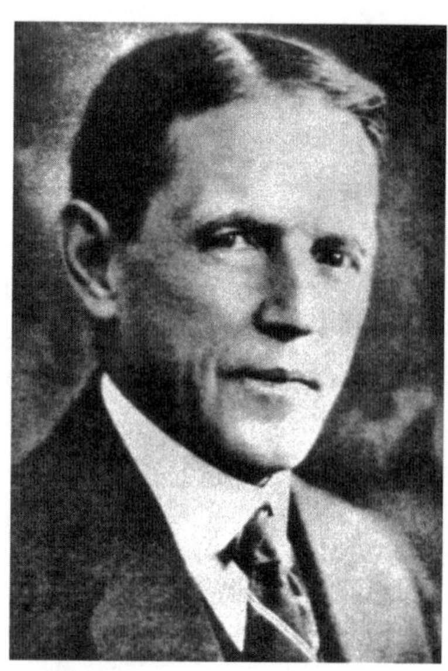

This book is dedicated to ophthalmologist Dr. William H. Bates, M.D., who discovered the principles and habits of natural, clear vision.

ACKNOWLEDGMENTS

I gratefully acknowledge my teachers Janet Goodrich, Ph.D., and the late Anna Kaye, who have gifted me with the knowledge and joy of the Bates method of natural vision improvement.

I acknowledge all of the wonderful students I have taught since 1983. They have enriched my life and work immeasurably, and have also been my teachers.

I wish to express appreciation to Kathy Glass for her monumental editing work and outstanding suggestions for making this a better book.

I also acknowledge Catherine Campaigne for her expert designing advice and patience, and the staff at North Atlantic Books for guiding this author through a maze of variables in order to successfully complete this work.

Thanks especially to my parents for all their support of my work.

Table of Contents

List of Illustrations

* Graphic not shown.

* Graphic not shown.

List of Plates

Introduction

Most people in this society obtain glasses or contact lenses when their eyesight becomes blurred. These crutches, or "machines of seeing," are not necessary. Nor are they natural. "Corrective" lenses do not correct the real problem. A person wearing glasses or contact lenses still has blurred vision.

Ophthalmologist Dr. William H. Bates, M.D. (1860–1931), discovered the principles and habits underlying natural eyesight. Concurrently, Bates discovered the interferences to normal sight. Bates then taught students to stop interfering with their clear vision; they were literally relearning to see.

Bates rejected contemporary theories about blurred vision because he found too much evidence in his practice as an ophthalmologist that contradicted them. Bates' decades of research on natural vision and the real causes of nearsightedness, farsightedness, astigmatism, crossed eyes, and many other vision problems went far beyond the ideas of his contemporaries. Today, most orthodox vision specialists still do not support his discoveries. Unfortunately, Bates was forced to leave his teaching post as instructor of ophthalmology at the New York Post-Graduate Medical School and Hospital and was ostracized from the conventional medical community because of his revolutionary discoveries.

Someone once asked Bates what technique he was using. Bates' reply was that he did not use any technique, but if it was a technique, it would be *nature's* technique. Bates wrote in his June 1923 *Better Eyesight* magazine, "... my methods are the methods employed by the normal eye."

Blurred vision is a message from the mind and body that a person's visual system is out of balance with nature.

Clarity is a connection; blur is a disconnection. Blur is created primarily in the mind; it is much more a disconnection from ourselves than from the world. The processes involved in improving eyesight naturally are an opportunity to reconnect with ourselves. The Bates educational method is an opportunity for internal change.

The great majority of attendees at my introductory lectures say they have seen their vision improve spontaneously. Vision fluctuates for all people. For many people in industrialized societies, sight generally becomes worse over time. Yet sometimes people see better. Most people know, either intuitively or experientially, that there is a way to improve their sight.

How is it people accept a theory that says blurry sight is due to old age when many people—especially in non-industrialized cultures—have excellent eyesight at 40, 50, 60, 70, 80, and even 90 years of age? The idea that age and genetics determine blurry vision is also contradicted by the fact that many students have improved their sight by relearning correct vision habits. And, I have watched many children improve their vision along with their parents in my classes.

Many people experience a lowering of their sight during a period of high stress. Bates showed that when vision (excluding pathologies) lowers, it is due to acquiring incorrect vision habits. When vision improves, it is due to the person relearning relaxed vision habits. Relaxation is the key to normal, clear sight.

Broken bones heal. Burns and cuts heal. Stomach aches get better. Are we to believe that eyesight, the most important sense perception we have and one that has evolved over millions of years, is the only part of the human body that cannot heal itself? Are artificial glasses, contact lenses, drugs, and surgeries the only solutions to the functional vision problems, including nearsightedness, farsightedness, astigmatism and strabismus? Bates concluded the answer was "no."

Personally, I had several good reasons to pursue the possibility of improving my sight: 1) I suffered physically from wearing heavy glasses and painful contact lenses every day; 2) I began to experience improvement in all parts of my health once I began receiving natural healing and education from many holistic health practitioners. Could vision improvement be the only natural healing process I investigated that did not work? 3) I experienced a dramatic improvement in my eyesight for approximately one hour while participating in a stress reduction program; this occurred *before* I knew about the Bates method. So, I knew there was a way vision could improve naturally.

In the beginning, I read several eyesight improvement books. I did all of the "exercises" and "drills," but did not notice any improvement. Looking back, I realize I had almost no real understanding of the Bates method. The processes—especially the more subtle aspects—are difficult to understand from books. I had continuing improvement of my eyesight only after receiving instructions from a Bates teacher.

Contrary to popular belief, the Bates method is not *about* "eye exercises." Many natural eyesight improvement books present this topic in a relatively ineffective, left-hemisphere eye exercise manner. This issue is discussed further in Chapter 19, "Brains and Vision." Since vision is primarily a right-hemisphere activity, lessons are best presented in an integrative, holistic manner, with the emphasis on the correct vision habits (or skills) to be used automatically and subconsciously our entire lifetime.

Along with improvement of clarity, many *qualities* of the vision system improve, e.g., color brightness and variations, contrast, spatial/depth perception, and texture awareness. There is a high correlation between memory and concentration improvement and natural eyesight improvement.

Since poor vision habits strain the neck and shoulders, no one is truly healthy who has blurred sight.

Many of the important writings by Bates

are in his original 1920 book *Perfect Sight Without Glasses* and his monthly *Better Eyesight* magazine. A good deal of this material is reproduced and discussed in the present book. All indented quotations from *Perfect Sight Without Glasses* and the *Better Eyesight* magazines are indicated by vertical lines along the left and right sides. All material quoted from the *Better Eyesight* magazines are from Bates, unless otherwise noted.

I have watched eyesight improve naturally with hundreds of students from 1983 to 1997. Many of my students have freed themselves from glasses or have prevented moving into wearing glasses in the first place. If you are interested in vision re-education, study this book and other books on natural eyesight improvement to learn and apply as much as you are able; better yet, find a Bates teacher who understands and can teach you the key habits and principles of natural vision. Then, discover the joys and rewards of relearning to see—naturally. As the original jacket of Aldous Huxley's book *The Art of Seeing* says, this process of improving vision is "An Adventure in Re-education."

A few more notes are necessary before beginning this book.

Because Dr. Bates was a medical doctor and eye surgeon (ophthalmologist), and because much of his work is discussed in this book, some terms used herein are medical. After Bates died in 1931, his wife Emily and other Natural Vision teachers have taught the "Bates method" in an educational manner. The Bates method, as presented in this book, is solely educational in nature—it is not medical or optometric.

Since most Bates method teachers are not eye doctors, some words in Bates' original text, and in some other quoted materials, have been changed or modified to reflect the educational nature of the modern Bates method. As an example, the term "patient" has often been changed to "person" or "student." Such changes are not necessarily indicated in this book.

The term "blur" as used in this book refers to nearsightedness, farsightedness, presbyopia, or astigmatism as determined by an eye doctor. Some individuals have eye damage due to accidents or diseases, and the term "blur" as used in this book does *not* refer to such conditions. Such individuals should seek the care of an eye doctor. All vision problems referred to in this book do *not* refer to any type of pathology or disease unless specifically stated.

The case histories of my students in this book are true, but most of their names have been changed and/or abbreviated.

PART ONE

Fundamentals

Chapter One

Relearning to See

This book presents a formal, educational approach to improving vision naturally. This approach was discovered by ophthalmologist William H. Bates, M.D.

First, we study basic anatomy of the eye. Next, we gain an understanding of prescription glasses. Then, we explore the research of Bates.

Understanding the cause of, and the solution to, blurred vision has been helpful to many students. With sufficient knowledge, students can not only take measures to improve their vision, but often become highly motivated and enthusiastic about the process of relearning to see naturally.

Then we study the three key principles underlying natural, clear sight—movement, centralization, and relaxation. The student who desires to return to natural, clear vision will need to re-establish the same correct principles of seeing he learned automatically and subconsciously early in life.

Next we explore the three habits of natural seeing—sketching (shifting), breathing, and blinking. These habits are based on the three principles of vision.

Practicing correct vision habits removes the incorrect habits which created the blurred vision. Bates referred to the incorrect habits as "interferences" to normal, clear vision. Strained vision habits create nearsightedness, farsightedness, astigmatism, and many other vision problems. What the natural vision student is *un*learning is more the issue than what the student is relearning.

As the student relearns natural vision habits, a "spotlight" begins to shine on the areas of his life that are out of balance—at least those associated with incorrect vision habits. Correct vision habits are often associated with correct living habits. For some, the interferences may be poor posture or an unhealthy diet. For others the interferences may be overwork, fatigue, accidents, traumas, unhealthy attitudes, boredom, and so on.

If during a period of stress, a person interferes with the normal, relaxed habits of vision given to him by nature, the vision will lower. The principles and habits of natural vision were clearly identified by Bates.

Today we have an even better appreciation of his discoveries, because of advancements in our knowledge of the function of the mind and the body—especially right-brain/

left-brain concepts. The idea that blurred vision is only one of the many harmful consequences of living in an imbalanced, highly left-brain oriented society is explored in Chapter 19, "Brains and Vision," and Chapter 20, "The Two Sides of Health and Healing."

Natural vision education is part of a larger holistic movement in which many people in this society are seeking—and finding—solutions to many health problems—problems they have been told by the orthodox cannot improve. More and more people are moving away from artificial solutions to health problems, and seeking out a balance with nature. Normal sight is a reflection of a person's balance with nature.

Chapter Two

Anatomy

Studying the structure and functions of the various parts of the visual system is helpful in understanding how to use our vision in the naturally correct way.

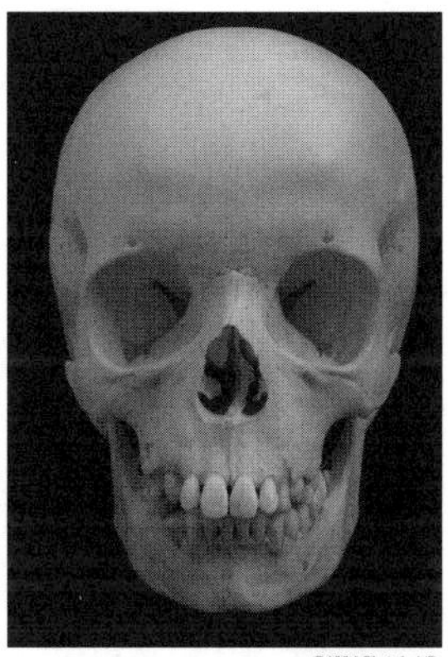

Figure 2–1: The Skull.

THE EYE ORBIT

The bony structure of the *eye orbit,* along with the fatty tissue surrounding the eye, protect the back and sides of the eye.

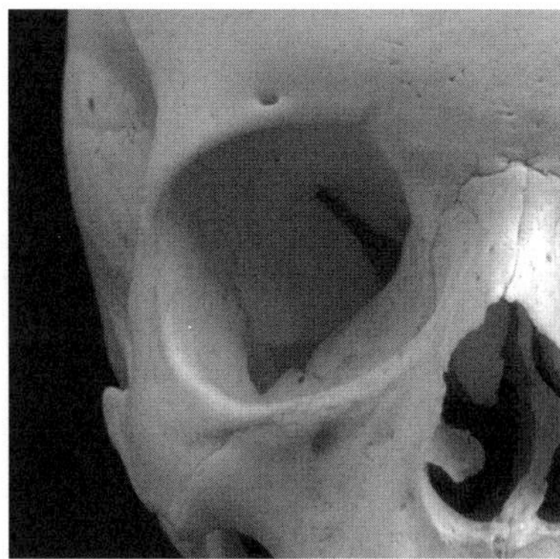

Figure 2–2: The Eye Orbit.

THE EYEBALL

See *Plate 1: The Eye.*

As the human embryo develops, two protrusions extend forward from the brain. The long, thin portions become the optic nerves, and the bulbs at the ends become the two eyeballs. Nerves from the brain travel through the optic nerve and "fan out" throughout the retina. The eyeball is literally an extension of the brain—a "mini-brain."

The *eyeball* is a soft round sphere filled with liquid. It grows from approximately 1.6 cm (about ⅔ inch) in diameter at birth to 2.3 cm at age three. Its diameter is about 2.4 cm at age thirteen and older—about the size of a ping-pong ball (1 inch = 2.54 cm).

THE THREE LAYERS OF THE EYE

See *Plate 2: The Three Layers of the Eye.*

The eye can be classified into three basic groups:

1. The three layers of the eye: The outer layer consists of the sclera and cornea; the middle layer consists of the choroid, ciliary body, lens, and iris; and the inner layer consists of the visual and non-visual portions of the retina.
2. The fluids and chambers of the eye: The anterior and posterior chambers are filled with aqueous humor; and the vitreous chamber is filled with vitreous humor.
3. The external parts of the eye: the optic nerve, eyelids and tear glands, and the six external muscles.

The Outer Layer: Sclera and Cornea

The Sclera

The *sclera* (pronounced skleh'-rah; from the Greek *skleros,* meaning "hard") is the eye's protective, leather-like outer layer. It is strong, thick, and opaque. This "white of the eyes" covers about ⅚ of the outer surface of the eyeball.

The Cornea

The clear, crystalline front of the eye is called the *cornea* (from the Latin *corneus,* meaning "horn-like"). The hard, tough cornea is the part of the sclera that has become transparent, and it allows light to enter the eye. The cornea bulges forward in a dome-like shape. In adults the cornea is about one-half inch in diameter—a little smaller than the size of a dime—and covers the remaining ⅙ of the eye's outer surface. The cornea consists of several dozen layers of epithelial cells, which are like the sheets of glass used to make safety glass in automobiles.

Because blood vessels are excluded from the cornea, light can pass through it more perfectly to the retina. The cornea receives nutrients on its inner surface from the *aqueous humor,* on its outer surface from tears and oxygen from the air, and along its circumference from blood vessels in the sclera.

The cornea is a convex lens and accounts for 80% of the curvature needed to focus light rays onto the retina. By bending light rays inward, the cornea and lens shrink the large image of the world down to the size of a nickel onto the retina.

The Middle Layer: Choroid, Ciliary Body, Lens, and Iris

The Choroid

The *choroid* lies between the sclera and the retina. The choroid consists of many blood vessels and provides nutrients to the entire eye, but especially to the retina.

The choroid is discussed further in Chapter 17, "The Retina."

The *ora serrata* is the notched junction between the choroid and the ciliary body.

The Ciliary Body

The ciliary body is a highly vascularized, enlarged continuation of the choroid that encircles the lens.

Within the ciliary body is the ciliary process, which produces aqueous humor. Suspensory ligaments extend between the ciliary process and the lens capsule, 360° around the lens.

The ciliary body contains a circular (parasympathetic) ciliary muscle, and a meridional-radial (sympathetic) ciliary muscle. The contraction of the circular muscle decreases the circumference of the ciliary body, like the narrowing of the iris in bright light. The contraction of the radial muscle expands the ciliary body, like the enlarging of the iris in dim light.

Most orthodox books on eyesight state that the contraction and expansion of the internal ciliary muscle changes the shape of the front side of the lens to give it more and less curvature, respectively. More on this theory in later chapters.

The Lens

Behind the iris and in front of the vitreous body lies the double convex, transparent *lens*. The front side of this "living crystal" touches the back side of the iris and is nourished by the aqueous humor. The back side of the lens contacts the vitreous body.

The lens is enclosed in a transparent membrane called the elastic capsule. The *suspensory ligaments* between the lens capsule and the ciliary body "suspend" the lens vertically, behind the iris.

The lens is composed of many microscopic, onion-skin-like layers, and accounts for the remaining 20% of the curvature needed to focus light rays onto the retina.

The lens grows slowly each year due to a constant addition of external layers. The older, inner layers, which cannot be absorbed or discarded, are compressed in the middle of the lens. The lens doubles in size between the ages of 20 and 80.

Orthodox textbooks state that the hardening of the lens into a relatively flat shape is the reason many people lose their ability to see clearly up close around age 40; this is called *presbyopia*, or "old-age" sight.

Theories of the role of the lens are discussed more in later chapters.

The Iris

In front of the lens lies the *iris*. The iris is a colored (pigmented), circular, and variable diaphragm. A pupillary sphincter muscle along the inner circumference of the iris surrounds the *pupil*. When the pupillary sphincter muscle contracts, the pupil becomes smaller. When the dilator muscle contracts, the pupil becomes larger. The pupil is not a physical structure; it is an opening in the center of the iris, through which light enters the eye.

The iris regulates the amount and distribution of light entering the eyeball. In the brightest light, the diameter of the pupil is about 1.5 mm (with an area of only 2 mm^2); in very low levels of light, the diameter expands to about 9 mm (with an area of 64 mm^2); the average diameter is about 4 mm (with an area of 13 mm^2).

Changes in the pupil size can easily be observed in a mirror while turning a light on and off; the iris constricts and dilates, respectively. The pupil normally appears black because most of the light entering the eyeball is absorbed by the retina and choroid. Very little light is reflected out through the pupil.

See *Plate 3: Suzie Q's Red Eyes.* Red pupils appear in some photographs. In dim light, the pupil is large. When the high-intensity bulb on the camera flashes, a lot of light enters the eye. The retina glows red because lights reflects from the blood vessels in the retina and choroid.

Modern cameras have been able to reduce "red eyes" by turning on a special "red-eye reduction lamp" before the picture is taken. The pupil has a chance to contract small and thus much less light enters the eye. The result is a picture with a normal, black pupil.

The Inner Layer: The Retina

The retina is the inner third layer, covering about 95% (back, sides, and part of the front) of the interior surface of the eye. The entire eyeball is designed for the retina.

There are two parts of the retina: the visual and non-visual portions.

The Visual Portion of the Retina

The rear 70% of the retina contains light receptors, called cones and rods.

The design of the visual portion of the retina is discussed in great detail in Chapter 17, "The Retina."

The Non-Visual Portion of the Retina

The other 30% of the retina, the non-visual portion, extends forward from the visual portion at the *ora serrata,* along the back part of the ciliary process and the back side of the iris up to the pupil. There are no light receptors in the non-visual portion of the retina.

THE FLUIDS AND CHAMBERS OF THE EYE

Aqueous Humor, and the Anterior and Posterior Chambers

See *Plate 4: Aqueous Humor.*

The anterior chamber lies between the back (inner) side of the cornea and the front side of the iris. The much smaller posterior chamber lies between the back side of the iris and the lens, lens capsule, suspensory ligaments, and ciliary body.

These two chambers contain *aqueous humor,* which means "watery fluid." Aqueous humor supplies the cornea and the lens with nutrients. Aqueous humor is referred to by an ophthalmologist consultant as "clear blood."

Aqueous humor is produced by the ciliary process and secreted into the posterior chamber. From there, it travels slowly around the iris through the pupil into the larger anterior chamber. The entire volume of the aqueous humor is replenished every hour. The aqueous humor's pressure helps maintain the cornea's convex shape.

Aqueous humor also "percolates" from the posterior chamber into the vitreous chamber.

Excess aqueous humor, along with dead cornea cells, drains away through the Canal of Schlemm, which encircles the cornea. The Canal of Schlemm discharges these fluids and cells into veins.

Vitreous Humor and Chamber

The *vitreous chamber* lies behind the lens and comprises the majority of the volume of the eye. It is almost completely surrounded by the visual portion of the retina. Filling the vitreous chamber is a "jelly-like" clear liquid called the *vitreous humor.*

Positive intraocular pressure created by the vitreous humor helps hold the rear four-fifths of the eye in its round shape.

THE EXTERNAL PARTS OF THE EYE

The external parts of the eye consist of the optic nerve, eyelids and tear glands, and the six external (extrinsic) muscles.

The eye socket is lined with fatty tissue which: 1) cushions the eye from blows to the head; 2) lubricates the continually moving eyeball; and 3) provides warmth.

The Optic Nerve

The optic nerve is the second cranial nerve and the second-largest nerve in the human body. This nerve transmits the signals from the 137 million light receptors in the retina to the brain. The central nervous system is directly exposed to light stimulation via the retina and optic nerve—the only part of the human body where this occurs.

The Eyelids and Tear Glands

The eyelids and tear glands are discussed in Chapter 14, "The Third Habit—Blinking."

The Six External Muscles

See *Plate 5: The Six External Eye Muscles.*

There are six external (extrinsic) muscles around each eye. One end of each muscle attaches to the sclera, while the other end attaches to the eye orbit.

The eye muscles are very powerful. Comparing on a weight basis, the eye muscles are some of the strongest in the human body.

The top (superior) and bottom (inferior) oblique muscles wrap over the top and bottom of the eye, respectively. They form almost a complete belt wrapping around the eyeball. The superior oblique muscle passes through a small loop called the *trochlea.* The trochlea is located at the inner, upper, forward part of the eye orbit.

The four external recti muscles are attached to the top (superior), bottom (inferior), outer (lateral), and inner (medial) parts of the eye. When contracting, a rectus muscle shortens and pulls backward on the part of the eye where it is attached. For example, when the superior rectus muscle contracts, the eye rotates upward. When the medial rectus muscle contracts, the eye rotates inward, and so on.

Much of Bates' research was directed toward the role of these muscles in errors of refraction and accommodation.

Chapter Three

Understanding Lenses and Prescriptions

In this chapter we discuss various types of refractive, or "corrective," lenses that are commonly used in prescription glasses and contact lenses. In this book, the term "lense" refers to an artificial lense, while "lens" refers to the natural lens inside the eye.

FOUR TYPES OF REFRACTIVE LENSES

Figure 3–1 shows a plano lense and four types of refractive, or "corrective," lenses commonly used in glasses or contact lenses—concave, convex, cylindrical, and prismatic.

Of course, the term "corrective" does not mean that the lense corrects the *cause* of the vision problem; only the angle of light rays entering the eyes changes. As Bates stated, "corrective" lenses are more correctly referred to as "compensating" lenses.

Figure a shows a *plano* lense. Since a plano lense has no curvature, parallel light rays continue in straight paths through the lense; it is not really a "corrective" lense. A plano lense has no focal point. Notice the image seen through the lense on the right is the same as the original image on the left.

Plano lenses are often used in safety glasses to protect the eyes from injury. They are also used for cosmetic reasons. For example, if one eye has no sight, but the other eye uses a corrective lense, a plano lense can be placed in glasses in front of the sightless eye.

Figure b–1 shows a double *concave* lense, which can compensate for the refractive error in nearsightedness. A double concave lense is a *diverging* lense because the light rays "spread out" after passing through the lense. A diverging lense has a "virtual" focal point in front of the lense.

A meniscus lense is concave on one side and convex on the other. Notice how the front side of the meniscus lense in *Figure b–2* is convex, while the back side has a higher degree of concavity. This type of meniscus lense is a diverging lense. Contact lenses are often meniscus lenses.

In glasses for nearsightedness, a meniscus lense is usually used in place of a single or double concave lense, mainly for cosmetic reasons.

Figure c shows a double *convex* lense, which can compensate for the refractive error in farsightedness. A convex lense is a

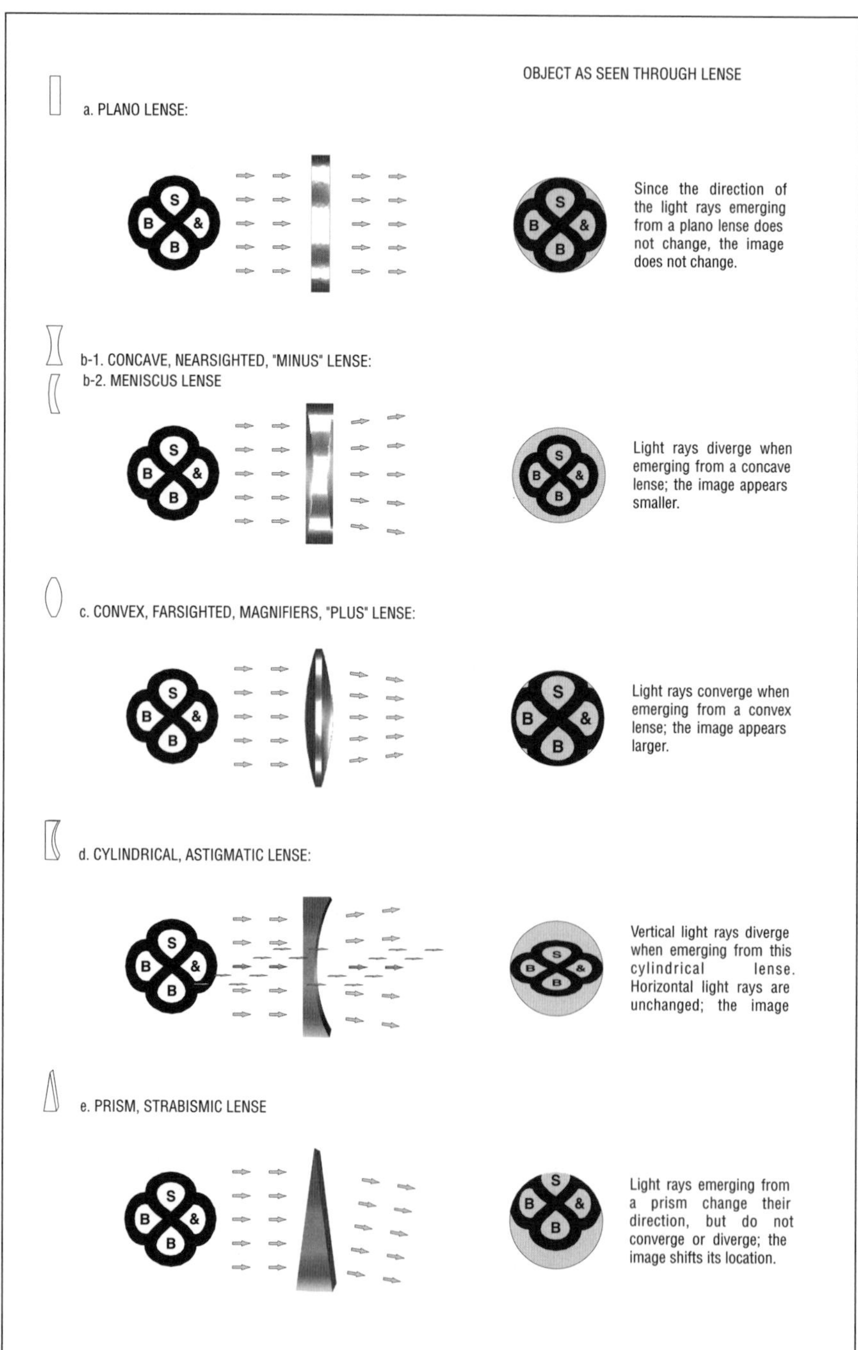

Figure 3–1: Four Types of Refractive Lenses.

converging lense because light rays converge to a point after passing through the lense. A converging lense has a focal point beyond the lense.

Figure d shows a *cylindrical* lense, which can compensate for the refractive error in astigmatism.

Figure e shows a *prismatic* lense, which can compensate for an eye with strabismus.

Glasses can have more than one "correction" combined into one lense. For example, a lense can be both diverging and cylindrical, compensating for nearsightedness and astigmatism.

UNDERSTANDING LENSES: DIOPTER, AXIS, AND BASE

DIOPTERS

A *diopter*, abbreviated "D," is a unit of measurement of the refractive power of a concave, convex, or cylindrical lense. The number of diopters indicates the light-bending ability of a lense. The more diopters, the more refractive power of a lense, and, generally, the more curvature in a lense.

When parallel light rays pass from air through a curved piece of glass or other transparent material, they change direction. When parallel light rays pass through a convex lense, the rays converge to a *focal point* at some distance beyond the lense. This distance, measured in meters, is called the *focal length*. The greater the curvature of the lense, the greater the change in direction of the emerging light rays, and the shorter the focal length.

Since it is convenient to have a system of measurement in which a lense with a higher refractive power corresponds to a higher value, the dioptric system was created. The mathematical definition of a diopter is the reciprocal (or inverse) of the focal length in meters.

When parallel light rays from a distant object travel through a typical (plano) window in a home, the light rays simply continue straight through—without changing direction. Diopters do not apply to plano lenses because there is no focal point.

Most corrective lenses are made in multiples of 0.25 D—for example, 0.50 D, 1.25 D, and 3.75 D. Some lenses are made in 0.125 D increments. A total correction of less than 0.25 D in one eye is seldom prescribed.

DIOPTERS AND DIVERGING LENSES

A diverging lense with a small amount of curvature and a long focal length of –2 meters is a –0.50 D lense; 1 ÷ –2 meters = –0.50 D.

The minus sign in front of the 0.50 D indicates there is a *virtual* focal point located in front of the diverging lense. Since parallel light rays emerging from a concave lense diverge, there is no focal point beyond the lense. However, there is a virtual focal point located in front of the lense. This focal point is determined by drawing rays in the opposite direction of the diverging rays, so that they converge at a point in front of the lense. Since the focal length is in the opposite direction of the direction of original light rays, the number of meters has a minus sign in front of it.

A diverging lense that has a little more curvature with a shorter focal length of –1 meter is a –1.00 D lense; 1 ÷ –1 meter = –1.00 D. A diverging lense that has much greater curvature with a much shorter focal length of –⅙ meter is a –6.00 D lense; 1 ÷ –⅙ meter = –6.00 D.

The nearsighted eye is too long from front to back. A "–" diverging lense is used to focus light rays farther back into the eyeball, onto the retina.

Some materials have a higher *index of refraction* than others. Therefore, a lense with a high index of refraction and low curvature may have the same refractive power as a lense with a low index of refraction and a high curvature. Lenses with a high index of refraction are sometimes used in glasses for people with high errors of refraction, i.e., very blurred vision. The thinner lenses are lighter and cosmetically pleasing. However, some people have difficulty adjusting to them.

Diopters and Converging Lenses

A converging lense with a small amount of curvature and a long focal length of 2 meters is a +0.50 D lense; 1 ÷ 2 meters = +0.50 D.

The plus sign indicates the focal point is beyond the converging lense.

A converging lense that has a little more curvature with a focal length of 1 meter is a +1.00 D lense; 1 ÷ 1 meter = +1.00 D. A much stronger convex lense with a focal length of only ⅕ meter is a +5.00 D lense; 1 ÷ ⅕ meter = +5.00 D.

The farsighted eyeball is too short from front to back. A converging lense is used to focus light rays closer to the front of the eye, onto the retina. Glasses made with converging lenses are often called "magnifiers" or "readers."

Diopters and Cylindrical Lenses

Diverging and converging lenses have equal curvatures in all planes. These lenses bend light equally in all planes and bring the rays to a focal point.

A cylindrical lense bends light rays in only one plane. Think of a lense in the shape of a can of soup that has been cut in half vertically. When a horizontal plane of parallel light rays passes through this cylindrical lense, the light rays come to a vertical "focal line" at some distance beyond the cylinder.

However, when a vertical plane of light rays passes through the same cylindrical lense, the light rays continue straight through the lense without converging. The direction of the original vertical plane of light rays is not affected by the lense.

Since a cylindrical lense brings a plane of parallel light rays to a "focal line," there is a dioptric measurement associated with the cylindrical lense. A cylindrical lense can have "+" or "–" diopters. The sign in front of cylindrical diopters is not a measure of nearsightedness or farsightedness, and it is not important for the discussion in this book. We will consider only the magnitude, or absolute value, of the number of diopters for astigmatism correction; the plus or minus sign in front of a cylinder diopter number is ignored here.

In nearsightedness and farsightedness, the eyeball is too long and too short, respectively, but it is still round from the front point of view. In astigmatism, the eyeball is oval, or lopsided, from the front point of view, like a teaspoon or football. The amount, or magnitude, of this "ovalness" is measured in the diopters.

The oval shape in astigmatism can be oriented at any angle. It can be horizontal (like a lemon lying on its side), vertical, or any other angle. The angle of astigmatism is called *axis.* The axis determines the angle, or orientation, of the cylindrical lense put into glasses that compensate for astigmatism. Axis is *not* a measure of the amount of the astigmatism—only its angle.

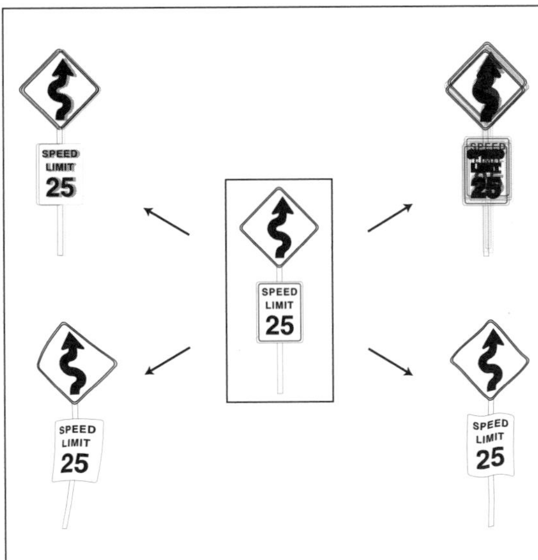

Figure 3–2: Images Distorted by Astigmatism.

the British physician Thomas Young, who did research with his own eyes between 1799 and 1801. Using a square piece of paper, Young found that horizontal lines were clear, while the vertical ones were blurry. Cylindrical lenses used to compensate for astigmatism were first used by the astronomer Airy in 1827.

Bases and Prism Lenses

A prism uniformly changes the angle of all incoming parallel light rays. The path of the light rays simply changes to a new direction. Since there is no focal point, the power of the prism is not measured in diopters.

Prism correction for strabismus is measured in units of *base,* and is indicated by the prism symbol, Δ. For example, 1^{Δ}BO, called "one prism base out," is a relatively small correction for an eye that turns slightly inward. 4^{Δ}BI, "four prism base in," is a larger correc-

In astigmatism, one plane of light can focus in back of the retina, as in farsightedness, while another plane of light can focus in front of the retina, as in nearsightedness. This is because one plane of the cornea can have too much curvature, while another plane has too little curvature.

In astigmatism, the shapes of objects at all distances or only at specific distances can be distorted. Astigmatism can also create multiple images of, or shadows around, an object.

With astigmatism, vertical lines on a piece of paper may appear to be darker or lighter than horizontal lines.

The discovery of astigmatism is attributed to

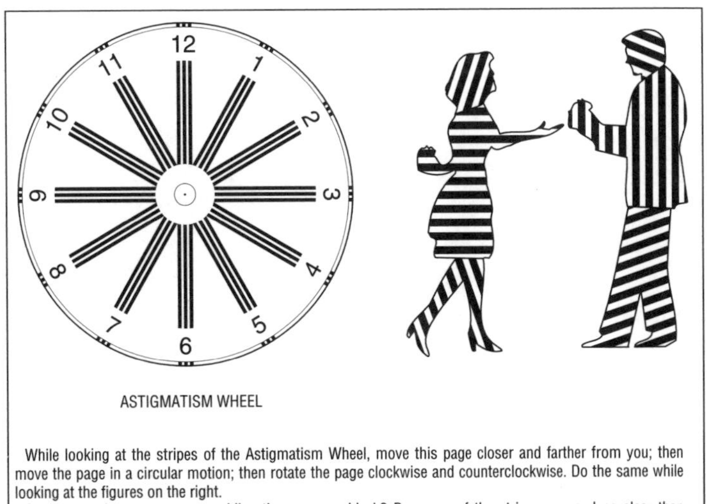

12
1
2
3
4
5
6
7
8
9
10
11
ASTIGMATISM WHEEL
While looking at the stripes of the Astigmatism Wheel, move this page closer and farther from you; then move the page in a circular motion; then rotate the page clockwise and counterclockwise. Do the same while looking at the figures on the right.
Do some stripes appear gray while others appear black? Do some of the stripes appear less clear than others? If so, you may have astigmatism.

Figure 3–3: Astigmatism Chart.

tion for an eye that turns outward. 2$^{\Delta}$BU, "two prism base up," is for an eye that turns down. 2$^{\Delta}$BD, "two prism base down," is for an eye that turns up.

Strabismus and prisms are discussed further in Chapter 18, "Stereoscopic Vision."

VISUAL ACUITY AND EYE CHARTS

Distance "20/20" Vision

In 1864, a test for visual acuity was devised by the Dutch ophthalmologist Herman Snellen. Using the sight of an anonymous young Dutch man (actually, Snellen's assistant) as his standard for normal vision, Snellen created a chart with letters on it. The "Snellen" chart was used to test the sight of children reading the chalkboard from the back of a classroom.

The Snellen chart has different-size letters on it.

A black letter E, which is ⅜" in height and width, placed twenty feet away, occupies a 5° area in the macula. The macula is the area in the center of the retina with a high concentration of cones. Cones pick up sharp detail (acuity). If the three black horizontal lines and the two horizontal white spaces in the letter E are of equal width, a horizontal stroke or white space occupies a 1° area in the center of the macula, called the fovea. The fovea contains the highest concentration of cones within the macula (and the retina). The letter E's three horizontal black strokes plus the two horizontal white spaces, at 1° each, equal 5°.

The distance of twenty feet is important, because, for all practical purposes, the eye accommodates only within the first twenty feet. If an object at twenty feet is clear, (usually) objects farther away will also be clear.

Snellen placed several ⅜" letters, like the letter E described above, in a row. Snellen's

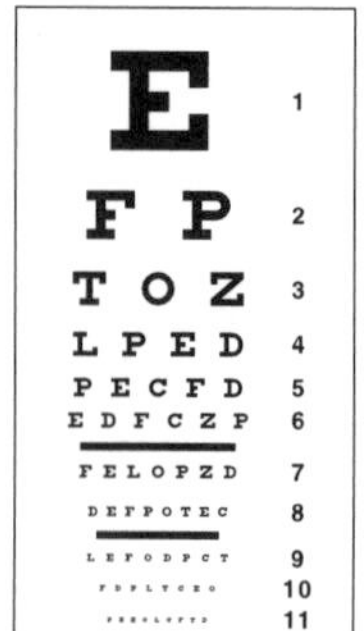

Figure 3–4: Snellen Eye Chart.

assistant could read this line, so Snellen called it the "20/20" line. When all of the letters on the 20/20 line can be read with one eye, without correction, you are said to have "normal," "perfect," or "20/20" sight for distance vision in that eye.

Larger letters on the eye chart correspond to vision less than 20/20 sight. For example, if you can read all of the ½" letters, you have at least 20/30 sight; reading the line with 11⁄16" letters is 20/40 sight. The line with a 3½" letter is 20/200. This is usually the largest (top) letter, the letter E on the Snellen chart.

If you can read all of the letters on the 20/30 line, but only most of the letters on the 20/20 line, you may have slightly less than 20/20, or $20/20^{-}$, vision. If you read all of the letters on the 20/100 line and some of the letters on the 20/80 line, you may have slightly better than 20/100 vision, or $20/100^{+}$ sight.

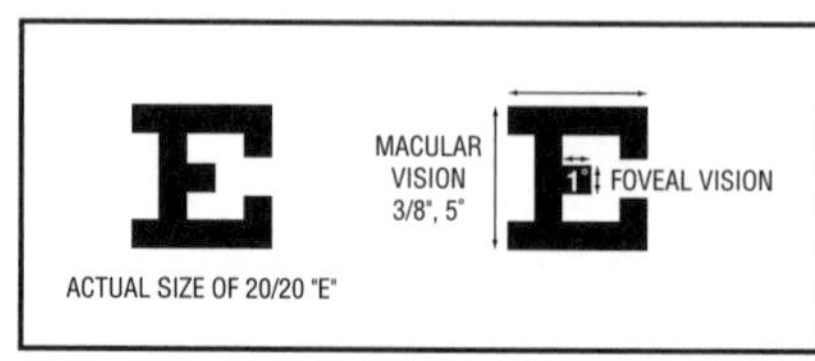

Figure 3–5: The 20/20 " E" for Distance.

What do the xx/yy Top and Bottom Numbers Refer To?

One way to think about the xx/yy numbers on an eyeglass prescription or an eye chart is to consider xx to be the number of feet a person with xx/yy vision is standing from the eye chart, while yy is the number of feet a person with 20/20 vision is standing from the same chart. Both people are looking at the same xx/yy line.

For example, a person with 20/200 sight would need to stand at twenty feet to see the same 3½" letters a person with 20/20 sight could see at 200 feet. A person with 20/40 sight would need to stand at twenty feet to see the same 11⁄16" letters a person with 20/20 sight could see at 40 feet.

Letters smaller than ⅜" on the eye chart correspond to better than 20/20 sight. For example, a person with 20/15 sight can read at twenty feet the same ¼" letters a person with 20/20 sight would need to stand at 15 feet to see. Reading the 3⁄16" letters at twenty feet is 20/10 vision; 3⁄32" letters is 20/5 vision, which is four times better than "normal" 20/20 sight. A person with 20/5 vision can see at twenty feet what a person with 20/20 sight would need to stand at 5 feet to see!

Another way to think of the xx/yy numbers is to consider the ratio: 20/20 is 1/1, or "normal" sight. 20/200 sight is 1⁄10th of 20/20 sight. 20/10 is two times better than normal sight.

How can a person see better than 20/20 if the cones in the fovea pick up the ⅜" letters? The cones in the fovea are not distributed evenly. As the center of the fovea is approached, the density (cones/mm^2) increases to it maximum density. People with superior vision have their attention in a very tiny central area—a key natural vision principle called *centralization*. This will be explained further in Chapter 17, "The Retina."

People are typically given corrective lenses that bring the eyes back to "normal" 20/20 sight, or better. The more the refractive error, the more diopters of correction are needed to let that person see 20/20 again. For example, a person with 20/40 uncorrected vision might need only –1 D to read the 20/20 line, but a person with 20/200 might need –4.00 D to read the same 20/20 line.

Height of Letter	Vision Acuity (at 20 feet)
3½"	20/200
1¾"	20/100
1¼"	20/70
⅞"	20/50
11⁄16"	20/40
½"	20/30
⅜"	**20/20**
¼"	20/15
3⁄16"	20/10
3⁄32"	20/5

***Figure 3–6:** Table for Distance Eye Chart.*

Bates offers the following suggestion to those with nearsightedness in *Perfect Sight Without Glasses:*

> It will be well . . . to have two . . . cards, one to be used at the near point, where it can be seen best, and the other at ten or twenty feet. The student will find it a great help to shift from the near card to the distant one, as the unconscious memory of the letters seen at the near point helps to bring out those seen at the distance.

The opposite approach can be used by those with farsightedness. Both approaches can be used by those with astigmatism.

There are identical Distance and Near Eye Charts in Appendix F.

Driving Requirements

20/40 sight is the driving requirement for eyesight in most states. Although 20/40 is "half" of normal sight, this is still quite functional sight. Your eye doctor can tell you the vision requirement for your state.

Bates and the Snellen Eye Chart

Here Bates discusses the limitations of testing vision with the subjective Snellen eye chart, and the advantages of objective simultaneous retinoscopy.

Quoting from *Perfect Sight Without Glasses:*

> Much of my information about the eyes has been obtained by means of simultaneous retinoscopy. The retinoscope is an instrument used to measure the refraction of the eye....
>
> This exceedingly useful instrument has possibilities which have not been generally realized by the medical profession. Most ophthalmologists depend upon the Snellen[a] card, supplemented by trial lenses, to determine whether the vision is normal or not, and to determine the degree of any abnormality that may exist. This is a slow, awkward, and unreliable method of testing the vision, and absolutely unavailable for the study of the refraction of the lower animals, of infants, and of adult human beings under the conditions of life.
>
> [a] Herman Snellen (1835–1908). Celebrated Dutch ophthalmologist, professor of ophthalmology in the University of Utrecht, and director of the Netherlandic Eye Hospital. The present standards of visual acuity were proposed by him, and his test types became the model for those now in use.
>
> The Snellen card and trial lenses can be used only under certain favorable conditions, but the retinoscope can be used anywhere. It is a little easier to use it in a dim light than in a bright one, but it may be used in any light.... It may also be used under many other unfavorable conditions.
>
> It takes a considerable time, varying from minutes to hours, to measure the refraction with the Snellen card and trial lenses. With the retinoscope, however, it can be determined in a fraction of a second. By the former method it would be impossible, for instance, to get any information about the refraction of a baseball player at the moment he swings for the ball, at the moment he strikes it, and at the moment after he strikes it. But with the retinoscope it is quite easy to determine whether his vision is normal, or whether he is myopic, hypermetropic, or astigmatic, when he does these things; and if any errors of refraction are noted, one can guess their degree pretty accurately by the rapidity of the movement of the shadow.
>
> With the Snellen card and trial lenses conclusions must be drawn from the person's statements as to what he sees; but the person often becomes so worried and confused during the examination that he does not know what he sees, or whether different glasses make his sight better or worse; and, moreover, visual acuity is not reliable evidence of the state of the refraction. One person with 2 D of myopia may see twice as much as another with the same error of refraction. The evidence of the Snellen card is, in fact, entirely subjective; that of the retinoscope is entirely objective, depending in no way upon the statements of the person.
>
> In short, while the testing of the refraction by means of the Snellen card and trial lenses requires considerable time, and can be done only under certain artificial conditions, with results that are not always reli-

able, the retinoscope can be used under all sorts of normal and abnormal conditions on the eyes both of human beings and the lower animals; and the results, when it is used properly, can always be depended upon. This means that it must not be brought nearer to the eye than six feet; otherwise the subject will be made nervous, the refraction, for reasons which will be explained later, will be changed, and no reliable observations will be possible. In the case of animals it is often necessary to use it at a much greater distance.

Near "20/20" Vision

A different chart is used by eye doctors to test the near vision of farsights. The Near Eye Chart has different sizes of type and is held 14 inches away.

When a person can read the line consisting of 3-point type letters, she has normal 20/20 near vision. Reading 7-point type is 20/40 near vision, half of normal near vision. If the small letters cannot be read, the eye doctor may prescribe converging lenses, "magnifiers," to focus near objects onto the retina.

Type Size	Visual Acuity (at 14")
23 point	20/200
14 point	20/100
13 point	20/90
12 point	20/80
11 point	20/75
10 point	20/70
9 point	20/65
8 point	20/50
7 point	20/40
6 point	20/35
5 point	20/30
4 point	20/25
3 point	**20/20**

Figure 3–7: Table for Near Eye Chart.

There is a Near Eye Chart in Appendix F, "Eye Charts." There are also samples of small print in Chapter 22, "Reading—For All Ages."

Over-Correction: A Strain; Under-Correction: A Relief

Prescription glasses are sometimes "over-corrected" to give sharper acuity than 20/20—for example, 20/10 correction. Unfortunately, 20/10 lenses create a greater strain on the eyes than 20/20 lenses.

Glasses can be "under-corrected" to give functional but not 20/20 sight—for example, 20/30 or 20/40 correction. Some eye doctors intuitively under-correct prescriptions to prevent 20/20 glasses from straining a person's eyes.

Students improving vision often choose to get glasses that are weaker than 20/20. Over- and under-corrections are discussed further in the next two chapters.

Understanding Prescriptions

NOTE: *Prescriptions are always obtained from an eye doctor. Bates teachers do not prescribe, diagnose, treat, or determine function.*

Many people who wear glasses have seen numbers associated with their glasses. The numerical description of the lenses made for glasses or contact lenses by an eye doctor is called a *prescription.*

Figure 3–8 is a theoretical sample single lense (non-bifocal) prescription for nearsightedness and astigmatism in both eyes, and strabismus (crossed eye) in the right eye.

In nearsightedness the eye is too long; in farsightedness the eye is too short. In both cases, the eye is not spherical when viewed from the side. Diverging and converging

		Spherical	Cylindrical	Axis	Prism	Base
Distance	O. D. (Right Eye)	− 7.25	− 1.25	x 170	1Δ	OUT
	O. S. (Left Eye)	− 6.75	− 1.75	x 145	—	—
Near/Add	O. D. (Right Eye)					
	O. S. (Left Eye)					

Figure 3–8: Theoretical Sample Single Lense Prescription for Nearsightedness, Astigmatism, and Crossed Eye.

lenses compensate for the nearsighted and farsighted eye's "non-spherical" shape, respectively. This correction is indicated in the "Spherical" column of a prescription. Spherical corrections for nearsightedness and farsightedness are measured in diopters.

Unlike the nearsighted and farsighted eye, the astigmatic eye is oval (not spherical) from the front point of view. The amount of correction for astigmatism is indicated in the "Cylindrical" column, in diopters. The angle of the astigmatism correction is indicated in the "Axis" column, in degrees. The axis is sometimes preceded by an "X"; a degree symbol is usually not written.

In strabismus, an eye turns away from the point of interest. The amount of correction for strabismus is indicated in the "Prism" column. The direction of the correction is indicated in the "Base" column.

"O. D." stands for *oculus dexter,* which means "right eye." "O. S." stands for *oculus sinister,* which means "left eye."

The top two rows indicate corrections for "Distance" vision. Distance vision correction is commonly given to nearsights. Distance vision correction may also be given to farsights if their distance vision becomes sufficiently blurred.

The bottom two rows are for "Near" vision correction, commonly given to farsights.

In bifocals, the bottom two rows indicate a correction that has been "Added" to the Distance/Spherical diopters (in the top two rows) to create the prescription in the bottom part of bifocals. For nearsights, the correction on the bottom part of the bifocal is less than the distance correction. For farsights, the correction on the bottom part is greater than the distance correction.

Sometimes the correction given by the prescription, e.g. 20/20 or 20/40, is written on the prescription. The uncorrected visual acuity may also be indicated, e.g. "WOG 20/400"; "WOG" means without glasses.

Prescriptions for Nearsightedness

Refer to *Figure 3–8: Theoretical Sample Single Lense Prescription for Nearsightedness, Astigmatism, and Crossed Eye.*

A prescription for nearsightedness has a negative (–) number in the Spherical column. Usually this is the number of diopters needed to correct the nearsighted eye back to 20/20 normal sight. If less diopters are given, the sight can be corrected to less than 20/20, e.g. 20/40.

In our example, the Distance vision has a

correction of –7.25 D for the right eye, and –6.75 D for the left eye. This is not a bifocal prescription because there is no Near/Add diopter measurement in the bottom two rows.

Sometimes the prescription is written with "DS" after the number of diopters, e.g. –7.25 DS, or –7.25 D. S. DS means diopters of spherical correction. The plus or minus sign in front of the number of diopters indicates whether the correction is for nearsightedness or farsightedness.

Nearsights can also be given bifocals. In a bifocal prescription, there might be two +1.25 D Near/Add numbers in the bottom two rows. The bottom part of this bifocal would then be –6.00 D (–7.25 D "Add" +1.25 D) for the right eye, and –5.50 D (–6.75 D "Add" +1.25 D) for the left eye. Notice that the plus and minus signs of the diopters are taken into account when adding diopters in the Spherical column. The amount of nearsighted correction is less on the bottom part of the bifocal because the nearsighted eye does not need the full distance correction to see clearly up close. (In fact, there is usually a point up close where *no* correction is needed to see clearly up close.) Though the bottom part of a nearsighted bifocal prescription is reduced in power, a person could still have 20/20 or sharper near vision with this lower correction.

As your vision changes, a prescription adjusted originally for 20/20 correction would no longer correct a person to 20/20. When the vision improves, the prescription would be sharper than 20/20, i.e., too strong. When the vision lowers, the prescription would be less sharp than 20/20.

Diopters and 20/xx Distance Numbers: A Loose Correlation

Many students ask about the relationship between the number of diopters in their prescriptions and their acuity, e.g. 20/20, 20/40, 20/200, etc.

There is no absolute correlation. The number of diopters in a prescription relates to the refractive error of the eyeball. As Bates stated above, the Snellen eye chart test is a subjective test and can vary from individual to individual. Squinting can change acuity quickly and dramatically. One person with –3.00 D of nearsightedness may read the 20/100 line, while another person with –3.00 D may only be able to read the 20/200 line.

That being said, there is a loose correlation between diopters and 20/xx numbers. At approximately –1.00 D of nearsightedness, a person might have difficulty passing a "20/40" driver's test. –2.00 D might be 20/80; –3.00 D may be between 20/100 to 20/200. –5.00 D may be around 20/500 sight.

Beyond –3.00 D distant objects usually appear very blurry. When improving vision, the most pronounced experiences of sharper vision occur from –3.00 D to zero D.

Prescriptions for Astigmatism

Figure 3–8: Theoretical Sample Single Lense Prescription for Nearsightedness, Astigmatism, and Crossed Eye shows a prescription with –1.25 D of astigmatism correction for the right eye. The angle of the astigmatism (axis) is 170 degrees. The left eye has a correction of –1.75 D at an axis of 145 degrees.

Trying to correct for astigmatism can be a problem because not only can the magnitude (diopters) change (as with nearsightedness and farsightedness), but the angle (axis) can change as well. If either one changes, the original correction will be incorrect and can create a strain.

Prescriptions for Strabismus (Crossed Eye, Wall Eye, etc.)

Figure 3–8 also shows a correction for a crossed (inward turning) right eye.

1^{Δ}, called "one prism," in the Prism column is the amount of the prism correction. "OUT" in the Base column indicates this prism is correcting for a right eye that turns inward. (The direction of the correction is the *opposite* of the direction the eye is turning.)

In terms of eyestrain, one might equate 1^{Δ} with 1 D, 2^{Δ} with 2 D, and so on.

Prescriptions for Farsightedness

In *Figure 3–9,* we see that a theoretical sample prescription for farsightedness has a positive number in the Spherical column. This is the number of diopters needed to correct the farsighted eye, usually back to 20/20 near vision in a single lense prescription.

Since this is a bifocal prescription, there are two parts: the "Distance" and the "Near/Add."

The top part of this bifocal has a +1.50 D correction for the right eye and a +1.75 D correction for the left eye. Both of these corrections are for distance vision.

The bottom part of a bifocal is for near vision. In this prescription there is an "Add" of +1.25 D for each eye. The "Add" diopters are "added" to the diopters in the top (Distance) part of the bifocal. In this example, the right eye near prescription is +2.75 D (+1.50 D "Add" +1.25 D). The bottom part of a farsighted bifocal is stronger than the top part, because a farsight's near vision is more blurred than the far vision. A farsight with this prescription might have difficulty passing the driver's vision test without corrective lenses.

There is also –1.25 D of astigmatism correction in each eye. Sometimes astigmatism correction is indicated by DC, or D. C., e.g., –1.25 DC. DC means *d*iopters of *c*ylindrical correction. The axis in the right eye is 40°; the axis in the left eye is 95°. Remember, since the axis is not a measure of the magnitude of the astigmatism, 95° is *not* more blurred than 40°.

At about +1.00 D of farsightedness, a person often begins to need glasses for reading small print, especially in dim light. However, such a person might be able to pass the driver's vision test without glasses.

		Spherical	Cylindrical	Axis	Prism	Base
Distance	O. D. (Right Eye)	+ 1.50	– 1.25	x 40		
	O. S. (Left Eye)	+ 1.75	– 1.25	x 90		
Near/Add	O. D. (Right Eye)	+ 1.25				
	O. S. (Left Eye)	+ 1.25				

Figure 3–9: Theoretical Sample Bifocal Prescription for Farsightedness and Astigmatism.

Many people obtain "magnifiers" at the "5&10" store when their near vision first becomes blurry. Often the number of diopters of farsighted correction is written on the inside of one of the frame's temples. 5&10 glasses do not have astigmatism correction. Also, a prescription from an eye doctor is not needed to buy 5&10 "readers."

Mixed Prescriptions

The total correction for one eye is the sum of the absolute values (magnitudes) of the nearsighted (or farsighted) diopters, the astigmatism diopters, and the prism base. The plus or minus signs in front of the cylindrical diopters are ignored when adding diopters to determine the total correction in one eye. For example, if a person has –3.00 D of nearsightedness and +2.00 D of astigmatism for distance correction in the left eye, the total distance correction in the left eye is 5.00 D (3.00 D plus 2.00 D).

Interestingly, the sum of the spherical and cylindrical diopters for the right eye is often the same as, or close to, the sum in the left eye. For example, a person may have –3.00 D spherical/+1.00 D cylindrical correction in the right eye, and –2.25 spherical/+1.75 cylindrical in the left eye. In this case, the total correction in each eye is 4.00 D.

Inadequate Prescriptions

If there is too much blur, or if there are pathologies involved, like cataracts, lenses may not be able to correct a person to 20/20 or even usable vision.

CHAPTER FOUR

The Problem with Glasses and Contact Lenses

I am weary of glasses—
I have worn them so long,
I wonder as time passes
Will my eyes—ever be strong?
Time was when I
Could read in dim light;
Now even with glasses
That light must be bright....
Too many are wearing glasses,
They put them on too soon;
For looks, for sight, for pain and strain,
They wear them night and noon.
I've done my best to tell the rest
That of glasses I would beware;
You'll find it's true, I'm telling you
Glasses will not get you there.[1]

—Joseph J. Kennebeck, optometrist

GLASSES AND CONTACT LENSES: ARTIFICIAL SOLUTIONS TO BLUR

Rather than identifying the cause of their initial blur and reversing it, most people obtain glasses or contact lenses. Even stronger "crutches" are used when vision becomes worse. "Strong" glasses are those that correct one's eyes to 20/20 vision or stronger, for near or far vision.

BATES: "WHAT GLASSES DO TO US"

Contact lenses were not generally available when Bates taught his students how to improve their vision. Even though he limited his discussion to the problems with eyeglasses, many of these problems apply to strong contact lenses.

The opinions of Bates regarding the strain caused by wearing strong glasses are now being echoed by more and more eye doctors, including ophthalmologists.

From *Perfect Sight Without Glasses:*

> *On a tomb in the Church of Santa Maria Maggiore in Florence was found an inscription which read: "Here lies Salvino degli Armati, Inventor of Spectacles. May God pardon him his sins." Nuova Enciclopedia Italiana, Sixth Edition...*[2]
>
> WHAT GLASSES DO TO US
>
> The Florentines were doubtless mistaken in supposing that their fellow citizen ... was the inventor of the lenses now so commonly worn to correct errors of refraction. There has been much discussion as to the origin of these devices, but they are generally believed to have been known at a

> period much earlier than that of Salvino degli Armati. The Romans at least must have known something of the art of supplementing the powers of the eye, for Pliny tells us that Nero used to watch the games in the Colosseum through a concave gem set in a ring for that purpose. If, however, his contemporaries believed that Salvino of the Armati was the first to produce these aids to vision, they might well pray for the pardon of his sins; for while it is true that eyeglasses have brought to some people improved vision and relief from pain and discomfort, they have been to others simply an added torture, they always do more or less harm, and at their best they never improve the vision to normal.

The "relief from pain and discomfort" provided by glasses is not necessarily beneficial in the long term. A drug used to relieve stomach pain may cause serious problems if used continuously. A drug does not necessarily remove the cause of the stomach ache. A drug or mechanical crutch may even lead a person to ignore the real cause of a problem.

Continuing with Bates' words:

> That glasses cannot improve the sight to normal can be very simply demonstrated by looking at any color through a strong convex or concave glass. It will be noted that the color is always less intense than when seen with the naked eye; and since the perception of form depends upon the perception of color, it follows that both color and form must be less distinctly seen with glasses than without them. Even plane glass lowers the vision both for color and form, as everyone knows who has ever looked out of a window.
>
> . . . That glasses must injure the eye is evident from the facts given in the preceding chapter. One cannot see through them unless one produces the degree of refractive error that they are designed to correct. But refractive errors, in the eye which is left to itself, are never constant. If one secures good vision by the aid of concave, or convex, or astigmatic lenses, therefore, it means that one is maintaining constantly a degree of refractive error which otherwise would not be maintained constantly. It is only to be expected that this should make the condition worse, and it is a matter of common experience that it does. After people once begin to wear glasses their strength, in most cases, has to be steadily increased in order to maintain the degree of visual acuity secured by the aid of the first pair. Persons with presbyopia who put on glasses because they cannot read fine print too often find that after they have worn them for a time they cannot, without their aid, read the larger print that was perfectly plain to them before. A person with myopia of 20/70 who puts on glasses giving him a vision of 20/20 may find that in a week's time his unaided vision has declined to 20/200, and we have the testimony of Dr. Sidler-Huguenin, of Zurich,[a] that of the thousands of myopes [under his care] the majority grew steadily worse, in spite of all the skill he could apply to the fitting of glasses for them. When people break their glasses and go without them for a week or two, they frequently observe that their sight has improved. As a matter of fact the sight always improves, to a greater or lesser degree, when glasses are discarded, although the fact may not always be noted.
>
> [a] Archiv f. Augenh., vol. lxxix, 1915, translated in Arch. Ophth., vol. xlv, No. 6, 1916.

A person's sight would not necessarily improve if a person practiced *worse* vision habits—especially straining to see—than the ones he had before discarding glasses. This is why relearning *relaxed* vision habits is essential for improving eyesight. Still, many people have found that their vision improves by wearing glasses less.

Continuing from *Perfect Sight Without Glasses:*

> That the human eye resents glasses is a fact which no one would attempt to deny. Every oculist knows that people have to "get used" to them, and that sometimes they never succeed in doing so. People with high degrees of myopia and hypermetropia have great difficulty in accustoming themselves to the full correction, and often are never able to do so. The strong concave glasses required by myopes of high degree make all objects seem much smaller than they really are, while convex glasses enlarge them. These are unpleasantnesses that cannot be overcome. People with high degrees of astigmatism suffer some very disagreeable sensations when they first put on glasses, for which reason they are warned by one of the "Conservation of Vision" leaflets published by the Council on Health and Public Instruction of the American Medical Association to "get used to them at home before venturing where a misstep might cause a serious accident."[a] Usually these difficulties are overcome, but often they are not, and it sometimes happens that those who get on fairly well with their glasses in the daytime never succeed in getting used to them at night.
>
> All glasses contract the field of vision to a greater or lesser degree. Even with very weak glasses people are unable to see distinctly unless they look through the center of the lenses, with the frames at right angles to the line of vision; and not only is their vision lowered if they fail to do this, but annoying nervous symptoms, such as dizziness and headache, are sometimes produced. Therefore they are unable to turn their eyes freely in different directions. It is true that glasses are now ground in such a way that it is theoretically possible to look through them at any angle, but practically they seldom accomplish the desired result.
>
> The difficulty of keeping the glass clear is one of the minor discomforts of glasses, but nevertheless a most annoying one. On damp and rainy days the atmosphere clouds them. On hot days the perspiration from the body may have a similar effect. On cold days they are often clouded by the moisture of the breath. Every day they are so subject to contamination by dust and moisture and the touch of the fingers incident to unavoidable handling that it is seldom they afford an absolutely unobstructed view of the objects regarded.
>
> Reflections of strong light from eyeglasses are often very annoying, and in the street may be very dangerous.
>
> Soldiers, sailors, athletes, workmen, and children have great difficulty with glasses because of the activity of their lives, which not only leads to the breaking of the lenses, but often throws them out of focus, particularly in the case of eyeglasses worn for astigmatism.
>
> The fact that glasses are very disfiguring may seem a matter unworthy of consideration in a medical publication; but mental discomfort does not improve either the general health or the vision, and while we have gone so far toward making a virtue of what we conceive to be necessity that some of us have actually come to consider

[a] Lancaster: Wearing Glasses, p. 15.

glasses becoming, huge round lenses in ugly tortoise-shell frames being positively fashionable at the present time, there are still some unperverted minds to which the wearing of glasses is mental torture and the sight of them upon others far from agreeable....

Up to a generation ago glasses were used only as an aid to defective sight, but they are now prescribed for large numbers of persons who can see as well or better without them....The hypermetropic eye is believed to be capable of correcting its own difficulties to some extent by altering the curvature of the lens, through the activity of the ciliary muscle. [This topic is covered in Part Two, "Accommodation and Errors of Refraction."]

The eye with simple myopia is not credited with this capacity, because an increase in the convexity of the lens, which is supposed to be all that is accomplished by accommodative effort, would only increase the difficulty; but myopia is usually accompanied by astigmatism, and this, it is believed, can be overcome, in part, by alterations in the curvature of the lens. Thus we are led by the theory to the conclusion that an eye in which any error of refraction exists is practically never free, while open, from abnormal accommodative efforts. In other words, it is assumed that the supposed muscle of accommodation has to bear not only the normal burden of changing the focus of the eye for vision at different distances, but the additional burden of correcting for refractive errors. Such adjustments, if they actually took place, would naturally impose a severe strain upon the nervous system, and it is to relieve this strain—which is believed to be the cause of a host of functional nervous troubles—quite as much as to improve the sight that glasses are prescribed.

It has been demonstrated [by Bates], however, that the lens is not a factor, either in the production of accommodation, or in the correction of errors of refraction. Therefore under no circumstances can there be a strain of the ciliary muscle to be relieved. It has also been demonstrated that when the vision is normal no error of refraction is present, and the extrinsic muscles of the eyeball are at rest. Therefore there can be no strain of the extrinsic muscles to be relieved in these cases. *When a strain of these muscles does exist, glasses may correct its effects upon the refraction, but the strain itself they cannot relieve. On the contrary, as has been shown, they must make it worse.* [TQ emphasis] ... When glasses do not relieve headaches and other nervous symptoms it is assumed to be because they were not properly fitted, and some practitioners and their clients exhibit an astounding degree of patience and perseverance in their joint attempts to arrive at the proper prescription. A person who suffered from severe pains at the base of his brain was fitted sixty times by one specialist alone, and had besides visited many other eye and nerve specialists in this country and in Europe. He was relieved of the pain in five minutes by the methods presented in this book, while his vision, at the same time, became temporarily normal.

It is fortunate that many people for whom glasses have been prescribed refuse to wear them, thus escaping not only much discomfort but much injury to their eyes. Others, having less independence of mind, or a larger share of the martyr's spirit, or having been more badly frightened by the oculists, submit to an amount of unnecessary torture which is scarcely conceivable. One such person wore glasses for twenty-five years, although they did not prevent her from suffering continual misery and lowered her vision to such an extent that she had to look over the tops when she wanted to see anything at a distance. Her oculist assured her that she might expect the most serious consequences if she did not wear the glasses, and was very severe about her practice of looking over instead of through them.

As refractive abnormalities are continually changing, not only from day to day and from hour to hour, but from minute to minute, even under the influence of [the paralyzing drug] atropine, the accurate fitting of glasses is, of course, impossible. In some cases these fluctuations are so extreme, or the person so unresponsive to mental suggestion, that no relief whatever is obtained from correcting lenses, which necessarily become under such circumstances an added discomfort. At their best it cannot be maintained that glasses are anything more than a very unsatisfactory substitute for normal vision....

The idea that presbyopia is "a normal result of growing old" is responsible for much defective eyesight. When people who have reached the presbyopic age [forty] experience difficulty in reading, they are very likely to resort at once to glasses, either with or without professional advice. In some cases such persons may be actually presbyopic; in others the difficulty may be something temporary, which they would have thought little about if they had been younger, and which would have passed away if Nature had been left to herself. But once the glasses are adopted, in the great majority of cases, they produce the condition they were designed to relieve, or, if it already existed, they make it worse, sometimes very rapidly, as every ophthalmologist knows. In a couple of weeks sometimes, the person finds, as noted in the chapter *What Glasses Do to Us*, that the large print which he could read without difficulty before he got his glasses can no longer be read without their aid. In from five to ten years the accommodative power of the eye is usually gone; and if from this point the person does not go on to cataract, glaucoma, or inflammation of the retina, he may consider himself fortunate. Only occasionally do the eyes refuse to submit to the artificial conditions imposed upon them; but in such cases they may keep up an astonishing struggle against them for long periods. A woman of seventy, who had worn glasses for twenty years, was still able to read diamond type and had good vision for the distance without them. She said the glasses tired her eyes and blurred her vision, but that she had persisted in wearing them, in spite of a continual temptation to throw them off, because she had been told that it was necessary for her to do so.

If persons who find themselves getting presbyopic, or who have arrived at the presbyopic age, would, instead of resorting to glasses, follow the example of the gentleman mentioned by Dr. Holmes [see Chapter 6, "Accommodation and Errors of Refraction—The Orthodox View"] and make a practice of reading the finest print they can find, the idea that the decline of accommodative power is "a normal result of growing old" would soon die a natural death.

Tom's Personal Log: At age 10, I was given a prescription of –2.50 D for myopia. My glasses and contact lenses increased in power until at age 30 I had approximately –8 D and –1 D of astigmatism. At that time I could not see anything clearly more than a few inches from my nose. For over twenty years, I suffered with glasses and contact lenses, which made both my vision and my health worse.

Potential serious problems due to blurred vision are discussed in Chapter 27, "Serious Vision Problems."

"WHY GLASSES ARE HARMFUL FOR CHILDREN AND YOUNG PEOPLE" AND EVERYONE ELSE

In 1969, Joseph J. Kennebeck, O.D., a practicing optometrist for more than 50 years, wrote *Why Glasses Are Harmful for Children and Young People*. In this book, Kennebeck says that if a nearsight uses glasses that were given to him for distance (20+ feet) vision to see up close, he puts a strain on his eyes.

For nearsights, Kennebeck writes:

> Glasses fitted at twenty feet are harmful and habit-forming at twenty feet and beyond ... Inside of twenty feet the glasses are many times worse. Glasses are wrong at every foot inside of twenty feet. At ten feet the glasses are *twice wrong;* at five feet they are *four times wrong;* at one foot, they are *twenty times wrong* ... This is the reason glasses are not scientifically correct ... eyes cannot compensate through glasses made for twenty feet for all other distances, WITHOUT BEING HURT ... This is what brings on progressive myopia, which could have been prevented if the glasses had never been prescribed or worn....[3]
>
> Nearsighted eyes have to over-accommodate through nearsighted glasses to read at thirteen inches, as compared to normal eyes. Their over-accommodation adds up to the nearsighted lens power they wear for distance, say for example minus three diopters, plus the same three diopters that normal eyes use to see at thirteen inches, which makes six diopters of accommodation used by such nearsighted eyes through nearsighted glasses ... such terrific over-accommodation through nearsighted glasses causes the increased progressive nearsightedness....[4]
>
> ... Nearsighted and farsighted glasses will create more of the same problem for which the lenses were prescribed and worn. If left alone, without glasses, and the [incorrect] eye habits in all close work were stopped, the eyes would return toward normal.[5]
>
> ... Where glasses begin, good eyes end.[6]

Regarding nearsightedness, optometrist Bruce May states:

> Sadly, the most common approach to myopia is the least likely to prevent its further increase. Usually, corrective concave lenses are supplied for clearing distance seeing, along with advice that the lenses are to be worn all the time. This procedure can only increase the near point stress. It is almost certain that more myopia will develop.[7]

Similarly, a farsight who looks into the distance with his reading glasses on will also strain his sight.

Dr. Thomas H. David, in his booklet *Improve Your Vision with Television,* writes:

> To put on glasses when one has developed a strain may give temporary relief, however, if incorrect habits of using the eyes are not overcome, the wearer returns to the eye specialist for an increase in his lense.[8]

The scope of these problems increases when lighting factors are taken into consideration. Most people who have blurred vision have more blur in darkness than in bright light. Better vision in bright light is due to the pinhole effect, discussed in Chapter 14, "The Third Habit—Blinking." One reason eyesight is tested in darkness is to ensure you are given the *maximum* correction needed for all situations.

A nearsight's vision is checked at twenty feet in darkness—the "worst case scenario." When a 20/20 prescription is given for this situation, it will automatically be too strong, not only for close vision, but for distance vision in bright light.

Farsighted Glasses for Nearsights?

After wearing prescription glasses for many years, some nearsights lose the ability to see clearly up close while wearing their strong, distance glasses. (Since without corrective lenses a nearsight can still see clearly up close, the person is not truly "farsighted," as is often mistakenly stated.)

Many nearsights are given converging, "+" reading glasses to wear on top of their concave, "–" contact lenses for reading up close. For example, if the contact lense is –5 D, and the glasses are +2 D, the resultant combination contact lense/reading glasses correction is –3 D.

A person in this predicament could simply wear a –3 D pair of glasses for near vision, but without using the contact lenses. But a common motivation for using contact lenses is to not have to wear glasses in the first place. This scenario has led some people to enroll for natural vision classes.

The Monovision Solution

Another solution to the nearsight's loss of near vision while wearing strong "–" contact lenses is monovision. One eye is fitted with a lense to see in the distance, while the other is fitted with a reduced lense to see up close. The idea is to use only one eye at a time, like a chameleon. This can result in the loss of normal depth perception experience with binocular (two-eye) vision, as the brain tries to emphasize the picture from only one eye, and de-emphasize the picture from the other.

Nearsighted Glasses Can Double Peripheral Objects

As mentioned by Bates, when a person wears strong "–" diverging lenses, objects appear smaller through the lenses. As a result, nearsights who wear strong glasses can experience a doubling of objects, or parts of objects, around the frames. The stronger the prescription, the more the doubling.

Farsighted Glasses Can Lose Some Objects

When "+" converging lenses are used, objects appear larger through the lenses. "Magnifiers" literally magnify. As a result, farsights who wear strong glasses can experience loss of objects, or parts of objects, at the borders of the frames. The stronger the prescription, the more the loss.

Bifocals and "Bifocal Neck"

A common solution to the problem of strong, single prescriptions is the use of bifocals, or "progressive" lenses.

Bifocals are often provided as a convenience so that people will not need to switch between two different powers of glasses to see at different distances.

One problem with bifocals is that the neck becomes even more tense than when "singles" were used. Many people I have talked with acknowledge this fact. One eye doctor, who prescribes reduced-power glasses for natural vision students, refers to people wearing bifocals as having "bifocal necks."

Before wearing bifocals, a person would be more likely to move the head up and down naturally to see objects far and near, respectively. With bifocals, the tendency is to tilt the head back, lock the head and neck tight, and move the eyes down to see through the bottom portion of the bifocal lens. This can create a high strain on a person's neck.

Ophthalmologist R. S. Agarwal, in his book *Mind and Vision*, writes regarding bifocals:

> The upper glass is meant to see distant objects, while the lower glass is meant for reading. One is not able to see through the junction between the two glasses. Hence one has to raise the eyeball to see distant objects and lower the eyeball to see the near objects. The eye is forced to move up and down in an unnatural way. This unnatural movement causes great strain on the eyes.[9]

June Biermann and Barbara Toohey write in their book *The Woman's Holistic Headache Relief Book:*

> *Do you regularly hold your chin forward?* In this category we can put "bifocal headaches," headaches caused by sticking your chin forward to peer better through the reading [lower] portion of your glasses. June suspects this was a contributing factor in her headaches.[10]

People with blurred vision have a tight neck because the same strained vision habits that tighten the eye muscles also tighten the neck muscles. Bifocals only increase that neck tension.

Clients with blurred vision can be a source of frustration for holistic health practitioners. The neck and shoulders cannot release their chronic tension completely unless vision is normalized.

Trifocals, Quadrafocals, even Dozenfocals!

Modern technology can create almost any type of lenses for glasses. The student of one vision teacher had been given dozenfocals! The more complex the lenses, the more unnatural the vision experience, and the greater the strain.

Problems with Contact Lenses

The painful "adaptation" period experienced by wearers of hard contact lenses is a message to stop putting foreign objects into the eyes!

Some problems experienced by some contact lense wearers include:

- Lenses not fitting the cornea properly
- Lenses are not durable
- Inconvenience of handling
- Non-compliance with hygienic measures in cleaning, disinfection, and storage
- Sudden pain and dizziness
- Distortion of the cornea
- Irritation of the eye and eyelids
- Cornea abrasion and infections
- Allergic reactions to cleaning solutions
- Protein buildup on lenses
- Restrictions from some occupations
- Continuous expense
- Allergic reactions
- Red eyes
- Scar tissue on the cornea
- Possible melting of the lense onto the cornea with certain types of accidents involving electrical sparks
- Risks of oxygen deprivation to the cornea, which can cause abrasions,

especially with hard and extended-wear contact lenses

- Extended-wear contact lenses causing corneal ulcers, abrasions, and inflammation; possible partial or complete vision loss
- Corneal transplant
- Serious infections
- Vision loss, including blindness
- Mucus trapped under the lense
- Interference with normal blinking and tearing
- Inflammation of the upper eyelid
- Drying out of the eyes
- Serious safety hazard if dust lodges between contact lense and cornea
- In 1986, contact lenses had the highest number of product-related injuries reported to the US Consumer Product Safety Commission for all medical devices; 33,458 injuries were linked to contact lenses.[11]

A VISUAL BIOFEEDBACK—IN THE WRONG DIRECTION

For most people, strong corrective lenses create a negative biofeedback loop:

1. The initial mental and physical strain of incorrect vision habits abnormally tightens the eye muscles, creating blur.
2. Corrective lenses lock the eye muscles tight. The mind and body are now confused. Clarity is supposed to be experienced only when a person has relaxed, natural vision habits. Blur is a message of imbalance from the mind and body telling you to return to the normal, relaxed way of seeing. Strong corrective lenses tell the mind and body that everything is now "fine"—but it's not! The mental and physical strain remains.
3. This increased strain tightens the eye muscles even more, creating additional blur. It's as if the mind and body *want to give* you blurred vision, no matter what artificial approaches you take. Blur is a *correct* message telling you to eliminate excessive strain.

   Unfortunately, most people in industrialized cultures do not listen to this message.

In the next chapter, we discuss how a person can minimize the strain caused by corrective lenses, thus giving room for vision to improve when relearning correct vision habits.

Notes

1 Joseph J. Kennebeck, *Why Eyeglasses are Harmful for Children and Young People* (New York: Vantage Press, 1969), pp. 119–21.

2 All quotes in this book which contain emphasis with italics are by the quoted author, unless otherwise noted.

3 Kennebeck, pp. 26–27.

4 Ibid., pp. 28–29.

5 Ibid., p. 29.

6 Ibid., p. 62.

7 Bruce May, *Rx for Nearsightedness: Stress-Relieving Lenses*, Optometric Extension Program Foundation pamphlet (1981).

8 Thomas H. David, *Improve Your Vision with Television!* (Los Angeles, California: DeVorss & Co., 1951), p. 7.

9 R. S. Agarwal, *Mind and Vision* (Pondicherry, India: Sri Aurobindo Ashram Press, 1983), p. 33.

10 June Biermann and Barbara Toohey, *The Woman's Holistic Headache Relief Book* (Los Angeles: J. P. Tarcher, Inc., 1979), p. 47.

11 MDDI Report (September 4, 1987).

Chapter Five

Reduced Prescriptions

People who wear strong "corrective" lenses for blurred vision have two interferences to normal vision: incorrect vision habits and the strong glasses.

The first interference is the original incorrect vision habits acquired when the vision initially blurred. The correct vision habits are discussed in Part Four, "The Three Habits of Natural Vision."

The other interference to normal sight is strong glasses. Unfortunately, some people are given glasses when they are not needed. This can strain the visual system.

Some people are confused about what Bates said regarding glasses. Bates stated that the *best* approach while improving vision is to discard glasses permanently. He also stated that in cases where this would be "too great a hardship," *glasses of reduced strength* can be used while improving, but it may take longer to succeed. Therefore, it is *not* necessary to completely eliminate glasses immediately to succeed. Many natural vision students have succeeded by using reduced glasses during the transition period.

It would be too stressful and impractical for many students with strong prescriptions to take off glasses altogether. Since relaxation is the key to normal sight, it is best to approach the vision improvement process in as reasonable and relaxed a way as possible.

WORKING WITH A SUPPORTIVE EYE DOCTOR

If a student is unable to eliminate glasses immediately, he can consult with a supportive or "neutral" eye doctor to obtain reduced prescriptions.

If your eye doctor is not supportive initially, you may be able to educate him or her that there are now ophthalmologists and optometrists who give natural vision students reduced prescriptions and some who even *teach* their students how to improve their vision naturally. There are even eye doctors, several of whom this author has met personally, who have improved their own eyesight with the Bates method. Most likely there is at least one eye doctor in your community who will support your vision improvement program. They are *your* eyes, and you want to take care of them the best way you know how.

THE IMPORTANCE OF REDUCED PRESCRIPTIONS

Bates wrote in May 8, 1915, issue of the *New York Medical Journal:*

> As a general rule it is best for the student to discard glasses. In some cases of extreme myopia, where going without glasses entails too great a hardship, good results have been obtained by gradually reducing the strength of the glasses worn as the vision improves, but the process is then prolonged.[1]

Most people were given glasses due to the mastery of staring and other poor vision habits. Therefore glasses, to some degree, "remind" the student to continue poor vision habits. Students *can* succeed with vision improvement by using reduced prescriptions or "transition" glasses, *if* they continue to practice correct vision habits while wearing them, and if they remove the glasses when they are not essential. In the long term, correct vision habits are more powerful than the negative effects of the reduced glasses.

DRIVING AND WORK GLASSES

If you need glasses for driving, you must obtain and use safe and legal driving glasses from your eye doctor. 20/40 is the driving requirement for eyesight in many states, while no state requires better than 20/25 sight for driving. Check with your eye doctor regarding the vision requirements for driving in your state.

If you have an occupation that requires safe work up close, wear glasses that are adequate for your task.

TWO PAIRS OF REDUCED GLASSES?

Many nearsights have obtained a reduced, legal, and safe prescription for driving. However, as Kennebeck emphasized in the last chapter, this prescription is too strong to wear up close. Wearing a distance prescription while seeing up close is a strain.

Nearsights have two options for their close vision: 1) If possible, do not use glasses; you may already be doing this, knowing intuitively that the glasses for distance sight are too strong for your eyes, and that you can function adequately up close without them. 2) If glasses for close vision are necessary, obtain a second, even weaker, pair of reduced glasses.

Bifocals create an even greater strain on the neck and visual system than single-prescription lenses. In the long term, increased blur and strain on the visual system is *less* convenient, especially if they lead to more serious vision problems. (See Chapter 27, "Serious Vision Problems.") If different corrective lenses are needed for more than one distance, it is better to have two pairs of reduced glasses. Besides, the more you improve your vision, the less you need them.

If you have some older, weaker pair of glasses, you can ask your eye doctor to check their power. They may be fine for your first pair of reduced glasses. If not, you may be able to put reduced lenses into the old frames.

Although there is usually an additional expense in obtaining two pairs of reduced glasses, it is not more expensive in the long term. This is because the weaker of the two pairs of reduced glasses can often be used for the other distance as the vision improves.

How much money have you spent already on corrective lenses? How much more would you spend for the rest of your life?

When vision with a pair of reduced glasses becomes crystal clear, they are no longer "reduced" prescriptions, because vision improved! It is then time to switch to an even weaker prescription. Many students are happy to pay their eye doctor for weaker glasses! And eye doctors who support natural vision students get *more* business!

"5&10" or EYE DOCTOR PRESCRIPTIONS?

Farsights who buy "reading" glasses at the "5&10" store need to decide whether inexpensive glasses are the correct choice when obtaining reduced glasses. Some authorities warn people to not "compromise" eyesight with "imperfect lenses." The implication given in some literature is that some glasses might not contain lenses of as high a quality as others, and that the difference could be based on cost.

Regardless of the cost, improperly made glasses can strain your eyes. There are many factors that go into making the correct prescription. You will need to decide whether inexpensive 5&10 glasses are the correct choice.

CAN VISION IMPROVE WHILE WEARING CONTACTS?

Wearing contact lenses while improving vision is not the best approach for several reasons:

- Contact lenses are a foreign object in the eye. While improving vision, the eyes increase circulation in many ways. The more life force energy that returns to your eyes, especially due to the release of neck tension, the more likely your eyes will "reject" these foreign objects.
- For nearsights, strong, single-prescription contact lenses are designed for distance vision. This means that reduced single-prescription 20/40 contacts would be too strong for close vision.
- It is important not to use any corrective lenses when they are not absolutely needed. Since it is impractical to constantly take contact lenses out and put them back in, using glasses is an obvious advantage.

Many students do not like the idea of returning to glasses after wearing contact lenses. Temporary sacrifices are sometimes necessary to reach wonderful goals.

Some people have told me they will never take my natural vision class because they are not willing to go back to wearing glasses. (Students *can* attend natural vision classes and continue to wear contact lenses.) If these people could remember the joys of beautiful, naturally clear vision, they might think differently. Students who have completely eliminated their need for both contact lenses and glasses are happy they were willing to use glasses temporarily.

One of my students held onto her contact lenses until she saw improvement of her sight, which occurred by the second class. She brought her contact lenses to that class and had a little ceremony in disposing of them into the trash can. After the course she became a Natural Vision teacher.

I have met some extraordinarily motivated individuals in the last thirteen years of teaching Natural Vision classes. The following is a most remarkable case.

A woman, T. B., called me and talked with me about my classes. She said she was a scuba diver, welding oil pipelines underwater off the shores of Alaska! Since she wore contact lenses while scuba diving, returning to glasses was not very practical for her—at least, not initially. She was extremely motivated to get rid of any corrective lenses, especially because none of her colleagues needed them. (People who are in occupations closely connected to nature appear less likely to have blurred vision.)

T. B., whom I later learned had healed her cancer by eliminating excessive stress from her life, requested temporary surface duty on a boat. She was then able to stop wearing contact lenses and obtained reduced glasses. She enrolled for my class in June 1988, when she had 20/200 uncorrected vision. In July 1988, her optometrist measured her uncorrected vision at 20/70. At this time she received –1.75 diopter glasses to correct her to 20/40. In October 1988, she was seeing 20/20– with the same reduced glasses. Eventually, she eliminated her need for corrective lenses and returned to her regular underwater scuba-diving, pipe-welding work.

BUILDING VISION CONFIDENCE

Some students, especially at the start of their natural vision re-education, are a bit nervous at the prospect of using reduced glasses.

If you are one of these students or potential students, consider the following:

1. Many, if not most, people already know what reduced glasses are like, because they have usually experienced "reduced" vision through their glasses after a period of time.
2. When a student relearns to see correctly, confidence in your natural vision can grow quickly. As we shall learn in Chapter 10, "The Second Principle—Centralization," only a small part of the visual picture we see is clearest, while most of the visual picture is "unclear"—even for those with perfect sight! People with blur tend to put their visual attention into the areas of the picture that are unclear. A person sees better—instantaneously—when he shifts attention from the unclear areas back to the clearer area.

Students are often surprised at how many activities they can do comfortably fairly soon—with and without glasses. Many activities they did not think they would be able to do without strong glasses.

"Where there is a will...."

Notes

[1] William H. Bates, "The Reversal of Errors of Refraction by Education Without Glasses" in the *New York Medical Journal*, May 8, 1915.

PART TWO

Accommodation and Errors of Refraction

In the next three chapters, we explore theories and facts relating to how the eyes adjust to see clearly from far to near—called accommodation—and the errors of refraction: nearsightedness, farsightedness, so-called presbyopia, and astigmatism.

CHAPTER SIX

Accommodation and Errors of Refraction—The Orthodox View

The universe is not to be narrowed down to the limits of understanding, which has been man's practice up to now, but the understanding must be stretched to take in the image of the universe as it is discovered.

—Sir Francis Bacon

BATES' "INTRODUCTORY"

Bates' "Introductory" is the first chapter in his seminal work on natural vision improvement, *Perfect Sight Without Glasses*.

> INTRODUCTORY
>
> Most writers on ophthalmology appear to believe that the last word about problems of refraction has been spoken, and from their viewpoint the last word is a very depressing one. Practically everyone in these days suffers from some form of refractive error. Yet we are told that for these ills, which are not only so inconvenient, but often so distressing and dangerous, there is not only no way to reverse them, and no palliative save those optic crutches known as eyeglasses, but, under modern conditions of life, practically no prevention.
>
> It is a well-known fact that the human body is not a perfect mechanism. Nature, in the evolution of the human tenement, has been guilty of some maladjustments.... But nowhere is she supposed to have blundered so badly as in the construction of the eye. With one accord ophthalmologists tell us that the visual organ of man was never intended for the uses to which it is now put. Eons before there were any schools or printing presses, electric lights or moving pictures, its evolution was complete. In those days it served the needs of the human animal perfectly. Man was a hunter, a herdsman, a farmer, a fighter. He needed, we are told, mainly distant vision; and since the eye at rest is adjusted for distant vision, sight is supposed to have been ordinarily as passive as the perception of sound, requiring no muscular action whatever. Near vision, it is assumed, was the exception,... necessitating a muscular adjustment of such short duration that it was accomplished without placing any appreciable burden upon the mechanism of accommodation. The fact that primitive woman was a seamstress, an embroiderer, a weaver, an artist in all sorts of fine and beautiful work, appears to have been generally forgotten. Yet women living

under primitive conditions have just as good eyesight as the men.

When man learned how to communicate his thoughts to others by means of written and printed forms, there came some undeniably new demands upon the eye,... affecting at first only a few people, but gradually including more and more, until now, in the more advanced countries, the great mass of the population is subjected to their influence. A few hundred years ago even princes were not taught to read and write. Now we compel everyone to go to school, whether he wishes to or not, even the babies being sent to kindergarten. A generation or so ago books were scarce and expensive. Today, by means of libraries of all sorts, stationary and traveling, they have been brought within the reach of practically everyone. The modern newspaper, with its endless columns of badly printed reading matter, was made possible only by the discovery of the art of manufacturing paper from wood, which is a thing of yesterday. The tallow candle has been but lately displaced by the various forms of artificial lighting, which tempt most of us to prolong our vocations and avocations into hours when primitive man was forced to rest, and within the last couple of decades has come the moving picture to complete the supposedly destructive process.

Was it reasonable to expect that Nature should have provided for all these developments, and produced an organ that could respond to the new demands? It is the accepted belief of ophthalmology today that she could not and did not,[a] and that, while the processes of civilization depend upon the sense of sight more than upon any other, the visual organ is but imperfectly fitted for its tasks.

There are a great number of facts which seem to justify this conclusion....

For the prevailing method of vision care, by means of compensating lenses, very little was ever claimed except that these contrivances neutralized the effects of the various conditions for which they were prescribed, as a crutch enables a lame man to walk. It has also been believed that they sometimes checked the progress of these conditions; but every ophthalmologist now knows that their usefulness for this purpose, if any, is very limited. In the case of myopia[b] (shortsight), Dr. Sidler-Huguenin of Zurich, in a striking paper recently published,[c] expresses the opinion that glasses and all methods now at our command are "of but little avail" in preventing either the progress of the error of refraction, or the development of the very serious complications with which it is often associated.

These conclusions are based on the study

---

[a] The unnatural strain of accommodating the eyes to close work (for which they were not intended) leads to myopia in a large proportion of growing children.—Rosenau: Preventive Medicine and Hygiene, third edition.

The compulsion of fate as well as an error of evolution has brought it about that the unaided eye must persistently struggle against the astonishing difficulties and errors inevitable in its structure, function and circumstance.—Gould: The Cause, Nature and Consequences of Eyestrain, Pop Sci Monthly, Dec., 1905.

With the invention of writing and then with the invention of the printing press a new element was introduced, and one evidently not provided for by the process of evolution. The human eye which had been evolved for distant vision is being forced to perform a new part, one for which it had not been evolved, and for which it is poorly adapted. The difficulty is being daily augmented.—Scott: The Sacrifice of the Eyes of School Children, Pop Sci Monthly, Oct., 1907.

[b] From the Greek *myein,* to close, and *ops,* the eye; literally a condition in which the subject closes the eye, or blinks.

[c] Archiv f. Augenh, vol. lxxix, 1915, translated in Arch. Ophth., vol. xlv, No. 6, Nov., 1916.

of thousands of cases in Dr. Huguenin's private practice and in the clinic of the University of Zurich, and regarding one group of individuals, persons connected with the local educational institutions, he states that the failure took place in spite of the fact that they followed his instructions for years "with the greatest energy and pertinacity," sometimes even changing their professions.

I have been studying the refraction of the human eye for more than thirty years, and my observations fully confirm the foregoing conclusions as to the uselessness of all the methods heretofore employed for the prevention and improvement of errors of refraction. I was very early led to suspect, however, that the problem was by no means an unsolvable one.

Every ophthalmologist of any experience knows that the theory of the irreversibility of errors of refraction does not fit the observed facts. Not infrequently such cases recover spontaneously, or change from one form to another. It has long been the custom either to ignore these troublesome facts, or to explain them away, and fortunately for those who consider it necessary to bolster up the old theories at all costs, the role attributed to the lens in accommodation offers, in the majority of cases, a plausible method of explanation. According to this theory, which most of us learned at school, the eye changes its focus for vision at different distances by altering the curvature of the lens; and in seeking an explanation for the inconstancy of the theoretically constant error of refraction the theorists hit upon the very ingenious idea of attributing to the lens a capacity for changing its curvature, not only for the purpose of normal accommodation, but to cover up or to produce accommodative errors.…in the case of the disappearance or lessening of hypermetropia, we are asked to believe that the eye, in the act of vision, both at the near point and at the distance, increases the curvature of the lens sufficiently to compensate, in whole or in part, for the flatness [short from front to back] of the eyeball. In myopia, on the contrary, we are told that the eye actually goes out of its way to produce the condition, or to make an existing condition worse.

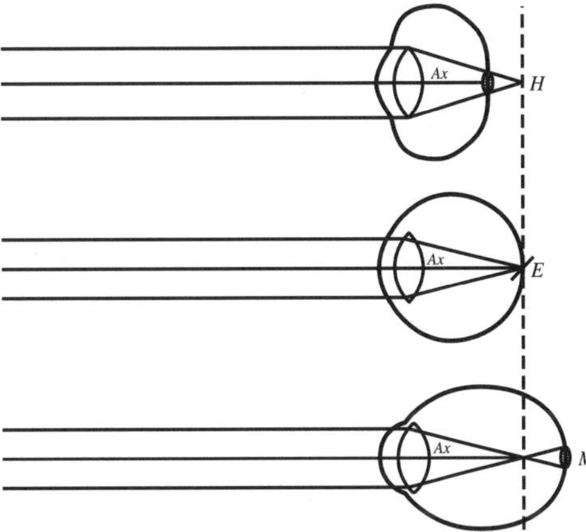

Figure 6–1: Diagram of the Hypermetropic, Emmetropic, and Myopic Eyeballs.[1] H, hypermetropia; E, emmetropia; M, myopia; Ax, optic axis. Note that in hypermetropia and myopia the rays, instead of coming to a focus, form a round spot upon the retina.

A normal, emmetropic eye is said to be "at rest"; it has a spherical shape and sees clearly in the distance. Light rays from a far object focus properly on the retina. In order for an emmetropic eye to see near objects clearly, there must be some mechanism by which the diverging light rays from a near object can be focused onto the retina. The changing of the eye to see clearly up close is called *accommodation*.

Conventionally, accommodation is attributed only to the lens, which supposedly acquires more curvature on its front side by the contraction of the ciliary muscle. Bates (and others) attributed accommodation to the action of the two oblique muscles producing an elongated eyeball.

A hypermetropic ("farsighted") eye is too short from front to back; it does not see clearly near. (Or far, but near objects are usually less clear than far objects. Many farsights are surprised to see their distance vision improve while improving their near vision.)

A myopic (nearsighted) eye is too long from front to back; it cannot see clearly in the distance. Light rays from near objects focus correctly on the retina of a myopic eye.

In a multitude of debates about eyesight, virtually all authorities agree on these three facts:

1. The normal, "at rest" eyeball is in a round shape; in this state, far objects are clear and close objects are not clear.
2. The myopic (nearsighted) eyeball is elongated; near objects are clear, and far objects are not clear.
3. The hypermetropic ("farsighted") eyeball is foreshortened; near objects are not clear.

Continuing with Bates' words from *Perfect Sight Without Glasses:*

> In other words, the so-called "ciliary muscle," believed to control the shape of the lens, is credited with a capacity for getting into a more or less continuous state of contraction, thus keeping the lens continuously in a state of [greater] convexity which, according to the theory, it ought to assume only for vision at the near point.

To clarify what Bates said about the conventional position on accommodation:

Normally, the lens is said to be in the flatter (less convex) shape when "at rest." As just discussed, the emmetropic (spherical) eyeball at rest sees clearly in the distance. When the ciliary muscle contracts, the front side of the lens is said to gain more curvature, which would allow the spherical eyeball to see clearly up close. This is the orthodox explanation of normal accommodation.

The hypermetropic (foreshortened) eyeball does not see clearly near. With a foreshortened eyeball, and an "at rest" lens in its normal flatter shape, light rays are focused "in back of" the retina; light rays on the retina are "out of focus." Theoretically, if the ciliary muscle contracts, the front side of the lens could gain greater curvature and would be able to focus light rays from far objects clearly onto the retina.

Bates again from *Perfect Sight Without Glasses:*

> These curious performances may seem unnatural to the lay mind; but ophthalmologists believe the tendency to indulge in them to be so ingrained in the constitution of the organ of vision that, in the fitting of glasses, it is customary to instill atropine—the "drops" with which everyone who has ever visited an oculist is familiar—into the eye, for the purpose of paralyzing the ciliary muscle and thus, by preventing any change of curvature in the lens, bringing out "latent hypermetropia" and getting rid of "apparent myopia."

In other words, when atropine is used, the ciliary muscle loses any possible contraction power to change the curvature of the lens, and, theoretically, the lens relaxes into its normal, "at rest," flatter shape for distance vision. The "true" condition of a person's sight, i.e., the amount of myopia or hypermetropia due to the eyeball being non-spherical, can then be determined.

From *Perfect Sight Without Glasses:*

> The interference of the lens [without the instillation of atropine], however, is believed to account for only moderate degrees of variation in errors of refraction, and that only during the earlier years of life. For the higher ones, or those that occur after forty-five years of age, when the lens is supposed to have lost its elasticity to a greater or lesser degree, no plausible explanation has ever been devised.

Above, Bates presents one of his primary arguments against the lens being the mechanism of accommodation. To recap:

The conventional explanation for hypermetropic (farsighted) young people improving their sight is not that the eyeball returns to its normal round shape, but that the lens gains greater (than normal) curvature to see clearly near and far again. Hypermetropia is considered to be congenital and irreversible.

A problem with this conventional position is it cannot explain how hypermetropia improves or is eliminated in elderly people, in whom the lens is said to become rigid and inflexible. A Natural Vision Center consultant, who has seen numerous elderly people who have natural clear vision near and far, refers to such people by quoting an ancient Chinese phrase—"Returning of Youth." This consultant states that conventional eye specialists have "no set answer" to explain how people can maintain clear vision well into their seventies. Are the elderly people who keep clear vision all of their lives keeping their "youth" somehow? I believe Bates, many Natural Vision teachers, and many natural vision students would say, "Yes."

Another consultant, an ophthalmologist, agrees that the multitude of people who have clear vision near and far long after the so-called presbyopic age is confusing to the orthodox. As Bates pointed out, nearly all experienced eye specialists have seen such cases.

If the lens is the only mechanism of accommodation, as stated conventionally, it should be easy to demonstrate that these older people are accommodating with the lens. In this case, the lens has obviously not become rigid enough to prevent normal accommodation.

If the lens has become so rigid the ciliary muscle can no longer produce accommodation, the two oblique eye muscles must be producing accommodation, in which case the lens is obviously not essential for accommodation.

Note that the refractive power of the lens of a camera remains fixed.

Continuing from *Perfect Sight Without Glasses:*

> Examining 30,000 pairs of eyes a year at the New York Eye and Ear Infirmary and other institutions, I observed ... many cases in which errors of refraction either recovered spontaneously, or changed their form, and I was unable either to ignore them, or to satisfy myself with the orthodox explanations, even where such explanations were available. It seemed to me that if a statement is a truth it must always be a truth. There can be no exceptions. If errors of refraction are irreversible, they should not recover, or change their form, spontaneously.
>
> In the course of time I discovered that myopia and hypermetropia, like astigma-

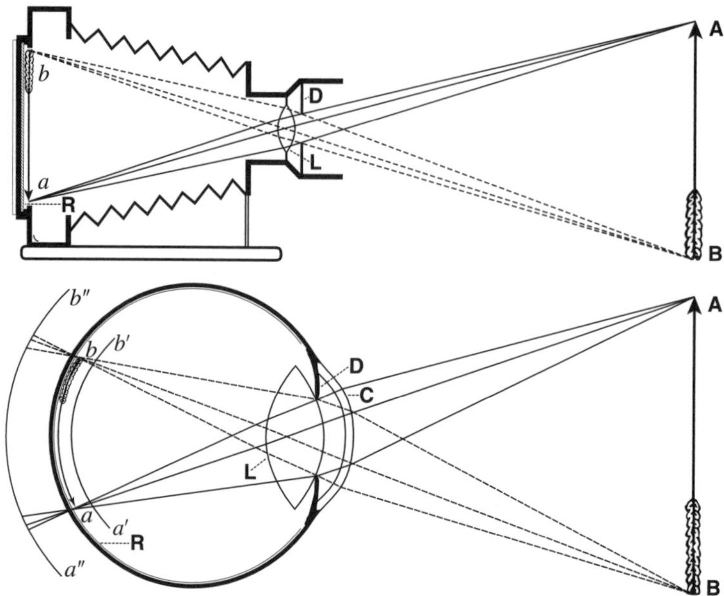

Figure 6–2: The Eye as a Camera.[2] *The photographic apparatus:* ***D****, diaphragm made of circular overlapping plates of metal by means of which the opening through which the rays of light enter the chamber can be enlarged or contracted;* ***L****, lens;* ***R****, sensitive plate (the retina of the eye);* ***AB****, object to be photographed; ab, image on the sensitive plate. The eye: C, cornea where the rays of light undergo a first refraction;* ***D****, iris (the diaphragm of the camera);* ***L****, lens, where the light rays are again refracted;* ***R****, retina of the normal eye;* ***AB****, object of vision; ab, image in the normal or emmetropic eye;* ***a'b'****, image in the hypermetropic eye;* ***a"b"****, image in the myopic eye. Note that in a'b' and a"b" the rays are spread out upon the retina instead of being brought to a focus as in ab, the result being the formation of a blurred image.*

tism, could be produced at will; that myopia was not, as we have so long believed, associated with the use of the eyes at the near point, but with a strain to see distant objects, strain at the near point being associated with hypermetropia; that no error of refraction was ever a constant condition....

In seeking for light upon these problems I examined tens of thousands of eyes, and the more facts I accumulated the more difficult it became to reconcile them with the accepted views. Finally, about half a dozen years ago, I undertook a series of observations upon the eyes of human beings and the lower animals, the results of which convinced both myself and others that the lens is not a factor in accommodation, and that the adjustment necessary for vision at different distances is effected in the eye, precisely as it is in the camera, by a change in the length of the organ, this alteration being brought about by the action of the muscles on the outside of the globe. [The focal length—the distance between the lense and the film—of a camera is increased to focus near objects clearly. The focal length is decreased to focus far objects clearly. As noted above, the curvature of a camera's lens never changes.] Equally convincing was the demonstration that errors of refraction [nearsightedness, astigmatism, and farsightedness], including presbyopia, are due not to an organic change in the shape of the eyeball or in the constitution of the lens, but to a functional and therefore reversible derangement in the action of the extrinsic muscles.

In making these statements I am well aware that I am controverting the practically undisputed teaching of ophthalmological science for the better part of a century;...but I have been driven to the conclusions which they embody by the facts, and that so slowly that I am now surprised at my own blindness. At the time I was improving high degrees of myopia; but I wanted to be conservative, and I differentiated between functional myopia, which I was able to reverse, or improve, and organic myopia, which, in deference to the orthodox tradition, I accepted as irreversible.

Note that the problem of the lens not being able to accommodate, from the conventional viewpoint, is only an issue *after* the age of forty, when supposedly the lens has become rigid. This is commonly referred to as presbyopia. This means that the *mechanism* of accommodation does not need to be known, and is irrelevant, if the elongated myopic eye is brought back to its normal shape. The same is true if the hypermetropic and astigmatic eyes are brought back to their normal shapes.

Stated another way: nearsightedness, farsightedness (at least before the age of forty), and astigmatism do not have anything to do with the front side of the lens not being able to acquire more curvature.

BATES AND SIMULTANEOUS RETINOSCOPY

One of the key principles of natural vision is motion, or movement. Most people's sight is tested when they are not moving. Bates showed that vision blurs when a person is still for too long. His advanced discoveries about natural vision were largely possible because he studied the vision of people and animals as they were moving.

In Chapter Two of the ground-breaking work, *Perfect Sight Without Glasses,* Bates discusses how the retinoscope made such research possible.

Much of my information about the eyes has been obtained by means of simultaneous retinoscopy. The retinoscope is an instrument used to measure the refraction of the eye. It throws a beam of light into the pupil by reflection from a mirror, the light being either outside the instrument—above and behind the subject—or arranged within it by means of an electric battery. On looking through the sight-hole one sees a larger or smaller part of the pupil filled with light, which in normal human eyes is a reddish yellow, because this is the color of the retina, but which is green in a cat's eye, and might be white if the retina were diseased. Unless the eye is exactly focussed at the point from which it is being observed, one sees also a dark shadow at the edge of the pupil, and it is the behavior of this shadow when the mirror is moved in various directions which reveals the refractive condition of the eye.... This exceedingly useful instrument has possibilities which have not been generally realized by the medical profession....

For thirty years I have been using the retinoscope to study the refraction of the eye. With it I have examined the eyes of tens of thousands of school children, hundreds of infants and thousands of animals, including cats, dogs, rabbits, horses, cows, birds, turtles, reptiles and fish. I have used it when the subjects were at rest and when they were in motion—also when I myself was in motion;...I have used it in the daytime and at night, when the subjects were comfortable and when they were excited; when they were trying to see and when they were not; when they were lying and when they were telling the truth; when the eyelids were partly closed, shutting off part of the area of the pupil, when the pupil was dilated, and also when it was contracted to a pin-point; when the eye was oscillating from side to side, from above downward and in other directions. In this way I discovered many facts which had not previously been known, and which I was quite unable to reconcile with the orthodox teachings on the subject. This led me to undertake the series of experiments already alluded to. The results were in entire harmony with my previous observations, and left me no choice but to reject the entire body of orthodox teaching about accommodation and errors of refraction.

A *SCIENTIFIC AMERICAN* REPORT ON THE BATES METHOD

Mary Dudderidge writes in the January 12, 1918, issue of *Scientific American:*

> The revelations regarding the physical condition of the American people which have resulted from the examination of men for military service under the Draft Law have come as a shock to the nation, but are no more than was expected by those who had previously been giving attention to such matters. Even under a liberal interpretation of the lowered standard which we adopted in 1909, when we abandoned the attempt to raise an army and navy with normal vision, defective eyesight has been one of the leading causes of rejection for service in both the Army and Navy, if it has not actually headed the list. In 1915 it was by far the most common of the defects found among applicants for enlistment in the Navy and Marine Corps. The total number refused for this cause among 106,392 was 12,374, while flat feet came next with only 8,188 cases. This too was under a standard which, while higher than that of the Army and Navy is only three-quarters normal.
>
> The fact is that defective sight is a world-wide plague, making its appearance along with civilization, and increasing just in proportion as modern modes of living are adopted....
>
> At the present time the general attitude of the medical profession toward this evil, which we have learned to take lightly only because it is so common, is one of hopelessness. Writers of books on the subject, practicing ophthalmologists and others, while admitting the inadequacy of the eyeglass, all assure us that it is the only [solution] for errors of refraction; while the only means of prevention they can suggest is that of sparing the eye as much as possible from the close application necessitated not only by the modern educational system, where most of the trouble begins, but by many of the employments upon which human life now depends. Some have even concluded that nature, who could not have been expected to provide for such a tremendous change as has taken place in the environment of the human animal, was not in a position to make the eye properly, while several scientists of repute have held that a moderate degree of myopia is a kind of a natural adaptation, and should not be

looked upon as abnormal....defects of vision are accepted as irreversible, and no means of alleviating them are suggested except the one, fraught with peril to the soldier, of placing convex or concave glasses before the eyes.[3]

...We were all taught at school that the accommodation of the eye depends upon an alteration in the curvature of the crystalline lens. Now defects of vision have been found to be associated with deviations from the normal in the shape of the eyeball, which ought to be a perfect sphere; and such deformations are always supposed to be permanent. In nearsightedness the sphere is elongated, so that it can be focused accurately only on near objects. Rays of light coming from a distance are focused in front of the retina instead of upon it. In farsightedness the eyeball is too short, and the light rays are focused behind the retina. In astigmatism the eyeball becomes lopsided, the deviation from the normal curvature not having been uniform. In an effort to overcome these conditions the crystalline lens is supposed to alter its curvature, through the agency of what is known as the ciliary muscle; on which theory the unfortunate muscle would have imposed upon it not only the ordinary labors of accommodation, but the duty of compensating for refractive errors; and from these labors it would practically never be free so long as the eye was open. The thought is really an appalling one, and is enough to drive the victim to eyeglasses, even if the physical discomfort of the situation did not do so.[4]

FUNCTIONAL PROBLEMS—ERRORS OF REFRACTION AND STRABISMUS

Bates referred to nearsightedness, farsightedness, presbyopia, astigmatism, and strabismus as functional problems. These problems, he said, are caused by chronically tense extrinsic eye muscles. Since these are not "organic" problems, he, and others, have said they are reversible.

Strain in one's eye muscles is similar to holding your fist tightly for a long time. The muscles are tense, there is less mobility, and the hand does not function properly. Holding the fist tight for many years, and putting a brace on it, would likely lead to more problems. The arm and shoulder become tight, and for some, the breathing becomes shallow or irregular. The tight fist becomes a holistic problem.

What is the solution? Letting go. Everything returns to its normal, relaxed, flexible state. Everything functions correctly again.

Errors of Refraction

When light rays do not focus on the retina correctly, the eye cannot see objects clearly at all distances. In this state the eye is said to have a refractive error. The three errors of refraction are nearsightedness, farsightedness (including presbyopia), and astigmatism.

Like the farsighted eye, the presbyopic eye has refractive error, but unlike the farsighted eye, presbyopic refractive error is said, conventionally, to be caused not by a foreshortened eyeball, but by the hardening of the lens. Bates said the cause of presbyopia is the same as the cause of farsightedness—tense recti muscles.

Strabismus, an Error of Convergence

Strabismus, e.g. crossed eye, is the abnormal turning of an eye away from the point of interest. Bates said that the abnormal tensing of one or more recti muscles can produce strabismus.

Strabismus, by itself, is not an error of refraction because light rays still focus on the retina to see clearly near and far. Of course if the strabismic eye is also nearsighted or farsighted, the eye cannot see clearly at all distances.

Strabismus and related issues are covered in Chapter 18, "Stereoscopic Vision."

ACCOMMODATION EXPLAINED FURTHER

Optical devices, e.g. cameras, binoculars, microscopes, and telescopes, require some way of changing in order to focus images at different distances clearly. In binoculars, microscopes, and telescopes the distance between the lenses is increased and decreased. In cameras the distance between the lens and the film is *increased* to focus a *near* object, and *decreased* to focus a *far* object.

As stated above, the eye, in its normal, round, "resting" state, sees clearly in the distance. If the eye did not change in some way, a near object could not be seen clearly. This is because light rays from the near object would come to a focus in back of the retina.

Accommodation is the ability of the eye to change from the state of seeing clearly in the distance to seeing clearly up close. When the eye is in the process of changing to see clearly up close, or when it is in the state of seeing clearly up close, it is said to be "accommodating." The reverse action of accommodation returns the eye to seeing clearly in the distance, when, once again, it is said to be "at rest," and no longer accommodating. Stated more simply, the eye accommodates to see clearly up close, and then "unaccommodates" to see clearly in the distance.

How the eye accommodates has been debated for many decades—long before Bates did his research on eyesight.

The Helmholtz Lens Theory of Accommodation

Hermann von Helmholtz (1821–1894) was a great German scientist and ophthalmologist. He developed the idea of the conservation of energy and made important contributions to the fields of optics and acoustics. The action of the ciliary muscle on the lens being the mechanism of accommodation is generally attributed to Helmholtz.

In 1943, ophthalmologist May stated the orthodox position on accommodation in his book *Diseases of the Eye:*

> During accommodation, the ciliary muscle (especially the circular fibers) contracts, drawing forward the choroid and relaxing the suspensory ligament; this diminishes the tension of the lens capsule and allows the inherent elasticity of the lens to increase its convexity. The change in curvature affects chiefly the anterior surface of the lens. This is Helmholtz's *theory* and the one *usually* accepted. [TQ emphasis.] Tscherning has advanced a different theory: He maintains that the ciliary muscle increases the tension of the suspensory ligament during contraction, and that this causes peripheral flattening of the lens with bulging anteriorly at its center.[5]

Bates writes in *Perfect Sight Without Glasses*, "Marius Hans Erik Tscherning (1854–) is a Danish ophthalmologist who for twenty-five years was co-director and director of the ophthalmological laboratory of the Sorbonne. Later he became professor of ophthalmology in the University of Copenhagen."

Although both of the theories of accommodation mentioned by May involve the changing of the front side of the lens, he presents two opposite mechanisms. It is interesting that as late as 1943, there were still questions as to the actual mechanism of accommodation. So, Helmholtz's explanation was still being referred to as a "theory" and this theory apparently was not accepted by everyone.

The 1980 edition of *Webster's New Collegiate Dictionary* defines visual accommodation as: "the automatic adjustment of the eye for seeing at different distances effected *chiefly* [TQ emphasis] by changes in the convexity of the crystalline lens."[6] The word "chiefly" seems to imply there is at least one other mechanism of automatically seeing at different distances.

In 1976 *University Physics* states:

> To see an object distinctly, a sharp image of it must be formed on the retina. If all the elements of the eye were rigidly fixed in position, there would be but one object distance for which a sharp retinal image would be formed, while in fact the normal eye can focus sharply on an object at any distance from infinity up to about 25 cm in front of the eye. This is made possible by the action of the crystalline lens and the ciliary muscle to which it is attached. When relaxed, the normal eye is focused on objects at infinity, i.e., the second focal point is at the retina. When it is desired to view an object nearer than infinity, the ciliary muscle tenses and the crystalline lens assumes a more nearly spherical [i.e., more convex] shape. This process is called *accommodation.*[7]

However, there seems to be some question as to whether the lens becomes rigid in presbyopia in the next paragraph in *University Physics* which is quoted later in this chapter.

Bates Questions the Accepted Theory of Accommodation

In *Perfect Sight Without Glasses,* in Chapter III, entitled "Evidence for the Accepted Theory of Accommodation," Bates discusses research by many scientists on the role, if any, of the lens in accommodation.

Much of the research on the lens was conducted by observing possible changes in the size of reflections of images on the front and back surfaces of the lens, using reflections of images from the cornea as a reference point.

Theoretically, the corneal reflections should remain constant in size because the eyeball and cornea are said (conventionally) not to change their shapes during accommodation.

Bates discusses research by Donders, and other scientists, on the lens. In regards to Donders, Bates writes in *Perfect Sight Without Glasses,* "Frans Cornelis Donders (1818–1889) was professor of physiology and ophthalmology at the University of Utrecht, and is ranked as one of the greatest ophthalmologists of all time." After discussing Donders' work, he discusses the work of the great ophthalmologist Helmholtz.

From *Perfect Sight Without Glasses:*

> Like Donders, Helmholtz found the image obtained by the ordinary methods on the front of the lens very unsatisfactory, and in his "Handbook of Physiological Optics" he describes it as being "usually so blurred that the form of the flame cannot be definitely distinguished."[a] So he placed two lights, or one doubled by reflection from a mirror, behind a screen in which were two small rectangular openings, the whole being
>
> [a] Handbuch der physiologischen Optik, edited by Nagel, 1909–11, vol. i, p. 121.

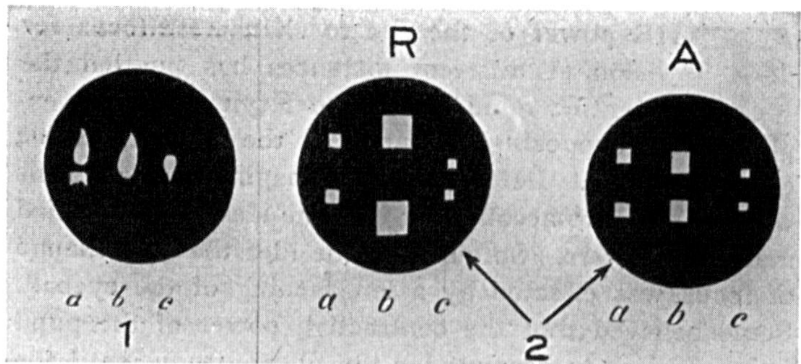

Figure 6–3: Diagram of the Images of Purkinje.[8] No. 1—Images of a candle: a, on the cornea; b, on the front of the lens; c, on the back of the lens. No. 2—Images of [two] lights shining through rectangular openings in a screen while the eye is at rest (R) and during accommodation (A): a, on the cornea; b, on the front of the lens; c, on the back of the lens (after Helmholtz). Note that in No. 2, A, the central images are smaller and have approached each other, a change which, if it actually took place, would indicate an increase of curvature in the front of the lens during accommodation.

so arranged that the lights shining through the openings of the screen formed two images on each of the reflecting surfaces. During accommodations, it seemed to him that the two images on the front of the lens became smaller and approached each other, while on the return of the eye to a state of rest [for distance clarity] they grew larger again and separated. This change, he said, could be seen "easily and distinctly."[b] The observations of Helmholtz regarding the behavior of the lens in accommodation, published about the middle of the last century, were soon accepted as facts, and have ever since been stated as such in every textbook dealing with the subject.

If an image reflecting from the front side of a convex lens becomes smaller, it could indicate the front side of that convex lens has increased its curvature. Helmholtz's research seemed to indicate that the images reflecting from the front side of the lens decreased in size when the eye accommodated to see clearly up close. An increase in the size of an image would indicate that the surface had become flatter, and vice versa.

However, the size of the images reflecting from the back side of the lens remained constant, indicating that the back side of the lens did not change in curvature during accommodation. How can a ciliary muscle change

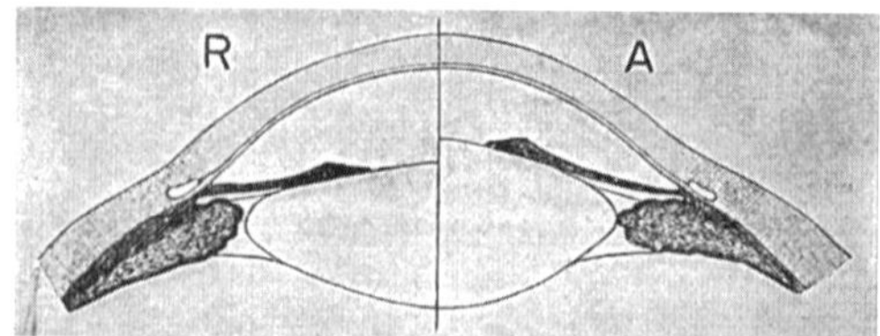

*Figure 6–4: Diagram By Which Helmholtz Illustrated His Theory of Accommodation.[9] **R** is supposed to be the resting state of the lens, in which it is adjusted for distant vision. In **A** the suspensory ligament is supposed to have been relaxed through the contraction of the ciliary muscle, permitting the [front side of the] lens to bulge forward by virtue of its own elasticity....*

[b] Ibid., vol. i, p. 122.

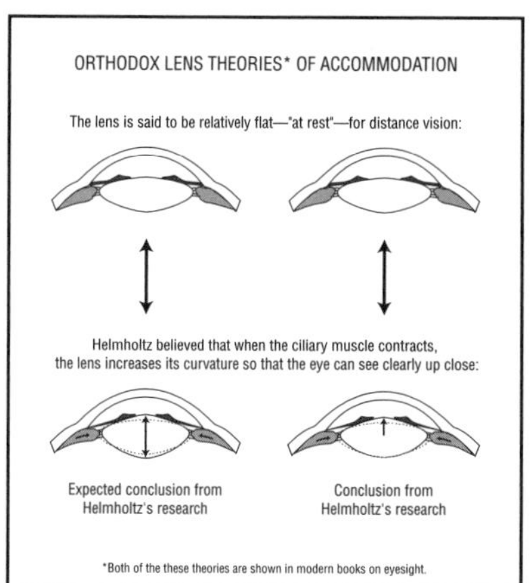

ORTHODOX LENS THEORIES* OF ACCOMMODATION
The lens is said to be relatively flat—"at rest"—for distance vision:
Helmholtz believed that when the ciliary muscle contracts,
the lens increases its curvature so that the eye can see clearly up close:
Expected conclusion from
Helmholtz's research
Conclusion from
Helmholtz's research
*Both of the these theories are shown in modern books on eyesight.

Figure 6–5: Expected Conclusion and Conclusion from Helmholtz's Research.

only the front side of a lens, without changing the back side?

According to the Helmholtz lens theory of accommodation, when the circular ciliary muscle contracts, it moves inward toward the lens. The suspensory ligaments, which span between the ciliary body and the lens capsule, relax their tension on the lens capsule. As a consequence, *the front side* of the lens is said to acquire more curvature. If this actually occurred, a person would then see clearly, or at least more clearly, up close; in other words, the person would be accommodating. When the ciliary muscle expands (relaxes) back to its normal state, the suspensory ligaments pull on the lens capsule, and *the front side* of the lens is said to return to its normal flatter shape for clear distant vision again.

Some contemporary books on eyesight have illustrations showing only the front side of the lens changing its curvature during accommodation, as attributed to Helmholtz. Others show *both* sides of the lens changing during accommodation. Helmholtz's research did not indicate that *both* sides of the lens change their curvature, which is what a person might expect when the ciliary muscle contracts and expands around the lens.

Lensless Accommodation—The "Grand Objection"

To continue from Bates' exposition from *Perfect Sight Without Glasses:*

> Yet in examining the evidence for the [Helmholtz's lens] theory we can only wonder at the scientific credulity which could base such an important department of medical practice as the [care] of the eye upon such a mass of contradictions. Helmholtz, while apparently convinced of the correctness of his observations indicating a change of form in the [front side

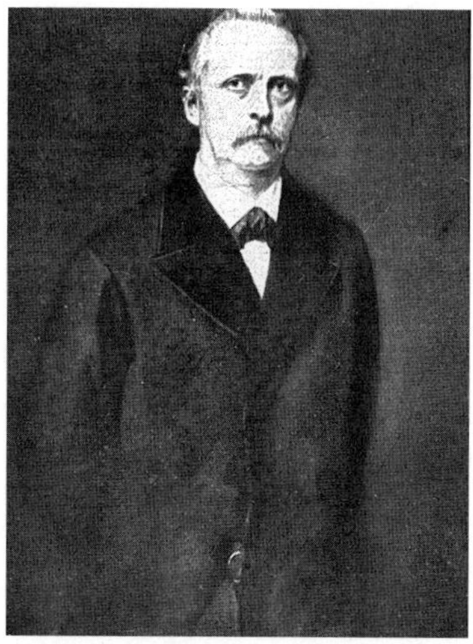

Figure 6–6: Hermann Ludwig Ferdinand von Helmholtz.[10] (1821–1894), whose observations regarding the behavior of images reflected from the front of the lens are supposed to have demonstrated that the curvature of this body changes during accommodation....

of the] lens during accommodation, felt himself unable to speak with certainty of the means by which the supposed change was effected,[a] and strangely enough the question is still being debated. Finding, as he states, "absolutely nothing but the ciliary muscle to which accommodation could be attributed,"[b] Helmholtz concluded that the changes which he thought he had observed in the curvature of the [front side of the] lens must be effected by the action of this muscle; but he was unable to offer any satisfactory theory of the way it operated to produce these results, and he explicitly stated that the one he suggested possessed only the character of probability. Some of his disciples, "more loyal than the king," as Tscherning has pointed out, "have proclaimed as certain what he [Helmholtz] himself with much reserve explained as probable,"[c] but there has been no such unanimity of acceptance in this case as in that of the observations regarding the behavior of the images reflected from the lens. No one except the present writer, so far as I am aware, has ventured to question that the ciliary muscle is the agent of accommodation; but as to the mode of its operation there is generally felt to be much need for more light. Since the lens is not a factor in accommodation, it is not strange that no one was able to find out how it changed its curvature. It is strange, however, that these difficulties have not in any way disturbed the universal belief that the lens does change.

[a] Handbuch der physiologischen Optik, vol. i, pp. 124 and 145.

[b] Ibid., vol. i, p. 144.

[c] Physiologic Optics, p. 166.

Bates then presents evidence of accommodation in people who are lensless:

When the lens has been removed for cataract the person usually appears to lose his power of accommodation, and not only has to wear a glass to replace the lost part [i.e., convex glasses for distance, compensating for the loss of the lens], but has to put on a stronger [convex] glass for reading. A minority of these cases, however, after they become accustomed to the new condition, become able to see at the near point without any change in their [distance] glasses. The existence of these two classes of cases has been a great stumbling block to ophthalmology. The first and more numerous appeared to support the theory of the agency of the lens in accommodation; but the second was hard to explain away, and constituted at one time, as Dr. Thomas Young observed, the "grand objection" to this idea. A number of these cases of apparent change of focus in the lensless eye having been reported to the Royal Society by competent observers. Dr. Young, before bringing forward his theory of accommodation, took the trouble to examine some of them, and considered himself justified in concluding that an error of observation had been made. While convinced, however, that in such eyes the "actual focal distance is totally unchangeable," he characterized his own evidence in support of this view as only "tolerably satisfactory." At a later period Donders made some investigations from which he concluded that "in aphakia[a] not the slightest trace of accommodative power remains."[b] Helmholtz expressed similar

[a] Absence of the lens.

[b] On the Anomalies of Accommodation and Refraction of the Eye, p. 320.

views, and von Graefe, although he observed a "slight residuum" of accommodative power in lensless eyes, did not consider it sufficient to discredit the theory of Cramer and Helmholtz. It might be due, he said, to the accommodative action of the iris, and possibly also to a lengthening of the visual axis through the action of the external muscles.[a]

For nearly three-quarters of a century the opinions of these masters have echoed through ophthalmological literature. Yet it is today a perfectly well-known and undisputed fact that many persons, after the removal of the lens for cataract, are able to see perfectly at different distances without any change in their glasses. Every ophthalmologist of any experience has seen cases of this kind, and many of them have been reported in the literature.

In 1872, Professor Forster of Breslau reported[b] a series of twenty-two cases of apparent accommodation in eyes from which the lens had been removed for cataract. The subjects ranged in age from eleven to seventy-four years, and the younger ones had more accommodative power than the elder. A year later Woinow of Moscow[c] reported eleven cases, the subjects being from twelve to sixty years of age. In 1869 and 1870, respectively, Loring reported[d] to the New York Ophthalmological Society and the American Ophthalmological Society the case of a young woman of eighteen who, without any change in her glasses, read the twenty line on the Snellen test card at twenty feet and also read diamond type at from five inches to twenty. On October 8, 1894, a client of Dr. A. E. Davis who appeared to accommodate perfectly without a lens consented to go before the New York Ophthalmological Society. "The members," Dr. Davis reports,[e] "were divided in their opinion as to how the person was able to accommodate for the near point with his distance glasses on"; but the fact that he could see at this point without any change in his glasses was not to be disputed.

[This person] was a chef, forty-two years old, and on January 27, 1894, Dr. Davis had removed a black cataract from his right eye, supplying him at the same time with the usual outfit of glasses, one to replace the lens, for distant vision, and a stronger one for reading. In October he returned, not because his eye was not doing well, but because he was afraid he might be "straining" it. He had discarded his reading glasses after a few weeks, and had since been using only his distance glasses. Dr. Davis doubted the truth of his statements, never having seen such a case before, but found them, upon investigation, to be quite correct. With his lensless eye and a convex glass of eleven and a half diopters, the chef read the ten line on the test card at twenty feet, and with the same glass, and without any change in its position, he read fine print at from fourteen to eighteen inches. Dr. Davis then presented the case to the Ophthalmological Society but, as has been stated, he obtained

[a] Archive. f. Ophth., 1855, vol. ii, part 1, p. 187 et seq. Albrecht von Graefe (1828–1870) was professor of ophthalmology in the University of Berlin, and is ranked with Donders and Arlt as one of the greatest ophthalmologists of the nineteenth century.

[b] Klin. Montasbl. f. Augenh., Erlangen, 1872, vol. x, p. 39 et seq.

[c] Archiv. f. Ophth., 1873, vol. xix, part 3, p. 107.

[d] Flint: Physiology of Man, 1875, vol. v, pp. 110–111.

[e] Davis: Accommodation in the Lensless Eye, Reports of the Manhattan Eye and Ear Hospital, Jan., 1895. The article gives a review of the whole subject.

no light from that source. Four months later, February 4, 1895, the chef still read 20/10 at the distance and his range at the near point had increased so that he read diamond type at from eight to twenty-two and a half inches. Dr. Davis subjected him to numerous tests, and though unable to find any explanation for his strange performances, he made some interesting observations. The results of the tests by which Donders satisfied himself that the lensless eye possessed no accommodative power were quite different from those reported by the Dutch authority [Cramer?], and Dr. Davis therefore concluded that these tests were "wholly inadequate to decide the question at issue." During accommodation the ophthalmometer[a] showed that the corneal curvature was changed and that the cornea moved forward a little. Under scopolamine, a drug sometimes used instead of atropine to paralyze the ciliary muscle (1/10 percent solution every five minutes for thirty-five minutes, followed by a wait of half an hour), these changes took place as before [paralysis of the ciliary muscle rules out the possibility of the ciliary muscle being the cause of the change of the corneal curvature]; they also took place when the lids were held up. With the possible influence of lid pressure and of the ciliary muscle eliminated, therefore, Dr. Davis felt himself bound to conclude that the changes "must have been produced by the action of the external muscles."

...These and similar cases have been the cause of great embarrassment to those who feel called upon to reconcile them with the accepted theories. With the retinoscope the lensless eye can be seen to accommodate; but the theory of Helmholtz has dominated the ophthalmological mind so strongly that even the evidence of objective tests was not believed. The apparent act of accommodation was said not to be real, and many theories, very curious and unscientific, have been advanced to account for it.

[a] An instrument for measuring the curvature of the cornea.

How is the Helmholtz Lens Theory Regarded Today?

The orthodox opinion remains the same today: the lens *is the only mechanism of accommodation, and it becomes irreversibly rigid in middle age. After that time accommodation is not supposed to be possible.*

Ironically, this position presents excellent support for the muscles being—at the very least—another mechanism of accommodation, due to the following four facts (some from above):

1. Many lensless people accommodate.
2. Many older people keep excellent vision both near and far.
3. Many so-called presbyopes have improved their vision with the Bates method of re-education.
4. An eye with a paralyzed ciliary muscle, which rules out accommodation by the lens, can still accommodate.

The only rational explanation for these four facts is that the two oblique muscles accommodate the eyeball. Other physical factors have been ruled out.

These four facts indicate that whether or not the lens and/or ciliary muscle play any role in accommodation, they are not *necessary* for accommodation.

Could Presbyopia Be Caused by a Strained or Atrophied Ciliary Muscle?

Could a strained or atrophied ciliary muscle, unable to contract, be the reason a lens no longer accommodates? Could the normalization of the ciliary muscle be the reason presbyopes improve vision?

Some have taken the position that the ciliary muscle can lose its ability to change the shape of the lens as the person becomes older. The "sluggish" ciliary muscle is not functioning correctly, but after being "toned up" again, the ciliary muscle is said to regain its ability to accommodate the lens.

This position appears to require that:

1. the lens has not become rigid; or
2. the lens became semi-rigid, but kept sufficient flexibility to still accommodate; or
3. the lens became completely rigid, but regained its flexibility when the ciliary muscle was "toned up" again.

These theories are not supported by the orthodox.

The ciliary muscle "revitalization" theory still does not explain how a lensless eye, and an eye with a paralyzed ciliary muscle, can still accommodate.

In fact, Bates *agreed* with orthodox science that the lens becomes less flexible as a person ages. But for Bates the lens was "immaterial," because his research indicated that only the two oblique muscles are involved in accommodation.

Presbyopia, an Age-Old "Old-Age" Myth

When the eye cannot see clearly up close—*after the age of forty*—a person is said to have presbyopia (from Greek: *presby,* meaning "older," and *opia,* meaning "eye"). Presbyopes often hear or read that their near blur is due to the inflexibility of the lens, due to the "natural aging process."

Presbyopia is said to be the result of the lens becoming rigid, in its "non-accommodating" flatter shape. According to the Helmholtz lens theory of accommodation, the presbyope can see clearly only in the distance, not up close. Supposedly the lens loses its flexibility and therefore the front side of the lens loses its ability to have more curvature to focus clearly on near objects. Conventional textbooks do *not* state that presbyopia is caused by foreshortening of the eyeball, which was Bates' position.

Quoting again from *University Physics:*[11]

> The extremes of the range over which distinct vision is possible are known as the *far point* and the *near point* of the eye. The far point of a normal eye is at infinity. The position of the near point *evidently* [TQ emphasis] depends on the extent to which the curvature of the crystalline lens may be increased in accommodation. The range of accommodation gradually diminishes with age as the crystalline lens loses its flexibility. For this reason the near point gradually recedes as one grows older. This recession of the near point with age is called presbyopia, and should not be considered a defect of vision, since it proceeds at about the same rate in all normal eyes. The following is a table of the approximate position of the near point at various ages:

Age, years	Near point, cm [2.54 cm = 1 inch]
10	7
20	10
30	14
40	22
50	40
60	200

In using the word "evidently," the authors seem to suggest some doubt as to the relationship between the inflexibility of the lens' curvature and a person's near point with aging.

Bates believed presbyopia is *hypermetropia occurring at middle age,* and is caused by strained recti muscles foreshortening the eyeball.

Bates proved the two oblique muscles can elongate the eyeball, in which state a person sees clearly up close. When the oblique muscles release, the eye returns to the normal shape for distance vision. For Bates, accommodation occurs only by the action of the two, oblique, external eye muscles.

Bates felt there was ample evidence to support the position that the oblique muscles produce accommodation. Following is his view on presbyopia, from Chapter XX of *Perfect Sight Without Glasses.* According to Bates, this condition is not inevitable, and it can be reversed when it occurs.

> Among people living under civilized conditions, the accommodative power of the eye gradually declines, in most cases, until at the age of sixty or seventy it appears to have been entirely lost, the subject being absolutely dependent upon his glasses for vision at the near point. As to whether the same thing happens among primitive people or people living under primitive conditions, very little information is available. Donders[a] says that the power of accommodation diminishes little, if at all, more rapidly among people who use their eyes much at the near point than among agriculturists, sailors and others who use them mainly for distant vision; and Roosa and others[b] say the contrary. This is a fact, however, that people who cannot read, no matter what their age, will manifest a failure of near vision if asked to look at printed characters, although their sight for familiar objects at the near point may be perfect. The fact that such persons, at the age of forty-five or fifty, cannot differentiate between printed characters is no warrant, therefore, for the conclusion that their accommodative powers are declining. A young illiterate would do no better, and a young student who can read Roman characters at the near point without difficulty always develops symptoms of imperfect sight when he attempts to read, for the first time, old English, Greek, or Chinese characters.
>
> When the accommodative power has declined to the point at which reading and writing become difficult, the person is said to have "*presbyopia*," or, more popularly, "*old sight*"; and the condition is generally accepted, both by the popular and the scientific mind, as one of the unavoidable inconveniences of old age. "Presbyopia," says Donders, "is the normal quality of the normal, emmetropic eye in advanced age,"[c]
>
> [a] On the Anomalies of Accommodation and Refraction of the Eye, p. 223.
>
> [b] Roosa: A Clinical Manual of Diseases of the Eye, 1894, p. 537; Oliver: System of Diseases of the Eye, vol. iv, p. 431.
>
> [c] On the Anomalies of Accommodation and Refraction of the Eye, p. 210.

and similar statements might be multiplied endlessly. De Schweinitz calls the condition "a normal result of growing old";[d] according to Fuchs it is "a physiological process which every eye undergoes";[e] while Roosa speaks of the change as one which "ultimately affects every eye."[f]

The decline of accommodative power with advancing years is commonly attributed to the hardening of the lens, an influence which is believed to be augmented, in later years, by a flattening of this body and a lowering of its refractive index, together with weakness or atrophy of the ciliary muscle; and so regular is the decline, in most cases, that tables have been compiled showing the near point to be expected at various ages. From these it is said one might almost fit glasses without testing the vision of the subject; or, conversely, one might, from a man's glasses, judge his age within a year or two. The following table is quoted from Jackson's chapter on "The Dioptrics of the Eye," in Norris and Oliver's "System of Diseases of the Eye,"[g] and does not differ materially from the tables given by Fuchs, Donders and Duane. The first column indicates the age, the second diopters of accommodative power, the third the near point for an emmetropic[h] eye, in inches.

Age	Diopters	Inches
10	14.00	2.81
15	12.00	3.28
20	10.00	3.94
25	8.50	4.63
30	7.00	5.63
35	5.50	7.16
40	4.50	8.75
45	3.50	11.25
50	2.50	15.75
55	1.50	26.25
60	0.75	52.49
65	0.25	157.48
70	0.00	

According to these depressing figures one must expect at thirty to have lost no less than half of one's original accommodative power, while at forty two-thirds of it would be gone, and at sixty it would be practically nonexistent.

There are many people, however, who do not fit this schedule. Many persons at forty can read fine print at four inches, although they ought, according to the table, to have lost that power shortly after twenty. Worse still, there are people who refuse to become presbyopic at all. Oliver Wendell Holmes mentions one of these cases in *The Autocrat of the Breakfast Table.*

"There is now living in New York State," he says, "an old gentleman who, perceiving his sight to fail, immediately took to exercising it on the finest print, and in this way fairly bullied Nature out of her foolish habit of taking liberties at five-and-forty, or thereabout. [Some Natural Vision teachers would have preferred the word "coaxed" instead of "bullied," as effort is never associated with normal vision.] And now this old gentleman performs the most extraordinary feats with his pen, showing that his eyes must be a pair of microscopes. I should

[d] Diseases of the Eye, p. 148.

[e] Text-book of Ophthalmology, authorized translation from the twelfth German edition by Duane, 1919, p. 862. Ernst Fuchs (1851–). Professor of Ophthalmology at Vienna from 1885 to 1915. His Text-book of Ophthalmology has been translated into many languages.

[f] A Clinical Manual of Diseases of the Eye, p. 535.

[g] Vol. i, p. 504.

[h] An eye which, when it is at rest, focuses parallel rays upon the retina is said to be emmetropic or normal.

be afraid to say how much he writes in the compass of a half-dime—whether the Psalms or the Gospels, or the Psalms and the Gospels, I won't be positive."[i]

There are also people who regain their near vision after having lost it for ten, fifteen, or more years; and there are people who, while presbyopic for some objects, have perfect sight for others. Many dressmakers, for instance, can thread a needle with the naked eye, and with the retinoscope it can be demonstrated that they accurately focus their eyes upon such objects; and yet they cannot read or write without glasses.

So far as I am aware no one but myself has ever observed the last-mentioned class of cases, but the others are known to every ophthalmologist of any experience. One hears of them at the meetings of ophthalmological societies; they are even reported in the medical journals; but such is the force of authority that when it comes to writing books they are either ignored or explained away, and every new treatise that comes from the press repeats the old superstition that presbyopia is "a normal result of growing old." ... German science still oppresses our intellects and prevents us from crediting the plainest evidence of our senses ... German ophthalmology is still sacred, and no facts are allowed to cast discredit upon it.

Fortunately for those who feel called upon to defend the old theories, myopia postpones the advent of presbyopia, and a decrease in the size of the pupil, which often takes place in old age, has some effect in facilitating vision at the near point. Reported cases of persons reading without glasses when over fifty or fifty-five years of age, therefore, can be easily disposed of by assuming that the subjects must be myopic, or that their pupils are unusually small. If the case comes under actual observation, the matter may not be so simple, because it may be found that the subject, so far from being myopic, is hypermetropic, or emmetropic, and that the pupil is of normal size. There is nothing [for the orthodox] to do with these cases but to ignore them. Abnormal changes in the form of the lens have also been held responsible for the retention of near vision beyond the prescribed age, or for its restoration after it has been lost, the swelling of the lens in incipient cataract affording a very convenient and plausible explanation for the latter class of cases. In cases of premature presbyopia, "accelerated sclerosis"[j] of the lens and weakness of the ciliary muscle have been assumed; and if such cases as the dressmakers who can thread their needles when they can no longer read the newspapers had been observed, no doubt some explanation consistent with the German viewpoint would have been found for them.

The truth about presbyopia is that it is not "a normal result of growing old," being both preventable and reversible. It is not caused by hardening of the lens, but by a strain to see at the near point. It has no necessary connection with age, since it occurs, in some cases, as early as ten years, while in others it never occurs at all, although the subject may live far into the so-called presbyopic age. It is true that the lens does harden with advancing years, just as the bones harden and the structure of the skin changes; but since the lens is not a factor in accommodation, this fact is immaterial, and while in some cases the lens may

[i] Everyman's Library, 1908, pp. 166–167.

[j] Fuchs: Text-book of Ophthalmology, p. 905.

become flatter, or lose some of its refractive power with advancing years, it has been observed to remain perfectly clear and unchanged in shape up to the age of ninety. Since the ciliary muscle is also not a factor in accommodation, its weakness or atrophy can contribute nothing to the decline of accommodative power. [In this last paragraph, Bates completely discounts the role of the lens and ciliary muscle as having anything to do with accommodation.] Presbyopia is, in fact, simply a form of hypermetropia in which the vision for the near point is chiefly affected, although the vision for the distance, contrary to what is generally believed, is always lowered also ... In both conditions the sight at both points is lowered, although the person may not be aware of it.

It has been shown that when the eyes strain to see at the near point the focus is always pushed farther away than it was before, in one or all meridians; and by means of simultaneous retinoscopy it can always be demonstrated that when a person with presbyopia tries to read fine print and fails, the focus is always pushed farther away than it was before the attempt was made, indicating that the failure was caused by strain. Even the thought of making such an effort will produce strain, so that the refraction may be changed, and pain, discomfort and fatigue produced, before the fine print is regarded. [Relaxation of the mind is the most important principle Bates discovered about natural, clear vision.] Furthermore, when a person with presbyopia rests the eyes by closing them, or palming, he always becomes able, for a few moments at least, to read fine print at six inches, again indicating that his previous failure was due, not to any fault of the eyes, but to a strain to see. When the strain is permanently relieved the presbyopia is permanently reversed, and this has happened, not in a few cases, but in many, and at all ages, up to sixty, seventy and eighty.

Physician, Heal Thyself

Continuing from *Perfect Sight Without Glasses,* Bates explains how he reversed his own presbyopia:

> The first person that I reversed of presbyopia was myself. Having demonstrated by means of experiments on the eyes of animals that the lens is not a factor in accommodation, I knew that presbyopia must be reversible, and I realized that I could not look for any very general acceptance of the revolutionary conclusions I had reached so long as I wore glasses myself for a condition supposed to be due to the loss of the accommodative power of the lens. I was then suffering from the maximum degree of presbyopia. I had no accommodative power whatever, and had to have quite an outfit of glasses, because with a glass, for instance, which enabled me to read fine print at thirteen inches, I could not read it either at twelve inches or at fourteen. The retinoscope showed that when I tried to see anything at the near point without glasses my eyes were focused for the distance, and when I tried to see anything at the distance they were focused for the near point. My problem, then, was to find some way of reversing this condition and inducing my eyes to focus for the point I wished to see at the moment that I wished to see it. I consulted various eye specialists, but my language was to them like that of St. Paul to the Greeks, namely, foolishness. "Your lens is as hard as a stone," they said. "No one can do anything for you." Then I went to a nerve specialist. He used the retinoscope on me, and confirmed my own

observations as to the peculiar contrariness of my accommodation; but he had no idea what I could do about it. He would consult some of his colleagues, he said, and asked me to come back in a month, which I did. Then he told me he had come to the conclusion that there was only one man who could [reverse my presbyopia] . . . , and that was Dr. William H. Bates of New York.

"Why do you say that?" I asked.

"Because you are the only man who seems to know anything about it," he answered.

Thus thrown upon my own resources, I was fortunate enough to find a non-medical gentleman who was willing to do what he could to assist me, the Rev. R. B. B. Foote, of Brooklyn. He kindly used the retinoscope through many long and tedious hours while I studied my own case, and tried to find some way of accommodating when I wanted to read, instead of when I wanted to see something at the distance. One day, while looking at a picture of the Rock of Gibraltar which hung on the wall, I noted some black spots on its face. I imagined that these spots were the openings of caves, and that there were people in these caves moving about. [As with many great scientific discoveries, Bates accidentally stumbles upon two of the three key principles of normal sight: movement and centralization (attention to detail).] When I did this my eyes were focused for the reading distance. Then I looked at the same picture at the reading distance, still imagining that the spots were caves with people in them. The retinoscope showed that I had accommodated, and I was able to read the lettering beside the picture. I had, in fact, been temporarily reversed by the use of my imagination. Later I found that when I imagined the letters black I was able to see them black, and when I saw them black I was able to distinguish their form. My progress after this was not what could be called rapid. It was six months before I could read the newspapers with any kind of comfort, and a year before I obtained my present accommodative range of fourteen inches, from four inches to eighteen; but the experience was extremely valuable, for I had in pronounced form every symptom subsequently observed in other presbyopic people.

[Even if Bates had erred in his research, it still allowed him to find a way to reverse his own presbyopia.]

Fortunately for others, it has seldom taken me as long to reverse other people as it did to reverse myself. In some cases a complete and permanent reversal was effected in a few minutes. Why, I do not know. I will never be satisfied till I find out. A person who had worn glasses for presbyopia for about twenty years reversed in less than fifteen minutes . . . .

. . . In nine cases out of ten progress has been much slower, and it has been necessary to resort to all the methods of obtaining relaxation. [Relaxation is the third and most important principle of normal vision.]

. . . Their [the presbyopes'] sight for the distance is often very imperfect and always below normal, although they may have thought it perfect; and just as in the case of other errors of refraction, improvement of the distant vision improves the vision at the near point. . . .

[Repeating from Chapter 4, "The Problem With Glasses and Contact Lenses":] If persons who find themselves getting presbyopic, or who have arrived at the presbyopic age, would, instead of resorting to glasses, follow the example of the gentleman mentioned by Dr. Holmes and make a practice of reading the finest print they can find, the idea that the decline of accommodative power is "a normal result of growing old" would soon die a natural death.

More Problems with the Conventional Presbyopia Theory

Another problem with the presbyopic/lens-hardening theory is that some people who have had clarity for the first forty years of their life become nearsighted! I have met several such individuals. In nearsightedness the eyeball is too long. Since the eyeball can become too long at age forty, is it unreasonable to believe the eyeball can become too short, creating hypermetropia (farsightedness)? Bates said, "No."

In addition, some people who have had nearsightedness for many years return to normal, clear vision, near and far, after the age of forty. These people are told this occurs because their nearsightedness is being "balanced" by presbyopia. This is not a satisfactory explanation, because these people accommodate clearly both near and far. If nearsightedness could be "balanced" by presbyopia, a person would be unable to accommodate. Only one distance would be seen clearly.

For seventy-five years, Bates teachers have watched people with so-called presbyopia improve their vision. Many so-called presbyopic students have been able to improve their near vision and read, once again, without any corrective lenses.

Some people improve so-called presbyopia spontaneously. One of my students, who had presbyopic glasses for many years, told me she went on a three-month vacation on a cruise ship many years ago. At the end of this relaxing vacation, she could read books without her glasses. She did not know anything about the Bates method, or natural vision improvement. Her presbyopic vision improved automatically by relaxation. Her so-called "presbyopia" returned when she returned to her stressful job.

The father of one of my students is eighty-two years old. He has never needed glasses. He still reads books and drives a car without glasses.

A fifty-seven-year-old woman in one of my recent classes began to experience "presbyopia" at age forty-one. At age forty-seven she was given bifocals. She stated she has a tight neck and headaches. During vision classes she said she was once again beginning to be able to read books without her glasses.

One of the motivations for enrolling in natural vision classes is that some parents of students have had normal vision at ages seventy and eighty. These students know there is a way vision can be clear—at any age—and that blurred vision is not hereditary.

Regardless of the physical mechanisms involved, there is a way to see clearly up close, including reading books, at any age.

Acquiring farsightedness in mid-life is not due to "old age" any more than children acquiring nearsightedness is due to "young age." Bates showed that the habits of vision determine how well a person sees near and far.

"Why Do So Many People Lose Near Vision around Age Forty?"

It is a fact that many people *in stressful industrialized societies* lose the ability to see clearly up close around the age of forty.

Presbyopia is so prevalent in older people in our society that we are told to expect it, as if it were a certainty. Referring to presbyopia, one ad states definitively that if you are over forty, "you've got it." At a local 5&10 store, the rack with "magnifiers" for presbyopes provides a reading card with different-size letters to help you determine which power of glasses to buy. As the print gets smaller, this card educates you on how nature does not provide enough secretions to keep the lenses soft and flexible, and therefore the power of accommodation is lost. (Is this a new theory of lack of accommodation?) Further, it informs you that failure of sight is very common between the ages of thirty and forty. In our society, this last statement is true. Failure of sight is also common at many other ages!

Vision is very suggestible. If a person with normal sight for forty years is told she is going to lose her near vision, what do you think her response might be? Would she begin to not trust her eyesight anymore? (Trust is a key right-hemisphere characteristic of normal vision.) Would she consciously strain to see near objects? If she does, she will become farsighted according to Bates.

In industrialized societies, there appears to be a correlation between right-brain-dominant individuals who strain their near vision around age forty and then become farsighted. There also appears to be a correlation between left-brain-dominant individuals who strain their near vision at a young age and then become nearsighted. This is discussed more in Chapter 19, "Brains and Vision."

In the next chapter, we explore Bates' original and extensive research on the mechanism of accommodation and errors of refraction.

Notes

1 These graphics, caption, and text are from *Perfect Sight Without Glasses*.

2 Ibid.

3 Mary Dudderidge, "New Light Upon Our Eyes: An Investigation Which May Result in Normal Vision for All, Without Glasses" [or surgery], in *Scientific American* (January 12, 1918), p. 53.

4 Ibid.

5 Charles H. May, *Diseases of the Eye* (Baltimore, MD: William Wood and Company, 1943), p. 364.

6 H. B. Woolf, *Webster's New Collegiate Dictionary* (Springfield, MA: G & C Merriam Company, 1980).

7 F. W. Sears, M. W. Zemansky, and H. D. Young, *University Physics* (Springfield, MA: Addison-Wesley Publishing Company, Inc., May 1976), pp. 694–95.

8 These graphics, caption, and text are from *Perfect Sight Without Glasses.*

9 Ibid.

10 This graphic, caption, and text are from *Perfect Sight Without Glasses.*

11 Sears, Zemansky, and Young, *University Physics,* p. 695.

CHAPTER SEVEN

Accommodation and Errors of Refraction—Bates' View

This book aims to be a collection of facts and not of theories ... In the science of ophthalmology, theories, often stated as facts, have served to obscure the truth and throttle investigation for more than a hundred years. The explanations of the phenomena of sight put forward by Young, von Graefe, Helmholtz and Donders have caused us to ignore or explain away a multitude of facts which otherwise would have led to the discovery of the truth about errors of refraction and the consequent prevention of an incalculable amount of human misery....

—William H. Bates, 1920

BATES' RESEARCH ON THE ROLE OF THE SIX EXTRINSIC EYE MUSCLES

The theory that the eyeball elongates along the visual axis to accommodate did not originate with Bates. This idea had many supporters as early as the 1600s.

Due to many of the facts presented in the last chapter, Bates concluded that no one yet knew how the eyes accommodate. He believed that if he could discover the true mechanism of accommodation, and what interfered with it, he could then show people how to improve their sight.

Many parts of the body heal and normalize when the true cause of a problem is removed. Cuts and burns heal, broken bones heal, and so on.

Blurred vision is not a disease; it is a functional problem. Are the eyes the only parts of the human body that cannot heal or reverse a functional problem?

BATES: "THE TRUTH ABOUT ACCOMMODATION AS DEMONSTRATED BY EXPERIMENTS ON ANIMALS"

Perfect Sight Without Glasses contains much of Bates' research, including many photographs showing the production of errors of refraction and accommodation by the action of the extrinsic muscles. The following excerpt is from Chapter IV, "The Truth about Accommodation as Demonstrated by Experiments on Animals."

> The function of the muscles on the outside of the eyeball, apart from that of turning the globe in its socket, has been a matter of much dispute; but after the supposed demonstration by Helmholtz that accommodation

depends upon a change in the curvature of the lens, the possibility of their being concerned in the adjustment of the eye for vision at different distances, or in the production of errors of refraction, was dismissed as no longer worthy of serious consideration.

... In my own experiments upon the extrinsic eye muscles of fish, rabbits, cats, dogs and other animals, the demonstration seemed to be complete that in the eyes of these animals accommodation depends wholly upon the action of the extrinsic muscles and not at all upon the agency of the lens. By the manipulation of these muscles I was able to produce or prevent accommodation at will, to produce myopia, hypermetropia and astigmatism, or to prevent these conditions. Full details of these experiments will be found in the "Bulletin of the New York Zoological Society" for November, 1914, and in the "New York Medical Journal" for May 8, 1915; and May 18, 1918; but for the benefit of those who have not the time or inclination to read these papers, their contents are summarized below.

There are six muscles on the outside of the eyeball, four known as the "recti" and two as the "obliques." The obliques form an almost complete belt around the middle of the eyeball, and are known, according to their position, as "superior" and "inferior." The recti are attached to the sclerotic, or outer coat of the eyeball, near the front, and pass directly over the top, bottom and sides of the globe to the back of the orbit, where they are attached to the bone [a]round the edges of the hole through which the optic nerve passes. According to their position, they are known as the "superior," "inferior," "internal" and "external" recti. The obliques are the muscles of accommodation; the recti are concerned in the production of hypermetropia and astigmatism.

In some cases one of the obliques is absent or rudimentary, but when two of these muscles were present and active, accommodation, as measured by the objective test of retinoscopy, was always produced by electrical stimulation either of the eyeball, or of the nerves of accommodation near their origin in the brain. It was also produced by any manipulation of the obliques whereby their pull was increased. This was done by a tucking operation of one or both muscles, or by an advancement of the point at which they are attached to the sclerotic. When one or more of the recti had been cut, the effect of operations increasing the pull of the obliques was intensified.

After one or both of the obliques had been cut across, or after they had been paralyzed by the injection of atropine deep into the orbit, accommodation could never be produced by electrical stimulation; but after the effects of the atropine had passed away, or a divided muscle had been sewed together, accommodation followed electrical stimulation just as usual. Again when one oblique muscle was absent, as was found to be the case in a dogfish, a shark and a few perch, or rudimentary, as in all cats observed, a few fish and an occasional rabbit, accommodation could not be produced by electrical stimulation. But when the rudimentary muscle was strengthened by advancement, or the absent one was replaced by a suture which supplied the necessary countertraction, accommodation could always be produced by electrical stimulation.

After one or both of the oblique muscles had been cut, and while two or more of the recti were present and active,[a] elec-

[a] In many animals, notably in rabbits, the internal and external recti are either absent or rudimentary, so that practically, in such cases, there are only two recti, just as there are only two obliques. In others, as in many fish, the internal rectus is negligible.

trical stimulation of the eyeball, or of the nerves of accommodation, always produced hypermetropia, while by the manipulation of one of the recti, usually the inferior or the superior, so as to strengthen its pull, the same result could be produced. The paralyzing of the recti by atropine, or the cutting of one or more of them, prevented the production of hypermetropic refraction by electrical stimulation; but after the effects of the atropine had passed away, or after a divided muscle had been sewed together, hypermetropia was produced as usual by electrical stimulation.

It should be emphasized that in order to paralyze either the recti muscles, or the obliques, it was found necessary to inject the atropine far back behind the eyeball with a hypodermic needle. This drug is supposed to paralyze the accommodation when dropped into the eyes of human beings or animals, but in all of my experiments it was found that when used in this way it had very little effect upon the power of the eye to change its focus.

... Eyes from which the lens had been removed, or in which it had been pushed out of the axis of vision, responded to electrical stimulation precisely as did the normal eye, so long as the muscles were active; but when they had been paralyzed by the injection of atropine deep into the orbit, electrical stimulation had no effect on the refraction.

In one experiment the lens was removed from the right eye of a rabbit, the refraction of each eye having first been tested by retinoscopy and found to be normal. The wound was then allowed to heal. Thereafter, for a period extending from one month to two years, electrical stimulation always produced accommodation in the lensless eye precisely to the same extent as in the eye which had a lens. The same experiment with the same result was performed on a number of other rabbits, on dogs and on fish. The obvious conclusion is that the lens is not a factor in accommodation. [Rather, the obvious conclusion is that the lens is not a *necessary* factor in accommodation.]

In most text-books on physiology it is stated that accommodation is controlled by the third cranial nerve, which supplies all the muscles of the eyeball except the superior oblique and the external rectus; but the fourth cranial nerve, which supplies only the superior oblique, was found in these experiments to be just as much a nerve of accommodation as the third. When either the third or the fourth nerve was stimulated with electricity near its point of origin in the brain, accommodation always resulted in the normal eye. When the origin of either nerve was covered with a small wad of cotton soaked in a two percent solution of atropine sulphate in a normal salt solution, stimulation of that nerve produced no accommodation, while stimulation of the unparalyzed nerve did produce it. When the origin of both nerves was covered with cotton soaked in atropine, accommodation could not be produced by electrical stimulation of either or both. When the cotton was removed and the nerves washed with normal salt solution, electrical stimulation of either or both produced accommodation just as before the atropine had been applied. This experiment, which was performed repeatedly for more than an hour by alternately applying and removing the atropine, not only demonstrated clearly what had not been known before, namely, that the fourth nerve is a nerve of accommodation, but also demonstrated that the superior oblique muscle which is supplied by it is an important factor in accommodation. It was further found that when the action of the oblique muscles was prevented by dividing them, the stimulation of the third nerve produced not accommodation, but hypermetropia.

In all the experiments all sources of error are believed to have been eliminated. They were all repeated many times and always with the same result. They seemed, therefore, to leave no room for doubt that neither the lens nor any muscle inside the eyeball has anything to do with accommodation, but that the process whereby the eye adjusts itself for vision at different distances is entirely controlled by the action of the muscles on the outside of the globe.

[Fig. 7–1 graphics not shown][1]

Figure 7–1: Demonstration Upon the Eye of a Rabbit that the Inferior Oblique Muscle is an Essential Factor in Accommodation.[2] *No. 1—The inferior oblique muscle has been exposed and two sutures are attached to it. Electrical stimulation of the eyeball produces accommodation as demonstrated by simultaneous retinoscopy. No. 2—The muscle has been cut. Electrical stimulation produces no accommodation. No. 3—The muscle has been sewed together. Electrical stimulation produces normal accommodation.*

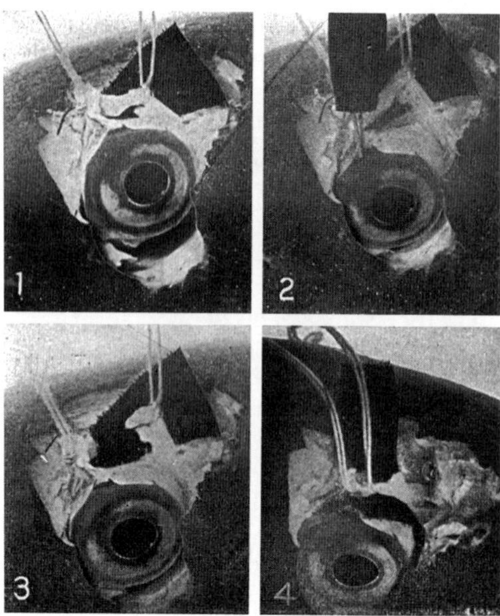

Figure 7–2: Demonstration Upon the Eye of a Carp that the Superior Oblique Muscle is Essential to Accommodation.[3] *No. 1—The superior oblique is lifted from the eyeball by two sutures, and the retinoscope shows no error of refraction. No. 2—Electrical stimulation produces accommodation, as determined by the retinoscope. No. 3—The muscle has been cut. Stimulation of the eyeball with electricity fails to produce accommodation. No. 4—The divided muscle has been reunited by tying the sutures. Accommodation follows electrical stimulation as before.*

[Fig. 7–3 graphics not shown]

Figure 7–3: Demonstration Upon the Eye of a Rabbit that the Production of Refractive Errors Is Dependent Upon the Action of the External Muscles.[4] *The string is fastened to the insertion of the superior oblique and rectus muscles. No. 1—Backward pull. Myopia is produced. No. 2—Forward pull. Hypermetropia is produced. No. 3—Upward pull in the plane of the iris. Mixed astigmatism is produced.*

The production of errors of refraction by the action of the extrinsic muscles in a rabbit does not prove, by itself, that errors of refraction cannot be produced by other means in the human eye. Bates proved here that the extrinsic muscles *can* produce errors of refraction.

[Fig. 7–4 graphic not shown]

Figure 7–4: Demonstration Upon the Eye of a Fish that the Production of Myopic and Hypermetropic Refraction Is Dependent Upon the Action of the Extrinsic Muscles.[5] A suture is tied to the insertion of the superior rectus muscle. By means of strong traction upon the suture the eyeball is turned in its socket, and by tying the thread to a pair of fixation forceps which grasp the lower jaw, it is maintained in this position. A high degree of mixed astigmatism is produced, as demonstrated by simultaneous retinoscopy. When the superior oblique is divided the myopic part of the astigmatism disappears, and when the inferior rectus is cut the hypermetropic part disappears, and the eye becomes normal—adjusted for distant vision—although the same amount of traction is maintained. It is evident that these muscles are essential factors in the production of myopia and hypermetropia.

Bates proved that the extrinsic muscles can produce myopia and hypermetropia.

[Fig. 7–5 graphic not shown]

Figure 7–5: Rabbit With Lense Removed.[6] The animal was exhibited at a meeting of the Ophthalmological Section of the American Medical Association, held in Atlantic City, and was examined by a number of ophthalmologists present, all of whom testified that electrical stimulation of the eyeball produced accommodation, or myopic refraction, precisely as in the normal eye.

Bates demonstrated the oblique muscles can produce accommodation. But he was not satisfied in just demonstrating the role of the extrinsic muscles in accommodation and the errors of refraction. He spent considerable time, energy, and ingenuity re-examining Helmholtz's research on the lens. If Bates could prove the lens did not play a role in accommodation, then action of the oblique muscles must be the only mechanism of accommodation.

Bates: "The Truth About Accommodation as Demonstrated by a Study of Images Reflected from the Lens, Cornea, Iris, and Sclera"

The above heading, "The Truth About Accommodation ..." is how Bates titled Chapter V of *Perfect Sight Without Glasses.* Following are excerpts from that chapter.

> As the conclusions to which the experiments described in the preceding chapter pointed were diametrically opposed to those reached by Helmholtz in his study of the images reflected from the front of the lens, I determined to repeat the experiments of the German investigator and find out, if possible, why his results were so different from my own. I devoted four years to this work, and was able to demonstrate that Helmholtz had erred through a defective technique, the image obtained by his method being so variable and uncertain that it lends itself to the support of almost any theory.
>
> I worked for a year or more with the technique of Helmholtz, but was unable to obtain an image from the front of the lens which was sufficiently clear or distinct to be measured or photographed. With a naked candle as the source of light, a clear and dis-

tinct image could be obtained on the cornea; on the back of the lens it was quite clear; but on the front of the lens it was very imperfect. Not only was it blurred, just as Helmholtz stated, but without any ascertainable cause it varied greatly in size and intensity. At times no reflection could be obtained at all, regardless of the angle of the light to the eye of the subject, or of the eye of the observer to that of the subject. With a diaphragm I got a clearer and more constant image, but it still was not sufficiently reliable to be measured. To Helmholtz the indistinct image of a naked flame seemed to show an appreciable change, while the images obtained by the aid of the diaphragm showed it more clearly; but I was unable, either with a diaphragm or without it, to obtain images which I considered sufficiently distinct to be reliable.

Men who had been teaching and demonstrating Helmholtz's theory repeated his experiments for my benefit; but the images which they obtained on the front of the lens did not seem to me any better than my own. After studying these images almost daily for more than a year I was unable to make any reliable observation regarding the effect of accommodation upon them. In fact, it seemed that an infinite number of appearances might be obtained on the front of the lens when a candle was used as the source of illumination. At times the image became smaller during accommodation and seemed to sustain the theory of Helmholtz; but just as frequently it became larger. At other times it was impossible to tell what it did.

With a thirty-watt lamp, a fifty-watt lamp, a 250-watt lamp and a 1000-watt lamp, there was no improvement.... To sum it all up, I was convinced that the anterior [front] surface of the lens was a very poor reflector of light, and that no reliable images could be obtained from it by the means described.

After a year or more of failure I began to work at an aquarium on the eyes of fish. It was a long story of failure. Finally I became able, with the aid of a strong light—1000 watts—a diaphragm with a small opening and a condenser, to obtain, after some difficulty, a clear and distinct image from the cornea of fish. This image was sufficiently distinct to be measured, and after many months a satisfactory photograph was obtained. Then the work was resumed on the eyes of human beings. The strong light, combined with the diaphragm and condenser, the use of which was suggested by their use to improve the illumination of a glass slide under the microscope, proved to be a decided improvement over the method of Helmholtz, and by means of this technique an image was at last obtained on the front of the lens which was sufficiently clear and distinct to be photographed. This was the first time, so far as published records show, that an image of any kind was ever photographed from the front of the lens. Professional photographers whom I consulted with a view to securing their assistance assured me that the thing could not be done, and declined to attempt it. I was therefore obliged to learn photography, of which I had previously known nothing, myself, and I then found that so far as the image obtained by the method of Helmholtz is concerned the professionals were right.

The experiments were continued until, after almost four years of constant labor, I obtained satisfactory pictures before and after accommodation and during the production of myopia and hypermetropia, not only of images on the front of the lens, but of reflections from the iris, cornea, the front of the sclera (white of the eye) and the side of the sclera. I also became able to obtain images on any surface at will without reflec-

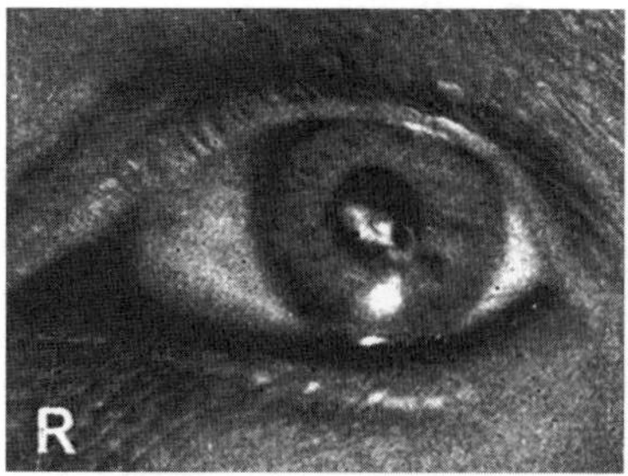

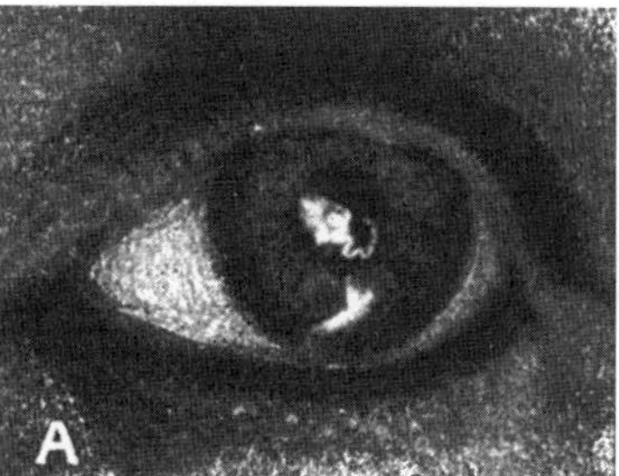

Figure 7–6: Image of Electric Filament on the Front of the Lens.[7]

R, rest; A, accommodation. Under the magnifying glass no change can be observed in the size of the two images. The image at the right looks larger only because it is more distinct. To support the theory of Helmholtz it ought to be smaller. The comet's tail at the left of the two images is an accidental reflection from the cornea. The spot of light beneath is a reflection from the light used to illuminate the eye while the photographs were being taken. It took two years to get these pictures.

tions from the other parts. Before these results were obtained, however, many difficulties had still to be overcome....

The results of these experiments confirmed the conclusions drawn from the previous ones, namely, that accommodation is due to a lengthening of the eyeball, and not to a change in the curvature of the lens. They also confirmed, in a striking manner, my earlier conclusions as to the conditions under which myopia and hypermetropia are produced.[a]

The images photographed from the front of the lens did not show any change in size or form during accommodation. The image on the back of the lens also remained unchanged, as observed through the telescope of the ophthalmometer; but as there is no dispute about its behavior during accommodation [Helmholtz never claimed the back side of the lens changed its curvature during accommodation], it was not photographed. Images photographed from the iris before and during accommodation were also the same in size and form, as was to be expected from the character of the lens images. If the lens changed during accommodation, the iris, which rests upon it, would change also.

[a] Bates: The Cause of Myopia, N. Y. Med. Jour., March 16, 1912.

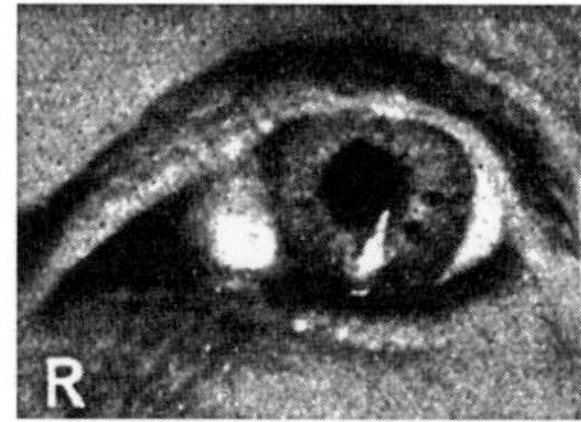

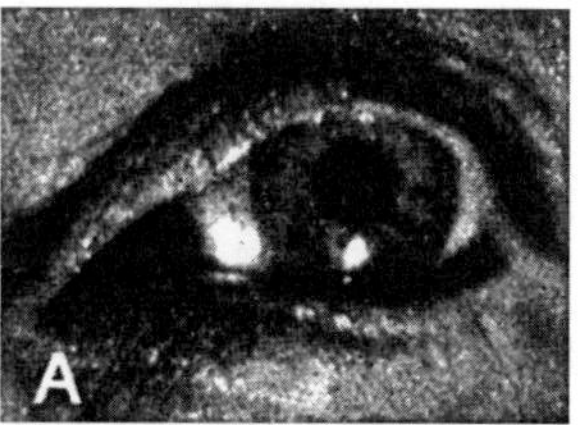

Figure 7–7: Image of Electric Filament on the Front of the Sclera.[8]

R, rest; A, accommodation. During accommodation the front of the sclera becomes more convex, because the eyeball has elongated, just as a camera is elongated when it is focused upon a near object. The spot of light on the cornea is an accidental reflection.

Bates: The Lens Does Not Change Its Curvature During Accommodation

Bates then states that his experiments have proven that the lens does not change its curvature during accommodation.

> The images photographed from the cornea and from the front and side of the sclera showed, however, a series of four well-marked changes, according to whether the vision was normal or accompanied by a strain. During accommodation the images from the cornea were smaller than when the eye was at rest, indicating elongation of the eyeball and a consequent increase in the convexity of the cornea. But when an unsuccessful effort was made to see at the near point, the image became larger, indicating that the cornea had become less convex, a condition which one would expect when the optic axis was shortened, as in hypermetropia. When a strain was made to see at a distance the image was smaller than when the eye was at rest, again indicating elongation of the eyeball and increased convexity of the cornea.
>
> The images photographed from the front of the sclera showed the same series of changes as the corneal images, but those obtained from the side of the sclera were found to have changed in exactly the opposite manner, being larger where the former were smaller and vice versa, a difference which one would naturally expect from the fact that when the front of the sclera becomes more convex the sides must become flatter.
>
> When an effort was made to see at a distance the image reflected from the side of the sclera was larger than the image obtained when the eye was at rest, indicating that this part of the sclera had become less convex or flatter, because of elongation of the eyeball. The image obtained during normal accommodation was also larger than when the eye was at rest, indicating again a flattening of the side of the sclera. The image obtained, however, when an effort was made to see near was much smaller than any of the other images, indicating that the sclera had become more convex at the side, a condition which one would expect when the eyeball was shortened, as in hypermetropia.
>
> The most pronounced of the changes were noted in the images reflected from the front of the sclera. Those on the side of the sclera were less marked, and, owing to the difficulty of photographing a white image on a white background, could not always be readily seen on the photographs. They were always plainly apparent, however, to the observer, and still more so to the subject, who regarded them in a concave mirror. The alterations in the size of the corneal image were so slight that they did not show at all in the photographs, except when the image was large, a fact which explains why the ophthalmometer, with its small image, has been thought to show that the cornea did not change during accommodation. They were always apparent, however, to the subject and observer.
>
> The corneal image was one of the easiest of the series to produce and the experiment is one which almost anyone can repeat, the only apparatus required being a fiftycandlepower lamp—an ordinary electric globe—and a concave mirror fastened to a rod which moves back and forth in a groove so that the distance of the mirror from the eye can be altered at will. A plane mirror might also be used; but the concave glass is better, because it magnifies the image. The mirror should be so arranged that it reflects the image of the electric filament on the cornea, and so that the eye of the subject can see this reflection by

looking straight ahead. The image in the mirror is used as the point of fixation, and the distance at which the eye focuses is altered by altering the distance of the mirror from the eye. The light can be placed within an inch or two of the eye, as the heat is not great enough to interfere with the experiment. The closer it is the larger the image, and according to whether it is adjusted vertically, horizontally, or at an angle, the clearness of the reflection may vary. A blue glass screen can be used, if desired, to lessen the discomfort of the light. If the left eye is used by the subject—and in all the experiments it was found to be the more convenient for the purpose—the source of light should be placed to the left of that eye and as much as possible to the front of it, at an angle of about forty-five degrees. For absolute accuracy the light and the head of the subject should be held immovable, but for demonstration this is not essential. Simply holding the bulb in his hand the subject can demonstrate that the image changes according to whether the eye is at rest, accommodating normally for near vision, or straining to see at a near or a distant point.

In the original report were described possible sources of error and the means taken to eliminate them.

Bates: "The Truth About Accommodation as Demonstrated by Clinical Observations"

This is how Bates titled Chapter VI of *Perfect Sight Without Glasses,* excerpts of which are reprinted below:

The testimony of the experiments described in the preceding chapters to the effect that the lens is not a factor in accommodation is confirmed by numerous observations on the eyes of adults and children, with normal vision, errors of refraction, or amblyopia, and on the eyes of adults after the removal of the lens for cataract.

It has already been pointed out that the instillation of atropine into the eye is supposed to prevent accommodation by paralyzing the muscle credited with controlling the shape of the lens. That it has this effect is stated in every text-book on the subject,[a] and the drug is daily used in the fitting of glasses for the purpose of eliminating the supposed influence of the lens upon refractive states.

In about nine cases out of ten the conditions resulting from the instillation of atropine into the eye fit the theory upon which its use is based; but in the tenth case they do not, and every ophthalmologist of any experience has noted some of these tenth cases. Many of them are reported in the literature, and many of them have come under my own observation. According to the theory, atropine ought to bring out latent hypermetropia in eyes either apparently normal, or manifestly hypermetropic, provided, of course, the person is of the age during which the lens is supposed to retain its elasticity. The fact is that it sometimes produces myopia, or changes hypermetropia into myopia, and that it will produce both myopia and hypermetropia in persons over seventy years of age, when the lens is

[a] Certain substances have the power of producing a dilation of the pupil (mydriasis) and hence are termed mydriatics. At the same time they act upon the ciliary body, diminishing and, when applied in sufficient strength, completely paralyzing the power of accommodation, thus rendering the eye for some time unalterably focused for the farthest point.—Herman Snellen, Jr.: *Mydriatics and Myotics, System of Diseases of the Eye,* edited by Norris and Oliver, 1897–1900, vol. ii, p. 30.

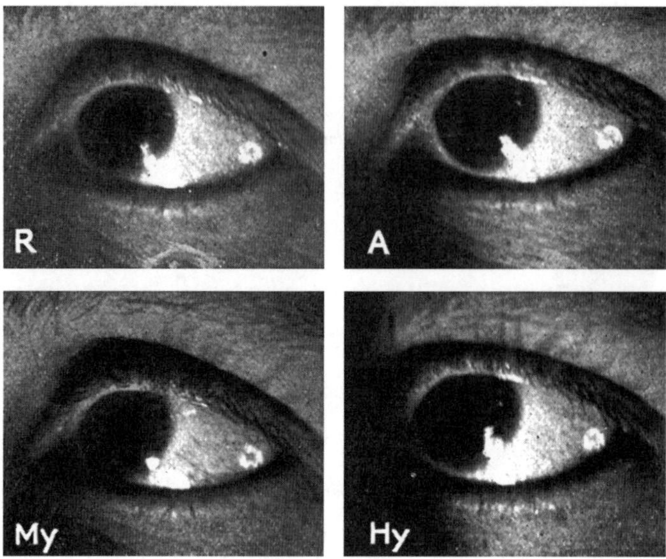

Figure 7–8: Image on the Side of the Sclera.[9]

***R**, rest; **A**, accommodation. The image in A is the larger, indicating a flattening of the side of the sclera as the eyeball elongates. **My**, Myopia. The eye is straining to see at the distance and the image is larger, indicating that the eyeball has elongated, resulting in a flattening of the side of the sclera. **Hy**, Hypermetropia. The eye is straining to see at two inches. The image is the smallest of the series, indicating that the eyeball has become shorter than in any of the other pictures, and the side of the sclera more convex. The two lower pictures confirm the author's previous observations that farsight is produced when the eye strains to see near objects and nearsight when it strains to see distant objects.*

supposed to be as hard as a stone, as well as in cases in which the lens is hard with incipient cataract. People with eyes apparently normal will, after the use of atropine, develop hypermetropic astigmatism, or myopic astigmatism, or compound myopic astigmatism, or mixed astigmatism.[a] In other cases the drug will not interfere with the accommodation, or alter the refraction in any way. Furthermore, when the vision has been lowered by atropine the subjects have often become able, simply by resting their eyes, to read diamond type at six inches. Yet atropine is supposed to rest the eyes [for distance vision] by affording relief to an overworked muscle.

In the treatment of squint and amblyopia I have often used atropine in the better eye for more than a year, in order to encourage the use of the amblyopic eye; and at the end of this time, while still under the influence of atropine, such eyes have

[a] In simple hypermetropic astigmatism one principal meridian is normal and the other, at right angles to it, is flatter. In simple myopic astigmatism the contrary is the case; one principal meridian is normal and the other, at right angles to it, more convex. In mixed astigmatism one principal meridian is too flat, the other too convex. In compound hypermetropic astigmatism both principal meridians are flatter than normal, one more so than the other. In compound myopic astigmatism both are more convex than normal, one more so than the other.

become able in a few hours, or less, to read diamond type at six inches (see Chapter XXII). The following are examples of many similar cases that might be cited:

A boy of ten had hypermetropia in both eyes, that of the left or better eye amounting to three diopters. When atropine was instilled into this eye the hypermetropia was increased to four and a half diopters, and the vision lowered to 20/200. With a convex glass of four and a half diopters the boy obtained normal vision for the distance, and with the addition of another convex glass of four diopters he was able to read diamond type at ten inches (best). The atropine was used for a year, the pupil being dilated continually to the maximum. Meantime the right eye was being addressed by methods to be described later. Usually in such cases the eye which is not being specifically addressed improves to some extent with the other, but in this case it did not. At the end of the year the vision of the right eye had become normal; but that of the left eye remained precisely what it was at the beginning, being still 20/200 without glasses for the distance, while reading without glasses was impossible and the degree of the hypermetropia had not changed. Still under the influence of the atropine and still with the pupil dilated to the maximum, this eye was now addressed separately; and in half an hour its vision had become normal both for the distance and the near point, diamond type being read at six inches, all without glasses. According to the accepted theories, the ciliary muscle of this eye must not only have been completely paralyzed at the time, but must have been in a state of complete paralysis for a year. Yet the eye not only overcame four and a half diopters of hypermetropia, but added six diopters of accommodation, making a total of ten and a half. It remains for those who adhere to the accepted theories to say how such facts can be reconciled with them.

Equally if not more remarkable was the case of a girl of six who had two and a half diopters of hypermetropia in her right or better eye, and six in the other, with one diopter of astigmatism. With the better eye under the influence of atropine and the pupil dilated to the maximum, both eyes were addressed together for more than a year, and at the end of that time, the right being still under the influence of the atropine, both became able to read diamond type at six inches, the right doing it better, if anything, than the left. Thus, in spite of the atropine, the right eye not only overcame two and a half diopters of hypermetropia, but added six diopters of accommodation, making a total of eight and a half. In order to eliminate all possibility of latent hypermetropia in the left eye—which in the beginning had six diopters—the atropine was now used in this eye and discontinued in the other, the eye education being continued as before. Under the influence of the drug there was a slight return of the hypermetropia; but the vision quickly became normal again, and although the atropine was used daily for more than a year, the pupil being continually dilated to the maximum, it remained so, diamond type being read at six inches without glasses during the whole period. It is difficult for me to conceive how the ciliary muscle could have had anything to do with the ability of this person to accommodate after atropine had been used in each eye separately for a year or more at a time.

According to the current theory, atropine paralyzes the ciliary muscle and thus, by preventing a change of curvature in the lens, prevents accommodation. When accommodation occurs, therefore, after the pro-

longed use of atropine, it is evident that it must be due to some factor or factors other than the lens and the ciliary muscle. The evidence of such cases against the accepted theories is, in fact, overwhelming; and according to these theories the other factors cited in this chapter are equally inexplicable. All of these facts, however, are in entire accord with the results of my experiments on the eye muscles of animals and my observations regarding the behavior of images reflected from various parts of the eyeball. They strikingly confirm, too, the testimony of the experiments with atropine, which showed that the accommodation could not be paralyzed completely and permanently unless the atropine was injected deep into the orbit, so as to reach the oblique muscles, the real muscles of accommodation, while hypermetropia could not be prevented when the eyeball was stimulated with electricity without a similar use of atropine, resulting in the paralysis of the recti muscles. [TQ emphasis.]

As has already been noted, the fact that after the removal of the lens for cataract the eye often appears to accommodate just as well as it did before is well known. Many of these cases have come under my own observation. Such people have not only read diamond type with only their distance glasses on, at thirteen and ten inches and at less distance, but one man was able to read without any glass at all. In all these cases the retinoscope demonstrated that the apparent act of accommodation was real, being accomplished not by the "interpretation of circles of diffusion," or by any of the other methods by which this inconvenient phenomenon is commonly explained, but by an accurate adjustment of the focus to the distances concerned.

The reversal of presbyopia (see Chapter XX) must also be added to the clinical testimony against the accepted theory of accommodation. On the theory that the lens is a factor in accommodation such reversals would be manifestly impossible. The fact that rest of the eyes improves the sight in presbyopia has been noted by others, and has been attributed to the supposed fact that the rested ciliary muscle is able for a brief period to influence the hardened lens; but while it is conceivable that this might happen in the early stages of the condition and for a few moments, it is not conceivable that permanent relief should be obtained by this means, or that lenses which are, as the saying goes, as "hard as a stone" should be influenced, even momentarily.

A truth is strengthened by an accumulation of facts. A working hypothesis is proved not to be a truth if a single fact is not in harmony with it. The accepted theories of accommodation and of the cause of errors of refraction require that a multitude of facts shall be explained away. During more than thirty years of clinical experience, I have not observed a single fact that was not in harmony with the belief that the lens and the ciliary muscle have nothing to do with accommodation and that the changes in the shape of the eyeball upon which errors of refraction depend are not permanent. My clinical observations have of themselves been sufficient to demonstrate this fact. They have also been sufficient to show how errors of refraction can be produced at will, and how they may be reversed, temporarily in a few minutes, and permanently by continued practice.

Bates: "The Variability of the Refraction of the Eye"

From *Perfect Sight Without Glasses,* Chapter VII:

The theory that errors of refraction are due to permanent deformations of the eyeball leads naturally to the conclusion not only that errors of refraction are permanent states, but that normal refraction is also a continuous condition. As this theory is almost universally accepted as a fact, therefore, it is not surprising to find that the normal eye is generally regarded as a perfect machine which is always in good working order. No matter whether the object regarded is strange or familiar, whether the light is good or imperfect, whether the surroundings are pleasant or disagreeable, even under conditions of nerve strain or bodily disease, the normal eye is expected to have normal refraction and normal sight all the time. It is true that the facts do not harmonize with this view, but they are conveniently attributed to the perversity of the ciliary muscle, or if that explanation will not work, ignored altogether.

When we understand, however, how the shape of the eyeball is controlled by the external muscles, and how it responds instantaneously to their action, it is easy to see that no refractive state, whether it is normal or abnormal, can be permanent. This conclusion is confirmed by the retinoscope, and I had observed the facts long before the experiments described in the preceding chapters had offered a satisfactory explanation for it. During thirty years devoted to the study of refraction, I have found few people who could maintain perfect sight for more than a few minutes at a time, even under the most favorable conditions; and often I have seen the refraction change half a dozen times or more in a second, the variations ranging all the way from twenty diopters of myopia to normal. Similarly I have found no eyes with continuous or unchanging errors of refraction, all persons with errors of refraction having, at frequent intervals during the day and night, moments of normal vision, when their myopia, hypermetropia, or astigmatism wholly disappears. The form of the error also changes, myopia even changing into hypermetropia, and one form of astigmatism into another. [See Chapter 23, "Children and Schools," for Bates' discussion of school children.]

Among babies a similar condition was noted. Most investigators have found babies hypermetropic. A few have found them myopic. My own observations indicate that the refraction of infants is continually changing. One child was examined under atropine on four successive days, beginning two hours after birth. A three percent solution of atropine was instilled into both eyes, the pupil was dilated to the maximum, and other physiological symptoms of the use of atropine were noted. The first examination showed a condition of mixed astigmatism. On the second day there was compound hypermetropic astigmatism, and on the third compound myopic astigmatism. On the fourth one eye was normal and the other showed simple myopia. Similar variations were noted in many other cases.

What is true of children and infants is equally true of adults of all ages. Persons over seventy years of age have suffered losses of vision of variable degree and intensity, and in such cases the retinoscope always indicated an error of refraction. A man eighty years old, with normal eyes and ordinarily normal sight, had periods of imperfect sight which would last from a few minutes to half an hour or longer. Retinoscopy at such times always indicated myopia of four diopters or more.

A sudden exposure to strong light, or rapid or sudden changes of light, are likely to produce imperfect sight in the normal eye, continuing in some cases for weeks and months (see Chapter XVII) [of *Perfect Sight Without Glasses*].

Noise is also a frequent cause of defective vision in the normal eye. All persons see imperfectly when they hear an unexpected loud noise. Familiar sounds do not lower the vision, but unfamiliar ones always do. Country children from quiet schools may suffer from defective vision for a long time after moving to a noisy city. In school they cannot do well with their work, because their sight is impaired. It is, of course, a gross injustice for teachers and others to scold, punish, or humiliate such children.

Under conditions of mental or physical discomfort, such as pain, cough, fever, discomfort from heat or cold, depression, anger, or anxiety, errors of refraction are always produced in the normal eye, or increased in the eye in which they already exist.

The variability of the refraction of the eye is responsible for many otherwise unaccountable accidents. When people are struck down in the street by automobiles, or trolley cars, it is often due to the fact that they were suffering from temporary loss of sight. Collisions on railroads or at sea, disasters in military operations, aviation accidents, etc., often occur because some responsible person suffered temporary loss of sight.

To this cause must also be ascribed, in a large degree, the confusion which every student of the subject has noted in the statistics which have been collected regarding the occurrence of errors of refraction. So far as I am aware it has never been taken into account by any investigator of the subject; yet the result in any such investigation must be largely determined by the conditions under which it is made. It is possible to take the best eyes in the world and test them so that the subject will not be able to get into the Army. Again, the test may be so made that eyes which are apparently much below normal at the beginning may in the few minutes required for the test acquire normal vision and become able to read the test card perfectly.

Bates: "The Cause and Reversibility of Errors of Refraction"

This topic Bates engaged in Chapter IX of *Perfect Sight Without Glasses,* excerpted below:

> It has been demonstrated in thousands of cases that all abnormal action of the external muscles of the eyeball is accompanied by a strain or effort to see, and that with the relief of this strain the action of the muscles becomes normal and all errors of refraction disappear. The eye may be blind, it may be suffering from atrophy of the optic nerve, from cataract, or disease of the retina; but so long as it does not try to see, the external muscles act normally and there is no error of refraction. This fact furnishes us with the means by which all these conditions, so long held to be irreversible, may be reversed.
>
> It has also been demonstrated that for every error of refraction there is a different kind of strain. The study of images reflected from various parts of the eyeball confirmed what had previously been observed, namely, that myopia (or a lessening of hypermetropia) is always associated with a strain to see at the distance, while hypermetropia (or a lessening of myopia) is always associated with a strain to see at the near point; and the fact can be verified in a few minutes by anyone who

knows how to use a retinoscope, provided only that the instrument is not brought nearer to the subject than six feet.

In an eye with previously normal vision, a strain to see near objects always results in the temporary production of hypermetropia in one or all meridians. That is, the eye either becomes entirely hypermetropic, or some form of astigmatism is produced of which hypermetropia forms a part. In the hypermetropic eye the hypermetropia is increased in one or all meridians. When the myopic eye strains to see a near object, the myopia is lessened and emmetropia[a] may be produced, the eye being focused for parallel rays while still trying to see at the near point. In some cases the emmetropia may even pass over into hypermetropia in one or all meridians. All these changes are accompanied by evidences of increasing strain, in the form of eccentric fixation (see Chapter XI) and lowered vision; but, strange to say, pain and fatigue are usually relieved to a marked degree. ["Eccentric fixation" is "diffusion." Diffusion is a harmful, "spread out" mental way of seeing; it is the opposite of "centralization," discussed later in Chapter 10, "The Second Principle—Centralization."] If, on the contrary, the eye with previously normal vision strains to see at the distance, temporary myopia is always produced in one or all meridians, and if the eye is already myopic, the myopia is increased. If the hypermetropic eye strains to see a distant object, pain and fatigue may be produced or increased; but the hypermetropia and the eccentric fixation are lessened—and the vision improves. This interesting result, it will be noted, is the exact contrary of what we get when the myope strains to see at the near point. In some cases the hypermetropia is completely relieved, and emmetropia is produced, with a complete disappearance of all evidences of strain. This condition may then pass over into myopia, with an increase of strain as the myopia increases.

[a] Emmetropia (from the Greek *emmetros*, in measure, and *ops*, the eye) is that condition of the eye in which it is focused for parallel rays. This constitutes normal vision at the distance but is an error of refraction when it occurs at the near point.

In other words, the eye which strains to see at the near point becomes flatter than it was before, in one or all meridians. If it was elongated to start with, it may pass from this condition through emmetropia, in which it is spherical, to hypermetropia, in which it is flattened; and if these changes take place unsymmetrically, astigmatism will be produced in connection with the other conditions. The eye which strains to see at the distance, on the contrary, becomes longer than it was before in one or all meridians, and may pass from the flattened condition of hypermetropia, through emmetropia, to the elongated condition of myopia. If these changes take place unsymmetrically, astigmatism will again be produced in connection with the other conditions.

What has been said of the normal eye applies equally to eyes from which the lens has been removed. This operation produces usually a condition of hypermetropia; but when there has previously been a condition of high myopia the removal of the lens may not be sufficient to correct it, and the eye may still remain myopic. In the first case a strain to see at the distance lessens the hypermetropia, and a strain to see at the near point increases it; in the second a strain to see at the distance increases the myopia, and a strain to see at the near point lessens it. For a longer or shorter period after the removal of the lens many aphakic eyes strain to see at the near point, producing so much hypermetropia that the subject cannot read ordinary print, and the power of accommodation appears to have been completely lost. Later, when the subject becomes accustomed to the situation, this strain is often relieved, and the eye becomes able to focus accurately upon near objects. Some rare cases have also been observed in which a measure of good vision both for distance and the near point was obtained without glasses, the eyeball elongating sufficiently to compensate, to some degree, for the loss of the lens.

The phenomena associated with strain in the human eye have also been observed in the eyes of the lower animals. I have made many dogs myopic by inducing them to strain to see a distant object. One very nervous dog, with normal refraction, as demonstrated by the retinoscope, was allowed to smell a piece of meat. He became very much excited, pricked up his ears, arched his eyebrows and wagged his tail. The meat was then removed to a distance of twenty feet. The dog looked disappointed, but didn't lose interest. While he was watching the meat it was dropped into a box. A worried look came into his eyes. He strained to see what had become of it, and the retinoscope showed that he had become myopic. This experiment, it should be added, would succeed only with an animal possessing two active oblique muscles. Animals in which one of these muscles is absent or rudimentary are unable to elongate the eyeball under any circumstances.

Primarily the strain to see is a strain of the mind, and, as in all cases in which there is a strain of the mind, there is a loss of mental control. Anatomically the results of straining to see at a distance may be the same as those of regarding an object at the near point without strain; but in one case the eye does what the mind desires, and in the other it does not.

These facts appear sufficiently to explain why visual acuity declines as civilization advances. Under the conditions of civilized life men's minds are under a continual strain. They have more things to worry them than uncivilized man had, and they are not obliged to keep cool and collected in order that they may see and do other things upon which existence depends. If he allowed himself to get nervous, primitive man was promptly eliminated; but civilized man survives and transmits his mental characteristics to posterity. The lower animals when subjected to civilized conditions respond to them in precisely the same way as do human creatures. I have examined many domestic and menagerie animals, and have found them, in many cases, myopic, although they neither read, nor write, nor sew, nor set type.

A decline in visual acuity at the distance, however, is no more a peculiarity of civilization than is a similar decline at the near point. Myopes, although they see better at the near point than they do at the distance, never see as well as does the eye with normal sight; and in hypermetropia, which is more common than myopia, the sight is worse at the near point than at the distance.

The solution is not to avoid either near work or distant vision, but to get rid of the mental strain which underlies the imperfect functioning of the eye at both points; and it has been demonstrated in thousands of cases that this can always be done.

Bates' research begins to answer many questions about eyesight, especially the multitude of eyesight problems experienced in industrialized societies.

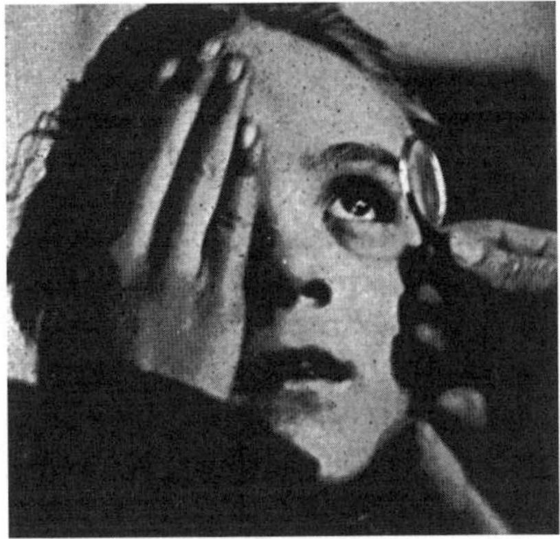

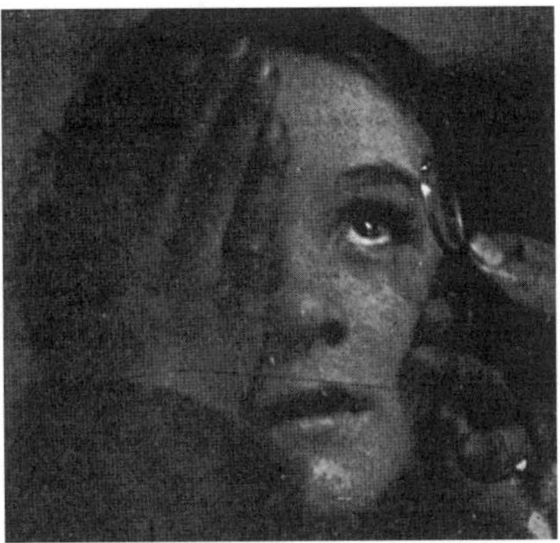

Figure 7–9: Straining to See at the Near Point Produces Hypermetropia.[10]

No. 1—Subject reading fine print in a good light at thirteen inches, the object of vision being placed above the eye so as to be out of the line of the camera. Simultaneous retinoscopy indicated that the eye was focused at thirteen inches. The glass was used with the retinoscope to determine the amount of the refraction. No. 2—When the room was darkened the subject failed to read the fine print at thirteen inches, and the retinoscope indicated that the eye was focused at a greater distance. When a conscious strain of considerable degree was made to see, the eye became hypermetropic, the object of vision being placed above the eye so as to be out of the line of the camera. Simultaneous retinoscopy indicated that the eye was focused at thirteen inches. The glass was used with the retinoscope to determine the amount of the refraction.

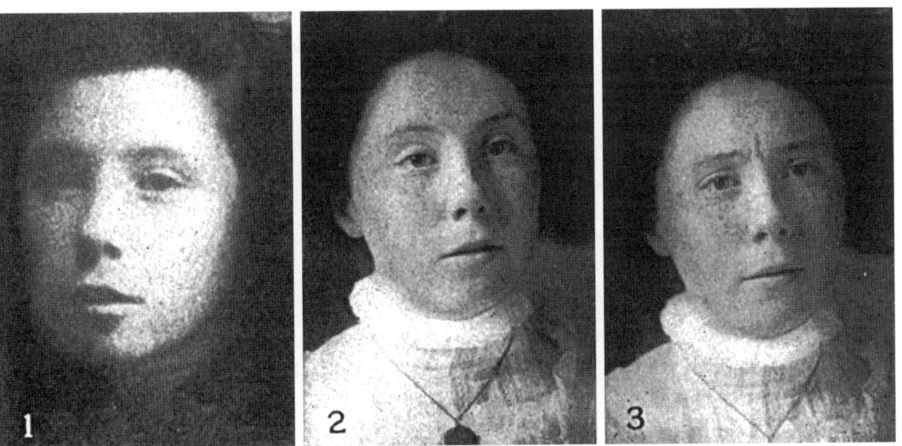

Figure 7–10: Myopia Produced by Unconscious Strain to See at the Distance is Increased by Conscious Strain.[11]

No. 1—Normal vision. No. 2—Same subject four years later with myopia. Note the strained expression. No. 3—Myopia increased by conscious effort to see a distant object.

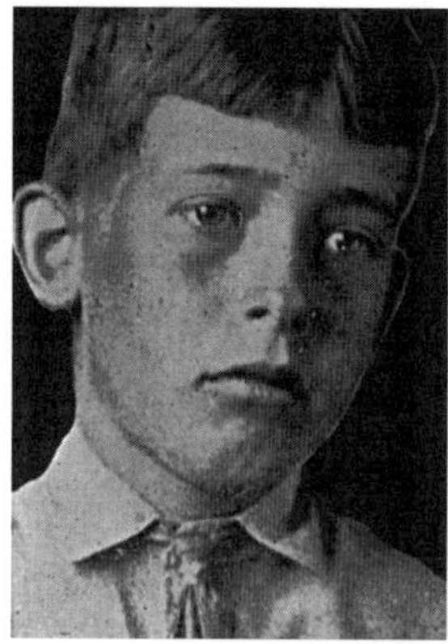
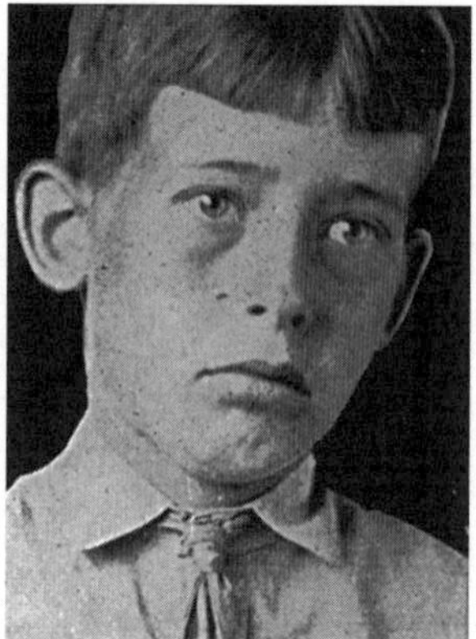
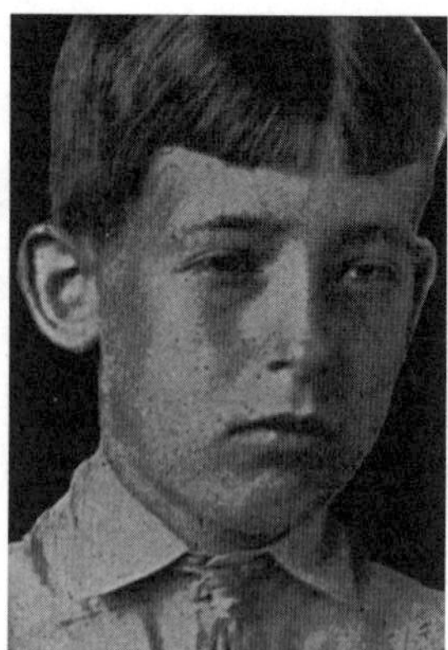

Figure 7–11: Immediate Production of Myopia and Myopic Astigmatism in Eyes Previously Normal by Strain to See at the Distance.[12]

***Left**—Boy reading the Snellen test card with normal vision. Note the absence of facial strain. **Middle**—The same boy trying to see a picture at twenty feet. The effort, manifested by staring, produces compound myopic astigmatism, as revealed by the retinoscope. **Right**—The same boy making himself myopic voluntarily by partly closing the eyelids and making a conscious effort to read the test card at ten feet.*

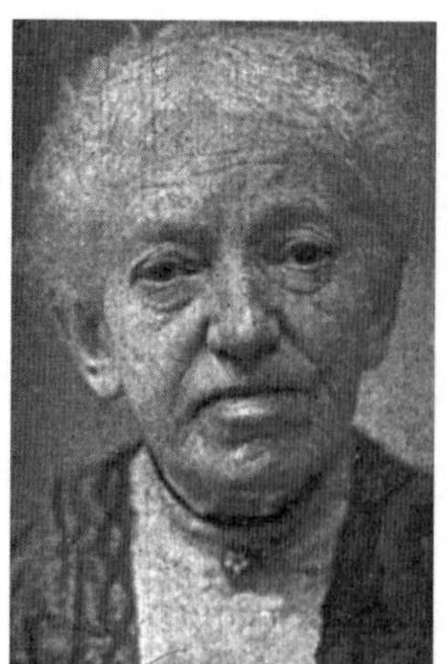
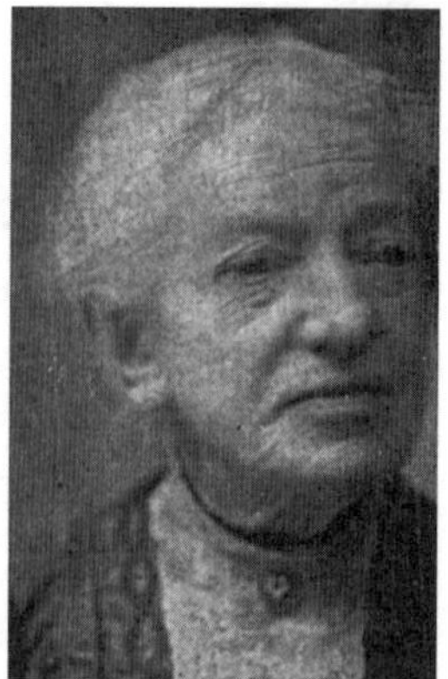

Figure 7–12: Myopic Astigmatism Comes and Goes as the Subject Looks at Distant Objects With or Without Strain.[13]

***No. 1**—Subject regarding the Snellen card at ten feet without effort and reading the bottom line with normal vision. **No. 2**—The same subject making an effort to see a picture at twenty feet. The retinoscope indicated compound myopic astigmatism.*

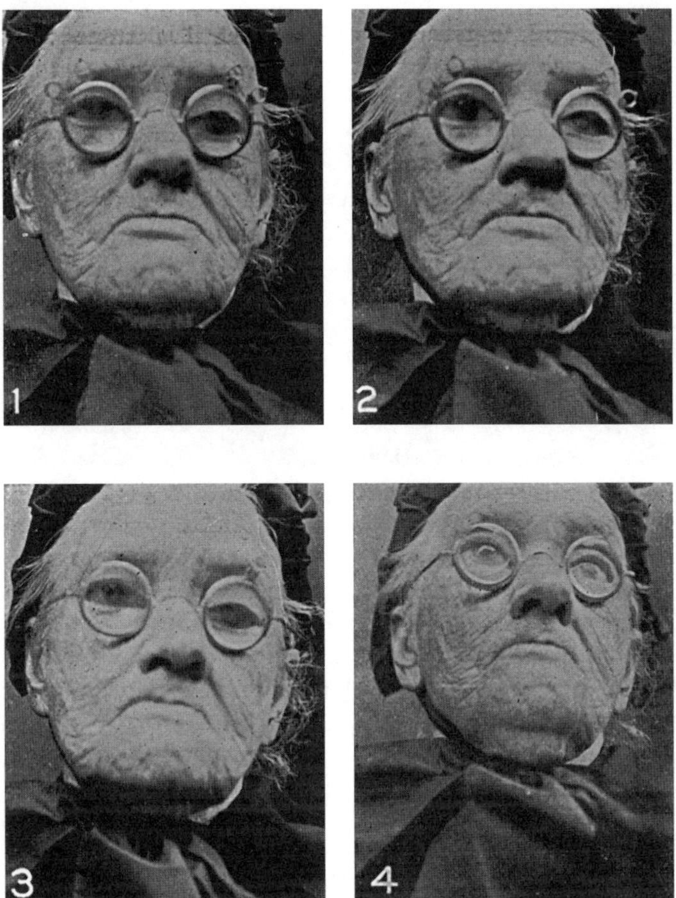

Figure 7–13: Subject Who Had the Lens of the Right Eye Removed for Cataract Produces Changes in the Refraction of this Eye by Strain.[14]

This subject had had the lens of the right eye removed for cataract and was wearing an artificial eye in the left socket. The removal of the lens created a condition of hypermetropia which was corrected by a convex glass of ten diopters. No. 1—The subject is reading the Snellen card at twenty feet with normal vision. No. 2—She is straining to see the card at the same distance, and her hypermetropia is lessened by two diopters so that her glass now overcorrects it and she cannot see the card perfectly. No. 3—With a convex reading glass of thirteen diopters the right eye is focused accurately at thirteen inches. No. 4—The subject is straining to see at the same distance and her hypermetropia is so increased that in order to read she would require a glass of fifteen diopters. On the basis of the accepted theory that the power of accommodation is wholly destroyed by the removal of the lens, these changes in the refraction would have been impossible. The experiment was repeated several times and it was found that the error of refraction produced by straining to see varied, being sometimes more and sometimes less than two diopters.

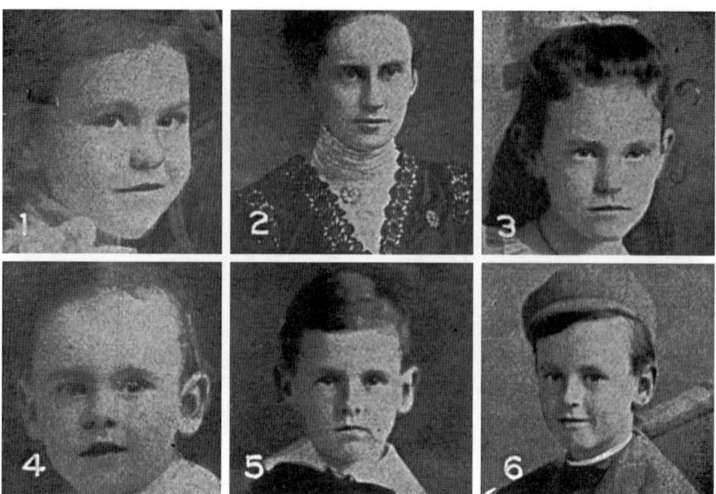

Figure 7–14: A Family Group Strikingly Illustrating the Effect of the Mind Upon the Vision.[15] *No. 1—Girl of four with normal eyes. No. 2—The child's mother with myopia. No. 3—The same girl at nine with myopia. Note that her expression has completely changed, and is now exactly like her mother's. Nos. 4, 5, and 6—The girl's brother at two, six, and eight. His eyes are normal in all three pictures. The girl has either inherited her mother's disposition to take things hard, or has been injuriously affected by her personality of strain. The boy has escaped both influences. In view of the prevailing theories about the relation of heredity to myopia, this picture is particularly interesting.*

How Long Does It Take?

Continuing in Chapter IX of *Perfect Sight Without Glasses,* Bates addresses the question of how much time is required to improve sight naturally:

> The time required to effect a permanent reversal varies greatly with different individuals. In some cases five, ten, or fifteen minutes is sufficient, and I believe the time is coming when it will be possible to improve everyone quickly. It is only a question of accumulating more facts, and presenting these facts in such a way that the student can grasp them quickly. At present, however, it is often necessary to continue the practice for weeks and months, although the error of refraction may be no greater nor of longer duration than in those cases that are improved quickly. In most cases, too, the practice must be continued for a few minutes every day to prevent relapse. Because a familiar object tends to relax the strain to see, the daily reading of the Snellen test card is usually sufficient for this purpose. It is also useful, particularly when the vision at the near point is imperfect, to read fine print every day as close to the eyes as it can be done. When an improvement is complete it is always permanent; but complete improvement, which means the attainment not of what is ordinarily called normal sight, but of a measure of telescopic and microscopic vision, is very rare. Even in these cases, too, the education can be continued with benefit; for it is impossible to place limits to the visual powers of man, and no matter how good the sight, it is always possible to

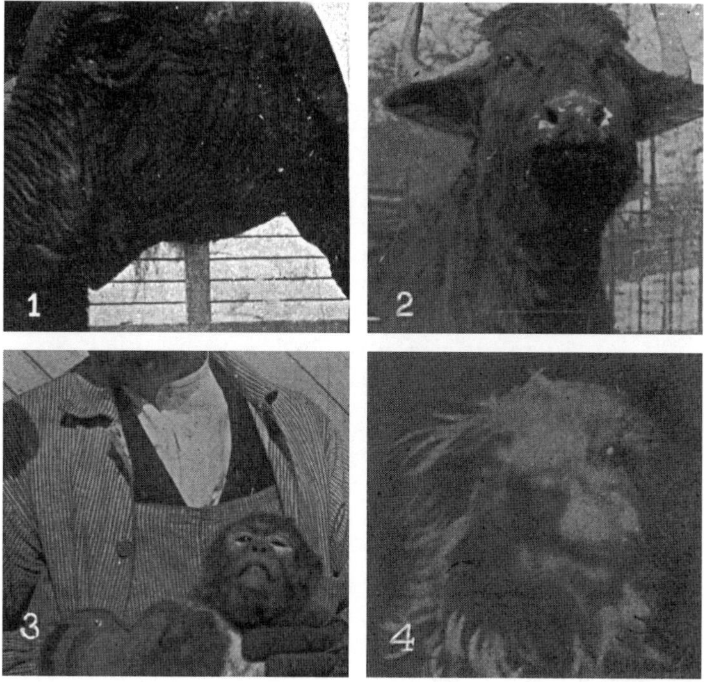

Figure 7–15: Myopes Who Never Went to School, or Read in the Subway.[16]
***No. 1**—Myopic elephant in the Central Park Zoo, New York, thirty-nine years old. Young elephants and other young animals were found to have normal vision. **No. 2**—Cape buffalo with myopia, Central Park Zoo. **No. 3**—Myopic monkey, also in the Central Park Zoo. **No. 4**—Pet dog with myopia which progressed from year to year.*

improve it. Daily practice of the art of vision is also necessary to prevent those visual lapses to which every eye is liable, no matter how good its sight may ordinarily be. It is true that no system of training will provide an absolute safeguard against such lapses in all circumstances; but the daily reading of small, distant, familiar letters will do much to lessen the tendency to strain when disturbing circumstances arise, and all persons upon whose eyesight the safety of others depends should be required to do this.

Generally persons who have never worn glasses are more easily improved than those who have, and glasses should be discarded at the beginning of the practice. When this cannot be done without too great discomfort, or when the person has to continue his work during the practice and cannot do so without glasses, their use must be permitted for a time; but this always delays the improvement. Persons of all ages have been benefited by this practice ... by relaxation; but children usually, though not invariably, respond much more quickly than adults. If they are under twelve years of age, or even under sixteen, and have never worn glasses, they are usually reversed in a few days, weeks, or months, and always within a year, simply by reading the Snellen card every day.

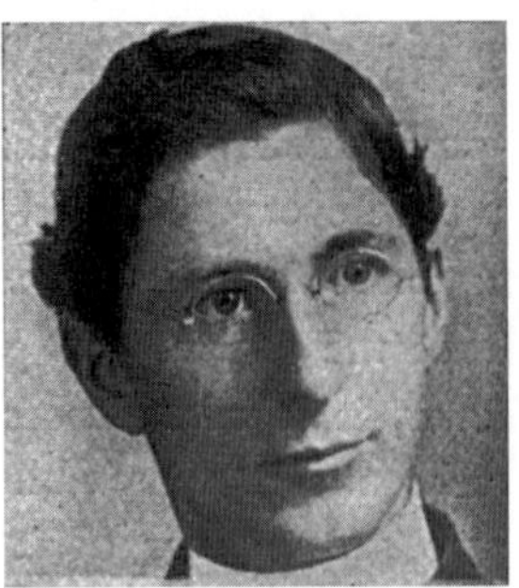
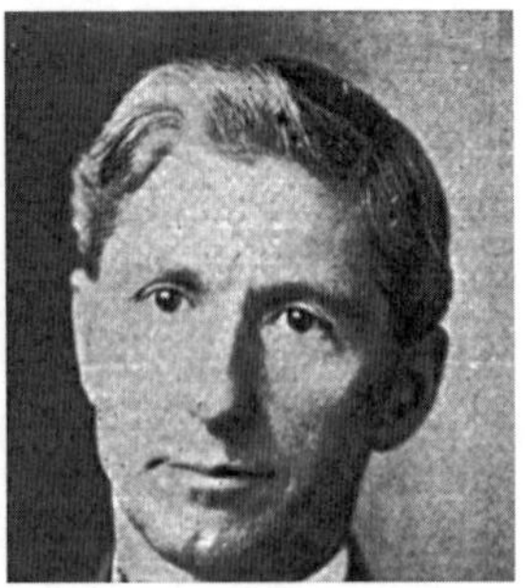

Figure 7–16: One of Many Thousands of People Who Eliminated Errors of Refraction by the Methods Presented in this Book.[17]
No. 1—Man of thirty-six, 1902, wearing glasses for myopia. Note the appearance of effort in his eyes. He was relieved in 1904 . . . and obtained normal sight without glasses. No. 2—The same man five years later. No relapse.

WHAT ARE THE FUNCTIONS OF THE LENS AND CILIARY MUSCLE?

Bates stated unequivocally the lens is not a factor in accommodation. Yet, this author is not aware of any role attributed to the lens by Bates. If the lens does not accommodate, what is its role?

The Ciliary Muscle Pumps Aqueous Humor

The contraction and relaxation of the ciliary muscle pumps aqueous humor into the posterior chamber of the eye. Does the ciliary muscle have other functions? Does it change the shape of the lens for a reason other than accommodation?

A Brightness/Darkness Lens Theory

A book[18] I read many years ago suggested that one function of the ciliary muscle might be to alternately flatten and give more curvature to the lens to aid in night and day vision, respectively.

Could the erratic fluctuations in the sizes of reflected images from the front side of the lens in Helmholtz's research, confirmed by Bates' research, be caused by changes in intensity of the original light source or other changes in lighting during Helmholtz's experiments?

Is there a reason that the iris and the ciliary muscles are both circular muscles that are nearly parallel to each other?

When the iris dilates in darkness, we see a larger picture, by about 10%. Could it be the ciliary muscle dilates simultaneously with the iris? This could pull on the edges of the lens, giving the lens its flatter shape as stated in the Helmholtz lens theory.

In true[19] nighttime vision, the cones do not function, and there is no central vision. Since only the rods function in true nighttime vision, the best vision possible is 20/400, and only in the peripheral vision. Peripheral vision constitutes about 99% of the visual field.

The maximum concentration of rods is located in a circle, 18° around the fovea. Does a flatter lens "spread out" the light rays onto the peripheral rods for better nighttime vision? Since it is not possible to see better than 20/400 with the peripheral rods, perhaps a spreading of light by a flatter lens is more important—to pick up as much peripheral movement as possible at nighttime—than focusing the light onto the retina for best acuity (20/400).

In the daytime the pupil is smaller because the iris contracts. If, simultaneously, the ciliary muscle contracts smaller around the lens, the lens could have more curvature, focusing the light more centrally into the fovea for sharp, 20/20+, cone vision.

Of course, a flexible lens is necessary for this theory.

Both the iris and the ciliary muscles are controlled by the same nerve from the brain. Richard G. Kessel and Randy H. Kardon state, "Both the [iris] sphincter muscle and the ciliary muscles are innervated [controlled] by the ciliary nerves and work in synchrony."[20]

The Johns Hopkins Atlas of Human Functional Anatomy states that, in addition to the third cranial nerve supplying the levator (eyelid) and four extraocular muscles, "The third nerve also sends off a motor root to the ciliary ganglion, which furnishes the autonomic innervation to the [ciliary] muscles within the globe, including the constrictor muscle of the iris."[21]

May in *Diseases of the Eye* states, "The act of accommodation is accompanied by contraction of the pupil."[22]

Do the iris and ciliary muscles contract and dilate in unison based on brightness and darkness?

MORE ON NEARSIGHTEDNESS (MYOPIA)

Nearsightedness is also called shortsightedness or myopia—from Greek *myops: my* means "to close;" *opia* means "eye."

*Near*sightedness means the person can see *near* objects clearly but not far objects. In nearsightedness, when the person is viewing a far object, light rays come to a focus in front of the retina. As a result, the far object appears blurry. Since light rays are not correctly "refracting" onto the retina, nearsightedness is an "error" of refraction.

In more than 99% of all cases of nearsightedness, the eyeball is abnormally elongated along the visual axis. In rare cases, the cornea may have too much curvature, causing the light rays from far objects to fall in front of the retina.

According to Bates: "In myopia it [the eye] is too long, and while the divergent rays from near objects come to a point upon the retina, the parallel ones from distant objects do not reach it."[23]

The following fact is universally agreed upon: *The eyeball can elongate, and, when in this shape, a person cannot see clearly in the distance; only near vision is clear.*

The orthodox explanation of what causes elongation of the eye in myopia is often omitted or ignored. When an explanation is offered it is usually stated that myopia is hereditary—the eyeball simply deforms. But *there is now sufficient evidence showing nearsightedness is not hereditary.*

NEARSIGHTEDNESS IS NOT HEREDITARY

The theory that nearsightedness is determined by heredity has been one of the greatest obstacles to discovering the truth about nearsightedness, and therefore discovering a way to improve vision. Once nearsights are told myopia is genetic, many stop looking for a way to improve their sight.

One of the most dramatic studies presenting evidence against the heredity theory of nearsightedness was conducted in Alaska in 1970. Wendy Murphy writes:

> ... for years ophthalmologists have insisted that nearsightedness stems from an innate anatomical problem. The experts may have been wrong. In 1970, for example, Francis A. Young of Washington State University checked the eyesight of the inhabitants of the village of Nuvuk in Point Barrow, Alaska, an isolated community of people of Eskimo ancestry. He found that parents and grand parents, who were generally illiterate, had almost no nearsightedness, while among the villagers less than 25 years old, who all had been taught to read, about 60 percent suffered from this impairment.[24]

Many of my students have been told that the reason they cannot improve their nearsightedness or farsightedness is because these problems are "structural." The physical causes of nearsightedness *are* anatomical and structural. But they are not "innate."

Natural vision students change the structure of their eyes when they improve their vision. Bates' research showed that the eye muscles let go of their chronic strain—strain which is squeezing the eyeball out of shape—when correct vision habits are relearned.

Murphy also discusses how it has been shown that the more education, from elementary through graduate school, a person receives in the US or Canada, the greater percentage of those students become nearsighted. Fifty percent of graduate students are nearsighted, "a proportion far greater than among people of the same age who do not attend graduate school."[25]

Rita Rubin, discussing the work of MIT Department of Brain and Cognitive Science's researcher Jane Gwiazda, writes:

> Until scientists discover ways to prevent myopia, Gwiazda says, parents might want to advise kids not to sit too close to the TV or read for hours without taking a break—activities that scientists speculate could contribute to nearsightedness, which is practically nonexistent in preliterate societies ... She theorizes that the children's eyes might react to prolonged close-up work by elongating ....[26]

The "TV and reading for hours without taking a break" is not the cause of nearsightedness. According to Bates, the cause of nearsightedness is the formation of strained, incorrect vision habits. It is *more likely*—but not essential—a person will form incorrect vision habits during these activities compared to some other, more mobile, activities. By "taking a break," the person simply has more mobility. Movement is the first principle of natural vision.

An article entitled "In Debate on Myopia's Origins, The Winner Is: Both Sides?" in *The New York Times* states:

> Yet in primitive cultures, where hunting and gathering is commonplace and illiteracy prevails, myopia is practically nonexistent ... Upwards of 70 percent of Taiwanese schoolchildren are now reported to be nearsighted. Myopia skyrocketed among Eskimos when their children first started going to school ....[27]

Kennebeck states:

> There are those ... who insist that one is born nearsighted, that it is hereditary ... But it is not so. ... It is not hereditary. It would make no difference if the parents, grandparents, uncles or aunts were or were not nearsighted. Each and every one who

> is nearsighted had to acquire it himself. There are parents having normal eyes whose children might be nearsighted, and there are nearsighted parents whose children's eyes are normal or farsighted.[28]

The blurred vision of a parent can, *and often does,* make a difference, because a child can emulate the parent's strained vision habits. Still, the point is blurred vision is not genetic. It is caused by the formation of abnormal, strained vision habits.

Due to the above studies and other research, some orthodox are now saying that nearsightedness is only "probably hereditary."

The fact that thousands of students have improved their nearsightedness naturally is additional indication nearsightedness is not hereditary. I have watched several children improve their vision *along with their parents* in my classes.

A holistic practitioner told me that when she was a child, during a period of high stress, she became nearsighted and was given glasses. She refused to wear them. Several months later, after the stress had passed, her vision returned to clarity, and she has never needed glasses since. I have heard similar stories from other people.

The fact that people improve their eyesight—without even knowing why it improves—is important. Other than diseases and accidents, Bates showed that a person's vision depends upon correct vision habits—whether the person is aware of them consciously or not.

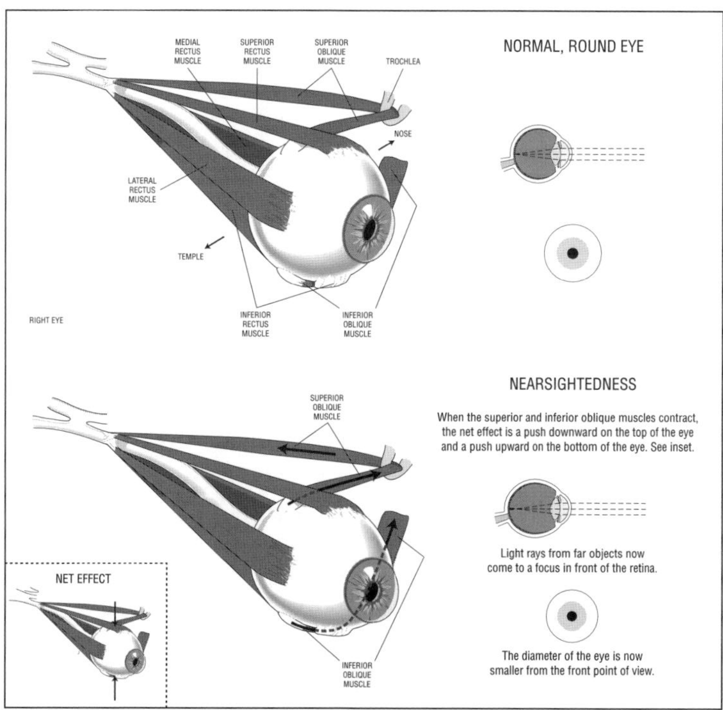

Figure 7–17: The Production of Nearsightedness.

Bates Explains Nearsightedness

In normal vision, it is conventionally stated that the front side of the lens changes from a flatter shape for distant clarity to a more curved shape for near clarity.

As stated above, it is universally agreed that, in nearsightedness, the eyeball is too long—and that nearsightedness is not determined by age. In the US, nearsightedness occurs very often at a young age. An explanation for this is offered in Chapter 19, "Brains and Vision."

Since the elongated myopic eyeball sees clearly up close, and since the lens is in the flatter shape, a lens that accommodates into a more curved shape would only create a greater amount of nearsightedness. This is why the nearsights are told they cannot see clearly in the distance.

Through the use of a diverging (–) lense, the image of a distant object is thrown farther back into the elongated eyeball. The distant object is now seen clearly through the corrective lense. Theoretically, the eye's lens can now continue to accommodate "normally," i.e., when the lens is flatter, the eye sees distant objects clearly, and when the lens accommodates, its front side gains more curvature and sees close objects clearly.

Bates said that when the superior oblique muscle contracts, it applies pressure on the top of the eyeball, pushing downward. When the inferior oblique muscle contracts, it applies pressure on the bottom of the eyeball, pushing upward. Acting independently, each oblique muscle would rotate the eye clockwise or counterclockwise. (You can watch this rotation by tilting your head in front of a mirror.) When both oblique muscles contract, the eye is squeezed into a long shape. When the two oblique muscles relax, the eyeball returns to its normal round shape. This is Bates' explanation of accommodation of the normal eye. This explanation for accommodation originated many years before Bates' research was performed.

In nearsightedness the two oblique muscles contract and the person sees clearly up close—but the oblique muscles *stay* contracted chronically. They do not release, and the eyeball remains elongated.

When the two oblique muscles release the chronic tension they hold in nearsightedness, myopia is reversed. The reversal of myopia and the subsequent return to normal vision is clearly—and only—an issue of the release of chronically tight oblique muscles.

Since age, heredity, and the lens are not the issues involved in nearsightedness, the question for Bates now became, "*Why* do the oblique muscles become chronically tense, and how do I remove the cause of this chronic tension?" Finding the answers to these questions was the real brilliance of Bates. Chronic tension is caused by strain, and removal of that strain is achieved by relaxation.

Artificial Corneal Refraction Procedures: Radial Keratotomy (RK) Surgery, Ortho-Keratology, etc.

A nearsighted eyeball, because it is elongated, has a cornea with too much curvature.

There are various artificial methods of making the cornea flatter to focus the light rays from distant objects more clearly onto the retina. Some of these include:

1. Ortho-keratology, in which a series of contact lenses is used to flatten the cornea;

2. Radial keratotomy (RK) surgery, in which deep incisions are made in the peripheral parts of the cornea to flatten it;
3. Photorefractive keratectomy (PRK) laser, in which the top central layers of the cornea are vaporized to flatten it;
4. Plastic ring, which is surgically implanted into the cornea;
5. Enzymes (under research), in which the top layers of the cornea are digested to flatten it.

Of course, all of these procedures have risks, some of which can be, and have been, very serious.

In all of these artificial, cornea-flattening procedures the original cause of nearsightedness is not addressed. The refractive error changes, but the eyeball remains chronically elongated. The oblique muscles remain chronically contracted, and they are chronically tight due to mental strain. The real cause of the nearsightedness remains.

Bruce May, O.D., writes:

> When processes like keratotomy or orthokeratology produce improved distance acuity without the use of glasses, they do not change the basic problem of myopia, only the refractive status. The change involves only the cornea, while the depth of the vitreous chamber remains increased, and so does the eyeball length. Thus, the [person] still has myopia and remains subject to all the risks of myopia.[29]

One reason corneal surgery has become popular is because it is a "quick fix." Improving vision naturally takes a longer time because *the real cause* of the problem is being addressed.

Improvement of Nearsightedness

Clara Hackett, in her book *Relax and See,* writes about her nearsighted students. Many students were referred to her by eye doctors to received natural vision education.

The following numbers include students who only had a few lessons and stopped, and students who were not diligent in relearning the proper vision habits.

Clara Hackett writes:

> There were 1,584 nearsighted people, or myopes, with vision ranging from 20/30 to 20/1000. The majority had 20/400, or one-twentieth of normal sight. Five hundred and sixty-nine regained at least 20/40, or half normal sight; 210 achieved 20/70; 163 attained 20/100 or one-fifth normal sight; 211 improved to 20/200 or one-tenth normal sight. In other cases there was lesser or only temporary improvement. All of those who achieved 20/20 vision could dispense with glasses as could most of those who gained 20/40, the sight required for passing drivers' tests in the states of New York, California and Washington.[30]

Many of my students have passed their driver's test without glasses after having nearsightedness (or farsightedness) for many years. Of course, not all students improve; some students do not practice the correct vision habits, and continue their strained vision habits.

More on Farsightedness (Hypermetropia)

Farsightedness is also called hyperopia and hypermetropia (Greek: *hyper* means "far," or "over"; *metron* means "measure"; *opia* means "eye").

*Far*sightedness means a person sees *far* objects more clearly than near objects. In far-

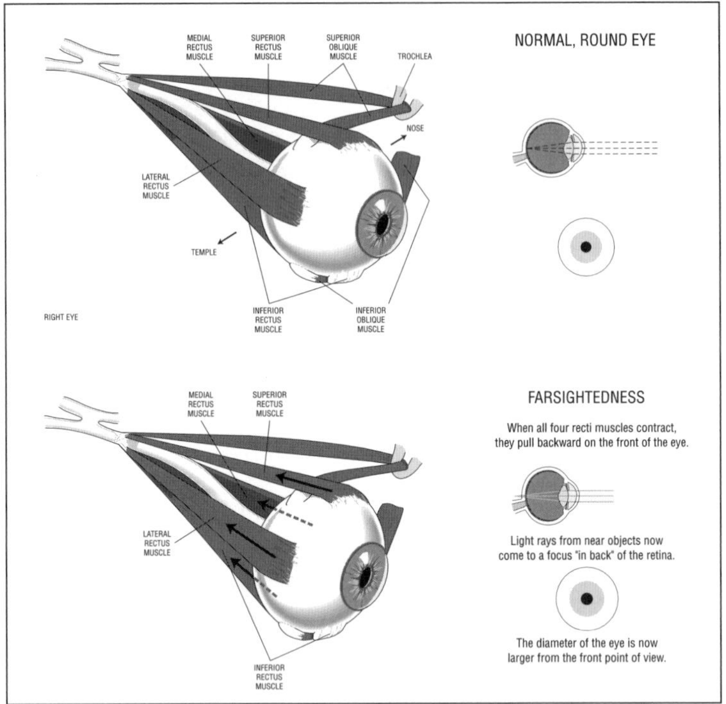

Figure 7–18: The Production of Farsightedness.

sightedness, when viewing a near object, light rays come to a focus "in back" of the retina. As a result, the near object appears blurry. Of course, the light rays do not actually penetrate the back of the eyeball and come to a focal point in back of it; but the light rays *would* come to a focus in back of the eyeball if the back of the eyeball were transparent. Since light rays are not correctly "refracting," in focus, onto the retina, farsightedness, like nearsightedness and astigmatism, is classified as an "error" of refraction.

Conventional books describe two types of farsightedness: 1) the eyeball is too short along the visual axis (hypermetropia); and 2) the lens is inflexible and locked in the flatter shape because of older age, an eye condition referred to as presbyopia.

From "Introductory" of *Perfect Sight Without Glasses:*

> ... In hypermetropia[a]—commonly but improperly called farsight[edness], although the person with such a defect can see clearly neither at the distance nor the near point—the eyeball is too short from the front backward, and all rays of light, both the convergent ones coming from near objects, and the parallel ones coming from distant objects, are focused behind the retina instead of upon it. Both these conditions [hypermetropia and presbyopia] are supposed to be permanent, the one
>
> [a] From the Greek *hyper,* over, *metron,* measure, and *ops,* the eye.

> congenital, the other acquired. When, therefore, persons who at one time appear to have hypermetropia, or myopia, appear at other times not to have them, or to have them in lesser degrees, it is not permissible to suppose that there has been a change in the shape of the eyeball. Therefore, in the case of the disappearance or lessening of hypermetropia, we are asked to believe that the eye, in the act of vision, both at the near point and at the distance, increases the curvature of the lens sufficiently to compensate, in whole or in part, for the flatness of the eyeball.

The reason Bates took exception to the term "farsightedness" is because a foreshortened eyeball cannot see clearly near *or far.* The eyeball needs to be in the "relaxed" round shape in order to see clearly in the distance. Bates felt the term "hypermetropia" was more accurate than "farsight."

This distinction is important, because Bates believed the eyeball elongates when it accommodates to see clearly up close. For Bates, an eyeball that remains in the round shape can only see clearly in the distance; it cannot see clearly up close.

In medium and high degrees of farsightedness where the eyeball is foreshortened and both the near and distance vision are blurred, the conventional point of view is that the front side of the lens cannot accommodate (curve) enough to focus the light rays of near objects onto the retina, but the lens *can* accommodate to see clearly *in the distance.*

Bates states above that in hypermetropia both distance and the near objects are not clear. This is true if the eyeball is foreshortened. However, if at first the eyeball simply is unable to change from the round shape into an elongated shape, a person will be able to see clearly in the distance but not up close. (This assumes, of course, that a person agrees with Bates that the lens is not a factor in accommodation.)

In any case, everyone agrees there is a way for the eyeball to become chronically short along the visual axis, causing farsightedness. It is also universally agreed that non-presbyopic farsightedness is not determined by age.

The conventional explanation of why the eyeball becomes foreshortened is that it is hereditary, and the eyeball deforms "somehow"—the same as for nearsightedness.

When one rectus muscles contracts, the eye turns. (If one rectus muscle contracts chronically, crossed eye can be produced.) Bates conclusively proved that when all four recti muscles contract, they pull the front of the eyeball backward, against the fatty tissue in the eye orbit, and thereby shorten it from front to back. Chronic tension of the recti muscles is a simple, logical, and straightforward explanation of the foreshortened eyeball in farsightedness. When these muscles let go of their chronic strain, the eyeball returns to its normal, round state, and with it, normal vision.

When the four recti muscles release the chronic tension they hold in farsightedness, hypermetropia is reversed—regardless of the mechanism of accommodation.

Since age, heredity, and the lens are not the issues involved in farsightedness, the question now is "*Why* do the recti muscles become chronically tense, and how do I remove the cause of this chronic tension?" The answers to these questions are the same as the answers to nearsightedness—strain is the cause of the tension, and relaxation is the solution.

Farsightedness is Not Hereditary

As with nearsightedness, Natural Vision teachers have observed farsights improving their sight for more than seventy-five years. Bates provided many examples of farsightedness improving. Farsightedness, like nearsightedness and astigmatism, is a functional problem and is due to stress. It is not genetic.

Improvement of Farsightedness

Clara Hackett, in her book *Relax and See,* writes about her farsighted students, "Three hundred and forty-eight of my students were farsighted; 116 discarded glasses entirely; 194 could wear weaker glasses for reading; 38 made no enduring improvement."[31]

ASTIGMATISM

From *Better Eyesight* magazine, October 1920:

> *Question:* Is astigmatism reversible with this method?
> *Answer:* Yes.

In most cases of astigmatism (Greek: *a* means "without"; *stigma* means "a point"; light rays do not come to a single point of focus) the eye is twisted in an oval, lopsided, or teaspoon shape from the front point of view. Since light rays do not focus on the retina clearly, astigmatism, like nearsightedness and farsightedness, is an "error" of refraction.

The conventional opinion about astigmatism is the same as for nearsightedness and

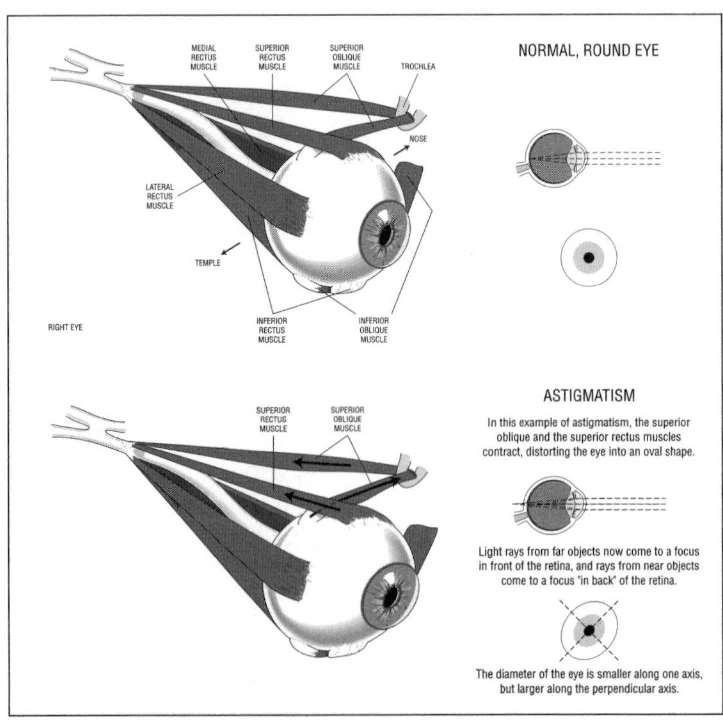

Figure 7–19: The Production of Astigmatism.

farsightedness—it cannot improve. This opinion does not agree with many case histories of improvement of astigmatism.

From Chapter I, "Introductory," of *Perfect Sight Without Glasses:*

> The disappearance of astigmatism,[a] or changes in its character, present an even more baffling problem. Due in most cases to an unsymmetrical change in the curvature of the cornea, and resulting in failure to bring the light rays to a focus at any point, the eye is supposed to possess only a limited power of overcoming this condition; and yet astigmatism comes and goes with as much facility as do other errors of refraction. It is well known, too, that it can be produced voluntarily. Some persons can produce as much as three diopters. I myself can produce one and a half.
>
> [a] From the Greek *a,* without, and *stigma,* a point.

From Chapter III, "Evidence for the Accepted Theory of Accommodation," of *Perfect Sight Without Glasses:*

> The voluntary production of astigmatism is another stumbling block to the supporters of the accepted theories, as it involves a change in the shape of the cornea, and such a change is not compatible with the idea of an "inextensible"[a] eyeball. ... It seems to have given them less trouble, however, than the accommodation of the lensless eye, because fewer of these cases have been observed and still fewer have been allowed to get into the literature. Some interesting facts regarding one have fortunately been given by Davis, who investigated it in connection with the corneal changes noted in the lensless eye. The case was that of a house surgeon at the Manhattan Eye and Ear Hospital, Dr. C. H. Johnson. Ordinarily this gentleman had half a diopter of astigmatism in each eye; but he could, at will, increase this to two diopters in the right eye and one and a half in the left. He did this many times, in the presence of a number of members of the hospital staff, and also did it when the upper lids were held up, showing that the pressure of the lids had nothing to do with the phenomenon. Later he went to Louisville, and here Dr. J. M. Ray, at the suggestion of Dr. Davis, tested his ability to produce astigmatism under the influence of scopolamine (four instillations, ⅕ percent solution). While the eyes were under the influence of the drug the astigmatism still seemed to increase, according to the evidence of the ophthalmometer, to one and a half diopters in the right eye and one in the left. From these facts, the influence of the lids and of the ciliary muscle having been eliminated, Dr. Davis concluded that the change in the cornea was "brought about mainly by the external muscles." What explanation others offer for such phenomena I do not know.
>
> [a] Inasmuch as the eye is inextensible, it cannot adapt itself for the perception of objects situated at different distances by increasing the length of its axis, but only by increasing the refractive power of its lens.—De Schweinitz: Diseases of the Eye, eighth edition, 1916, pp. 35–36.

Quoting Bates again:

> Astigmatism was usually produced in combination with myopic or hypermetropic refraction. It was also produced by various manipulations of both the oblique and recti muscles. Mixed astigmatism, which is a combination of myopic with hypermetropic refraction, was always produced by trac-

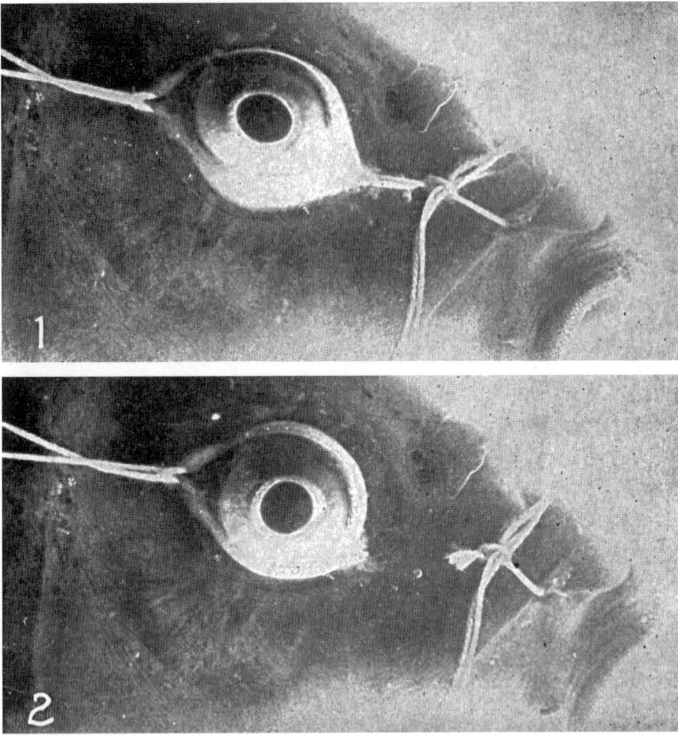

Figure 7–20: Production of Mixed Astigmatism in the Eye of a Carp.[32]
No. 1—Production of mixed astigmatism in the eye of a carp by pulling strings attached to the conjunctiva in opposite directions. Note the oval shape of the front of the eyeball. No. 2—With the cutting of the strings the eyeball returns to its normal shape, and the refraction becomes normal.

tion on the insertion of the superior or inferior rectus in a direction parallel to the plane of the iris, so long as both obliques were present and active; but if either or both of the obliques had been cut, the myopic part of the astigmatism disappeared. Similarly after the superior or the inferior rectus had been cut the hypermetropic part of the astigmatism disappeared. Advancement of the two obliques, with advancement of the superior and inferior recti, always produced mixed astigmatism.

From Bates' *Better Eyesight* magazine, November 1927:

> All persons who have astigmatism have eyestrain. When the eyestrain is relieved, the astigmatism disappears.

Bates' viewpoint on errors of refraction is convincing and his viewpoint on accommodation is reasonable.

Notes

[1] The author [TQ] wishes to minimize showing images of animals used in research.

[2] This caption and text are from *Perfect Sight Without Glasses.*

[3] These graphics, caption, and text are from *Perfect Sight Without Glasses.*

[4] This caption and text are from *Perfect Sight Without Glasses*.

[5] Ibid.

[6] Ibid.

[7] These graphics, caption, and text are from *Perfect Sight Without Glasses.*

[8] Ibid.

[9] Ibid.

[10] These graphics, caption, and text are from *Perfect Sight Without Glasses;* numbers have been added for clarification.

[11] Ibid.

[12] These graphics, caption, and text are from *Perfect Sight Without Glasses.*

[13] Ibid.

[14] Ibid.

[15] Ibid.

[16] Ibid.

[17] Ibid.

[18] Unfortunately, I have been unable to locate this reference to give the author proper credit.

[19] True nighttime vision is defined as any situation in which only the rods are functioning, but not the cones. This is discussed further in Chapter 17, "The Retina."

[20] Richard G. Kessel and Randy H. Kardon, *Tissues and Organs: a text-atlas of scanning electron microscopy* (New York: W. H. Freeman and Company, 1979), p. 101.

[21] Leon Schlossberg and George D. Zuidema, *The Johns Hopkins Atlas of Human Functional Anatomy* (Baltimore: The Johns Hopkins University Press, 1972), p. 55.

[22] Charles H. May, *Diseases of the Eye* (Baltimore: William Wood and Company, 1943), p. 364.

[23] From *Perfect Sight Without Glasses,* Chapter I, "Introductory."

[24] Wendy Murphy and the Editors of Time-Life Books, *Touch, Taste, Smell, Sight and Hearing* (Alexandria, VA: Time-Life Books Inc., 1982), p. 77.

[25] Ibid., p. 78.

[26] Rita Rubin, "Still in Diapers, and Off to the Eye Doctor," *U.S. News & World Report* (June 21, 1993), pp. 69–70.

[27] Jane E. Brody, "In Debate on Myopia's Origins The Winner Is: Both Sides?" *The New York Times,* June 1, 1994.

[28] Joseph J. Kennebeck, *Why Eyeglasses are Harmful for Children and Young People* (New York: Vantage Press, 1969), p. 34.

[29] Bruce May, *Rx for Nearsightedness: Stress-Relieving Lenses,* Optometric Extension Program Foundation pamphlet (1981).

[30] Clara A. Hackett and Lawrence Galton, *Relax and See* (London: Faber and Faber, Limited, 1957), p. 25.

[31] Ibid.

[32] These graphics, caption, and text are from *Perfect Sight Without Glasses.*

Chapter Eight

Accommodation and Errors of Refraction—Summary

[Bates'] basic view of the underlying causes of nearsightedness and other eye problems, and his approach to their remediation, have stood the test of time and new knowledge. He is, in a real sense, the spiritual grandfather of all who are involved in restoring functional vision.[1]

—Optometrist Ernest V. Loewenstein, Ph.D., O.D., 1982

BATES: NEARSIGHTEDNESS = FARSIGHTEDNESS = ASTIGMATISM = NO ACCOMMODATION

For Bates the issues of accommodation and errors of refraction are connected. To summarize:

If extrinsic eye muscles are chronically tight, producing nearsightedness, farsightedness, and/or astigmatism, the eye cannot accommodate to see clearly both near and far. When the external muscles are relaxed, the eye accommodates normally again by the action of the two oblique muscles.

Agreement with Bates' position that errors of refraction are caused by chronically tense external eye muscles has been echoed by some modern eye doctors. One of my students stated that her opthamologist said that this is the case. Recently another opthamologist stated publicly that nearsightedness, farsightedness, and astigmatism are caused by chronically tense external eye muscles, and that this tension can be reversed.

Bates' ideas regarding errors of refraction are simple, reasonable, and explain a multitude of facts that have not been adequately explained in any other way.

From the holistic perspective, there is no difference between nearsightedness, farsightedness (including presbyopia), astigmatism, and strabismus, because *strain* is the underlying cause of all of these problems.

The harmful vision habits a person acquires when creating functional problems are the same. As we shall discuss later, the type of blurred vision an individual acquires appears to be correlated to a person's hemisphere dominance (see Chapter 19, "Brains and Vision"). No matter what the hemisphere dominance, all students in natural vision education classes relearn the same correct vision habits.

Bates was too far ahead of his contemporaries for his advanced ideas to be accepted by the orthodox.

"MAN IS NOT A REASONING BEING"

Many people have asked Natural Vision teachers, "With such compelling research and evidence presented by Bates and others, why is Bates' work not embraced by the orthodox?" Perhaps the best answer comes from Bates in the last paragraph of *Perfect Sight Without Glasses:*

> The fact is that, except in rare cases, man is not a reasoning being. He is dominated by authority, and when the facts are not in accord with the view imposed by authority, so much the worse for the facts. They may, and indeed must, win in the long run; but in the meantime the world gropes needlessly in darkness and endures much suffering that might have been avoided.

Bates' biggest discovery may have been how the conventional system reacted to his research and discoveries.

From *Better Eyesight* magazine, April 1923:

> DR. BATES' LECTURE
>
> By L. L. Biddle, 2nd
>
> For the benefit of those who were unable to attend Dr. Bates' lecture, before the New York Association of Osteopaths, at the Waldorf Astoria on Saturday Evening, February 17th, I decided to take down a few notes which I will now try to compile.
>
> The chairman introduced Doctor Bates by stating that the Osteopaths take away the crutches and Doctor Bates takes away the glasses. . . .
>
> He then commenced by telling how he made his first discoveries and cited the opposition he had to buck against. He stated that his attitude of mind, ever since he was a little boy, was to find out all the facts possible about a subject and then work on these as a basis, rather than on a guess or theory. When he commenced practicing medicine in 1885, one of the first patients who came to him had a slight degree of myopia or nearsightedness. Upon examining his eyes with the ophthalmoscope, he found that the patient was not nearsighted all of the time. When the patient was looking at a blank wall and not trying to see anything, his eyes were for short periods, normal. He persuaded this patient to go without his glasses and his eyes finally reached a point where they stayed normal all the time.
>
> Doctor Bates said that he then started boasting around the hospital about this improvement. However, it got so on the house-surgeon's nerves that he brought up a ward patient who was nearsighted, and with him Doctor Bates managed to have equal success. Much to his surprise, instead of the rest of the doctors praising him, and trying to find out how he accomplished these heretofore impossible improvements, Dr. Bates suddenly became very unpopular with the rest of the staff. These successes nevertheless spurred him on in his experiments at the New York Aquarium and at the laboratory of the Columbia College for Physicians and Surgeons, and as a result he discovered that the accommodation of the eye is not brought about by a change in the shape of the lens, but by the lengthening and shortening [back to spherical] of the eyeball itself, as the bellows of a camera.
>
> When he explained and illustrated this to his doctor friends, it disturbed them greatly. The surgeon who had charge of the laboratory came to him and said: "Do you know that you have proven that Helmholtz is wrong and furthermore if you wish to be

accepted by scientific men you will have to show how or why he blundered?" This was quite a proposition, but Dr. Bates continued his experiments and for two years tried to prove that Helmholtz was *right,* but failed, and finally discovered how Helmholtz blundered; which Doctor Bates has illustrated in his book. As a reward for this, he was *expelled* from the University.

This was quite a handicap, but he obtained a small laboratory for himself and continued in his work.

[Biddle then states that Bates gave a case history.]

He then returned to his seat, but was so applauded and urged to continue that he finally stated that if anyone wished to remain and ask further questions, he would be glad to answer them.

While connected with the New York Post Graduate Medical School and Hospital, Dr. Bates improved myopia with many people in the clinic. Those who improved their sight included student doctors.

The May 1921 *Journal of the Allied Medical Associations* states:

> These facts came to the knowledge of the head of the institution (Dr. St. John D. B. Roosa), one of the most prominent ophthalmologists of the day, and were regarded as highly discreditable, since Donders and the other masters of ophthalmology had declared that myopia was [irreversible]. Dr. Bates was accordingly expelled from the faculty, even the privilege of resignation being denied to him.[2]

Mary Dudderidge writes in the January 12, 1918, issue of *Scientific American:*

> It is therefore not a little surprising to find one eye specialist who has actually been [reversing] errors of refraction without glasses for 30 years, and who as the result of a remarkable series of experiments has been able to present evidence which appears to invalidate most of the theories on which the present practice of ophthalmology is based. Dr. William H. Bates of New York is already well known as the discoverer of the properties of adrenaline, an extract from the suprarenal gland of the sheep which is now used all over the world as an astringent and haemostatic; but his remarkable experiments on the eyes of animals and the startling conclusions that he has drawn from them have, as yet, attracted comparatively little attention. Reported only in a few isolated articles, they have not yet found their way into the general literature of the subject and have scarcely been heard of by the lay public. Yet they promise to revolutionize the practice of ophthalmology and are at the present moment of tremendous import to the country.[3]

Another reason Bates' research has been ignored and rejected is because few people have studied his work deeply enough to understand it. Some of the principles involved are very subtle, and, on first encounter, even appear incorrect.

Optometrist Harris Gruman wrote in his book *New Ways to Better Sight:*

> Whether it was the result of such investigations that Dr. Bates hit upon his system of [improvement] or whether it was the other way around seems immaterial. In spite of his hypotheses and theories he did hit upon some worthwhile methods of aiding human sight. Time has proved their worth, and for this the world should be grateful.[4]

Aldous Huxley, after discussing the possible role of the external and internal muscles in accommodation, writes:

My own guess, after reading the evidence, would be that both the extrinsic muscles and the lens play their part in accommodation.

This guess may be correct; or it may be incorrect. I do not greatly care. For my concern is not with the anatomical mechanism of accommodation, but with the art of seeing—and the art of seeing does not stand or fall with any particularly physiological hypothesis. Believing that Bates' theory of accommodation was untrue, the orthodox have concluded that his technique of visual education must be unsound. Once again this is an unwarranted conclusion, due to a failure to understand the nature of an art, or psycho-physical skill....[5]

The proof of the pudding is in the eating, and the first and most convincing test of the system is that it works.[6]

ACCEPTING A NEW IDEA

With the limited information I had before investigating the Bates method, my vision became worse year after year. Glasses and contacts were not acceptable solutions to my vision problems. And the long-term consequences of continuing along the conventional path were grim.

When presented with a new philosophy or idea, I need to be shown how the new idea explains everything I have experienced so far, and how my previous experiences are only a limited subset of the new, more encompassing idea. I accept a new idea when these two conditions have been met.

The main ideas presented by Bates have met these two conditions, and the benefits to my vision—and health—have been immeasurable.

I am thoroughly convinced that strained external muscles squeeze the eyeball out of shape, producing nearsightedness, farsightedness, astigmatism, and strabismus—and that these functional problems are reversible.

I am also convinced that normally functioning external muscles can produce accommodation. If the lens and ciliary muscle have any role in accommodation, and if that mechanism is interfered with, I believe normally functioning external muscles can continue to accommodate the eye.

Bates' physical research makes sense to me. It answers a "multitude of facts," that have otherwise been ignored or explained away. Still, the physical mechanisms of accommodation and errors of refraction are secondary issues. If a person does not have any pathologies or diseases of the eyes, the physical mechanisms of vision do not matter. The primary issue is how to improve sight—naturally.

I am open to accepting any other model of vision, as long as it explains all of the facts I currently know about vision, and more.

THE PHYSICAL FOLLOWS THE IMAGINATION

The physical factors of accommodation and errors of refraction are only a part of the issues involved in seeing clearly and in relearning to see. Students do not need to know the physical mechanisms of eyesight to improve their vision. There are people (I have met several) who knew nothing about the Bates or any other method of natural eyesight improvement, and who returned to normal vision. In each case, these people removed the strain in their lives that created their blur.

Bates makes frequent references to strain, especially mental strain. The brilliance of Bates' work was not so much his studies with the eyeballs and eye muscles. This research simply allowed him to advance to more important questions.

How does the visual system become strained? What causes the eye muscles to tighten around the eyeball, creating errors of refraction? Bates unraveled the puzzle of the mind-body-vision connection. He discovered that functional vision problems are caused primarily by mental strain, and that they are relieved by relaxation.

In the next part, we discuss the three principles of natural vision discovered by Bates—Movement, Centralization, and Relaxation. In the subsequent part, we discuss the three habits of natural seeing—Sketching (Shifting), Breathing, and Blinking.

Notes

1. E. V. Loewenstein, "Yes! You Can Have Better Vision," *Whole Life Times,* March 1982, p. 16.
2. *Journal of the Allied Medical Associations,* Vol. 9, No. 2 (May 1921), p. 21.
3. Mary Dudderidge. "New Light Upon Our Eyes: An Investigation Which May Result in Normal Vision for All, Without Glasses," *Scientific American* (January 12, 1918), p. 53.
4. Harris Gruman, *New Ways to Better Sight* (New York: Hermitage House, 1950), pp. 176–77.
5. Aldous Huxley, *The Art of Seeing* (New York: Harper & Brothers Publishers, 1942), pp. 33–34.
6. Ibid., p. 36.

PART THREE

The Three Principles of Natural Vision

No one has as good sight as he might have. Therefore everyone can be benefited by practicing the principles presented in this magazine.

—William H. Bates, M.D.,
Better Eyesight, July 1920

The three principles of natural vision are Movement, Centralization, and Relaxation.

Chapter Nine

The First Principle—Movement

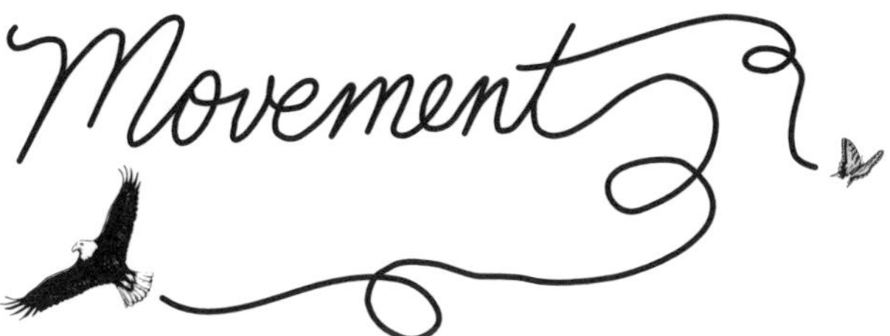

Figure 9–1: "Movement."
Reprinted with permission from Annie Buttons.

> *...there is no perception without movement.*[1]
>
> —T. Ribot

MOVEMENT

Movement is the first of the three principles of natural vision. All living creatures move. We have a visual system to see the world, both physically and mentally, and that process includes movement. The principle of movement is one of the key concepts Bates discovered about vision, and is a subset of the universal principle of continual change: "The only constant is change."

All sense perceptions are based on movement. Hearing involves sound waves, which vibrate the eardrum. The semi-circular canals in the ear require head and body movement to maintain equilibrium and balance. Molecules flowing through the nose allow us to smell. Taste involves molecules moving over the taste buds on the tongue.

In using only the sense of touch, if you rest your hand on a piece of cloth or metal for a long time, it will be difficult to tell which of the two objects your hand is on—until you move either your hand or the object.

Hot and cold temperatures on the skin are perceived not by the absolute temperature, but by *changes* in temperature. An interesting experiment is to put the right hand in a bucket of cold water, and the left in a bucket of hot water. Then put both hands in the same bucket of room-temperature water. To the right hand the water feels hot, but to the left hand the water feels cold!

We sense *changes*—and changes are based on movements.

Even supposed stationary objects are always changing. Researchers have found that very old windows in the churches in Europe are thicker at the bottom than at the top. This is due to gravity pulling downward, albeit very slowly, on the molecules in the glass. Technically, glass is a liquid! Glass is constantly changing its shape.

The best teachers of natural vision are children. Children move, exploring and learning

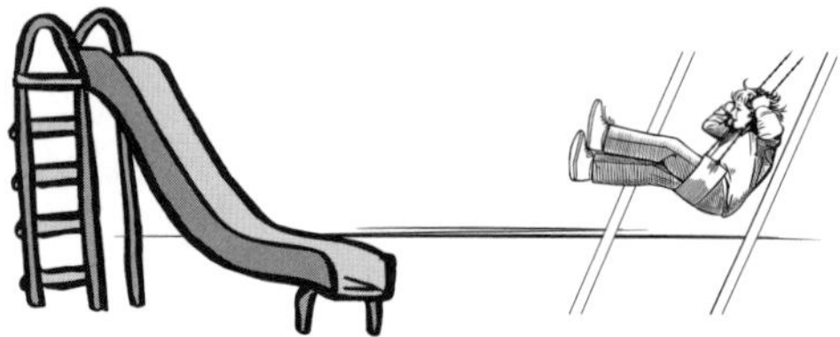

about the world with infinite interest and curiosity. We are meant to grow and learn physically, emotionally, mentally, and spiritually our entire lives. Movement is necessary for this natural process.

If you would like to watch what natural vision students relearn, go to a playground and watch the children. They are continually moving. Notice that no one *tells* the children to move. It is simply natural. You may also notice their parents sitting on the bench staring rigidly.

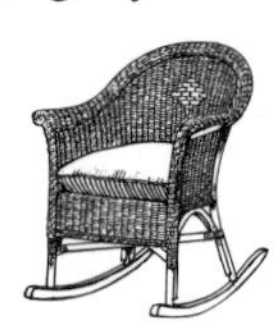

A mother rocks her baby to sleep. Bates said it is a mistake to dispose of cradles and rocking chairs and other methods of promoting the "swing."

Have you ever watched the continuous and even large movements of the blind musicians Ray Charles, Stevie Wonder, and George Shearing? Do we think to ourselves, "It is OK for them to move because they don't know any better?" Why do they move so much, when they cannot see with their physical eyes? The answer is: movement is natural, relaxing, and healthy.

One student, a massage therapist, told me she almost did not enroll for my course because I was always moving during the Introductory Lecture. She now moves.

People who have clear vision move. At times, this movement may be subtle and imperceptible to others, but they move much more than people who have blurred vision. To those who have blur, movement by people who have clarity is annoying and irritating, consciously and/or subconsciously.

Natural vision movement is not a hyper movement; it is a relaxed, casual movement.

An acquaintance of mine told me he was considered to be the only "hyper" member of his family. He could not "sit still, like everyone else." He is the only member of his family who has normal sight. People who have learned to not move often conclude that people who move are hyper.

Another student who has normal vision—and plans to keep it that way—said in class, "I'm squirmy."

Aldous Huxley uses the phrase "dynamic relaxation"[2] to describe natural vision—movement without effort. The opposite of dynamic relaxation is "static stress." Bates discovered static stress creates blurred vision.

BATES ON MOVEMENT

Quoting from *Perfect Sight Without Glasses:*

> It is impossible to see, remember, or imagine anything, even for as much as a second, without shifting from one part to another, or to some other object and back again; and the attempt to do so always produces strain.

> ...When shifting is not done unconsciously, students must be encouraged to do it consciously.
>
> ...A line of small letters on the Snellen test card may be less than a foot long by a quarter of an inch in height; and if it requires seventy shifts to a fraction of a second to see it apparently all at once, it must require many thousands to see an area of the size of the screen of a moving picture, with all its detail of people, animals, houses, or trees, while to see sixteen such areas to a second, as is done in viewing moving pictures must require a rapidity of shifting that can scarcely be realized. Yet it is admitted that the present rate of taking and projecting moving pictures is too slow. The results would be more satisfactory, authorities say, if the rate were raised to twenty, twenty-two, or twenty-four a second. The human eye and mind are not only capable of this rapidity of action, and that without effort or strain, but it is only when the eye is able to shift thus rapidly that eye and mind are at rest, and the efficiency of both at their maximum. It is true that every motion of the eye produces an error of refraction; but when the movement is short, this is very slight, and usually the shifts are so rapid that the error does not last long enough to be detected by the retinoscope, its existence being demonstrable only by reducing the rapidity of the movements to less than four or five a second. The period during which the eye is at rest is much longer than that during which an error of refraction is produced. Hence, when the eye shifts normally no error of refraction is manifest. The more rapid the unconscious shifting of the eye, the better the vision; but if one tries to be conscious of a too rapid shift, a strain will be produced.
>
> Perfect sight is impossible without continual shifting, and such shifting is a striking illustration of the [automatic] mental control necessary for normal vision. It requires perfect mental control to think of thousands of things in a fraction of a second; and each point of fixation has to be thought of separately, because it is impossible to think of two things, or of two parts of one thing, perfectly at the same time. The eye with imperfect sight tries to accomplish the impossible by looking fixedly at one point for an appreciable length of time; that is, by staring. When it looks at a strange letter and does not see it, it keeps on looking at it in an effort to see it better. Such efforts always fail, and are an important factor in the production of imperfect sight.
>
> One of the best methods of improving the sight, therefore, is to imitate consciously the unconscious shifting of normal vision, and to realize the apparent motion produced by such shifting. Whether one has imperfect or normal sight, conscious shifting and swinging are a great help and advantage to the eye; for not only may imperfect sight be improved in this way, but normal sight may be improved also...

The last few paragraphs come close to summarizing Bates' life work on natural vision improvement. People with normal sight unconsciously "shift" constantly with movement and centralization (attention to detail). This is nature's design for the visual system. Interference with these principles lowers sight. Other than vision problems caused by diseases and accidents, Bates found that vision habits determine a person's sight.

From *Better Eyesight* magazine, January 1924: "The normal eye is only at rest when it is moving...."

Better Eyesight magazine, February 1924: "*Question:* What one method of improving sight is best? *Answer:* Swinging and blinking."

Swinging is the same as shifting.

Better Eyesight magazine, March 1925: "Never look at an object for more than a few seconds at a time. Shift your gaze."

Better Eyesight magazine, June 1925:

"Question: When I look at an object and blink, it appears to jump with each blink. Would this be considered the short swing?

Answer: Yes. You unconsciously look from one side to the other of the object when blinking."

Better Eyesight magazine, November 1925:

> MOVING
>
> The world moves. Let it move. People are moving all day long. It is normal, right, proper that they should move. Just try to keep your head or one finger or one toe stationary, or keep your eyes open continuously. If you try to stare at a small letter or part of it without blinking, note what happens. Most people who have tried it discover that the mind wanders, the vision becomes less, pain and fatigue are produced.

People with blurred vision subconsciously imagine stationary objects to be stationary.

Better Eyesight magazine, December 1925:

> SHIFTING
>
> The point regarded changes rapidly and continuously...All persons with imperfect sight make an effort to stare with their eyes immovable. The eyes have not the ability to keep stationary. To look intently at a point continuously is impossible. The eyes will move, the eyelids will blink, and the effort [to lock on a point] is accompanied by an imperfect vision of the point regarded. In many cases the effort to concentrate on a point often causes headache, pain in the eyes, and fatigue. All persons with normal eyes and normal sight do not concentrate or try to see by any effort. Their eyes are at rest, and when the eyes are at rest, they are constantly moving. When the eyes move, one is able to imagine stationary objects, in turn, to be moving in the direction opposite of the head and eyes. It is impossible to imagine, with equal clearness, a number of objects to be moving at the same time, and an effort to do so is a strain which impairs the vision, the memory, or the imagination. To try to do the impossible is a strain which always lowers the mental efficiency. This fact should be emphasized. Many students have difficulty in imagining stationary objects to be moving opposite to the movements of the eyes or head...When pain, fatigue or other symptoms are present, it always means that the individual is consciously or unconsciously trying to imagine stationary objects are not moving. The effect is a strain...Very few people with normal sight...ever notice that they are constantly shifting correctly...One may shift in the wrong way and fail to improve the vision. What is the right way? The right way to shift is to move the eyes [and head] from one point to another slowly, regularly, continuously, restfully or easily without effort or without trying to see. The normal eye with normal sight has the habit of always moving or shifting, usually an unconscious habit. When, by practice, the eye with imperfect sight acquires the conscious habit of shifting [again], the habit may become unconscious. When the shifting is done properly, the memory, imagination, mental efficiency and vision are improved until they become normal. It often happens that when one consciously, or intentionally [sees objects] in the wrong way, a better knowledge of the right way to shift may be obtained. When the eyes are moved to the

right, stationary objects should appear to move to the left. And when the vision is good, all objects not regarded are seen less distinctly than those regarded [centralization]. When the vision is imperfect, objects not observed may be seen better, or an effort is made to see them better than those directly observed. In fact, it is always true, that in all cases of imperfect sight, the eyes do not see best where they are looking and centralization is lost. To shift properly requires relaxation or rest. To shift improperly and lower the vision requires an effort. When one stares at a point without blinking or shifting, fatigue, distress or pain is felt. To continue to stare without shifting is hard work. To see imperfectly is difficult...Imperfect sight or a failure to see requires much trouble and hard work. This fact should be demonstrated repeatedly...until thoroughly convinced that rest of the eyes, mind or body can only be obtained by shifting easily, continuously, and without effort....

[One student did not] look at any object for more than a fraction of a second. His vision after that improved from 20/50 to 20/10. He became able to imagine the movement of objects and demonstrated that all his pain and mental depression was caused by a stare or an effort to see all things stationary...He was comfortable when he imagined objects moving or swinging, but very uncomfortable when he made an effort or imagined them to be stationary.

Recently, I tested the sight of a girl about 10 years old. She read the Snellen card at 10 feet with normal vision. She was asked, "Do you see any of the small letters moving from side to side?" "Yes," she answered, "they are all moving." "Now can you imagine one of the small letters is stationary?" At once she quickly looked away and frowned. "Why did you look away?" her father asked her. She replied, "Because it gave me a pain in my eyes and the letters became blurred. Don't ask me to do it again!"

The experience of this child is the same as that of everyone young or old with perfect or imperfect sight. When the sight is normal and continuously good, to stop the swing of a letter or other object necessitates a strain, an effort which always lowers the vision and produces discomfort or pain in one or both eyes. It has been repeatedly demonstrated that a letter or other object cannot be remembered or even imagined perfectly and continuously unless one can imagine it to be moving or swinging. Not only does the sight become imperfect, but also the memory, imagination, judgment, and other mental faculties are temporarily lost....

Better Eyesight magazine, September 1927: "Your head and eyes are moving all day long."

From *Better Eyesight* magazine, September 1923:

BLINKING

...Usually unconsciously the normal eye closes and opens quite frequently and at irregular intervals and for very short spaces of time. Most people can demonstrate that when they regard a letter that they are able to see quite clearly, it is possible for them to consciously close their eyes and open them quick enough and see the letter continuously. This is called Blinking and it is only another name for dodging. Dodging what? Dodging the tendency to look steadily at things all the time. All the methods which have been recommended for the improvement of the vision, ...[centralizing]..., swinging, blinking, can all be grouped under the one word—dodging.

While teaching students to improve their vision, Bates emphasized head movement. People who have blurred vision have a tight neck, eye muscles, head, and shoulders. These tensions are caused by rigid staring and shallow, or even stopped, breathing.

TOM'S PERSONAL LOG: During my first vision lessons, I resisted the movement concepts and habits I was being taught. I kept objecting, "If I keep moving, how am I ever going to see anything?!" I thought, like many people with blurred vision, that it was necessary to lock fixedly on an object to see it; in other words, I felt it was necessary that stationary objects must appear to be stationary to see them. I discovered this idea is not only incorrect, it lowered my vision.

THE PROBLEM OF RIGIDITY

In a left-hemisphere-oriented society, body movement is often taboo. Children are frequently told, "Sit still." Even worse—"Be still," command the adults who have mastered rigidity and blurred vision themselves. "Pay attention when I speak to you," the child is told sternly—and the child freezes. "Don't fidget!" Children chide other children, "Ants in your pants?" One of my students was told by his teacher in grade school, "Head straight. Eyes down!"

Maurice Sendak's charming children's book, *Where the Wild Things Are,* tells of a boy named Max taming monsters. Maurice writes, "... till Max said 'BE STILL!' and tamed them with the magic trick of staring into all their yellow eyes without blinking once and they were all frightened...."[3]

One version of the Bible, 1st Kings, Chapter 14, Verse 4, states, "But Ahijah could not see, for his eyes were set." Curiously, this sentence has been changed in another version to "Now Ahijah could not see, his eyes were dimmed with age."[4] It appears that the presbyopia old-age theory has found its way into scriptures.

In our society, physical movement is generally not acceptable when two people are talking—it is considered rude. Supposedly, the moving person is not interested in what is being said. Ironically, since movement and circulation are essential for normal health, two individuals may be able to communicate *less* well by being rigid. They can become fatigued, and even irritable, from their rigidity. Movement while conversing can lead to *more* interest, e.g., by noticing the kind of clothes a person is wearing.

More than a few students have told me they could never catch a baseball. This can be due to "freezing" when the ball is hit toward them. They tighten up their body and *mind* at the time flexibility and movement are most needed.

I have observed many students who, when sitting in class, lean forward with their arms and legs crossed. Not only are the legs crossed, they are wrapped all the way around each other very tightly.

One video that demonstrates "eye exercises" teaches the student to try to stop an object on the TV screen, which is continually moving, from moving. This video continually reminds the subject to "keep the head still" and only move the eyes. This is incorrect, unnatural, and harmful.

If you want to watch what natural vision students are unlearning, take a ride on a big-city bus Friday at 5 P.M. and observe how rigid the passengers are.

One of my students was telling me about her travels to Nigeria. On one trip, one of the natives said to her, "You white people don't move your heads!"

At one of my review/support group classes, a student who had taken my course about two years earlier was in attendance. During the entire class, he was as rigid as anyone still living could be, and it was obvious he was not practicing correct vision habits. Toward the end of the class, he volunteered that he had not experienced any vision improvement. At the end of the review class, four students sitting near him immediately and simultaneously informed him that he never moves. This was a quite dramatic event to behold. Students who do not improve their vision are not relearning natural movement. They are holding on to the tight, tense way of using their body and mind—the way that created their blurred vision in the first place.

TOM'S PERSONAL LOG: After two years of teaching, while still improving my own vision, the simple realization came to me, "If *I* remain rigid, the eye muscles will also remain rigid; if *I* become flexible again, so will the eye muscles."

As someone once stated, "You are not in the problem. The problem is in you!"

One of my students says she can model for a much longer time by incorporating small movements into her poses. She says she is more relaxed and has more energy with less fatigue. Previously she would try to remain as motionless as possible.

"Don't lock life!" says P. B., natural vision student and yoga teacher.

"There is only one disease, called stagnation."

OPPOSITIONAL MOVEMENT— A VISUAL MASSAGE

One of the consequences of natural vision movements is that objects appear to move. This idea is alluded to above and is discussed in depth in this section.

From *Better Eyesight* magazine, July 1920:

> SEE THINGS MOVING
>
> When the sight is perfect the subject is able to observe that all objects regarded appear to be moving. A letter seen at the near point or at the distance appears to move slightly in various directions. The pavement comes toward one in walking, and the houses appear to move in a direction opposite to one's own. In reading, the page appears to move in a direction opposite to that of the eye. If one tries to imagine things stationary, the vision is at once lowered and discomfort and pain may be produced, not only in the eyes and head, but in other parts of the body.
>
> This movement is so slight that it is seldom noticed till the attention is called to it, but it may be so conspicuous as to be plainly observable even to persons with markedly imperfect sight. If such persons, for instance, hold the hand within six inches of the face and turn the head and eyes rapidly from side to side, that hand will be seen to move in a direction opposite to that of the eyes. If it does not move, it will be found that the person is straining to see it in the eccentric [peripheral] field. By observing this movement it becomes possible to see or imagine a less conspicuous movement, and thus the person may gradually become able to observe a slight movement in every object regarded. Some persons with imperfect sight have reversed it simply by imagining that they see things moving all day long.
>
> The world moves. Let it move. All objects

> move if you let them. Do not interfere with this movement, or try to stop it. This cannot be done without an effort which impairs the efficiency of the eye and mind.

Better Eyesight magazine, November 1921:

> [Students should practice] seeing things moving all day long from the time the eyes are opened in the morning until they are closed at night, and going to sleep finally with the imagination of the swing....
>
> The best thing for a busy person is to form a habit of constant shifting and to imagine that everything seen is moving. It is the habit of staring that spoils your sight. If you can correct this by constant shifting and the realization of the movement produced by the shift, you can get well without so much palming and you will also be able to do your school work better.

Better Eyesight magazine, September 1922:

> [While improving your vision, the] most important of all is to see things moving, or rather to be conscious that stationary objects are moving, in the opposite direction to the movement of the eyes. Unless this is done continuously one is apt to imagine stationary objects are stationary which is very injurious to the eyes....[Some people] complain that moving objects make them uncomfortable. It can always be demonstrated that it is not seeing things move which is uncomfortable but rather it is trying to stop the movement which causes the discomfort...One of the first things I have my students demonstrate is that it is impossible to keep the attention fixed on a point and imagine it stationary for any length of time, and that the effort to do so is disagreeable and lowers the memory and imagination and sight.

Better Eyesight magazine, July 1927:

> Acquire a continuous habit of imagining stationary objects to be moving easily, until it becomes an unconscious habit.

Better Eyesight magazine, September 1927:

> Imagine that stationary objects are moving in the direction opposite to the movement of your head and eyes. When you walk about the room or on the street, notice that the floor or pavement seems to come toward you, while objects on either side appear to move in the direction opposite to the movement of your body.

Better Eyesight magazine, December 1927:

> The importance of practicing certain parts of the routine habits at all times, such as...imagining stationary objects to be moving opposite to the movement of his head and eyes, is stressed.

A key concept intimately connected to the principle of movement is *oppositional movement*. The theme of oppositional movement is one example of Bates' teachings at first seeming contradictory, or even incomprehensible. Bates discovered vision cannot be normal without the experience of oppositional movement.

Whichever direction we move with our sight, stationary objects appear to move in the opposite direction.

When a person is driving a car, the road, trees, hills, and houses all seem to be moving in the opposite direction of the car's movement. Specifically, if the car (and you!) are moving north, all stationary objects outside of the car appear to be moving south. Conversely, when a person is *backing* his car out of the garage, the garage seems to be moving *forward*. These are examples of forward and backward oppositional movement.

As the child moves upward on a trampoline or on a teeter-totter, the world seems to move downward; as the child comes back down, the world seems to move upward—in the opposite direction.

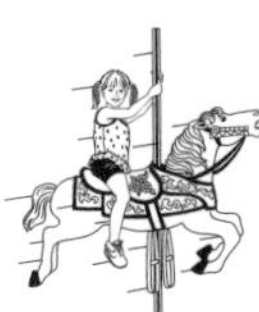

When we spin round and round on a merry-go-round or carousel, the world seems to spin in the opposite direction.

When our attention is on a moving object, oppositional movement is an even more subtle concept because our primary attention is on the moving object, and *not* on the objects that appear to be moving in the opposite direction. For example, when watching a bird fly across a field, the illusion of the trees moving in the opposite direction is experienced primarily subconsciously.

If our attention is on a house across a street, and a car drives by, the house seems relatively stationary, and the car "moves" by. But if our attention is on the car when it drives by, the house does not appear stationary—rather, it seems to move in the opposite direction of the car's movement.

We call evening "sunset," but shouldn't it really be called "earthrise," and "sunrise" called "earthset"?! The sun is not "setting"; the Earth is rotating. The stationary sun appears to move in the opposite direction of the Earth's rotation.

Of course, stationary objects do not *actually* move—but they *seem* to move. Bates discovered that this illusion—stationary objects appearing to move in the opposition direction of the head movement—is essential for clear, normal sight. Movement and the illusion of oppositional movement are meant to be occurring all day long.

The experience of oppositional movement is a natural, automatic consequence of head and body movement. Usually, oppositional movement is a secondary, subconscious experience. Still, it is an essential part of normal seeing.

While improving sight, people with high blur or serious vision problems may take a longer time before experiencing oppositional movement. This is because of the high degree of staring they have learned.

Better Eyesight magazine, January 1924: "The failure to imagine that stationary objects are moving is always due to a stare or strain." Later Bates wrote, "Staring is a strain...," so the problem is strain.

After several years of teaching natural vision, I began referring to the effect of the illusion of oppositional movement as a *visual massage*. When a person has normal vision, light rays move across the retina in the back of the eyeball and create a continuous, subtle, energetic massage for the eyes and the mind.

Movement and Oppositional Movement are Fun!

I once observed a father swinging his daughter around him many times. When he finished swinging her, she was dizzy and would even fall down on the grass. Then she ran back to him for more fun swinging!

Amusement parks have many "rides" we enjoy: roller coasters, bumper cars, carousels,

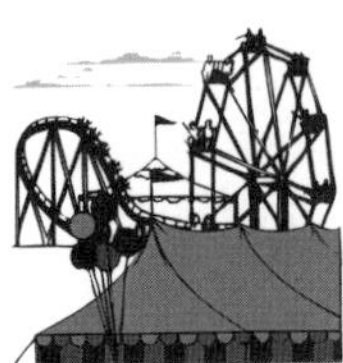

etc. Disneyland has spinning teacups. All of these experiences involve movement. Movement and oppositional movement are fun!

Experiencing Oppositional Movement of Stationary Objects

The following activities are demonstrations of the importance of *movement* and *oppositional movement*. They are not eye exercises. They are examples or demonstrations of natural movements students need all day long in order to have normal, clear vision. Ultimately, the movements can be large, medium, small, fast, or slow but *movement* is the key.

The better the vision, the more subtle the movements become, and vice versa. Larger movements are usually emphasized in the beginning to be certain the students do not slip back into the staring habit.

If you do not experience the effects described below, you may not be doing the activities correctly. Find a vision teacher to show you how to do them correctly.

Often, the mind resists the correct, natural vision experiences because of many years of ingrained, incorrect habits. If you do not experience oppositional movement in the activities described below, continue practicing them until you do. The experience *will* occur with sufficient practice.

Also, there are levels or "degrees" of experiences. Oppositional movement becomes more "fluid" with the practice of better vision habits each day.

Unless you have normal vision, you probably will not experience the following activities to the fullest extent the first time you do them. That is fine for now. I often remind my students that no one experiences everything I teach the first time they are taught. You are in the process of relearning to see. All of the following activities are experienced perfectly only when the vision is clear and normal. If you experience all of these activities perfectly the first time, you probably do not need this book or classes!

What we see in the world is mostly a *conscious* process, but *how* we see the world is a *subconscious* process. Therefore, there is some tendency for the mind to avoid correct vision habits when practiced consciously. Vision, and vision habits, cannot be perfectly normal until they are subconscious. Of course, the idea is to practice them consciously until they become automatic, subconscious habits—exactly like they used to be when you used to have clarity.

How to see clearly is fairly simple to understand, but it is not obvious. If it were obvious, many people would improve their vision without a book or teacher.

If you have health problems, all vision activities in the beginning should be done very slowly and for brief periods. As mentioned in the beginning of this book, the student—and not the teacher, author, or publisher—assumes responsibility for any responses generated by doing these activities. You may want to read the section on *reversal processes* in Chapter 20, "The Two Sides of Health and Healing," before doing any activities in this book.

Most students will find it valuable to receive instruction from an experienced Natural Vision teacher.

The Variable Swing—Simple Oppositional Movement

TO EXPERIENCE:

Hold your right forefinger vertical, six inches in front of your head, and six inches to the right. While moving your eyes *and head* to the right, notice how the finger appears to move to the left in the opposite direction. While moving your eyes and head to the left, notice how the finger appears to move to the right in the opposite direction. Repeat several times.

Do not look at the finger while moving your head left and right. Let your attention sweep along objects in the distance.

This effect and illusion of the stationary finger appearing to move in the opposite direction of your head movement is called *oppositional movement.*

Object Shifting

TO EXPERIENCE:

Notice three objects in front of you, one on the right, one in the center, and one on the left.

Let's call the object on the left Object L, the object in the center Object C, and the object on the right Object R.

Notice Object C. It is in the center of your visual field. Now, shift your attention to Object L. Notice that Object C is no longer in the center of your visual field. It appears as if Object C *moved* from the center to the right.

Now, shift your attention from Object L to Object R. Object C appears to have *moved* from the right, through the center of your visual field, to the left. Of course, Object C did not move; only the light rays from Object C moved across the retina, placing object C in its new location on the left.

When you shift your attention from Object R to Object L, Object C again appears to *move* from left to right.

Repeat this activity several times until you experience the oppositional movement of Object C.

Do this all day long with all objects! The idea is simple—continue to move, and never stare. In this way, stationary objects will always appear to be moving.

Some students say, "Of course Object C moved in the opposite direction of my movement; it is obvious." It may be obvious when the student thinks about it, but it is usually not obvious when the student is not thinking about it. The problem is that a person who has blurred vision returns to rigid staring during much of the day. Stationary objects do *not* appear to move when a person is staring, and this strains the visual system.

The principle of oppositional movement is, in truth, very subtle. It is one of the greatest keys to natural vision, and is one of the subconscious consequences of moving the eyes and the head all day long.

Better Eyesight magazine, November 1925:

> MOVING
>
> ...Stand facing a window and note the relative position of a curtain cord to the

OBJECT L	**OBJECT C**	**OBJECT R**

> background. Take a long step to the right. Observe that the background has become different. Now take a long step to the left. The background has changed again. Avoid regarding the curtain cord. While moving from side to side it is possible to imagine the cord moving in the opposite direction... Never imagine stationary objects to be stationary. To do this is a strain, which lowers the vision.

Oppositional Movement—The Pencil

TO EXPERIENCE:

Hold a pencil in front of you vertically, with the eraser at the top. Hold the bottom of the pencil near your mouth; the top of the pencil should now be near the forehead. Move the pencil out 8–10 inches from your head.

Now, as if your pencil (and hand) were attached to your head, move the pencil and the head together slowly to the left. Keep your attention on the pencil. Do not tilt the pencil or your head. Do not look into the distance. While you are moving to the left, distant objects appear to move to the right.

Now move the pencil and the head slowly to the right. Remember to keep your attention on the pencil as you move! Distant objects now appear to move to the left.

As you move your pencil and head slowly upward together, distant objects appear to move downward. As you move your pencil and head slowly downward, distant objects appear to move upward.

Stated again, the illusion of stationary objects appearing to move in the opposite direction of the head and pencil's movement is called *oppositional movement*.

While your attention is on the pencil, you might notice there are *two* of each object in the background! This is due to stereoscopic vision, discussed in Chapter 18, "Stereoscopic Vision."

The enjoyment of the following Sway, Long Swing, and Infinity Swing can be enhanced by listening to relaxing music while doing these activities.

The Sway

TO EXPERIENCE

Part A: **Swaying with Open Eyelids**

See *Figure 9–2: The Sway, a-1, a-2,* and *a-3*.

Stand with your arms relaxed by your sides and your feet separated about shoulder-width apart. Relax your kneecaps. Breathe abdominally. Blink frequently. The neck is buttery soft, and the head is balanced normally. Pretend you have a feather attached to your nose. The nose-feather extends out to whatever objects are in front of you.

Now, sway your body slowly and smoothly approximately 3–4 inches to the left while sweeping the nose-feather to the left a small distance. Keep your attention on whatever objects the nose-feather sweeps along in the distance. Do not *tilt* your body or head as in *Figure 9–2, b*. The weight of your body simply shifts over to one leg and then to the other. While swaying to the left, pretend that objects in front of you are moving to the right.

Now, sway your body slowly and gently to the right, moving the head and nose-feather to the right. While swaying to the right, pretend that objects are moving to the left.

Alternate swaying from left to right and back, allowing the distant objects, which your

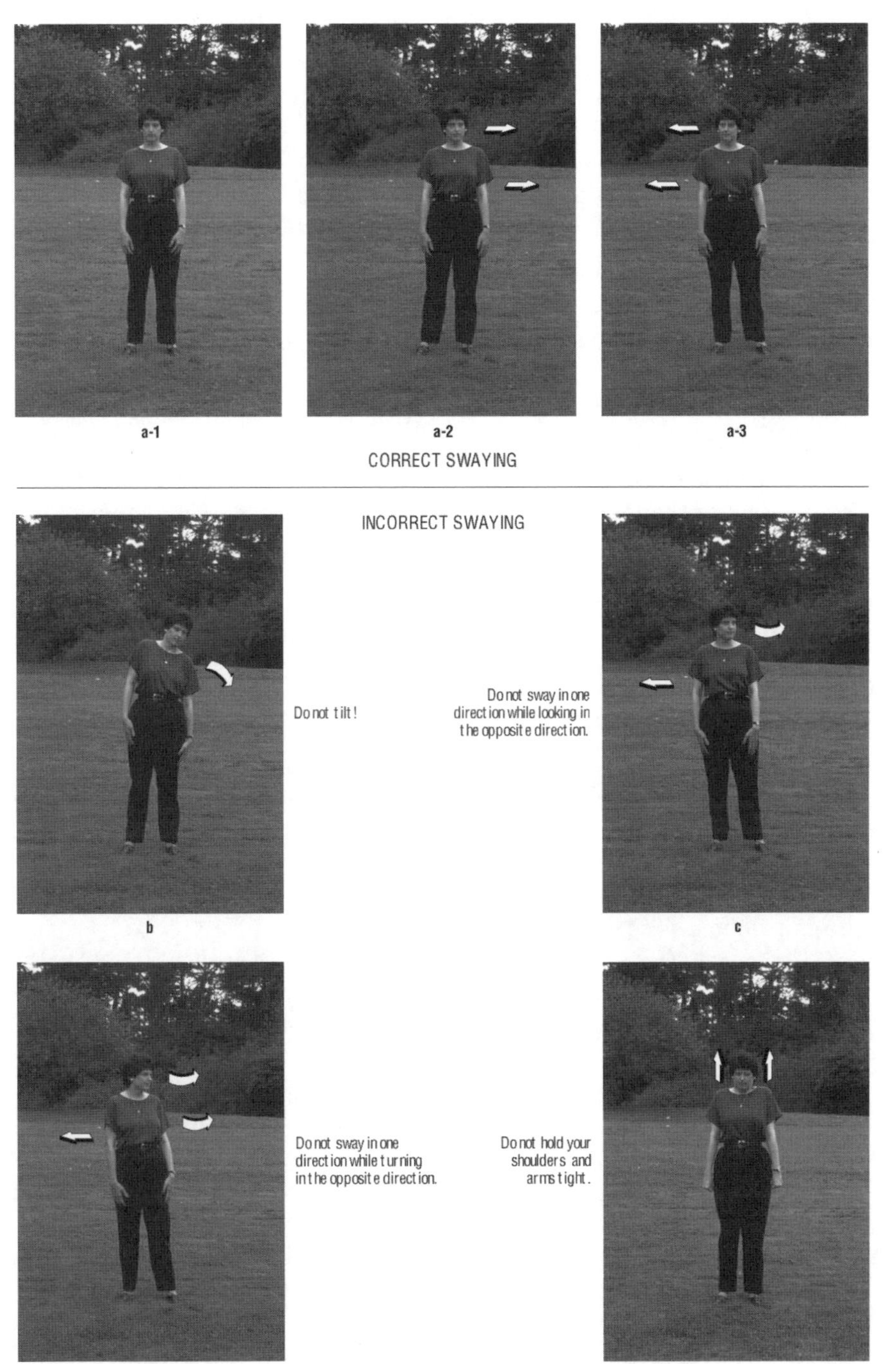
a-1
a-2
a-3
CORRECT SWAYING
INCORRECT SWAYING
Do not tilt!
Do not sway in one direction while looking in the opposite direction.
b
c
Do not sway in one direction while turning in the opposite direction.
Do not hold your shoulders and arms tight.
d
e

Figure 9–2: The Sway.

nose-feather is sweeping along, to move in the opposite direction of that of your body and head.

Part B: Swaying with Closed Eyelids:
The above sway can be repeated with the eyelids closed.

Pretend you are standing in a nice sunny meadow with many redwood trees in the distance, about 100 feet in front of you. The trees are aligned in a row from left to right. When you are swaying to the left, the nose-feather taps the trunks of the trees as they appear to move to the right. When swaying to the right, the tree trunks appear to move to the left.

Some students incorrectly move their head and nose-feather to the left while swaying to their right (see *Figure 9–2, c* and *d*), and move their head and nose-feather to the left while swaying to the right.

When a person walks down a hallway and turns to walk through a door on the left, both the body and the head turn and move naturally to the left. The body should move in the same direction as the head and nose-feather.

Also, do not tighten your shoulders as shown in *Figure 9–2, e*. The shoulders and arms should be relaxed.

From *Better Eyesight* magazine, February 1930:

THE SWAY

When one imagines stationary objects to be moving in the same or opposite direction to the movement of the head or eyes when both heels are resting on the floor, it is called "the sway." When both heels are lifted from the floor, it is not called the sway, but "the swing." The apparent movement of stationary objects may be horizontal, vertical or at any angle. The sway is a very valuable thing to use, because it promotes relaxation, or rest, much better than other methods. In fact, so general is this conclusion that I always try to have every student practice the sway immediately upon starting lessons.

The sway may be practiced rapidly or slowly, and with a wide or a narrow motion. When the sway is practiced, distant objects are covered more or less completely, which explains why rest is obtained. When the sway is used properly, all stationary objects regarded appear to be moving. Whether the sway is short or long, if practiced properly, the vision is usually improved...

Most people with imperfect sight have a constant strain and tension of nearly all the muscles of the body. The nerves are also under a strain and their efficiency is frequently lost. By practicing the sway properly, fatigue is relieved as well as pain, dizziness and other symptoms.

The sway always brings about a relief from the effort of trying to see, staring, or concentration. The normal eye needs relaxation or rest. It does not always have normal sight. When it is at rest it always has normal sight.

Things which are done by the student to improve the sight do not always succeed. There are many ways of improving the sight by the sway, provided it is practiced correctly....[One student] practiced the sway with her eyes moving in one direction and her head in the opposite direction.....This method of practicing the sway is to be condemned.

Better Eyesight magazine, June 1925: Emily C. Lierman, "The head should turn in the same direction with the eyes."

The Long (or Elephant) Swing

> *"It Don't Mean a Thing, If It Ain't Got That Swing." (title of a song)*

The image of an elephant's trunk swinging left and right is helpful to many students.

The Long, or Elephant, Swing is simply an "extended" Sway. See *Figure 9–3: The Long (Elephant) Swing.*

Part A:

The Long Swing With Open Eyelids

Instead of swaying the body left and right, turn your whole body gently to the left, *b,* and then to the right, *c.* When you are turning to the left, the right back of the heel raises slightly; similarly, when turning to the right, the left heel raises slightly. The head and nose-feather "swing" softly around the room (or scenery, if you are outdoors). The arms remain relaxed by your sides; any movement of the arms is due to the turning of the entire body.

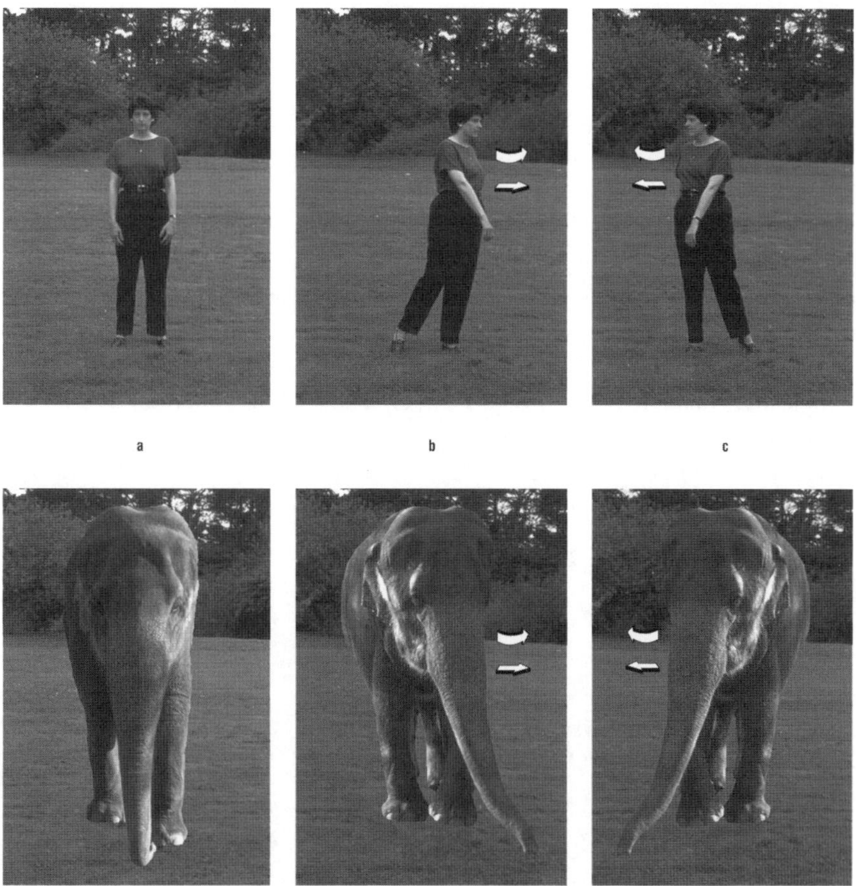

Figure 9–3: The Long (Elephant) Swing.

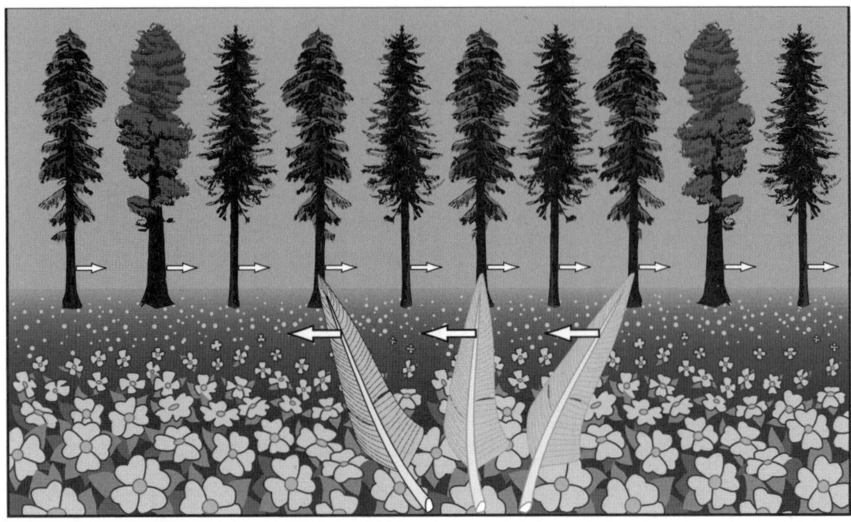

"Brush" the objects with your nose-feather like a searchlight sweeping across clouds in the sky at night.

This is not a physical workout. It is an easy, floating visual experience.

Many students try to lock onto objects while doing the Long Swing. This is due to the staring habit. Do not lock onto objects as they move past you. Allow all objects to "float" past you. Do not "space out" or diffuse.

Part B:

The Long Swing With Closed Eyelids

Same as above, except now pretend you are a hundred feet tall, standing in a beautiful, sunny meadow. Many redwood trees approximately fifty feet away extend around you in a circle. While swinging casually to the left let your nose-feather tap the trunks of the trees. Imagine a tap-tap-tap-tap-tap-tap-tap sensation as the feather touches the trunks. Pretend the trees are moving toward the right. While swinging to the right, pretend the trees

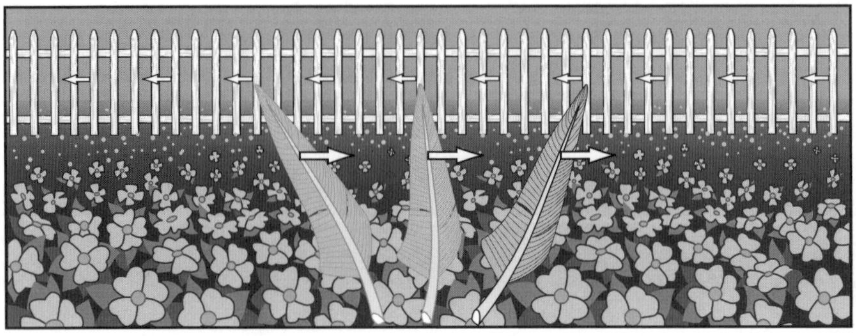

are moving to the left. Tap-tap-tap-tap-tap-tap-tap! The sun warms your body as you swing. Breathe in the fresh, clean air.

After swinging for a few minutes, sweep your nose-feather along the many beautiful and vibrant flowers in the field in front of you. Continue to swing left and right with your nose-feather.

About twenty feet away, there is a tall, white picket fence that extends all the way around you. Sweep the nose-feather along the pickets from left to right and back, tapping the pickets with the tip of the nose-feather. Tap-tap-tap-tap-tap-tap-tap. When you are swinging to the right, all of the pickets sprout little feet and run to the left. When you are swinging to the left, all the pickets run back to the right.

Do the Long Swing for several minutes. Remember to blink frequently and breathe abdominally. The more a person practices the Long Swing, the more fluidly the distant objects will flow in the opposite direction. The student can use the degree of fluidity as a gauge of progress.

The Long Swing can also be done with closed eyelids while remembering the image in *Plate 6: Long Swing Lake,* or any other beautiful, expansive scenery. Swing your nose-feather from one side of the lake, along the mountains, and to the other of the lake. Pretend you are enjoying the fresh mountain air and the warmth of the sun.

The purpose of the Sway and the Long Swing is to encourage, not force, stationary objects to appear to be moving in the opposite direction of your head and body movement.

Brush with the nose-feather as a habit all day long!

Some students feel small vibrations in their eyes, eyelids, and/or nose when swinging the feather along the pickets. This is a positive sign, because normal eyes have many different types of movements, oscillations, and vibrations. The rigid habit of staring causes the eyes to slow down their movements and become locked tight. Staring causes the eye muscles to lock the eyeball into a rigid, distorted shape.

Tom's Personal Log: When I first did the Long Swing, I did not want objects in the room to move at all. As I turned my head to the left, I would lock my eyes on an object (in a diffused way) on the right side of the room, trying to keep everything from moving. Eventually, the eyes have to turn with the head! Finally, my eyes would jump to the front part of the room and lock there, while my head continued turning to the left. When my head had turned all the way to the left, my eyes would once again jump to the left and lock on that part of the room.

I discovered I had a very high resistance to movement and oppositional movement. The thick, coke-bottle glasses I worn were proportional to my rigidity.

Become a Sharpshooter with Oppositional Movement!

Tom's Personal Log: When in basic training in the service, I was taught by experts how to shoot a rifle.

I was instructed to align the front sight[5] and the rear sight of the rifle with the stationary target, the "bull's eye" in the distance. One's initial inclination might be to try to lock the front sight onto the target with no movement.

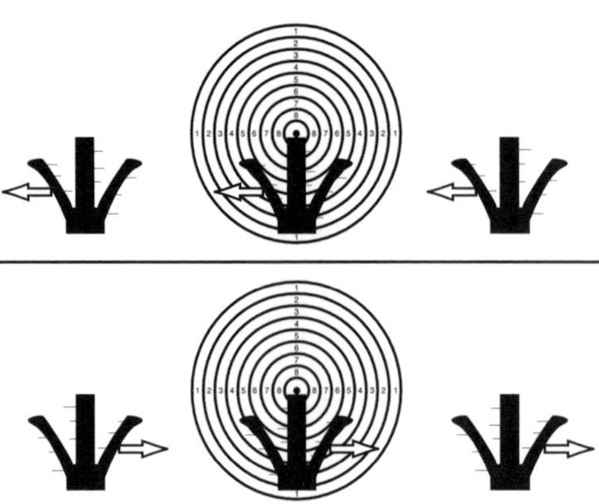

Figure 9–4: Movement During Target Practice.

Keeping my attention on the front sight, I was told to move the front sight smoothly through the target—first slightly to the left of the target. While moving to the left, the target appeared to move to the right. Then I was told to move the front sight smoothly back through the center of the target, and continue to move slightly to the right. The target then appeared to move to the left. "Breathe normally," they said.

Continuing this left-and-right movement of the front sight through the target, they then instructed me to slowly squeeze the trigger as I *moved* the front sight through the center of the target. There was a continual movement of the sight through the target at all times. The rifle never stops moving!

Not knowing any better, I followed their instructions exactly. I scored 58 out of a possible 60 points.

To quote again from Bates and his *Better Eyesight* magazine, January 1926:

> SWINGING
>
> When the eyes move slowly or rapidly from side to side, stationary objects appear to move opposite to the movement of the head and eyes. People with normal vision are not always conscious of the swing. When called to their attention, however, they can always demonstrate it, and are always able to imagine all stationary objects to be moving. In imperfect sight, the swing is modified or absent. This is a truth that has been demonstrated over a long period of years by a great many people and no exceptions have been found. The normal or perfect swing is slow, short, easy and continuous. When the swing is normal, it is always true that not only is the vision normal or perfect, but also the memory, the imagination or the mental efficiency corresponds. When the memory is imperfect, the imagination and mental efficiency and the sight are also imperfect. . .Severe pain, fatigue, or worry often prevent the demonstration of the swing. . .[and the illusion of oppositional movement.]. . .Make no effort to imagine stationary objects to be moving. . . .
>
> LONG SWING
>
> . . .The long swing when done before retiring lessens eyestrain during sleep.

Simply *allow* stationary objects to move—naturally. Do not try to force the illusion of oppositional movement. This will slow down, or defeat, progress.

Better Eyesight magazine, October 1923:

> *Question:* When does the long swing fail to produce relaxation?
>
> *Answer:* When one stares at objects [that appear to be] moving.

In other words, when a person locks onto an object, trying to stop the illusion of oppositional movement.

Swinging, when done correctly, is relaxing.

One Bates teacher had a history of migraine headaches until one day, while doing the Long Swing, her headaches stopped and never returned again.

The Infinity ∞ (or Figure-8) Swing

The Infinity, or Figure-8, Swing is an excellent variation of the Long Swing.

See *Figure 9–5: The Infinity Swing.*

In the Infinity Swing, the nose-feather brushes the tip of the middle finger of each hand as they alternately move in the shape of an infinity sign, ∞, or the shape of a horizontal "figure-8."

Continue the basic Long Swing movement, with the following changes:

Begin with the two middle fingers touching each other in front of your body, approximately sixteen inches from your nose. With the nose-feather brushing the tip of the middle finger of the left hand, begin moving the left hand upward and to the left in a counter-clockwise direction. The movement is very graceful and easy, like the graceful movements of a ballerina or Tai-Chi master. The head and the nose-feather follow the middle finger's movement around this circle. The body turns to the left during the upper half of this circle, just as in the regular Long Swing, and returns to the middle at the completion of the circle. Remember to lift the opposite heel when beginning the turn of your body. Breathe abdominally and blink softly and frequently.

When the circle is completed, the two middle fingers touch once again in front of the body as you return to the starting position.

Now follow the tip of the middle finger of the right hand upward and to the right in a clockwise direction, turning the body to the right and then back to the middle as you complete the circle, where the fingers touch again.

Notice that when you move your hands in the correct direction, you will always be moving the hands upward in the middle of the infinity sign, and downward on the outsides of the loops. If you are moving in the incorrect direction, you will be moving downward in the middle, and upward on the outsides.

Do *not* go clockwise on the left loop and do *not* go counter-clockwise on the right loop. This is imbalancing. The proper directions are important.

Not a few students forget, and later, when doing the Infinity Swing, go in the incorrect directions. Going in the incorrect directions is an indication you are not balanced. It is important to remember to move in the correct directions—even if you feel like the incorrect direction feels more "natural" to you.

Tom's Personal Log: When I first did the Infinity Swing, it was very difficult for me to go the proper directions. In fact, it would make me nauseated. Moving in the incorrect direction—down in the middle of the infinity sign—was more "comfortable" and felt more "natural."

The reason for this is I was very unhealthy at that time. When a person is out of balance, the incorrect directions seem correct. The "comfort" of moving in the incorrect directions only matched my imbalance.

In time, especially with benefit of years of natural healing, the correct directions began to feel comfortable and the incorrect directions began to make me nauseated. Today, I begin to feel nauseated just to *think* about going in the incorrect direction. This, of

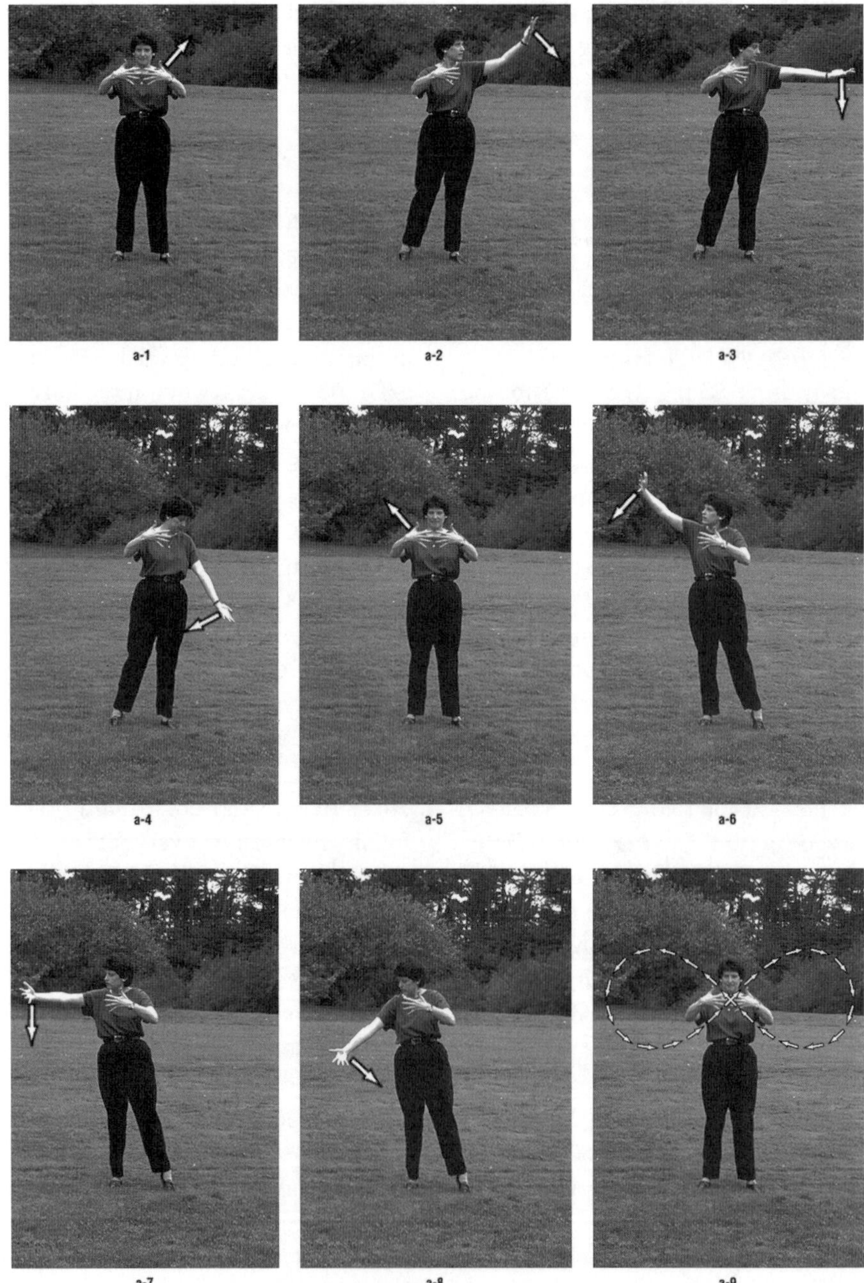

Figure 9–5: The Infinity Swing.

course, is a very good sign of progress, not just for my vision, but for all of my health.

I like (or should I say dislike) to think of going downward in the middle of the infinity sign as "depressing." I like to think of going upward in the middle of the infinity sign as "uplifting." Here is yet is another way to gauge your progress. The more comfortable the correct direction feels, the more progress you are making.

It is also important to keep your attention brushing the middle finger. If the attention goes into the distance, distant objects will most likely *not* appear to move in the opposite direction.

The Infinity Swing is an especially powerful variation of the Long Swing and most students find it very enjoyable, relaxing, and even energizing. Some students have uncomfortable sensations when doing the swings in the beginning. This is because they are not used to natural movements, and allowing stationary objects to move in the opposite direction.

The Infinity pattern (in the correct directions) helps to activate and balance the right and left hemispheres. Another advantage is the continual flow of movement, even at the right and left extremes.

Some students feel more comfortable on one side of the swing than the other. This is very common, and the movement becomes more balanced with practice.

In time, the student can comfortably experience objects moving in exactly the opposite direction of the finger's movement all the way along the infinity shape. When the finger is moving upward, background objects seems to move downward; when the finger moves left, background objects seem to move right; when the finger moves down, background objects seem to move upward, and so on. No matter which direction the finger is moving, background objects will seem to be moving in exactly the opposite direction.

One advantage of the Infinity Swing is the neck releases in more directions than the basic Long Swing.

One of my students, who was a cello musician with the San Francisco Symphony, demonstrated in one class how, when he moves the bow forward and backward, he includes a small looping pattern with his hand at the end of each stroke. There is no stopping at the end of each stroke. There is a continual flow of movement in the shape of an infinity sign.

The above Sway and Swings are used to teach students the important principle of movement. The Sway is a "subtle" Long Swing.

From Bates, *Better Eyesight* magazine, March 1928:

> Since a short swing improves the vision more than a long swing, the benefit of the short swing of the period [or any other small object] at the distance is manifest.

Ultimately, the Sway is more powerful than the Long Swing, because the feeling of oppositional movement is more subtle. In the beginning, however, the Long Swing may be more beneficial, because the feeling of oppositional movement is more obvious as when doing the Sway (short swing).

The nose-feather, described in more detail in Chapter 12, "The First Habit—Sketching (Shifting)," *is* the Long Swing "all day long." Re-integration of the movement principle is the key. The purpose of all of the above, again, is to eliminate the staring habit.

Double Oppositional Movement

EXPERIENCE DOUBLE OPPOSITIONAL MOVEMENT

Perform the regular Long Swing, with objects far in the distance. The distant objects seem to move in the opposite direction of your head movement as usual.

Now place a tall thin vertical object, like a pole or stick, in front of you about eight feet away. While you are doing the Long Swing the pole will appear to move in the opposite direction. However, the objects in the distance now seem to move in the *same* direction as your head movement, relative to the pole's movement.

The distant object's oppositional movement relative to the pole's oppositional movement creates a "double oppositional movement" or "same-direction" movement! In reality, even the distant objects are moving in the opposite direction of your movement, but that illusion is diminished because of the pole or stick eight feet away.

OPPOSITIONAL MOVEMENT AND DEPTH PERCEPTION

A cue the brain uses to gauge relative distances is the observation of how fast stationary objects move past us as we move past them.

As the car moves from right to left, the tree seems to move from left to right. The house also "moves" from left to right, but more slowly than the tree's movement. Both the tree and the house seem to move faster than the hills behind them.

Because the tree is "moving" faster than the house, the brain assumes the tree is closer to us. The house must be between the tree and the hills because it seems to move more slowly than the tree, but faster than the hills.

In reality, all stationary objects—near, middle distance, or far—move past you at the same speed.

John P. Frisby writes in his book *Seeing—Illusion, Brain and Mind:*

> Objects at different depths produce retinal images which move at different rates

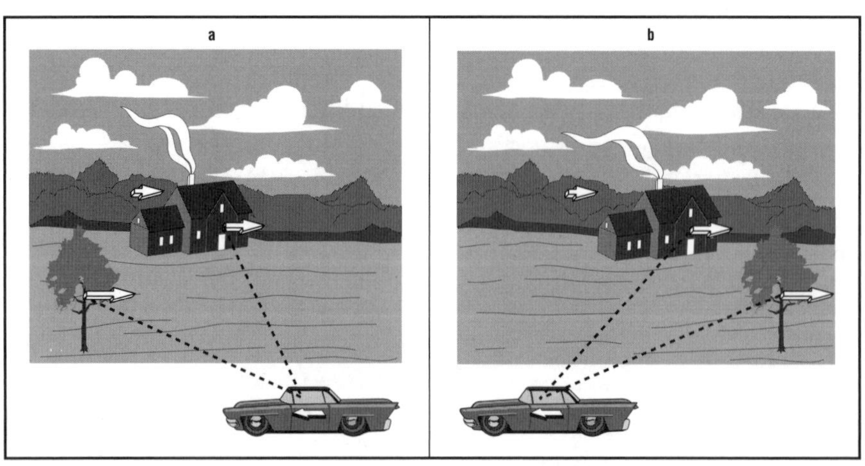

Figure 9–6: Oppositional Movement and Depth Perception.

> across the retina when the head is moved, a clue (or "cue") to depth called *head-movement parallax*. The brain is quite up to the task of using this cue to generate vivid depth perceptions which can appear equally as good as stereopsis. This is why in the opening paragraph you were invited to *walk* around the room with one eye covered, rather than looking at it from a single stationary position. Walking ensures that the depth cue of head-movement parallax is available to the visual system....[6]

While waiting to receive the ball from the server, professional tennis players move constantly to the left, to the right, forward, backward, up and down. Movement is essential for normal depth perception.

THE NEAR-TO-FAR/FAR-TO-NEAR SWING

Another important application of the movement principle is in near and far vision. Not only do we look right and left and up and down, we also notice objects up close and in the distance. Since the head is not normally moving forward or backward when we change our attention from far to near, respectively, the movement of vision from near to far and back occurs primarily in the mind. Usually there is a small, natural, up and down head movement when looking far and near, respectively.

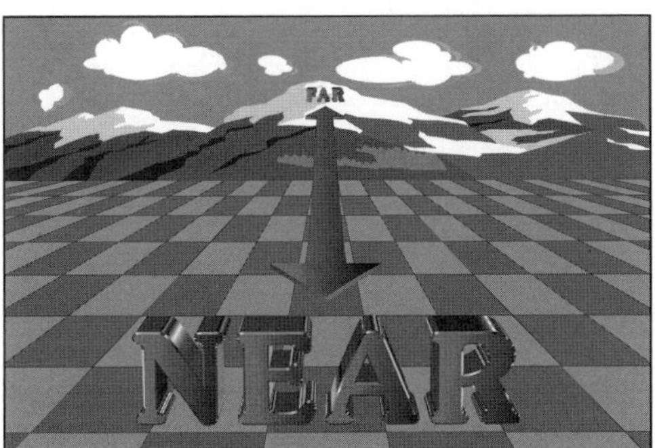

It is mainly our *interest* that moves from far to near and back. There is no "picture" out in the world—only light rays enter our eyes. The picture we see occurs primarily in the mind. The eye sees, and the mind perceives.

EXPERIENCE THE NEAR-TO-FAR/FAR-TO-NEAR SWING

Sit in a comfortable chair with your arms propped on a table or cushion.

Close your eyelids and pretend you are sitting in a cozy chair on a nice, sunny, island beach. You are holding a rope in your hands, which extends out over the sea to another island.

Brush the rope at your hands in a figure-8 pattern. Feel the texture of the rope with your nose-feather. Breathe abdominally. The neck is very soft and mobile.

Take a breath in. While exhaling, begin to sweep out along the rope: five feet, ten feet, twenty feet, feeling the rope with your nose-feather as you slide out over the sea. Continue to sweep out along the rope over the sea: 100 feet, 500 feet, 1000 feet, a mile, until finally you reach the end of the rope, where it is tied to a palm tree on a neighboring island.

You have just completed the Near-to-Far Swing!

Now, slide back along the rope over the sea: back to 1000 feet, 500 feet, 100 feet, and slowly back to twenty feet, ten feet, five feet, finally reaching the rope in your hands once again. Brushing the rope at your hands, you have just completed the Far-to-Near Swing!

Continue this swing along the rope from near to far, far to near, at your own pace for a few minutes. The neck is released and you are breathing abdominally.

This swing can also be practiced with the eyelids open and blinking frequently. Simply pretend you are holding a colorful yarn in your hands, and the other end is attached to the other side of the room you are in. Swing from near-to-far and back in the same manner.

One of my students had about 20/40 sight when he started the vision classes. In the third week he had a dream in which he was sitting on the side of a hill observing a waterfall on the other side of the valley. He could see the waterfall with 20/40 sight. As he was listening to the sound of water, he thought to himself that if he could *hear* the sound of the water clearly, he should obviously be able to *see* the water clearly. At that moment in the dream, his vision became clear, and he could see the waterfall with perfect clarity!

In the above Near-to-Far/Far-to-Near Swing, be sure to stop if you feel any discomfort or fatigue. Always associate better vision with pleasure, and not discomfort and pain.

Integration of movements from near-to-far and far-to-near throughout the day is the purpose of the near-to-far/far-to-near story above.

For example, when walking down the street, you can brush or sketch flowers along the path. Then, you can sweep out to the distant trees. When driving, you can shift from near cars or road signs to distant cars or road signs.

Nearsights have better vision habits when doing activities up close. They tend to stare and strain when their attention is in the distance. Nearsights are learning to have better vision habits when seeing objects in the distance.

Conversely, farsights have better vision habits when regarding objects in the distance. They tend to stare and strain when their attention is up close. Farsights are learning to have better vision habits more with close objects.

As we shall discuss later in Chapter 19, "Brains and Vision," seeing clearly up close is one of the functions of the left hemisphere. Seeing clearly in the distance is one of the functions of the right hemisphere. So, in one respect, seeing clearly near and far re-establishes a balance between the two hemispheres.

MOTION SICKNESS AND DIZZINESS? MOVE!

Bates discovered that one cause of "motion sickness" and dizziness is the unnatural strain and effort to try to stop objects from moving. A person in a rocking boat who gets "seasick" oftentimes is trying to stop the horizon from tilting. Trying to do the impossible is stressful(!), and when applied to the visual system, interferes with normal eyesight.

Similarly, some people get uncomfortable when attempting to read while in a moving car or train; they are straining to keep the words in the book stationary. People who are uncomfortable with movement need *movement*. The attitude that movement is not only OK, but essential and healthy, needs to replace the mainly subconscious desire to freeze moving objects. The person with blurred vision wants to become comfortable with natural movements.

Several of my students have commented on how uncomfortable the Long Swing is when we first do it in the class. This is due to many years of staring. The mind and body have become accustomed to non-movement.

In vision classes, these students sometimes react, temporarily, to what would normally be experienced as enjoyable movements. This discomfort diminishes as the student relearns natural, healthy movements all day long.

Better Eyesight magazine, December 1922:

> One student came to me complaining that never in her life had she been able to ride in an elevator without becoming very ill. Her vision for the distance was normal and she was able to read fine print without trouble. I at once took a ride with her in the house elevator and told her to look at a bell which was stationary in the elevator and to pay no attention to the floors which appeared to be moving opposite to the movement of the elevator. We rode up and down and had a good time because when she did not strain to see the moving floors she was just as comfortable and happy as she was when she did not ride in the elevator.

(In the 1920s, many elevators had iron gates, which you could "see through.")

Bates rode with the student up the elevator, and she acquired a headache during the ride. Bates then told her to notice the buttons inside the elevator on the ride down. The headache vanished on the way down. Bates explained to her that the reason for her headache was that she was mentally trying to keep the floors of the building from moving downward (the illusion of oppositional movement) when she was going up in the elevator. When she had her attention on the buttons inside the elevator on the way down, she was not trying to keep the floors from moving, and therefore the strain was relieved.

Better Eyesight magazine, December 1925: Bates relates the elevator story again:

> DIZZINESS
>
> Dizziness is caused by eyestrain...Usually the dizziness is produced unconsciously. It can be produced consciously, however, by staring or straining to see some distant or near object. Some persons while riding in an elevator are always dizzy, and suffer from attacks of imperfect sight, nausea and other nervous discomforts. An old lady, age 60, told me that riding in an elevator always made her dizzy, and produced headaches, with pain in her eyes. I tested her vision and found it to be normal both for distance and for reading without glasses. To obtain some facts, I rode in an elevator with her from the top to the bottom of the building and back again. I watched her eyes closely and found that she was staring at the floors [seen through the iron gate] which appeared to moving opposite to the movement of the elevator. I asked her the question, "Why do you stare at the floors which appear to be moving by?" She answered, "I do not like to see them move, and I am trying to correct the illusion by making an effort to keep them stationary. The harder I try, the worse I feel." I suggested to her that she look at one part of the elevator and avoid looking at the floors. Her discomfort was at once relieved....

MOVEMENT—THE PHYSICAL CONNECTIONS

When a person becomes rigid by staring, not only do the eye muscles contract tight, but many head, neck, and shoulder muscles become chronically tight. Many people have enrolled for my classes as soon as I mention the neck is tight for all people who have blurred vision. They know, experientially, the truth of this statement.

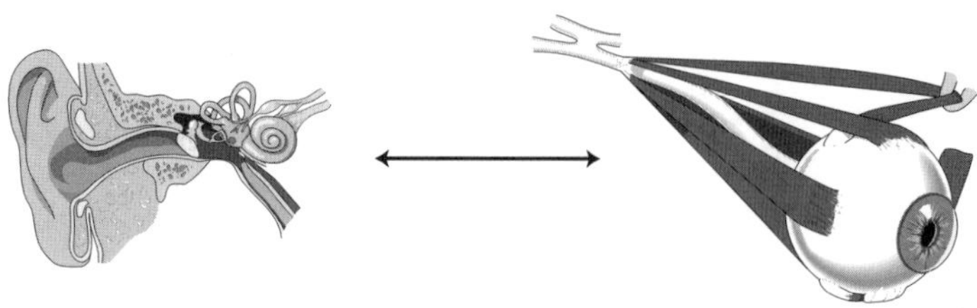

Figure 9–7: The Vestibulo-Ocular Connection.

The Vestibulo-Ocular Connection

The three semi-circular canals in the ear register movement along ciliary hairs to orient us in 3–D space. The lack of head movement, i.e., staring, slows down the normal functioning of the vestibulo-ocular system.

The Human Body states:

> Most complex of all eye movements is the vestibulo-ocular system; it works to keep the image of an object on the high-definition fovea while the head and body are moving. This action is assisted by the vestibular apparatus in the inner ear, which provides the brain with a continuous flow of information about the way in which the head is moving.[7]

Non-Movement Creates Tension

Tom's Personal Log: Last year I ruptured my Achilles tendon playing racquetball. My leg was in many casts for several months. When the last cast was removed, I was surprised to discover how *tight* and *tense* many of the muscles were in my foot and leg. Many months of physical therapy were needed to bring back normal flexibility to these muscles.

Non-movement made my eye and neck muscles chronically tight.

Light Receptors Need Change

The light receptors in the retina are not designed to be stimulated continuously by the same color and intensity of light.

Several books on vision describe how an "after-image" can be created by *staring* at an image for a long period of time and then looking away toward a blank white wall or paper.

An American flag, with its colors reversed, is often used as an example. After a person locks the eyes on the flag for a long enough period, the true colors—red, white, and blue-of the flag are seen by moving to a white background. (Illustration of flag to practice staring not provided!)

Another type of after-image is experienced when a bright light is observed, like the flash of a camera. If the eyelids are closed immediately after the flash, a small glowing after-image of the light can be observed.

In her fascinating and beautiful book, *How Animals See,* Sandra Sinclair discusses how important movement is to vision:

> The first eyes could detect only light and dark. The next step in evolution was an eye that could also detect movement. In fact, movement is of major importance to all eyes. The human eye cannot focus on any

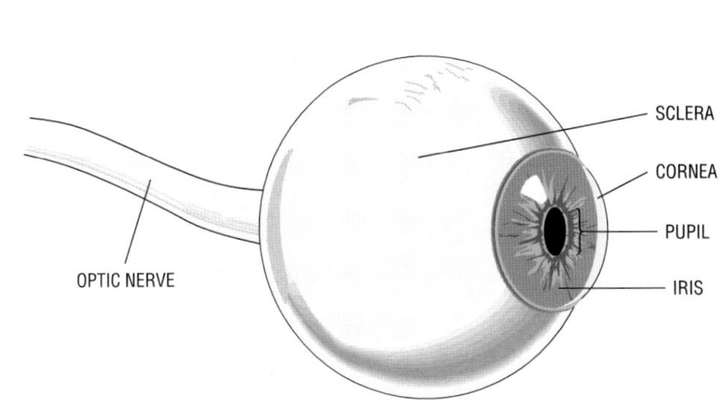

Plate 1. The Eye.

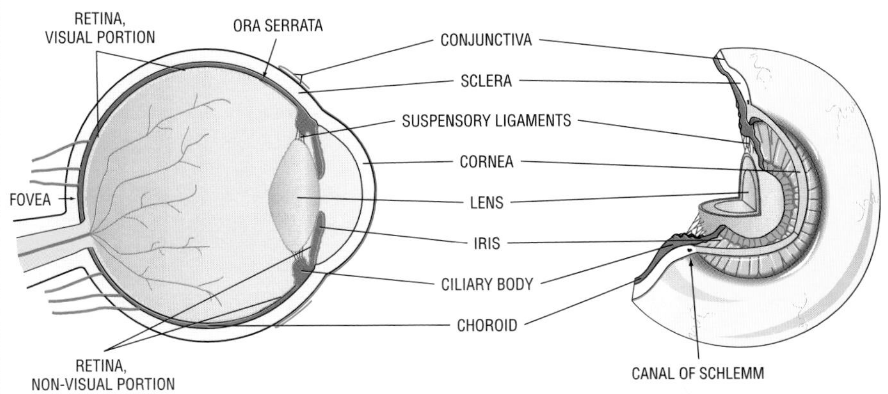

Plate 2. The Three Layers of the Eye.

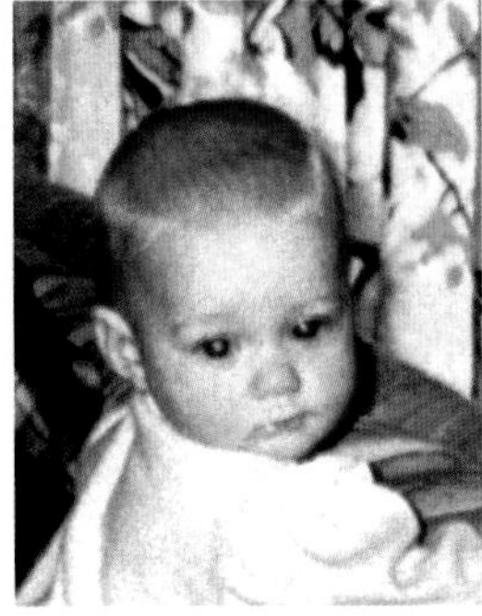

Plate 3. Suzie Q's Red Eyes.

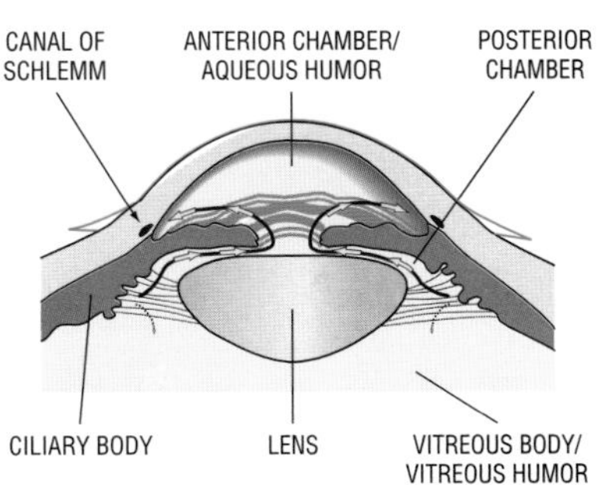

Plate 4. Aqueous Humor.

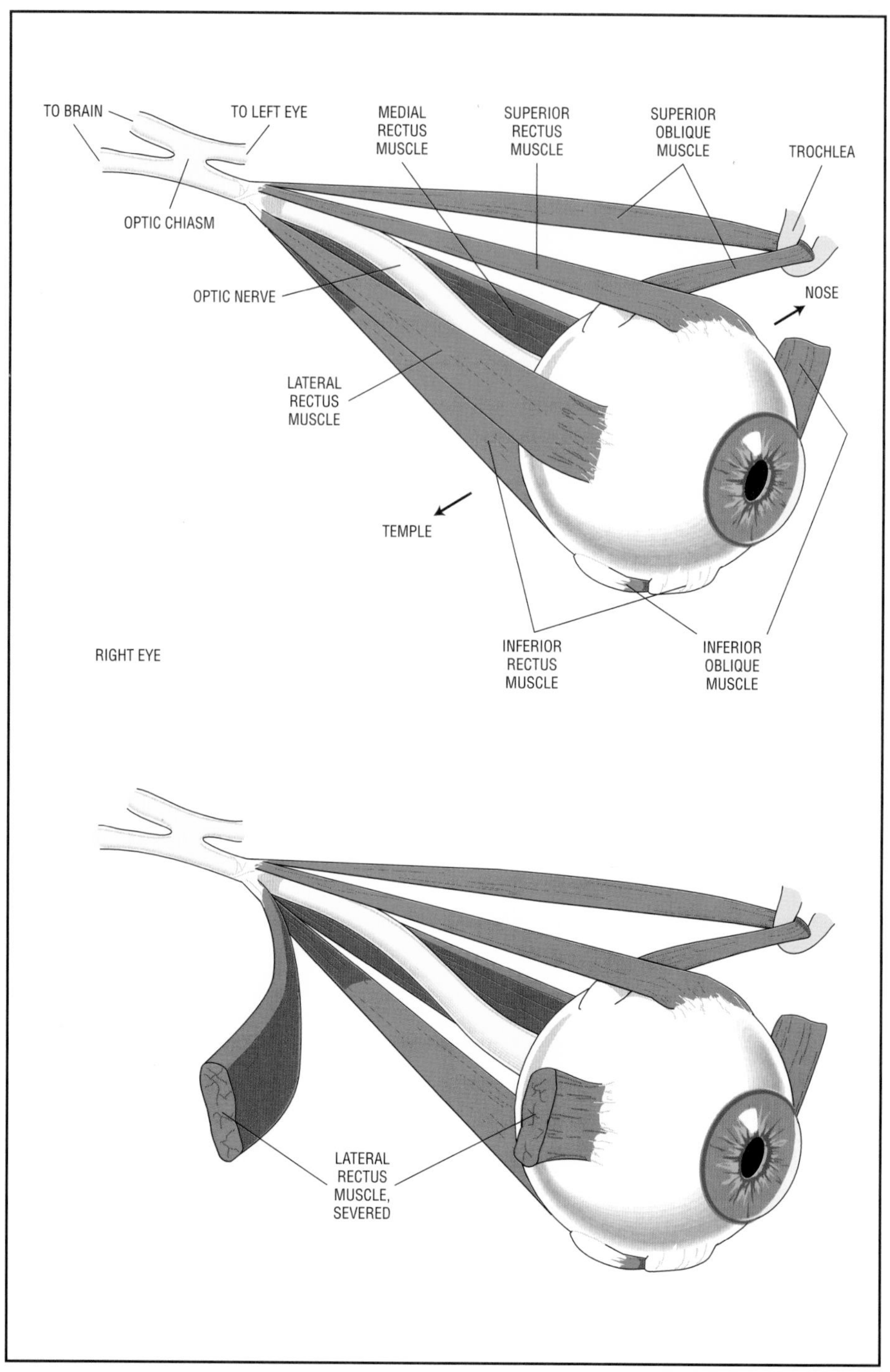

Plate 5. The Six External Eye Muscles.

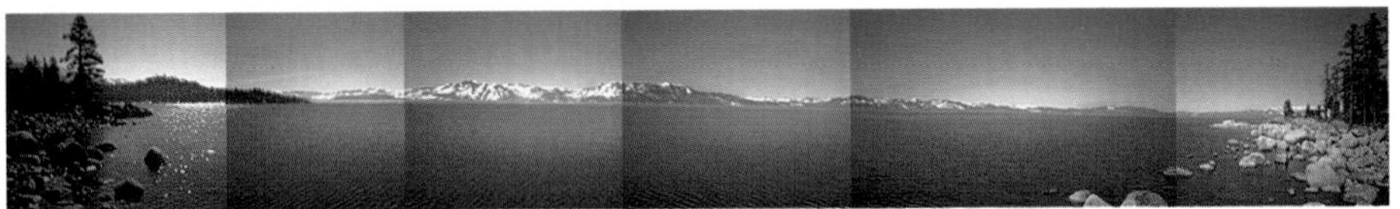

Plate 6. Long Swing Lake.

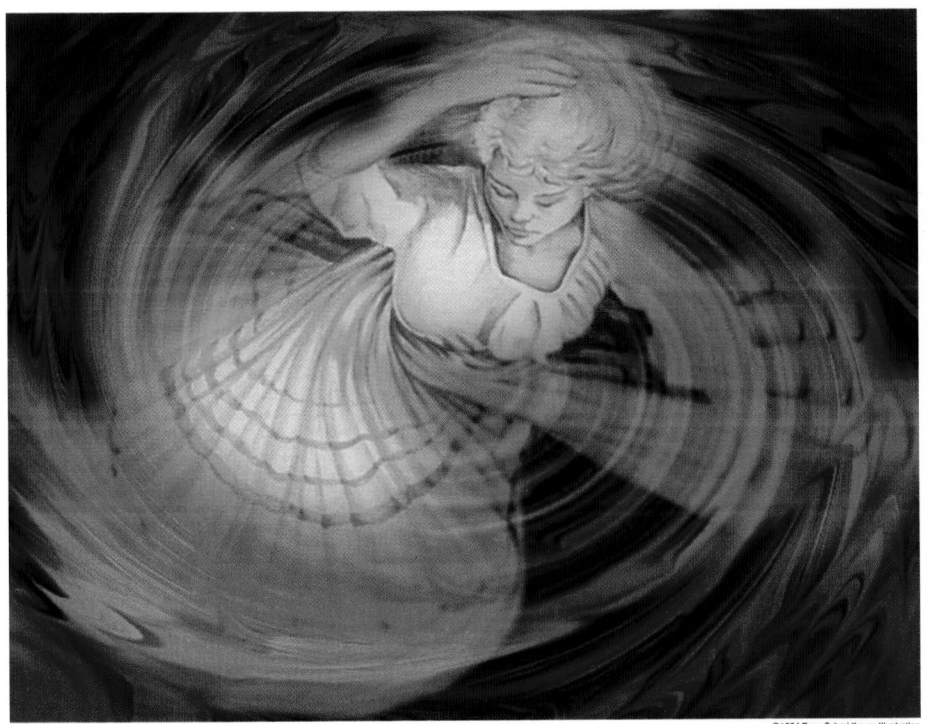

Plate 7. "Dancer."

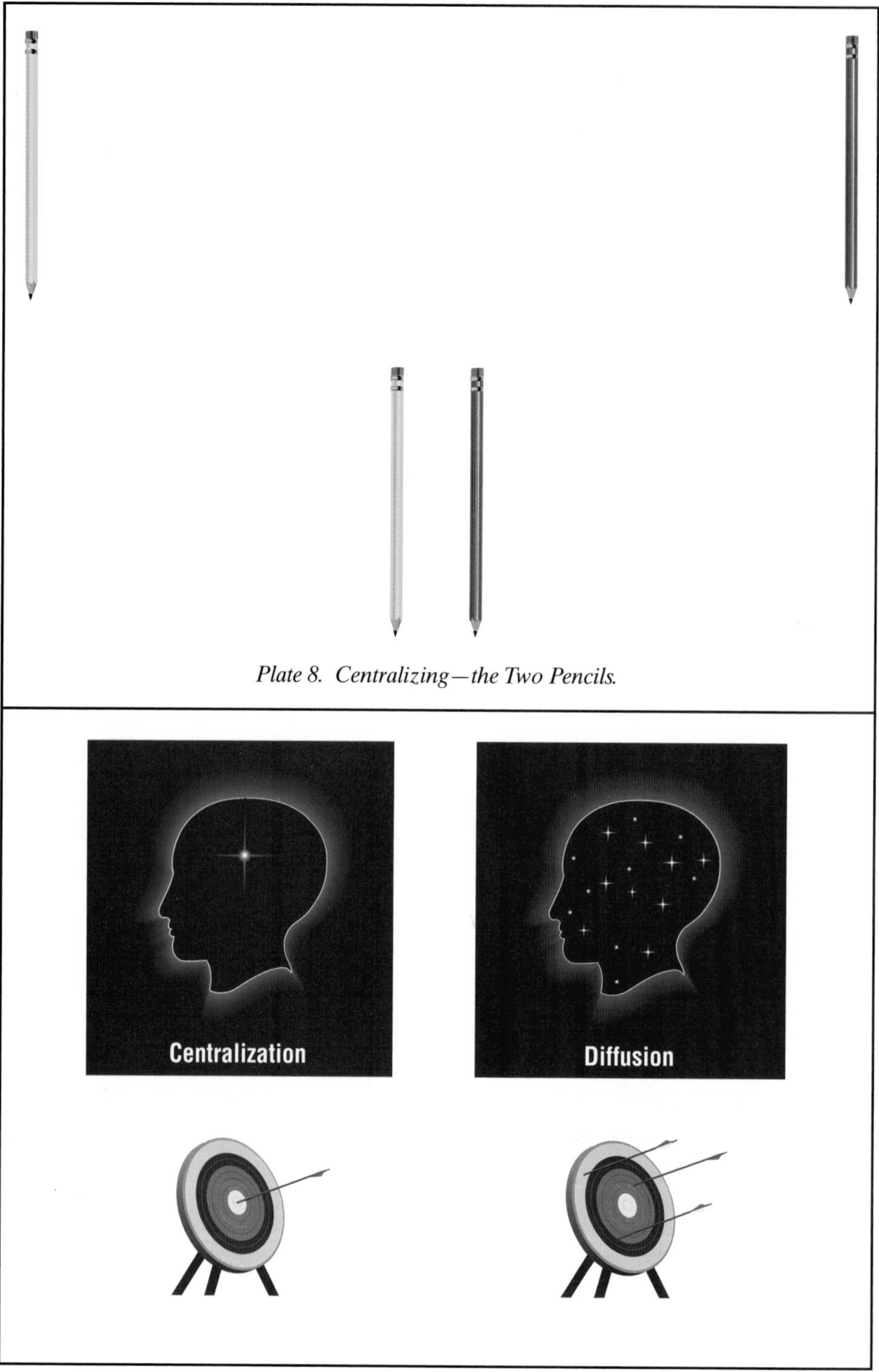

Plate 8. Centralizing—the Two Pencils.

Plate 9. Centralization vs. Diffusion.

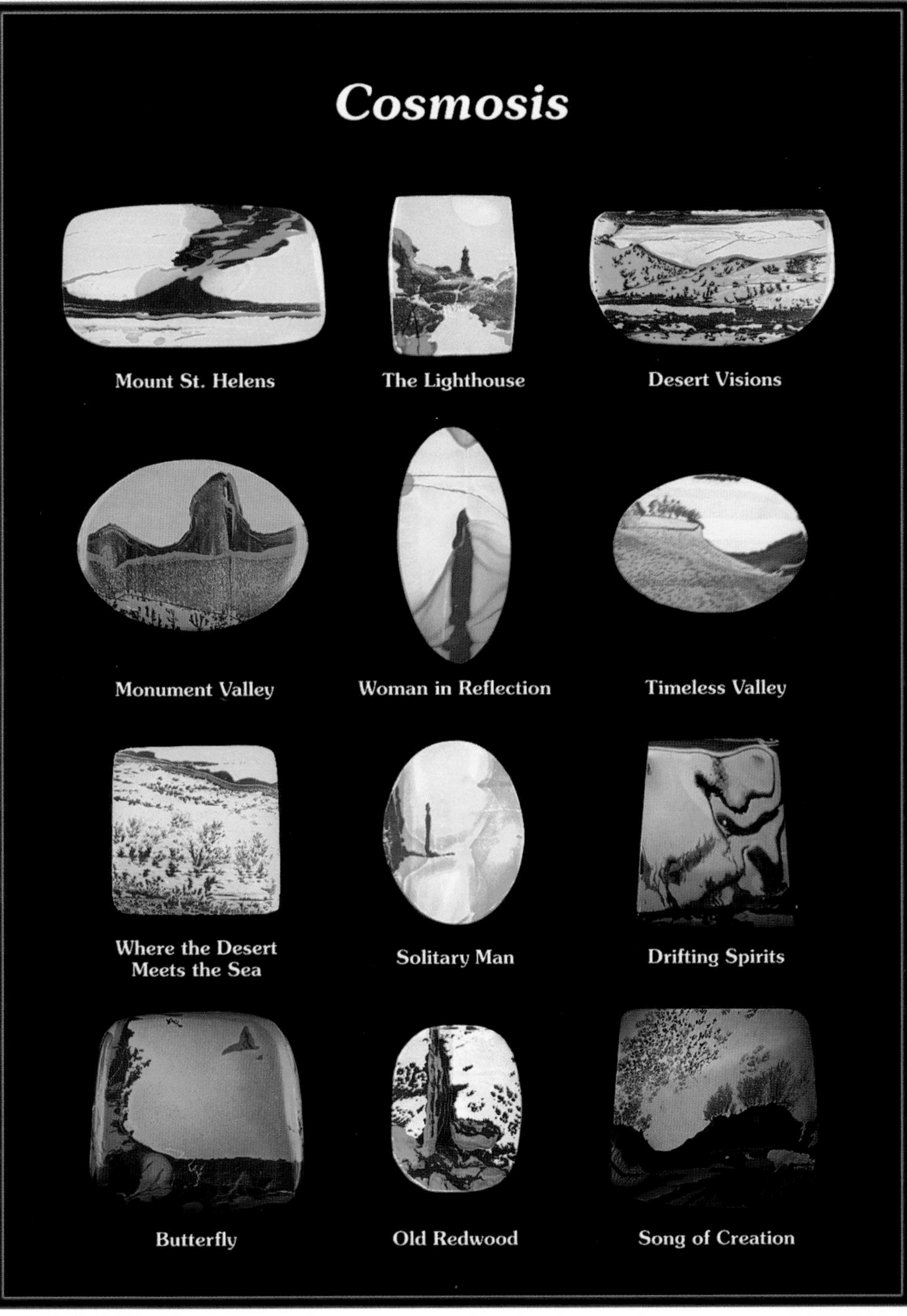

Plate 10. Cosmosis.

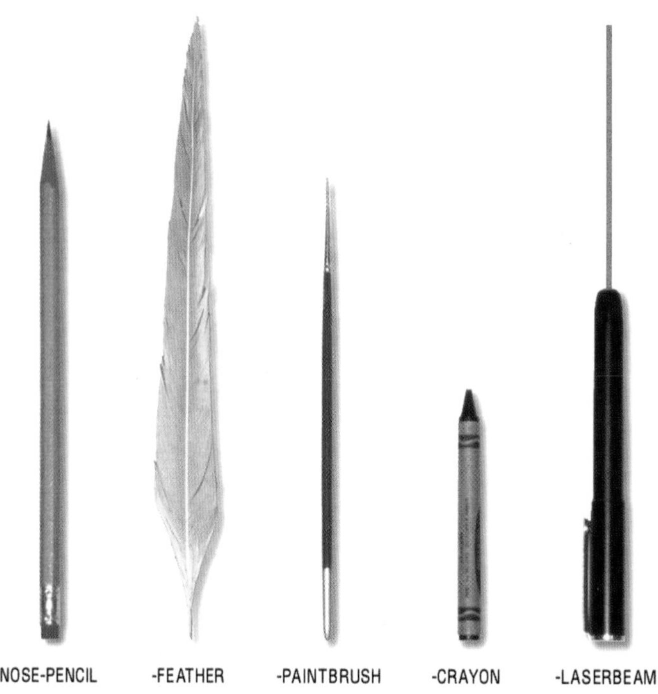

Plate 11. The Nose-Helpers.

Plate 12. The Edge.

INHALATION

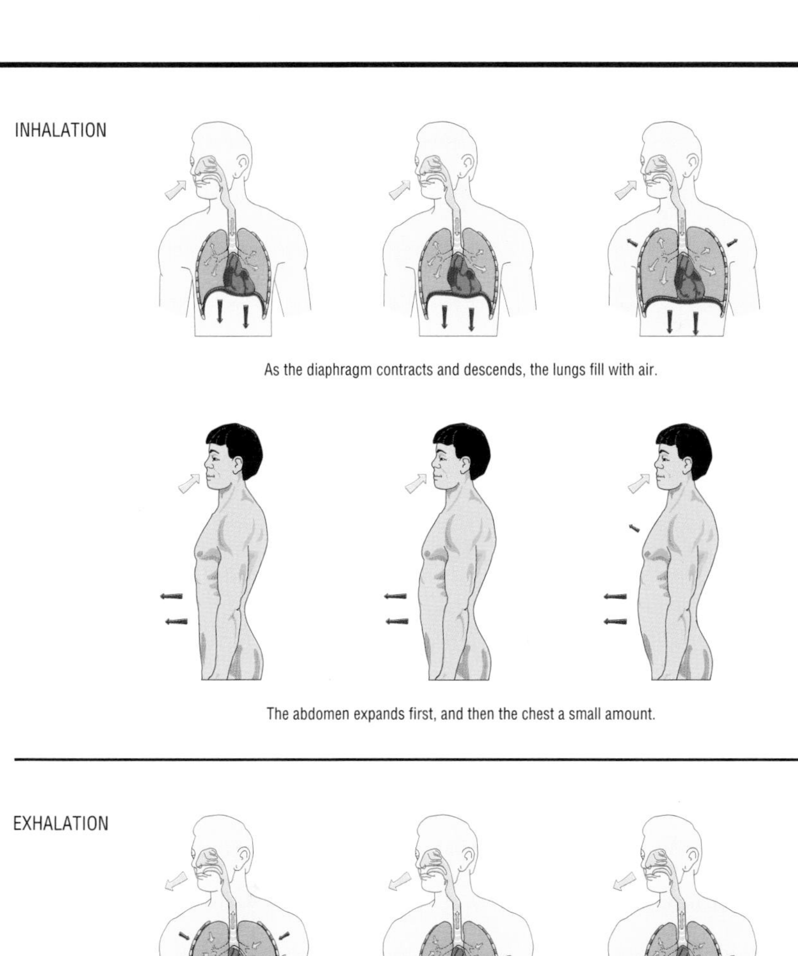

As the diaphragm contracts and descends, the lungs fill with air.

The abdomen expands first, and then the chest a small amount.

EXHALATION

As the diaphragm relaxes and rises, the lungs empty.

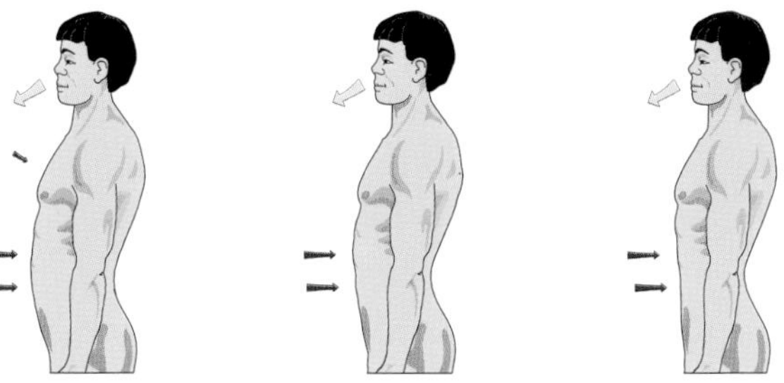

The chest contracts first, and then the abdomen.

Plate 13. Abdominal Breathing.

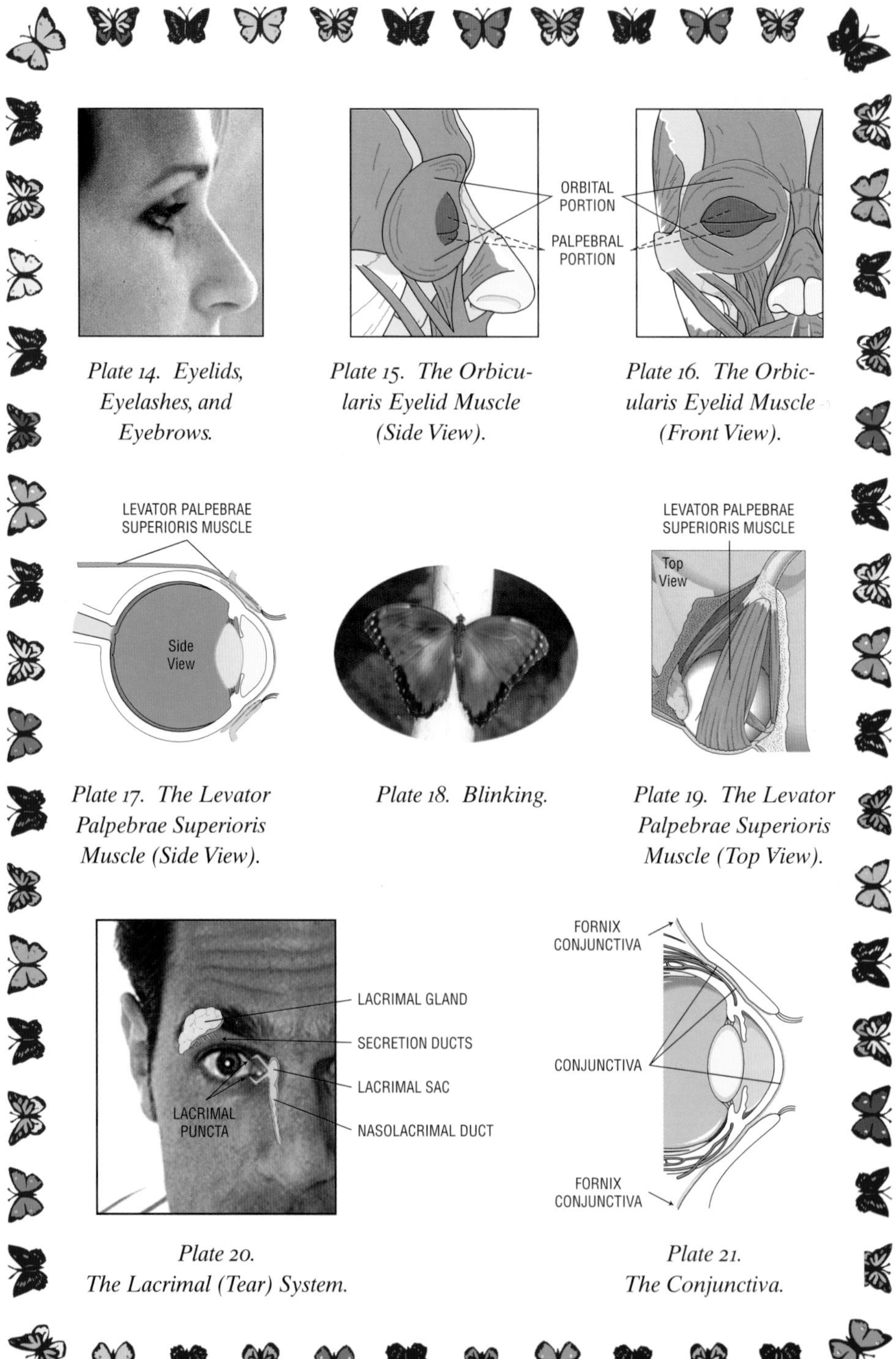

Plate 14. Eyelids, Eyelashes, and Eyebrows.

Plate 15. The Orbicularis Eyelid Muscle (Side View).

Plate 16. The Orbicularis Eyelid Muscle (Front View).

Plate 17. The Levator Palpebrae Superioris Muscle (Side View).

Plate 18. Blinking.

Plate 19. The Levator Palpebrae Superioris Muscle (Top View).

Plate 20. The Lacrimal (Tear) System.

Plate 21. The Conjunctiva.

image for longer than two to three seconds without the image fading. The image must move on the retina or it will disappear. The human eye jumps every three-tenths to five-tenths of a second in an involuntary tremor that nature seems to have designed to keep our eyes in motion. Although birds cannot move their eyes, they are constantly moving their heads...Moreover, if an object moves, the insect is able to see it even more clearly.[8]

R. L. Gregory writes:

> A simple way of optically stabilizing the retinal image. [Referring to an illustration of device not shown here.] The object (a small photographic transparency) is carried on the eye on a contact lens, and moved exactly with it. After a few seconds the eye becomes blind to the stabilised image, some parts fading before others.[9]

Mike Samuels, M.D., and Nancy Samuels write:

> Psychologists have found that if a person's gaze becomes absolutely fixed while looking at an object, the image of the object will extinguish within seconds. Most people are unfamiliar with this phenomenon because in the course of normal seeing they unconsciously move their eyes continuously. Studies have shown that people move their eyes in small, jerky scanning movements even when they are looking at an object that is not moving. If a person fixes his gaze on a mental image, it likewise tends to disappear. Whereas if a person scans a mental image as if it were a perception, he will find the image tends to be clearer and more stable....[10]

Researchers have independently confirmed Bates' discoveries about vision.

The light receptors in our eyes function best by variation in light rays, e.g. different intensities: bright, medium, and dark; and different frequencies (colors). *If the image we are viewing is not changing, e.g., a stationary chair, the only way the rods and cones can have the variations they need to function normally is if the person (or eye) moves.*

The visual system cannot tolerate the experience of stationary objects appearing to be stationary for more than a second or two. Continual movement is necessary for normal, clear vision.

T. Ribot, considered the "Father" of the new psychological era of experimental research, wrote in *The Psychology of Attention:*

> If we keep one of our eyes fixed upon any single point, after a while our vision becomes confused; a cloud is formed between the object and ourselves, and finally we see nothing at all. If we lay our hand flat upon a table, motionless, and without pressure (for pressure itself is a movement), by slow degrees the sensation wears off and finally disappears. The reason is, that there is no perception without movement, be it ever so weak. Every sensorial organ is at the same time both sensitive and motor. As soon as absolute immobility eliminates one of the two elements (motility), the functions of the other after a while is rendered null. In a word, movement is the condition of the change which is one of the conditions of consciousness. These well-known facts, of common experience, make us understand the necessity of these intermissions in attention, often imperceptible to consciousness, because they are very brief, and of a very delicate order....[11]
>
> As regards perceptions, there are no difficulties. All our organs of perception are at the same time sensorial and motor. To per-

> ceive with our eyes, ears, hands, feet, tongue, nostrils, movements are needed. The more mobile the parts of our body, the more exquisite is their sensibility; the less perfect their motile power, the more obtuse their sensibility. Nor is this all; without motor movements, perception is impossible. We will call to mind a previous statement that if the eye be kept fixed upon a given object without moving, perception after a while grows dim, and then disappears. Rest the tips of the fingers upon a table without pressing, and the contact at the end of a few minutes will no longer be felt. But a motion of the eye, or of the finger, be it ever so light, will re-arouse perception. Consciousness is only possible through change: change is not possible save through movement. It would be easy to expatiate at great length upon this subject; for although the facts are very manifest and of common experience, psychology has nevertheless so neglected the role sustained by movements that it actually forgot at least that they are the fundamental condition of cognition in that they are the instrument of the fundamental law of consciousness, which is, relatively, change. Enough has now been said to warrant the unconditional statement that where there is no movement, there is no perception.[12]

The irony of trying to lock-on and freeze objects is that you lose them. The fact is: *only when we are* moving *do we see best.*

An interesting consequence of normal sight being dependent on constant movement is the validity of conventional approaches to studying and measuring eyesight. Many conclusions drawn by researchers on, and measurements of, eyesight are based on the subject's head being held still—sometimes for long periods of time. When eyesight is checked or measured, the subject's head is often locked rigidly in a machine.

Many Types of Natural Eye Movements

The six external muscles keep the eyeball in constant movement. Various types of eye movements include high-frequency tremors, optical drift, microscopic twitches, saccadic vibrations, and, of course, larger eye movements for seeing different objects. Even during sleep the eyes have REMs, or "Rapid Eye Movements."

The Human Body states:

> ...These involuntary movements...make sure that the image constantly moves over fresh parts of the retina. As a result, the receptors at any spot do not get overloaded with input and effective vision is maintained.[13]

Eye movements also aid in circulation of fluids in and around the eyes.

Posture: The Eyesight Con-neck-tion

The neck is a key part of the body for vision. The neck is the pathway of nerve message between the head and the rest of the body. The second cervical vertebra (2C) is especially related to the visual system.

Cerebral spinal fluid travels from the head, through the neck, and up and down the spinal column. A tight neck interferes with this important flow.

The same incorrect vision habits that tense the eye muscles tense the neck muscles. Many students tell me they see better after chiropractic or osteopathic adjustments, massage therapy, or various forms of bodywork that release the neck muscles.

The neck cannot completely release its tension until the staring habit is eliminated.

Recently, after only one lesson, a student

told me her neck had released so much, she could turn it fully to the right and left. She was told by one authority that she would never have a full range of movement in her neck.

Tip: Use a shower head which "pulses" and gives your neck and shoulders a mini-massage.

The middle of the back of the neck is tight for many nearsights. The two back sides of the neck are tight for many farsights. A bifocal wearer has an especially tense "bifocal neck" and shoulders.

Do not tilt your head as a habit. This imbalance creates strain on the neck and whole body. It also makes the practice of normal head movements difficult.

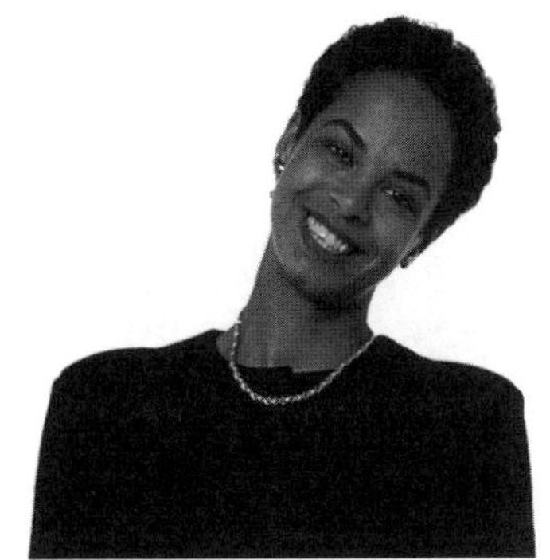

Figure 9–9: Head Tilt.

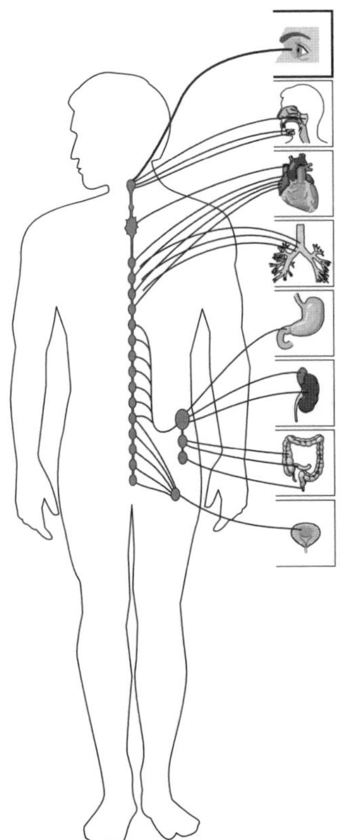

Figure 9–8: The Eyesight Con-neck-tion.

Telephones and Posture

If you use a telephone a large part of the day, a headset can relieve a lot of tension in the neck caused by tilting the head against the phone.

People with perfect sight who talk on a telephone constantly shift their visual attention, subconsciously, from one object to another, while their conscious attention is involved in the conversation.

People with blur stare "unseeingly," without moving. Subconsciously, their attention is not interested in their surroundings.

June Biermann and Barbara Toohey write in their book *The Woman's Holistic Headache Relief Book:*

> Are you a frequent telephone user and, if so, how do you hold the phone? One executive talked on the telephone most of his working day and had the habit of holding the telephone receiver between his left ear and his left shoulder. He developed a chronic headache on the left side of his head. His problem was solved by purchasing a telephone microphone....[14]

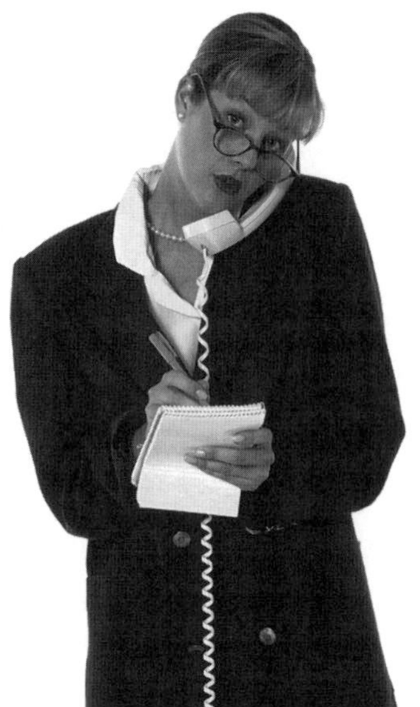

INCORRECT

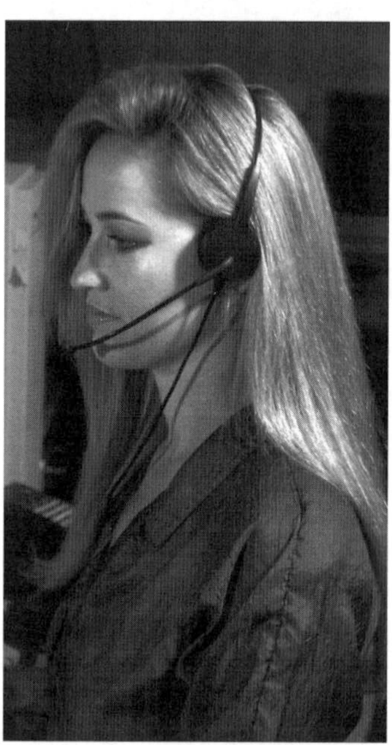

CORRECT

Figure 9–10: Use a Headset.

Chairs

Many Americans have desk jobs. Most chairs are not designed to support correct posture. Use a chair that is comfortable but also supports correct posture.

Posture During Sleep

Better Eyesight magazine, February 1923:

> Posture during sleep has been studied. Lying on the face has generally been accompanied by an increase of eye strain. Sleeping on the back with the arms and limbs extended with slight flexion is undoubtedly better than sleeping on the right or left side. A cramped [fetal] posture is always wrong. The person is not always conscious of his posture when asleep. In a number of cases observed by friends…one or both arms were held behind the head while asleep and strenuously denied by the person when awake.
>
> The correction of this and other strained positions of the arms and limbs has been followed by decided benefit to vision.

Biermann and Toohey write further:

> Do you always sleep on your stomach? If so, your head is turned to one side and one [neck] muscle is shortened. This stiffens the muscle to an extreme, especially if you sleep a regular eight hours nightly. The solution is to train yourself to sleep on your side or on your back.[15]

Don't lock your neck hard as stone! Move your head all day long—even while thinking!

Aldous Huxley writes:

> In myopes especially, posture tends to be extremely bad. This may be directly due in some cases to short sight, which encourages stooping and a hanging of the head.

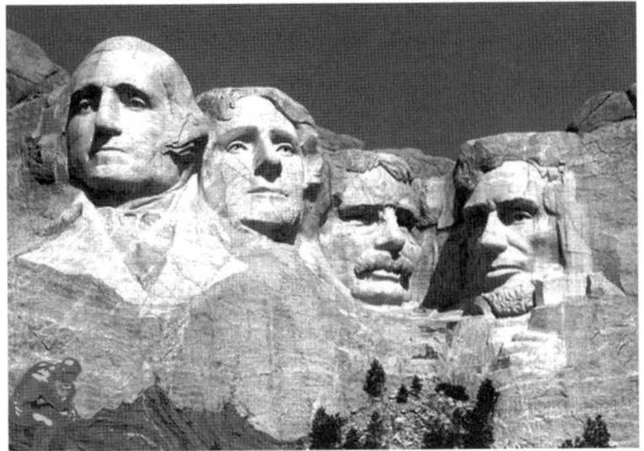

Figure 9–11: Don't Lock Your Neck...

> Conversely, the myopia may be due in part at least to the bad posture. F. M. Alexander records cases in which myopic children regained normal vision after being taught the proper way of carrying the head and neck in relation to the trunk.
>
> In adults, the correction of improper posture does not seem to be sufficient of itself to restore normal vision. Improvement in vision will be accelerated by those who learn to correct faulty habits....[16]

Note again that vision improvement is not about "eye exercises." Natural vision improvement involves the relearning of correct vision habits all day long.

Tom's Personal Log: When I began riding a motorcycle, I found the engine noise very annoying. I discovered I could lower this noise by swallowing hard and frequently. This tightened my neck and eardrums, and lowered the engine noise. I lost much of my high-frequency hearing ability by learning to do this.

It was also difficult to hold my head against the wind. So, I learned that by bending my body forward and angling my head upward I could take a lot of the pressure of the wind off of my head.

When I began improving my vision I became aware that while walking, I was seeing straight ahead, but my head was pulled upward and my eyes were looking downward relative to my head.

During my second visit to my chiropractor, I was shown an x-ray of how my neck and spinal column were severely out of alignment. The upper part of my body was curved, falling forward. My head was pulled upward and backward, creating a very large, unnatural angle in the vertebrae of my neck. I had severe, chronic headaches and neck tension for many years.

I asked her how long it would take to bring these distortions back to their normal positions. She said it would take about ten years. I think she was trying to be nice by not telling me it might take twenty or thirty years.

My high-frequency hearing is gradually returning to normal.

The tremendous strain in my neck is one of the factors in my vision improvement process taking much longer than for most students.

MOVEMENT—THE MENTAL/EMOTIONAL CONNECTIONS

St. Jerome wrote, "Eyes without speaking confess the secrets of the heart."

While physical movement is important for normal vision, "mental movement" is even more important. The natural interest and curiosity of children teaches us about seeing naturally.

A child first thinks about, or imagines, what he wants to do—in his mind—and then his body follows through with physical action. A girl who wants to play on the swings at the playground first *desires* to swing, and then she *moves* physically to the swing. A boy first *wants* to ride the bicycle, and then proceeds to ride down the street.

On one of the local cable TV channels,

there is a station called *The Discovery Channel.* Interest, curiosity, discovery, and exploration are key concepts for clear vision. They are natural and normal. These attitudes of natural seeing occur mostly subconsciously.

Ellen Raskin wrote a charming little booklet entitled *Nothing Ever Happens On My Block*[17]*;* it is all about interest and discovery. (This book is listed in the Bibliography.)

The average person who has lost a great deal of sight no longer looks around. He has a fixed stare.

So, instead of "checking out," "check it out!" Look around, with a head motion, in order to see. Point your nose at what you want to see. *Relearn* interest and curiosity!

Paul E. Dennison states, "The eyes must move in order to really see. Whole body movement aids the ability to internalize awareness and memory of objects in space."[18]

The issues involved in oppositional movement occur mainly in the mind. Some students find it difficult in the beginning stages of their vision improvement to allow stationary objects to move. The habit of rigid staring has become ingrained.

Oftentimes students remember a particularly stressful period of their life when they decided to "try" to stop objects from moving. This can occur for a child during a period of emotional stress (e.g. divorce, moving to another city, childhood abuse). The person who learned to stare often has issues of "trying to hold on tight." "If I try hard enough to keep everything from moving, then maybe the situation will not get worse." Fear is often a factor, especially for nearsights.

One of my students told me she could see clearly at all distances—except at 100 feet. Closer than 100 feet her sight was clear, and beyond 100 feet her sight was clear.

Initially, this was puzzling to me. For someone who has blur in the distance, usually everything from twenty feet out to infinity is not clear. This must have meant she was straining her sight with poor vision habits only at 100 feet. She told me that long ago, she had a very stressful experience with the events occurring at 100 feet.

TOM'S PERSONAL LOG: In the first grade I had excellent eyesight while attending playful Walt Disney Elementary School in Anaheim, California.

In the third grade, I switched to a very strict parochial school, where I was informed that if I moved in the classroom when I was not supposed to, I could die and go to hell and burn forever. Not preferring that outcome, I quickly mastered staring.

One of the few entertainments my fellow classmates and I had found involving no movement in the classroom was to choke ourselves and see how close we could come to passing out, without passing out.

In the third grade, I got my first pair of glasses. Comparing pictures of me from Walt Disney Elementary School and the new ("Martyr") school showed a dramatic change in expression from one of happiness and playfulness to one of seriousness and fear.

A holistic practitioner told me that, in Chinese health philosophy, the emotion most associated with kidney stones is fear. In 1982, I was hospitalized with an excruciatingly painful attack of kidney stones.

(I would like to add at this point that I have the most loving and caring parents anyone could hope for.)

TOM'S PERSONAL LOG: For a long time I felt my nearsightedness was related, in some respects, to fear of other people. (I was voted "the most shy" in grade school.) I did not want other people to come too close to me.

One of my farsighted students shared with me that she felt her (close) blur was related to not wanting other people to come too close to her.

This is very interesting. Both of us had come to the same conclusion, even though the vision problems were opposite of each other!

THE PROBLEM IS STARING

Out of sight, out of mind.

—Proverb

Seldom seen, soon forgotten.

—Proverb

A fixed position implies we are standing still, that even the eye is still. Yet we all know that our eyes move constantly and the only time they stop moving is when we're dead—or when we are staring. And if we are staring, we're not really looking.

—David Hockney

From *Better Eyesight* magazine, June 1923:

> When a person has normal sight the eye is at rest, and when the eye is at rest, strange to say, it is always moving to avoid the stare.

Better Eyesight magazine, September 1927:

> Staring is a strain and always lowers the vision.

Better Eyesight magazine, May 1928:

> THE STARE
>
> ...When a person stares, an effort is always made to hold the eyes still without moving them. It is impossible to hold the eyes perfectly still. Trying to do the impossible always requires a strain. This strain can be demonstrated to be a mental strain which affects all the nerves of the body as well as the eye. With a mental strain, the memory and imagination become imperfect and imperfect sight results. Pain, fatigue or dizziness are acquired or made worse. With relaxation of all the nerves, the sense of touch is improved, but with the stare or other efforts to see the sense of touch is lost while the sense of pain is increased...There are some people who have been using the stare to improve their vision for a sufficient length of time to acquire the habit without being conscious that an effort is being made.

Staring is defined as not moving the eyes, head, *and* interest (with centralizing) for more than a second or two. A person must also be blinking and breathing normally.

Why Do People Stare?

Since staring is one of the main causes of poor eyesight, it is valuable to explore some of the causes of staring. Staring can easily occur during periods of fatigue, boredom, worry, fear, injury, and pain.

Our society has become so fast-paced and complex that many people have forgotten about relaxation, and how to relax. "Time is money."

Mark Clements writes in his article "Sex in America Today" in *Parade Magazine:*

> "The population has gotten older, and people have gotten busier," notes Shirley Zussman. "Men and women today work harder than any other generation I've known. They're tired all the time...."[19]

The point is—many people, especially in industrialized countries, burn themselves out, and then due to fatigue, they stare.

Worrying is another common cause of staring. The person is not interested in the surrounding environment. He locks the neck and diffuses. I have mentioned issues of fear above.

Accidents and illnesses can cause a person to stare. As long as the person stops the staring after the excess stress, the vision can return to normal. But, if the staring becomes a habit, vision will lower. Also, if glasses are put on a person during the stress period and staring, the glasses will likely lower the vision and reinforce the strained vision habits.

How much of "Attention Deficit Disorder" (ADD) is caused by staring?

How many children are forced to do activities that bore them, especially in school? How many become "bored stiff?"

The Staring Trap

One of the problems with staring is that most individuals do not *know* they are staring while staring. They are "gone" or "spaced out." The mind is usually out of present time.

While staring, a person will not usually be aware that the vision is lowering during that time because he is "spaced out." He is not usually aware of the state of his vision, and therefore does not realize that staring is harmful to sight. Students become well aware of this relationship very early in vision classes.

One of the most important objectives in vision re-education is to bring the issue of correct and incorrect vision habits to the conscious level. In this way, the student is given the opportunity to relearn the correct way of using the mind and body, and to escape the harm of staring and straining to see. With practice, the correct vision habits become subconscious and continuous once again.

You Get What You Think

On a deeper level, visually, a person is *getting* what they are thinking of, or should we say, *not* thinking of. A person is not interested in the visual world, so it becomes blurred. It doesn't really matter *what* the vision is during staring, does it?!—because the person is not really seeing during staring. There is no reason for the vision to be clear during staring, because the person is not interested in seeing. Since the person is not *visually* interested in the environment, the person is not really "seeing" in a normal, visually connected way. The fact that the vision is blurred, or even clear, becomes irrelevant during staring. As stated before, people with blurry vision often look "unseeingly."

Staring "sneaks in" when a person is *least looking*. It is not usually the case that some consciously decide to stare, except for the infamous children's "staring contest," where the goal is to not blink! Those with the strongest glasses usually win!

If you want to see, *see!* In other words, *never* stare. See actively all day long, but never with an effort. This is normal and natural.

Staring While Moving

Better Eyesight magazine, January 1924: "...one can stare by trying to see with the sides of the retina, [called] eccentric fixation."

It is possible to be moving yet still staring. This is the case if a person is diffusing while moving. This is still a form of staring, because the student is not centralizing. Centralization is discussed in Chapter 10; centralization is attention to detail.

A person can move the head but still be "spaced out." In order for someone to not be staring, both movement and centralization are needed.

Non-Movement

One of my students said that her friends did not like her to move when they were talking with her. She decided that she was not going to relearn the vision principle of movement—and her vision stopped improving. Her sister decided to relearn natural movement and had excellent improvement of her sight.

One of my students told me that her husband's movement used to bother her when she was speaking with him. She thought he was rude because he was not giving her as much attention as he could if he would remain still. She stood as still as possible when talking with him. She wore strong prescription glasses. He has normal sight.

Another of my students, who had very strong prescription glasses, told me that some clients would tell him at work that when he talked with them, he never moved anything except his mouth. His rigidity was so pronounced, complete strangers would mention it to him.

Better Eyesight magazine, September 1922:

> Many persons, when they are talking to you, feel it the proper thing to keep their eyes fixed continuously on your face, that is to say, to stare at you. Instead of moving their eyes from one eye to the other or from one side of the nose to the other, they stare at one eye continuously, which lowers the vision and may cause headaches or some other discomfort. It is well to get into the habit of imagining the faces of the people are moving from side to side.

Movement does not need to be large when conversing with another person. One of the best ways to practice small movements is to nose-feather your face in a mirror. Practice shifting your nose-feather with small, slow movements.

Peripheral Rods for Movement

Sandra Sinclair writes, "We aren't really aware of what happens on the periphery of our vision until a movement there causes us to focus on that spot."[20]

As will be discussed in subsequent chapters, the rod light receptors in the peripheral part of our retina are designed to pick up movement—and they do so much better than the cones. The physical, and even more so the mental, attempt to make objects still—called staring—interferes with the ability of the rods to perceive movement in the peripheral vision.

Other Notes on Movement and Staring

Staring—and Blurred Vision—is Epidemic

In 1976, 51% of the US population (111 million people) needed corrective lenses. By 1986, the percentage had risen to 56%. These numbers will be more and more underestimated as more people say they do not need corrective lenses after doing corneal surgeries or other corneal procedures.

This is a 0.5% increase per year over a ten-year period. These numbers do not include people who have blurred vision but refuse to, or cannot, wear corrective lenses. There are many such people.

If this rate of 1% increase every two years continues, theoretically nearly every US citizen will need corrective lenses by the year 2100!

Blur is epidemic in this society. Anyone who has blurred vision stares. Staring is based on strain. Blurred vision is a reflection of the high strain most people experience in this society.

So, relax and dance!

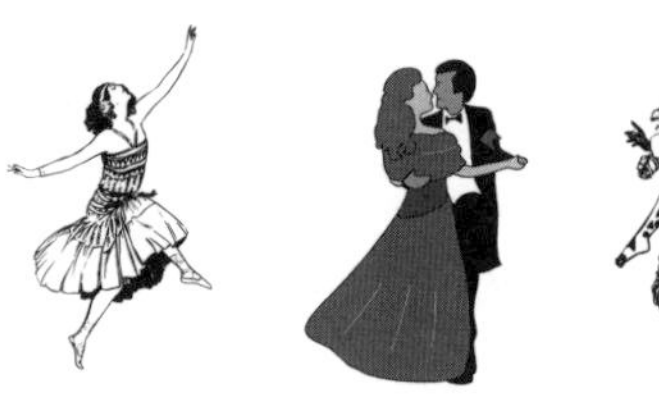

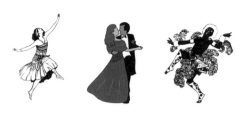

An 84-Year-Old Child

At my booth in a health fair in 1983, an elderly woman with a lot of spirit, interest, and positive energy came up to me and said, "What do you do here, sonny?" I said, "I teach students how to improve their vision by relearning relaxed vision habits." She said, "Very interesting. Do you know I have had perfect vision all of my life?" I answered, "No, but it would not surprise me." Then she said, "But you don't understand, sonny. I am 84 years old."

I think I do understand.

Then she left happily and energetically, moving her head and body with lots of curiosity down the aisle, exploring the other exhibits—like a six-year-old child.

This woman made a big impression on me. Bates taught all his students to see like children see, for their entire lifetime. "Unless ye become like children...."

Natural vision students want to become more accustomed to movement than they now are with staring and rigidity. They also want to become more accustomed to the illusion of oppositional movement than the experience of objects being fixed.

We had movement when we used to see clearly. Movement is not an exercise; it is the correct way of living naturally with the visual system, until 84 years old—at least!

If you relearn natural movements, you will never want to go back to staring. Staring is a manifestation of lowered health. No one is completely healthy—physically, emotionally, or mentally—who has blurred vision. If the reader is not interested relearning natural movements to improve her sight, I recommend relearning movement to improve her overall *health*.

THE SOLUTION IS MOVEMENT

See *Plate 7: "Dancer."*

The three key habits, discussed more in Part Four, "The Three Habits of Natural Vision," are all based on movements:

1. Sketching (shifting) includes both a physical movement of the head and eyes, but more importantly, a movement of the mind;
2. Breathing abdominally is a form of natural movement; and
3. Blinking is a natural movement of the eyelids.

In the next chapter we explore the one of the more subtle, mental principles of natural vision—centralization.

Notes

[1] T. Ribot, *The Psychology of Attention* (Chicago: The Open Court Publishing Company, 1890), p. 11.

[2] Aldous Huxley, *The Art of Seeing* (New York: Harper & Brothers, 1942), p. 37.

[3] Maurice Sendak, *Where the Wild Things Are* (New York: Harper & Row, 1963).

[4] Alexander Jones, *The Jerusalem Bible* (New York: Doubleday & Company, Inc., 1966), 1 Kings, Chapter 14, Verse 5, p. 439.

[5] The front sight is the one at the end of the barrel.

[6] John P. Frisby, *Seeing: Illusion, Brain and Mind* (Oxford: Oxford University Press, 1979), p. 141.

[7] John O. E. Clark, consultant editor, *The Human Body* (New York: Arch Cape Press, 1989), p. 258.

[8] Sandra Sinclair, *How Animals See* (New York: Facts on File Publications, 1985), p. xv.

[9] R. L. Gregory, *Eye and Brain: The Psychology of Seeing* (New York: McGraw-Hill Co., 1966), p. 46.

[10] Mike and Nancy Samuels, *Seeing with the Mind's Eye* (New York: Doubleday & Company, Inc., 1978), p. 59.

[11] Ribot, *The Psychology of Attention,* p. 11.

[12] Ibid., p. 46.

[13] Clark, *The Human Body,* p. 258.

[14] June Biermann and Barbara Toohey, *The Woman's Holistic Headache Relief Book* (Los Angeles: J. P. Tarcher, Inc., 1979), p. 47.

[15] Ibid.

[16] Huxley, *The Art of Seeing,* p. 273.

[17] Ellen Raskin, *Nothing Ever Happens On My Block* (New York: Macmillan Publishing Company, 1966).

[18] Paul E. Dennison, "Reading and Vision," *Brain Gym Magazine,* Vol. II, No. 3 (Fall, 1988), p. 1.

[19] Mark Clements, "Sex in America Today," *Parade Magazine* (August 7, 1994), pp. 5–6.

[20] Sinclair, *How Animals See,* p. 81.

CHAPTER TEN

The Second Principle—Centralization

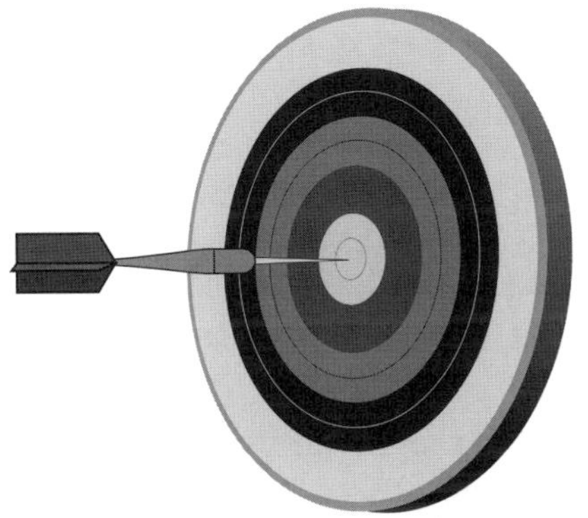

Shift your glance constantly from one point to another, seeing the part regarded best and other parts not so clearly. That is, when you look at a chair, do not try to see the whole object at once; look first at the back of it, seeing that part best and other parts worse.... shift your glance from the back to the seat and legs, seeing each part best, in turn. This is central[ization].[1]

—William H. Bates, M.D., *Better Eyesight,* September 1927

CENTRALIZATION

From *Perfect Sight Without Glasses:*

> It is impossible to see, remember, or imagine anything [clearly], even for as much as a second, without shifting from one part to another, or to some other object and back again; and the attempt to do so always produces strain.

Centralization is the second key principle of natural vision. The human eye can see only one point clearly at any moment. This is an anatomical fact. Since the point of clarity is only available in the center of the visual picture, it is impossible to see clearly without centralizing. The peripheral vision is never seen clearly. Several demonstrations of this fact are given below.

Centralization is the normal, natural, subconscious mental habit, or skill, of having one's primary visual attention, or interest, at one small, central point at any particular moment, and this central point of interest is the only place within the visual field that is clear and most colorful.

Better Eyesight magazine, December 1925 (Repeated from the previous chapter on Movement):

> SHIFTING
>
> . . . When the vision is good, all objects not regarded are seen less distinctly than those seen with centralization. When the vision is imperfect, objects not observed may be seen better, or an effort is made to see them better than those directly observed. In fact, it is always true, that in all cases of imperfect sight, the eyes do not see best where they are looking and centralization is lost.

When a person has normal centralization and normal sight, only the central object is seen clearly, and all peripheral objects are much less clear and less colorful. When a person has diffusion and imperfect sight, neither the central object nor the peripheral objects are seen clearly.

Centralization—The Searchlight

Have you ever seen a searchlight sweeping along clouds in the sky at night? Or have you ever shined a flashlight along objects in a dark room? If you have, you have an idea of centralization. Although there are lots of clouds in the sky, you can only see one small area of a cloud best with the searchlight; all the other clouds are seen less clearly. Similarly, one object is seen best at any moment when shining the flashlight along objects in the dark room. Adding the movement principle from the last chapter, the searchlight and flashlight are continually scanning or shifting to see different objects best—one at a time.

The human eye is capable of seeing only one point clearly at a time. The peripheral vision is never clear. It is impossible for humans to see clearly unless they are centralizing.

Peripheral vision is not ignored while centralizing; it is simply less clear and less colorful than the central vision. Since the peripheral vision is less clear and less colorful, it makes sense to have our visual attention where perception is best—and that place is only in the center. Peripheral vision is very important vision, *but* it is secondary to the central vision.

Generally, people who have blurred vision do not centralize—they diffuse. In fact, the instant a person diffuses away from the central point of the visual field, clarity lowers immediately—by definition. This is equally true for a person who has normal sight. The person with blur takes his attention away from the only place in the picture that is clear—the center. The peripheral vision is 20/400 unclear—at best! It will become apparent very soon that in order for a person to relearn to see, naturally and clearly, the individual must return the visual attention back to the center. There is no other possibility.

The Peripheral is "Not Clear"

Often, people who have perfect eyesight will *not* say that their peripheral vision is "blurry." Rather, some like to say it is "not clear." In normal vision, the light rays focus correctly on the retina. The rods, which pick up our peripheral vision, are incapable of picking up peripheral objects clearly. Only the cones in the fovea *centralis* pick up clarity.

Mary Dudderidge writes in *Scientific American:*

> The fundamental principle of this new system of eye training is what Dr. Bates calls central[ization.] The trouble with the

civilized eye, he says, is that we use it as though it were a photographic camera. The camera can see everything which falls upon its sensitive plate equally well, but the human eye is not built that way. The retina has more nerve cells in the center than anywhere else, and therefore is designed to see one point better than others in its field of vision. In other words, we see best in the direction in which we are looking. When we submit to this, the eye is at rest.... Central[ization] is attained by two methods, practice and rest, the latter coming first.[2]

See *Plate 44: How We See.*

CENTRALIZATION—THE PHYSICAL CONNECTION

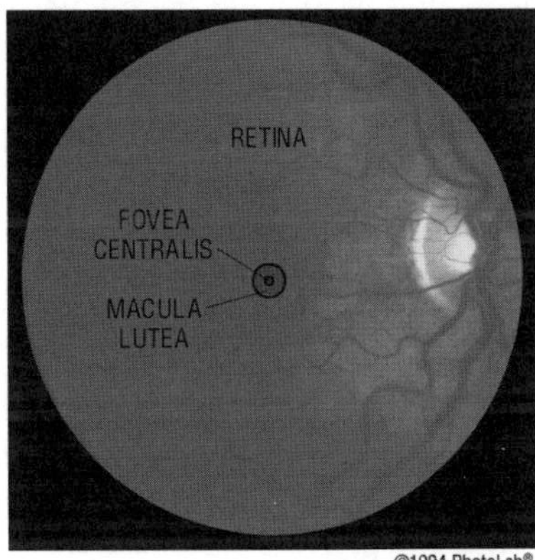

Figure 10–1: The Fovea Centralis.

See *Figure 10–1: The Fovea Centralis, Plate 30: The Retina (1),* and *Plate 31: The Retina (2).*

The explanation of why it is anatomically impossible to see clearly without centralizing is quite helpful to vision students. The principle of centralization is primarily mental, and is more subtle than the principle of movement. The intellectual agreement with the principle of centralization motivates students to relearn centralization faster.

As discussed earlier, there are two types of light receptors in the retina—cones and rods.

The cones are designed for clarity and color perception in medium or bright light. The great majority of the cones are located in center of the macula lutea at the fovea centralis. There are only cones exactly in the center of the fovea—no rods. There is a small number of cones extending out from the fovea. Unlike the cones in the fovea, these "peripheral" cones, like the rods, are buried under eight layers of retinal cells and blood vessels. Peripheral cones do not pick up the degree of clarity and colors that the high density of cones in the fovea do.

The rods pick up "unclear" movements, grays, and black/white shapes in our peripheral vision. Unlike the cones, they can function in very low levels of light. The rods are located outside of the center of the fovea centralis.

The cones and rods are discussed at length in Chapter 17, "The Retina."

THE STARING CONNECTION

Generally, when people stare, they diffuse. Diffusion is one of the worst habits of vision. *Diffusion is confusion.* During staring and diffusion, there is no *point* of interest—in fact, there is usually no visual interest at all—and therefore it is impossible to be seeing clearly during this time. This is true whether a person has normal sight, or the vision is artificially corrected to 20/20.

THE LARGER PROBLEM

When a person is given corrective lenses, or chooses any other artificial form of vision "correction," the strain of diffusion and rigidity has not necessarily been addressed, much less removed. Worse, strained vision habits are often reinforced. As stated in the Introduction, *blurred vision is a message from the mind and body that a person's visual system is out of balance with nature.* Bates proved this fact.

Until natural clarity returns, the imbalance continues. By approaching blurred vision with artificial methods, the imbalanced system is given the message that the imbalance is somehow "correct," because sharp acuity is available. This artificial sight can create more confusion and strain, and may well be one of the major reasons most people continue to need stronger glasses after they begin wearing them.

INITIALLY, CENTRALIZATION IS NOT OBVIOUS

People usually think about *what* they see, not *how* they see.

When asked, many people with normal vision will tell you they see everything clearly—*simultaneously.* Of course, this statement is incorrect. The principles of normal sight may not be obvious even to those who have normal sight! People with normal sight see objects clearly, of course, but only one at a time. They "shift constantly," as Bates stated, from one clear *point* to another clear *point.*

One reason people with normal sight *think* they see everything simultaneously clearly is because they have the *memory* of the objects they saw clearly before. For example, a person with normal sight could be noticing many objects in a room. Each individual object is clear, one by one. While seeing a chair, she knows that when she saw the door a few moments ago, it was clear. She can conclude subconsciously that the door in her peripheral vision is still just as clear as the chair she is currently noticing.

Another reason people with normal sight, and even more so those with imperfect sight, think the peripheral vision is clear is because they *want* it to be clear: "If everything is perfectly clear simultaneously, then I am better protected." It is an illusion of security.

EXPERIENCE CENTRALIZATION AND MEMORY

♥ ∞

If we notice the heart on the left, we see it clearly. Then, if we notice the infinity sign on the right we see it clearly. While interested in the infinity sign, we still have the memory of the *clear* heart on the left. Even though it is impossible to see the heart clearly while seeing the infinity sign clearly, the mind believes and wants to believe, the heart, out in the peripheral vision, is still clear.

CENTRALIZATION—ELUSIVE IN THE BEGINNING

After learning about the cones in the fovea and the rods in the peripheral vision, one of my students still thought that an object straight in front of him (Object C) was supposed to *remain* clear, even after he shifted his eyes (but not his head; the head is supposed to move, of course) to another object that was off to his right (Object R). He thought that even though his eyes moved to the right to see Object R, somehow the light rays from Object C were still able to enter the fovea for sharp clarity. No!

The point of clarity is always straight ahead of the direction of the *eyes*—along the visual axis from the *fovea centralis,* out through the center of the lens, iris and cornea, and straight out to the object of interest.

When a student shifts his attention to

Object R on the right, Object R is now the *central* object, and the light rays from Object R now enter the fovea for sharp clarity. Object C is now off to his left—in his peripheral vision. Object C is now much less clear.

Peripheral vision is whatever is outside the exact center of the visual field at any particular instant.

I have wondered for many years why many Bates teachers have not educated their students about the distribution of cones and rods in the retina.

INTERFERING WITH NORMAL CENTRALIZATION

Better Eyesight magazine, October 1923:

> When you have imperfect sight and look at the first letter of a line of letters on the Snellen Card which you cannot read, you can always note that you do not see the first letter or any other letter better than the rest. Usually the whole line looks pretty much the same shade of gray. Why is it? Because you are trying to see the whole line at once ... If you hold the card up close where you can readily read the same line you will notice, or you can get somebody with good eyesight to show you, that when you distinguish a letter you do not see any of the other letters so well. To see one letter at a time is much easier than to see a whole line of letters, in fact to see a number of letters all perfectly at the same time is impossible and trying to do it is a strain.... if you try to do the impossible, try to see the whole line of letters at once [clearly] you will always fail, because you will have to make an effort. It is not an easy thing at all to fail, it is difficult, you have to try, or you make an effort to do the impossible in order to fail. To prove that imperfect sight is more difficult and requires hard work, a great deal of trouble, and much effort, is a great benefit.

Centralizing is based on relaxation; diffusion is based on effort and strain.

Bates wrote in the May 8, 1915, issue of the *New York Medical Journal:*

> By eccentric fixation is meant the ability of the eye partially or completely to suppress the vision of the center of the fovea and to see best [but not clearly] with other parts of the retina.[3]

Mary Dudderidge writes in *Scientific American:*

> But when the eye attempts to see every point in its field of vision about as well as the central point, not only is its visual power lowered, but it is subjected to a severe strain, as anyone can observe for himself by trying to see every part of any surface of four or five inches in extent, or even much less, equally well at one time. This strain Dr. Bates believes to be at the bottom of most eye troubles.[4]

One of my students had normal sight in his first year at college. While playing basketball he recognized consciously that he saw only one point clearly at any moment. This, of course, is how a person with normal sight sees. Unfortunately, he began thinking about changing his natural way of seeing.

In discovering consciously that his peripheral vision was not clear, he decided to try to learn to see everything clearly simultaneously. He thought the entire picture could become clear if he practiced diffusing his visual attention throughout the picture. If he succeeded, he thought he would be able to see all of the other basketball players clearly at the same time, and then he would be able to play

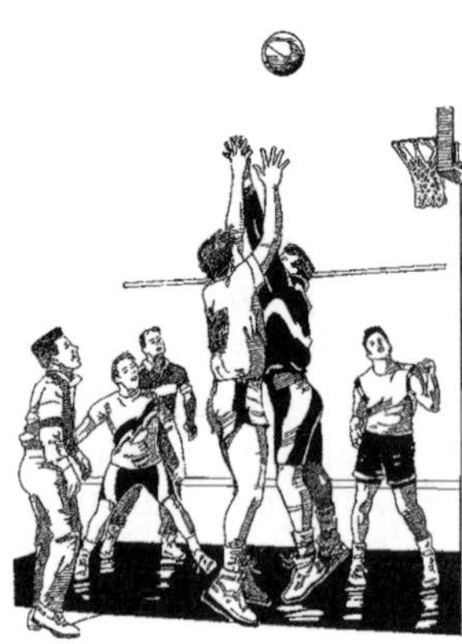

better basketball. He practiced diffusion and strained his vision. The result of his experiment was his vision blurred and he got glasses.

Notice this basketball player's motivation for trying to diffuse—to play better basketball. Some students assume that the circumstances present when their vision first blurred *must* have been unpleasant, maybe even traumatic. The basketball story shows this is not necessarily so. He formed strained vision habits, but his motivation and circumstances were positive.

Another student told me he was driving a big "semi" truck for many years while enjoying normal sight. One day he realized he was always moving his head to see the traffic and the road and scenery, one point at a time. He thought that if he diffused and saw everything at once, he would not need to move his head anymore! Not long after his mastery of diffusion and rigidity, his sight lowered, and he got his first pair of glasses. Notice how in this case diffusion was learned simultaneously with non-movement.

Another student said she remembered that, when in grade school, she thought about how she saw the world while walking home from school one day. She realized the peripheral vision was not clear; only the center was clear. She became very concerned about her lack of peripheral clarity, and concluded there was something wrong with her vision!

The memory of the specific interference to centralization often surfaces during natural vision classes. The interference to centralizing must be removed to improve sight.

One of my best students said, "I Choose to Refuse to Diffuse!"

The Vision Halo, also known as the "anti-diffusion halo," is described in Chapter 18, "Stereoscopic Vision."

RESISTANCE TO RELEARNING CENTRALIZATION

One of my students agreed that when her glasses were *off*, the peripheral vision was less clear than the central vision. However, when her glasses were *on*, for example, when driving her car, she said the peripheral vision was just as clear as the central vision.

I pointed out to her that, due to the distribution of cones and rods in the eye, it is impossible to see all objects clearly simultaneously—and there are *no* exceptions under any circumstances, with or without glasses. The following week she stated that when she drove home, she realized the peripheral vision was *not* as clear as the central vision.

Many students resist the truth of centralizing in the beginning. The vision could not have become blurred without acquiring diffusion. Diffusion becomes part of the personality.

There are various levels of acceptance students move through as they improve their vision. The process of improving vision takes time and patience.

CENTRALIZATION GOES WITH MOVEMENT; DIFFUSION GOES WITH RIGIDITY

In the last chapter, we discussed the importance of movement in regard to normal, clear vision. Centralization *goes with* movement. The person with clear vision is constantly moving from one point of interest to another. Both the head and eyes are moving.

Actually, it is the person's *interest* that shifts from one point to another, and the eyes and head simply follow the "mental movement."

Diffusion often *goes with* rigidity. Logically, when a person is trying to see everything at once, there is no reason to move. The problem with rigidity is the head, neck, and eye muscles become abnormally and chronically tight. The visual system cannot tolerate this strain—and blur results.

Fritz Kahn, in his outstanding two-volume set *Man in Structure and Function,* states:

> During the day one sees chiefly with the central part of the retina. Spatially, the central visual field is restricted, but everything contained in it is seen clearly and in all its colour. The spatial limitation [of central clarity] is compensated for by constant movement of the eyes.[5]

Conversely, locking the eyes and head still often goes with diffusion. A person with blur thinks, "If I lock my head still, I can just see everything at once. In fact, I don't need to move my head or my eyes when I diffuse." This attitude and practice is harmful to sight.

The above assumes the person is interested in seeing at all when the head is locked. A locked head and neck often go with "spaced out" staring.

Ultimately the natural vision student realizes head movement "goes with" centralizing. It is necessary to shift our attention from one point to another with a head movement. Head movement releases the neck.

Tom's Personal Log: When I was in Army basic training, we were taken to the base of a medium-size hill. This hill had many bushes, trees, and large rocks on it. There were about a dozen soldiers hiding on this hill. Some were more hidden than others, and some moving more than others, but all of them were at least partially visible. We were instructed to find as many of the men as we could while standing at the base of this hill.

Immediately, several of my fellow trainees began pointing to one soldier after another. I became frustrated, as I did not see any men at all. I tried as hard as I could to see the entire hill simultaneously in a very diffused, "spread out" manner.

It was only near the end of this training, when one soldier finally jumped up and started waving his hands back and forth high in the air, that I finally saw a soldier. I began to wonder about my fate if I should end up in combat.

CENTRALIZATION WITHOUT MOVEMENT; MOVEMENT WITHOUT CENTRALIZATION

Centralization Without Movement is Incorrect

Better Eyesight magazine, January 1924: "One can stare in looking straight ahead with the center of sight. . . ."

It is possible to centralize, i.e., to notice one point, without moving the head or eyes. It is not possible to lock onto one point for a long period of time without creating tension and possibly even pain. One problem is that people who have blurred vision often *try* to lock on one point for a long period of time.

One of my students had great difficulty with the centralizing principle of vision. In the last class of the eight-week course, he demonstrated how he had finally succeeded—with great effort and rigidity—to lock onto one point. Proud of his accomplishment, he asked, "Now what should I do?" I suggested he now shift to another point of interest, and then another, and another. He did not like my answer, since it had taken him eight weeks to finally *lock* onto one point.

Notice how this student wanted to continue his rigid way of seeing. This student did well to centralize, but now the movement principle needed to be added to the centralizing.

Natural vision is a process of "dynamic relaxation." Normal vision includes both movement and centralizing. In normal vision, the attention shifts (moves) to a new point (centralization) of interest about every one or two seconds.

One vision program that teaches its students eye exercises says to make a "conscious effort" to look at "the entire screen" of a TV, while holding the head still. Students in this program are also told to not blink. Unfortunately, this type of incorrect teaching is not uncommon; it is completely the opposite of Bates' teaching on natural vision.

Movement Without Centralization is Incorrect

Better Eyesight magazine, January 1924: "... and one can stare by trying to see with the sides of the retina, [called] eccentric fixation."

Eccentric fixation is diffusion.

As mentioned in the previous chapter, it is possible to move without centralizing. People with blur often move without centralizing. For example, a person can be walking along without noticing where they are going.

After thirteen years of teaching natural vision, I am convinced that staring and "spacing out" are the cause of many, if not most, accidents.

Centralization vs. Diffusion—The Emotional Connection

Diffusion can be a response to feelings of fear and being overwhelmed.

More than one of my students has told me they learned to diffuse in the subways and streets of New York City "to protect myself."

Some people had significant stress when their blur started. Several of my students have stated their vision blurred when they were children and moved to another city, state, or country.

One student said she began diffusing when, as a child, there was a swarm of bees around her.

The irony of trying to "grab" everything at once—clearly—is that clarity is lost. As stated before, the instant a person takes her attention away from where it is clear in the center, clear perception is lowered. The peripheral vision is far less clear than the central vision.

Tom's Personal Log: I found it extremely frustrating to centralize in my beginning vision lessons. It was scary. I thought it was essential to try to see everything at once clearly to be protected.

It seemed as if no one could possibly diffuse more than I did. This realization was the cause of extreme frustration.

Yet, my vision was improving, and I wanted

to continue my improvement, so I continued practicing centralizing better each day.

Centralizing becomes easier and better with practice. Remember, children centralize intuitively and naturally. They point.

Anyone can relearn to do something he used to do automatically and naturally—and this includes centralization.

CENTRALIZATION—THE MENTAL CONNECTION

Bates concluded that the process of seeing is primarily mental. *Whether a person is centralizing or diffusing is a mental choice.* Usually centralizing occurs subconsciously, but sometimes it is conscious. The same is true of the harmful practice of diffusion.

To a great extent, the principle of centralization has to do with how we live our lives. Do we try to do a dozen projects equally well at one time, or do we put our attention primary on one project at a time?

One of my students, while programming his computer at work, was being asked a question by a co-worker. Not wanting to be disturbed (diffused), this student stopped for a moment, looked at his co-worker and said, "Not right now. But, when I finish with my work, you will get my complete *foveal* attention!"

Notice that when children are deeply involved in a game, they do not like to be distracted. They are completely "absorbed" in the game. Children centralize—naturally.

Our society often emphasizes quantity (left brain) over quality (right brain). We produce many material goods, and people are encouraged to accumulate as many of these goods as they can. Our society also provides almost countless activities to participate in. Are we sacrificing some of the quality of our lives for quantity?

An Eastern yogi was visiting a big supermarket in the US for the first time. A sales clerk asked the yogi if he needed help in finding anything. The yogi answered, "No, I am just thanking God I don't need any of these things."

One man I met kept getting more and more degrees in school just to prove to himself he was smart. Quantity was more important than quality.

A great Eastern mystic once wrote, "Live a simple, happy, and relaxed life." In many years of teaching and healing my health, I have slowly realized these three adjectives are the same.

A person *can* have a lot of projects and goals in life, but he cannot do them all—with equally high quality—at one time.

The primary issue within the principle of centralization is the attitude in the mind. Trying to do many projects at one time is diffusing and creates tension. Doing one project *best* at a time is healthier and more relaxing. A person may not accomplish as many tasks, but the quality of each task will be higher. On the other hand, a person might accomplish *more* tasks, because the relaxation associated with centralizing gives her *more* energy.

With centralization, there is movement and flexibility. A person's energy is properly channeled and conserved.

Diffusion results in fatigue and a drain of energy. Fatigue is a major cause of staring.

Have you ever watched two people talking to each other *simultaneously?* Neither person is listening. This is an example of diffusion, and it is very common in this society.

CENTRALIZATION = RELAXED CONCENTRATION

Better Eyesight magazine, December 1922:

> *Question:* Has Dr. Bates' method anything to do with concentration?
> *Answer:* No, to concentrate is to make an effort. Dr. Bates' method is rest and relaxation, which cannot be obtained by concentration.

Centralization is *relaxed, involuntary* visual concentration. Like most other Natural Vision teachers, I rarely use the word "concentration" in my classes because most people in this society associate concentration with effort. Effort to see lowers natural vision. (Squinting is artificial vision.)

Better Eyesight magazine, April 1925:

> CONCENTRATION AND RELAXATION
>
> By Lawrence M. Stanton, M.D.
>
> I know of no writer who has clarified the murky philosophy of concentration and relaxation as has Dr. Bates, and yet the final word has not been said, as he himself would undoubtedly avow.
>
> Therefore, but with humblest intention, I offer a few thoughts upon the subject which is of the utmost importance to those who are striving for better eyesight.
>
> To my students I have forbidden the practice of concentration, saying that the very word suggests strain, or else I bid them modify the dictionary's definition. I have reasoned that if by concentration you mean, as Dr. Bates says, doing or seeing one thing better than anything else, you may speak of concentration; but if by concentration you mean, as the dictionary says, doing one thing continuously to the exclusion of all other things, then you must abandon the practice as an impossibility.
>
> Concentration, however, cannot psychologically be ignored, and recent psychology, I believe, has given us a new interpretation which is worthy of our consideration.
>
> Attention underlies concentration, as that word is commonly used, and Ribot's [See *Psychology of Attention* in Bibliography and additional excerpts in Chapter 23, "Children and Schools"] statement of attention is very enlightening. Ribot says "that the state of attention which seems continuous is in reality intermittent; the object of attention is merely a center, the point to which attention returns again and again, to wander from it as often on ever-widening circles. All parts of the object, and then the reflections inspired by these various parts, hold our interest by turns. Even when the attention is fixed on the most trifling material object, it works in just the same fashion." This is entirely in accord with Dr. Bates' statement; it is centralization.
>
> There are, however, two aspects of concentration to be considered—voluntary and involuntary. Voluntary concentration is an effort and, as Dr. Bates has so clearly shown, cannot be maintained without fatigue.
>
> The highest grades of attention, to which this brief consideration is confined, are involuntary, and involuntary concentration can be defined as "a psychological equivalent of attention minus effort." In ordinary attention—that is, in voluntary concentration—our thought holds the object in focus, whereas in involuntary attention (which we shall consider synonymous with involuntary concentration) the object holds our thought without our volition, perhaps even against our will. "Spontaneous attention is rooted at the very center of our being," and things that hold the attention captive, as in fascination, fixed contemplation, the

Hindu's meditation and revery are instances of involuntary concentration, and involuntary concentration is as effortless as the rising sun—it just happens. Then, there are those cases of [extraordinary quick reversals] of imperfect sight by one or another of Dr. Bates' methods, where it was enough for the person to see the better course in order to be able to follow it, the idea and its realization occurring simultaneously, without effort, without volition even. Contrast this with the attitude "No, I see the better course and approve it, but I follow the worse." Involuntary concentration is displayed in the case of the insect, related by Fabre and quoted by Dr. Bates, which in captivity hung downward for ten months, its whole life's span, and in this position performed all its functions, even to mating and laying of eggs, apparently without the least fatigue. Still another instance is that of Napoleon, who could work for eighteen hours at a stretch on one piece of work without the least fatigue. Napoleon speaks of his various affairs arranged in his head "as in a wardrobe." He says: "When I wish to put any matter out of my mind, I close its drawer and open the drawer belonging to another. The contents of the drawers never get mixed and they never worry me or weary me. Do I want to sleep? I close all the drawers, and then I am asleep."

The question, then, may be asked wherein does involuntary concentration differ from relaxation. If involuntary concentration and relaxation are not always one and the same thing, they often are psychological alternatives and not the opponents we think them.

To regard all phases of relaxation as purely passive is as erroneous as it is to say that concentration of the kind under consideration is associated with effort. Relaxation of the passive kind usually ends in sleep or sleepiness, as experienced by many people after palming. Relaxation combined with action, on the other hand, may also be absolutely free from effort and strain.

In any case it is the matter of effort and strain that concerns us most, rather than a question of concentration or relaxation ... surely nowhere is intensity so impressive as in calmness. To be calm is not to be oblivious, and to be intense need not be to strain.

Another thought about relaxation is this: Obstacles to relaxation may prove sources of relaxation. An instance of which is found in the noise that is keeping us awake when wishing to go to sleep. If we sufficiently relax, if we accept the disturbance and sleep in spite of it, not only is the obstacle overcome, but because overcome it in turn becomes rather pleasantly associated with going to sleep. When again we desire to sleep, we find the noise soothing rather than annoying, and really a source of relaxation instead of an obstacle to it....

Involuntary concentration without effort is equivalent to relaxation in action. If you can achieve such equilibrium; if you can perform your mental functions without strain as Fabre's little insect performed its physical; if you can, whatever your particular captivity, hang by your feet head downward without effort, then "be my friend and teach me to be thine."

[Stanton's] Note: Some of the quotations in this article and some of its material are from "The Power Within Us," Charles Baudouin.

From *Perfect Sight Without Glasses:*

As popularly understood, concentration means to do or think one thing only; but this is impossible, and an attempt to do the impossible is a strain which defeats its own

> end. The human mind is not capable of thinking of one thing only. It can think of one thing best, and is only at rest when it does so; but it cannot think of one thing only.

Trying to think of, or see, only one thing continuously is staring. To think of one thing *best* is centralization.

CENTRALIZATION—THE SOCIAL CONNECTION

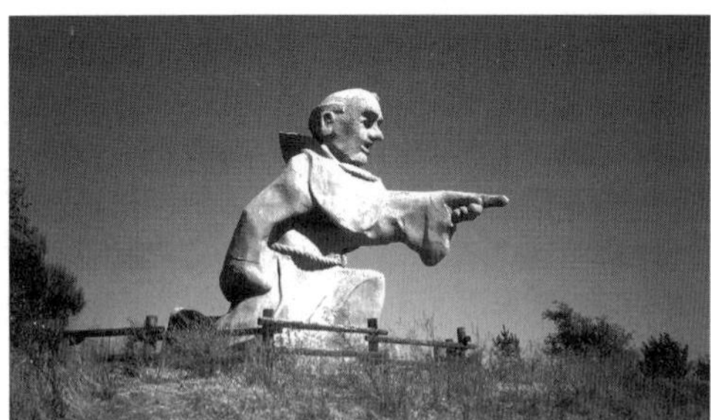

Figure 10–2: The Pointer.

Babies point. Pointing is natural. No one teaches a child to point, or to move. Centralization and movement are learned naturally and automatically.

In our society children are often told, "Don't point." Pointing is considered rude. A man from Africa once attended my introductory lecture. After the lecture he commented on how strange our culture is, not allowing children to point or yawn.

When we watch the documentaries on television about the natives who live in the forests of Brazil, we see that adults and children frequently point. Pointing is centralizing.

In the previous chapter, I stated that children are often told to "sit still." Add to this the warning to never point, and what we have is a society that teaches children not to move and not to centralize.

Regardless of Bates' opinions on accommodation, he proved that mental and physical principles of movement and centralization are essential for clear vision, and that if they are interfered with, vision will lower.

We unwittingly teach our children how to lose their sight by discouraging—even punishing them for—movement and centralization. After studying the principles of natural seeing, it is no wonder so many people have blurred vision in this society.

Oftentimes it is the rebellious children in this society who keep their normal sight. They keep moving and pointing, regardless of the consequences. This is a subconscious, primitive drive to maintaining normal vision and health.

CENTRALIZATION—THE HEARING CONNECTION

See *Figure 9–7: The Vestibulo-Ocular Connection.*

When hearing is normal, we hear one sound best at a time.

If you are attending a concert, you can selectively "tune in" to one instrument at a time to hear it the best. You listen most attentively to the violin, then the piano, then the drums, then the trumpet, etc. You continue to hear the entire orchestra, but one instrument is heard best.

You can be listening to the radio while driving a car, and hardly notice the noise from the engine. When a strange noise is heard from the engine, the auditory attention shifts from hearing the radio best to hearing the engine best. During this time, you may not even be aware of the words spoken or what tune is being played on the radio. After returning the attention to the radio, you are hardly aware of sound from the engine. This is called centralization.

Notice in both the above examples, the sound waves reaching the eardrum are the same. The mind has the ability to centralize on one particular sound and it is *designed* to do so.

Margaret Corbett, in her book *Help Yourself to Better Sight,* writes:

> Sounds that do not bother normal ears do bother the defective ear because it hears so many sounds, all distorted, confusing and irritating.[6]

The auditory system is designed to be used like the visual system.

EXPERIENCE CENTRALIZATION AND DIFFUSION

Close your eyelids, and pretend you are in a large auditorium. Imagine there are a hundred people around you in a large circle about fifty feet from you.

Now, imagine there are fifty conversations (two people per conversation) going on simultaneously.

Try to comprehend all of the conversations simultaneously. Do this now for about thirty seconds, if you can!

To comprehend fifty conversations simultaneously is, of course, impossible to do, and the attempt to do the impossible is stressful!

Reactions described by students include: strain, diffusion, confusion, scattering, effort, chaos, impossibility, freezing, locking, tension, breathing stops, the body freezes, and even blurred vision.

These reactions can occur just by *thinking* about diffusing hearing, showing how centralization and diffusion are primarily mental. Diffusion is confusion is stressful.

Now pretend you are listening to only one of the conversations best. Let it be a pleasant conversation! Do this now for about thirty seconds, and for the rest of your life!

Notice how much more "centered" you now feel compared to the diffused experience a few moments ago. Students often describe this experience as peaceful, relaxing, possible, easy, and so on.

The parallels are identical to vision.

CENTRALIZATION—THE UNIVERSAL CONNECTION

From Chapter XI, "Centralization," in *Perfect Sight Without Glasses:*

> ... Since centralization is impossible without mental control, centralization of the eye means centralization of the mind. It means, therefore, health in all parts of the body, for all the operations of the physical mechanism depend upon the mind. Not only the sight, but all the other senses—touch, taste, hearing and smell—are benefited by centralization. All the vital processes—digestion, assimilation, elimination, etc.—are improved by it.... The efficiency of the mind is enormously increased. The benefits of centralization already observed are, in short, so great that the subject merits further investigation.

Centralization is a universal principle. Living beings tend to organize and unify. For example, we have organs in the body that "specialize" in certain functions. The heart pumps blood, the digestive tract assimilates food, the lungs breathe, and so forth.

When any living being dies, entropy (diffusion) begins. The body dissolves into its elements and becomes diffused ashes.

Above, we discussed how centralization relates to sight and hearing. Centralization also applies to touch, smell, and taste. Movement and centralization apply to all sense perceptions. When either movement or centralization is interfered with, sense perception diminishes.

In nutrition there is a concept called "food combining." Certain types of foods do not digest well together with other types of foods. For example, starchy foods do not digest well with proteins. Different chemical environments are created in the stomach for starches and proteins. If starches are eaten with proteins, neither are digested well—the stomach is confused. Similarly, fruits are generally best eaten without starches or proteins. The concept is centralization.

In the game of chess, one of the key objectives is to gain control of the center of the board. Much of the strategy in chess is based on control of the four center squares. From the *center,* pieces have the greatest *mobility* and are more *powerful* because they are free to move to any other parts of the board quickly to attack or to defend.

Pieces placed on the *peripheral* parts of the board have much less mobility and are generally less powerful.

For example, a knight placed in the center of the board can move to eight different squares; when located in the corner, it can only move to two squares. The knight has four times as much mobility and power when placed in the center of the board. Control of the central squares often determines who wins the game.

Centralization allows greater movement. They go together.

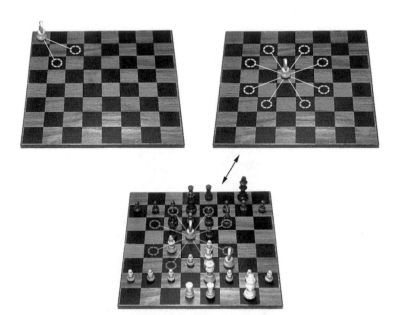

Figure 10–3: Strategic Centralization.

Centralization is powerful. Diffusion is weak. Centralization conserves energy. Diffusion wastes it. A martial arts master is powerful because he is centered. He does not waste energy. Many people who meditate say they feel more relaxed and centered.

The sun, which provides essential energy for life on Earth, is at the *center* of the solar system.

"The eye of the hurricane is calm."

CENTRALIZING—THE TWO PENCILS

Many students, before enrolling in the vision classes, would probably answer the question, "If you had perfect clarity right now, would everything be clear simultaneously?" with "Yes." The enrolling student may be thinking, "Wouldn't it be nice to see *everything* clearly *again?*" He thinks that when he had normal vision in the past, everything was clear simultaneously. This idea is incorrect, and needs to change to improve vision.

EXPERIENCE CENTRALIZING—THE TWO PENCILS

See *Plate 8: Centralizing—The Two Pencils*.

Hold two different colored pencils vertically, about 12 inches out in front of you. Place the erasers at the top. If there is lettering or designs on the pencil, face them toward you. Separate the pencils horizontally by about 16 inches. If you are a high myope, you can bring the pencils closer to you and closer together.

In this example, a yellow pencil is held on the left, and a green pencil is held on the right. Remember to breathe abdominally, blink frequently, and have a mobile neck as you do this activity.

Note: This is *not* an eye exercise. The purpose of this activity is to demonstrate the truth of centralization, which is the normal, correct way of seeing all day long.

Pretending you have an imaginary pencil attached to, and extending out from your nose, "sketch" the yellow pencil. "Sketching" is simply a movement of your visual interest from one point to another. See Chapter 12 for more on sketching. The cones in the fovea pick up the sharp detail and color of this pencil. Without shifting your attention to it, wiggle the peripheral green pencil. The rods pick up the unclear movement and shades of gray from the green pencil. If you did not already know that the peripheral pencil is green, you might not be able to say what its color is now.

Now shift your attention to the green pencil. Sketching the green pencil, notice its details and colors—*which you could not see when you were sketching the yellow pencil.* Now wiggle the peripheral yellow pencil. *The peripheral yellow pencil is now almost, or maybe even completely, gray and it has much less detail* compared to when you were sketching it in the beginning. No peeking!

Of course, in reality, the yellow pencil *has* detail and color, but you cannot *see* them while sketching the green pencil. Centralization is the acknowledgment, and the mental cooperation with the fact, that only the central object is clear and most colorful. Peripheral vision has little to no color, and is much less clear than the central vision.

There *is* some diminished color in the peripheral areas of the visual field because there are some cones in the peripheral part of the retina. Still, color perception is always best in the center. More on this in Chapter 17, "The Retina."

As stated above, people who have blurred vision diffuse; they try to see everything equally clearly simultaneously. As Bates pointed out many times, this is impossible to do. The *attempt* to do this strains the visual system, and always lowers sight.

Alternate sketching each pencil, proving to yourself that you see best—by far—only where you centralize.

Now *try* to see both pencils equally clear and sharp—*simultaneously.* The best you can do is to place the attention in the center, between the two pencils, and then spread out your attention, trying visually to grab both images at one time. Notice that neither pencil is clear now. It should now be obvious that sight lowers *instantaneously* when you are diffusing.

Now bring the pencils a little closer to each other and sketch one at a time as before. You may now notice *more* of the peripheral pencil, but it is *still* less clear and colorful than the pencil you are sketching.

Continue this activity, slowly bringing the pencils closer to each other and alternating sketching one pencil at a time. A person with excellent centralization skills will be able to notice the other pencil is less clear—even when they are touching!

Practice centralizing more and better each day until it becomes a habit.

CENTRALIZING—THE PEBBLE GAME

EXPERIENCE CENTRALIZING—THE TWO-PEBBLE GAME

Place two pebbles about 14 inches apart, one to the left and the other to the right. This is like the two pencils activity, except the area of centralization is smaller.

Sketch the left pebble with your nose-pencil. If you are a high myope, bring the pebbles closer to you so that the one you are sketching is seen more clearly than the peripheral pebble.

If you are a high farsight, you may want to use your reduced glasses for this game. The pebble you are sketching needs to be more clear than the peripheral pebble.

Remember to have a head movement. Breathe abdominally and blink frequently!

While noticing the left pebble's detail, texture, colors, three-dimensionality, and so on, say out loud, "The other pebble is less clear!" Is it? The right pebble should be significantly less clear than the left pebble you are sketching.

No peeking over to the right pebble! Some students peek, and then reply, "No, they both look the same to me!" This is not how the game is played!

Once you notice that the left pebble is more clear than the right pebble, shift over to the right pebble and sketch it. While noticing right pebble's detail, texture, colors, etc., say out loud, "The other pebble is less clear." Is it? The left pebble should now be significantly less clear than the right pebble you are sketching.

If the peripheral pebble seems equally or more clear than the central pebble, you are diffusing and need to practice this game frequently, until you experience the peripheral pebble as less clear than the one you are sketching.

If your vision is such that the pebble you are sketching is not clear at this time, do not be overly concerned. It is more important, at this point, that you notice *the other pebble is less clear* than the one you are sketching. If this is still not true because of serious vision problems, then pretend it is true. Remember, vision is primarily mental. Natural vision teachers have seen many types of vision problems improve.

Alternate back and forth three or four times, spending about 15–20 seconds on each pebble.

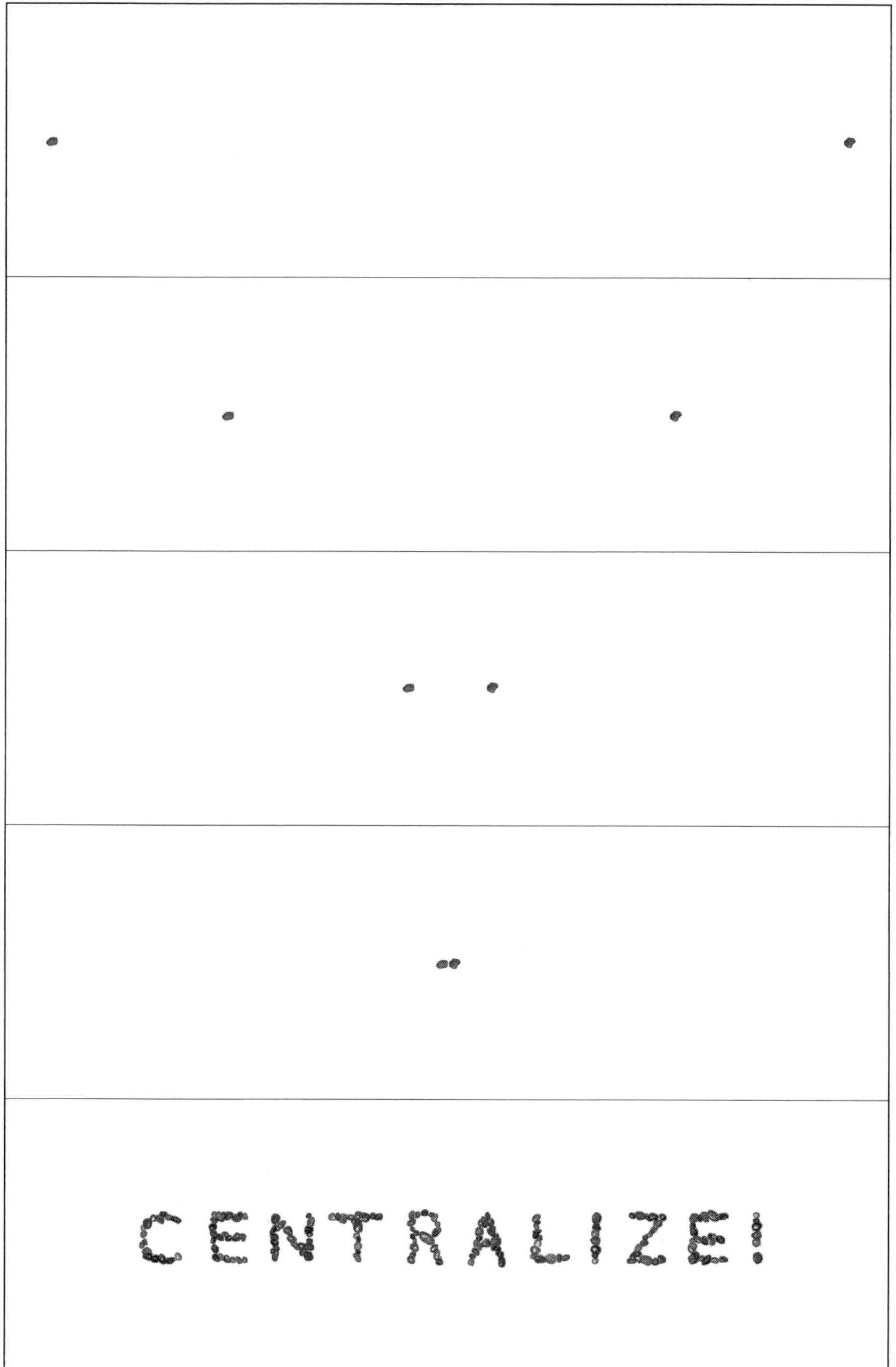

Figure 10–4: The Pebble Game.

Be sure to say out loud "The other pebble is less clear" each time you sketch a pebble.

The main principle in this game is centralization. Centralization is the attitude of mind that you see one central point best, and everything else out in the peripheral vision is significantly less clear. [I realize I am being repetitive, but this principle is extremely important.]

Notice we do *not* say "The other pebble is gone." Peripheral vision is essential vision, and we want to have excellent peripheral awareness with the rods. Rods pick up movement. However, since peripheral vision is much less clear than the central vision, peripheral vision is secondary to central vision.

You may agree that it only makes sense to have the primary visual attention where vision is best—and that place is exactly in the center of the visual field.

Continuing the pebble game:

Now move the pebbles about one inch closer to each other. Just like before, sketch the pebble on the left, saying out loud, "The other pebble is less clear! Wow!" (Enthusiasm is important!)

Is the other pebble less clear, even though the two pebbles are closer to each other? Do you notice *more* of the peripheral pebble than when the pebbles were farther apart?

"Hmmm," thinks the natural vision student, "I wonder what the ultimate outcome of this pebble game is going to be, as those two pebbles come closer and closer to each other?!"

Alternate sketching each pebble, spending 10–15 seconds with each pebble and saying, "The other pebble is less clear."

Once you notice the peripheral pebble is consistently less clear than the one you are sketching, move the pebbles another inch closer to each other. Sketch each pebble alternately, continuing the same theme.

At some point you will notice the peripheral pebble to be *more* clear than it was when you began this game. However, it will still be much less clear than the pebble you are sketching.

Do not continue this game if you become fatigued or feel any discomfort. Take a rest and come back to it later if necessary. It is important to associate natural vision habits and principles with pleasure and fun.

Continue playing this game, gradually moving the two pebbles closer to each other.

At some point you may feel your mind diffuse over the two pebbles equally. If you feel this tendency to diffuse, do one of the following:

1. Simply move the pebbles farther away from each other, and slowly move them closer together again playing the same game. The second time, you may be able to bring them a little closer together before the mind tries to grab both of them equally, i.e., before diffusing; or
2. Close your eyelids and play the same game in your mind. Move your head left and right alternately, exactly as if your eyelids were open. Say out loud, "The other pebble is less clear." Do this for at least one minute. Then, take a breath in, and open your eyelids, "zooming" to one pebble and sketching it. Some students feel a powerful "siphoning" or "funneling" effect con-

necting them to the pebble. If you feel this effect, it is a step forward in relearning centralization. If you do not feel this effect, you will with continued practice.

In time, you will be able to bring the pebbles close enough that they touch each other. Sketching one pebble, you will be able to notice that the peripheral pebble, even though it is much clearer, is *still less clear* than the pebble you are sketching! When you reach this point you have progressed a very long way in relearning centralization.

In the above Pebble Game, if the student does not continue to move, first the peripheral pebble will fade away, and then even the central pebble will begin to fade away. In the last chapter, we discussed how important movement is to natural vision.

EXPERIENCE CENTRALIZING—THE MULTI-PEBBLES GAME

Spread lots pebbles out in front of you. While sketching one pebble, say out loud, "All the other pebbles are less clear." Are they? The peripheral pebbles should be less clear than the one you are sketching. However, the pebbles closest to the one you are sketching will be *more clear* than the pebbles farther away.

Only the single pebble you are sketching can be absolutely clear. The light rays from that single pebble enter the very high density of cones exactly in the center of your fovea centralis. That is where you see with the sharpest acuity.

Now shift from one pebble to another, like stars in the night sky, saying out loud, "All the other pebbles are less clear." Not only is it OK for only one point to be the clearest, it is *desired.* We want to retrain the mind to have its primary visual attention where nature intended it to be—in the center. While relearning centralization, it is important to remember that you do not lose your peripheral vision (in this case, the other pebbles).

The study of the distribution of the cones and rods, in Chapter 17, "The Retina," will help you further understand and appreciate the many differences between your central and peripheral vision.

If you need assistance with the principle of centralization, seek out instructions from a Natural Vision teacher.

One of my students missed the class with the pebble game, so he played the "raisin game" at breakfast, receiving a delicious reward for each centralizing skill!

Another of my students, W. B., said he did not really "get" centralization until we played the pebble game. In the class following the pebble game, he said, "I have had *pebble* vision all week!" He had worn glasses and contact lenses since the seventh grade, increasing in strength to O.D. –2.50, with 0.50 D of astigmatism, and O.S. –3.00 by age 38. He had 20/70 sight in the right eye and 20/200 sight in the left eye. Within three months after completing the eight-week vision course, his optometrist told him his sight was 20/25 in his right eye. He has since passed the California driver's vision test without glasses, and is no longer required to wear corrective lenses when driving.

C. Y. reports that fish are much more vibrant, colorful, and three-dimensional while scuba diving in Hawaii.

Tom's Personal Log: After about two years of improving my vision, while exercising in a place that had lots of pebbles, I noticed I could centralize on a pebble about ten feet away, and the pebble touching it was less clear!

The Color Centralizing Game

An excellent form of centralization is picking out any color you like, e.g., green, and then finding that particular color throughout your environment and painting it with your nose-paintbrush. After painting the first color, select a second color, e.g., blue, and then find and paint that color everywhere you find it. Then paint a third color, and so on. Have a "visual feast." Vision loves variety, but, of course, one at a time.

The Counting Centralizing Game

Another simple centralization game is to count similar objects. For example, you can count the number of light posts along a street, the number of windows of a house or building, the number of trees in a field, and so on. This is excellent centralizing practice.

The idea is to form the habit of shifting from one point to another throughout the day. Never stare or diffuse. Centralize within a smaller area each day.

Have *laser beam* vision. Illuminate each place you are centralizing on with your nose-laser beam! Always have a head movement. Even a small movement is correct, as long as the neck is released and mobile.

Centralization Patterns

In *Figure 10–5: Centralization Patterns,* practice centralizing with the objects in the top rectangles. Then centralize on the smaller objects in the middle rectangles.

In the bottom rectangle, centralize on a small group of dots approximately the size of the circle shown in the bottom left corner. (Those with farsightedness and astigmatism may need to use corrective lenses to see this round area.) You may be able to see a small round area of sharp dots, while all of the peripheral dots are less clear.

Some students notice that the small round area of sharp dots appears to be three-dimensional, like a small mound. When you see this small round area of sharp dots you are experiencing the area of the fovea centralis and the macula lutea on your retina!

See *Plate 9: Centralization vs. Diffusion.*

But It Is *Not* Clear Everywhere I Centralize—Yet!

But that is why (most likely) you are reading this book!

Most likely, while improving your vision, the point of centralization will not be clear at all distances. For nearsights the distance is not clear; for farsights the near is not clear. It is the *concept* of centralization that is important at this time.

When centralizing at a point that is not clear, think to yourself, "I see *most* clearly and colorfully where I am centralizing. All peripheral objects are *less* clear and colorful." And, "If my vision were normal right now, where I am centralizing I would see perfectly clear only at this point. My peripheral vision would be 20/400, at best, if I had clear vision right now."

This attitude is essential for improving eyesight. Ultimately, it becomes true when the student has normal sight again. You are retraining your mind to centralize. It is the only way to return to clear sight; and it is exactly what you used to do when you used

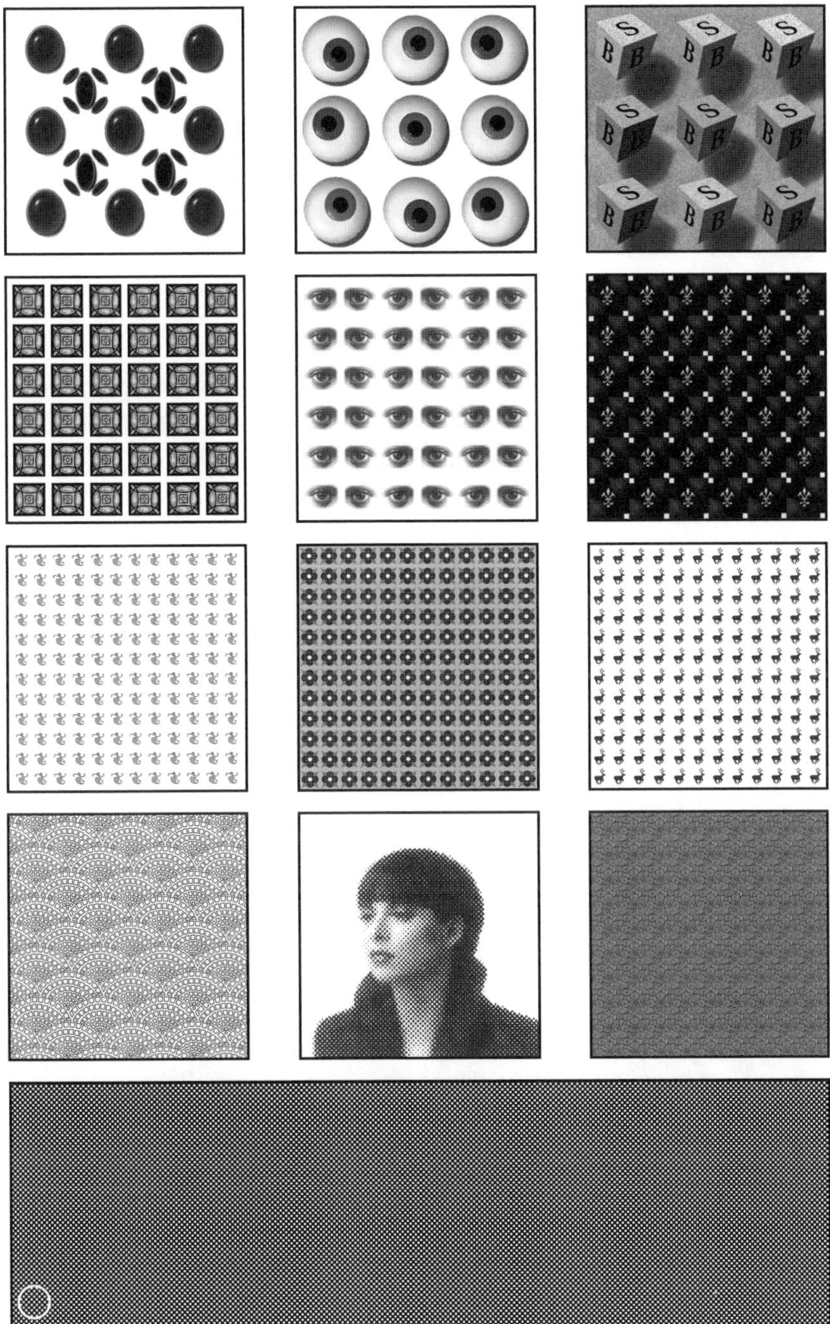

Figure 10–5: Centralization Patterns.

to have clear sight. Centralizing *is* clarity. Diffusion *is* blur. "Refuse to diffuse." Centralize more perfectly each day.

The practice of centralization relaxes the mind and body. This mental relaxation, along with the relaxation provided by relearning movement, allows the extrinsic eye muscles to release their chronic tension.

When the eyeball is squeezed out of shape, peripheral light rays fall into the fovea centralis. Peripheral light rays are not supposed to fall into the fovea centralis, and doing so creates blurred sight in the center of your visual field. As the eye muscles release their tension, all light rays are focused correctly again onto the retina. Peripheral light rays no longer fall incorrectly into the fovea; they land outside of the fovea. In normal vision, only light rays from the object you are centralizing on fall into the fovea. The central vision is then clear.

The mental process of relearning to centralize and its effect on the eye muscles is one of the most remarkable consequences of Bates' thirty-five years of research on natural vision. Bates created a holistic model of vision which says: if we have a stressful, mentally diffused lifestyle, our vision will be diffused and blurry. If we have a relaxed, centered lifestyle, our vision is centered and clear. The design of the retina, with its central cones and peripheral rods, teaches us how to live in cooperation with principles of nature. The benefits to the student are immeasurable.

Our vision is, in many ways, a barometer of the way we live.

It is Easier with Practice

As vision improves, the experience of better clarity in the center makes centralizing easier. When vision is perfectly clear, it is obvious that only the center is clear, and the student *wants* her visual attention to be at the point of best sight. Then, even the *thought* of diffusion becomes abhorrent.

See *Plate 10: Cosmosis* for more centralization practice with unique, natural art stones.

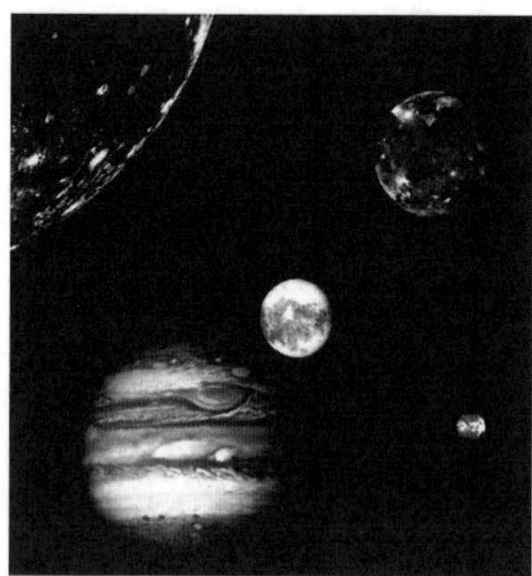

LIMITS TO VISION?

As students begin to understand that their best vision is in the center of the visual field, some ask, "Exactly how small is the area of centralization?" I do not believe anyone knows the answer to that question. Theoretical calculations of the limit of sight have been made based on the area of the cones in the fovea, but this does not take into consideration any other mental and physical aspects of sight.

Earlier we learned that 20/20 sight is vision which sees ⅜" letters twenty feet away. Much better vision than 20/20 is possible.

Quoting again from *Perfect Sight Without Glasses:*

> ... Complete reversals, which mean the attainment, not of what is ordinarily called normal sight, but of a measure of telescopic and microscopic vision, are very rare. Even

in these cases, too, the practice can be continued with benefit; for it is impossible to place limits to the visual powers of man, and no matter how good the sight, it is always possible to improve it.

" ... There is now living in New York State," [Oliver Wendell Holmes] says, "an old gentleman who, perceiving his sight to fail, immediately took to exercising it on the finest print, and in this way fairly bullied Nature out of her foolish habit of taking liberties at five-and-forty, or thereabout. And now this old gentleman performs the most extraordinary feats with his pen, showing that his eyes must be a pair of microscopes. I should be afraid to say how much he writes in the compass of a half-dime—whether the Psalms or the Gospels, or the Psalms and the Gospels, I won't be positive."[a]

... The primitive memory as well as primitive keenness of vision has been found among civilized people; and if the necessary tests had been made it would doubtless have been found that they always occur together, as they did in a case which recently came under my observation. The subject was a child of ten with such marvelous eyesight that she could see the moons of Jupiter with the naked eye, a fact which was demonstrated by her drawing a diagram of these satellites which exactly corresponded to the diagrams made by persons who had used a telescope. Her memory was equally remarkable.

[a] Everyman's Library, 1908, pp. 166–167.

Steve Richards writes:

"Keenness of sight has achieved instances transcending belief in the highest degree," wrote Pliny. "Cicero records that a parchment copy of Homer's *Iliad* was enclosed in a nutshell. He also records the case of a man who could see 123 miles. Marcus Varro also gives this man's name, which was Strabo, and states that in the Punic Wars he was in the habit of telling from the promontory of Lilybaeum in Sicily the actual number of ships in a fleet that was passing out from the harbour at Carthage."[a, 7]

Several people have told me they can read the copyright on the eye chart twenty feet away.

As mentioned earlier, the husband of one of my students has 20/5 vision. This is four times better than 20/20 sight.

Better than 20/20 vision is possible by refining the principles and habits of natural seeing—smaller centralizing, more subtle movements and oppositional movements, a more relaxed, receptive attitude of seeing, better abdominal breathing, and softer (and frequent) blinking.

TRUSTING PERIPHERAL VISION WHILE CENTRALIZING

1. DEMONSTRATE:

Hold this book in your hands and, while sketching the middle of *Figure 10–6: Concentric Circles* (next page), shake and tilt this page in a circular motion. Notice if Concentric Circles seems to spin!

Now, while sketching the word "TRUST," continue to move this book in a tilting and circular motion. Since the rods pick up movement better than the cones, you may notice much more spinning within the circles while they are in the peripheral vision.

[a] Pliny, Natural History. London: The Loeb Classical Library, 1958–1963, Book 7, Chapter 21.

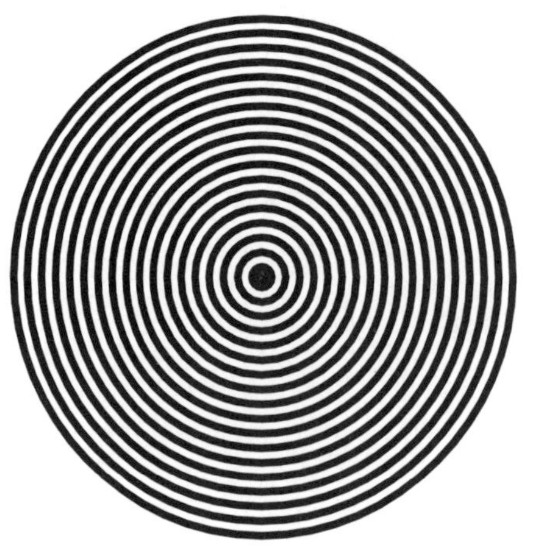

TRUST

Figure 10–6: Concentric Circles.

Trust your peripheral vision! The more you centralize and move, the better the rods pick up peripheral movements. Staring and straining to see lower the ability of the rods to pick up peripheral movements.

2A. GETTING THE CENTRALIZING WINDOW (OR GATE)

Notice a far object, Object F, straight out in front of you at least ten feet away. Hold a pencil in front of you vertically; the eraser should be at the top. Hold the bottom of the pencil near your mouth; the top of the pencil should be near the forehead. Move the pencil out about six inches from your head. For this activity do *not* bring your attention to the pencil!

Ideally, you should notice two partially transparent pencils, not one! One of the pencils is to the right of Object F; it is seen by the left eye. The other pencil is to the left of Object F; it is seen by the right eye.

Note: If you do not see two near pencils, you are either not doing this activity correctly, or the brain is switching off one of the pencils. For the former, ask a Natural Vision teacher to show you how to do this activity correctly. For the latter, see Chapter 18, "Stereoscopic Vision."

If the pencil is aligned exactly in front of your nose, Object F will be exactly in the middle of the two pencils. The two pencils form a "window" or "gate."

Move the pencil a little closer to your head, and then a little farther out. Notice that the closer the pencil, the wider the window; the farther the pencil, the narrower the window. Return the pencil to the original six inches distance from the nose.

2B. THE WINDOW (OR GATE) SWING FOR CENTRALIZING

Now, as if your pencil and hand were attached to your head, move the pencil, hand, arm, and head together slowly to the left, all in unison. Do not tilt the pencil or head—just turn them all together. As you move, keep your attention on the objects in the distance which are *within* the window. This may take some practice.

Notice that the objects in the center of the window are more clear than the objects outside of the window. The window reminds us to notice one point best at a time, and therefore is an excellent centralizing game. People who have blur try, mostly subconsciously, to see the objects outside of the window as clearly or equally as the objects that are in the center of the window. This strains vision.

To make a Vision Halo (a centralization halo) that moves a vertical bar automatically with your head, refer to Chapter 18, "Stereoscopic Vision."

THE CENTER CORRECTLY DISAPPEARS(!) IN TRUE NIGHTTIME VISION

In extremely low levels of light the cones do not register light. Only the rods function. Since there are no rods in the center of the fovea, there is no sight available exactly in the center of the visual field in "true nighttime" vision. This special situation is covered more in Chapter 17, "The Retina."

FINAL NOTES ON CENTRALIZATION

In this chapter, you have proven that it is impossible to see clearly without centralization. A person who wants to see clearly needs to relearn to have his visual attention where clarity is—in the center—all day long.

If you reflect on the ideas in this chapter for a few days, and if you do not have natural, clear vision, you will most likely discover that you diffuse your vision frequently and for long periods of time. You can now begin to change this strained, diffused way of seeing back to centralization. Remember, "Think small!"

Ultimately, only movement and centralization are relaxing; rigidity and diffusion are a strain. In the next chapter we study the most important principle of all—relaxation.

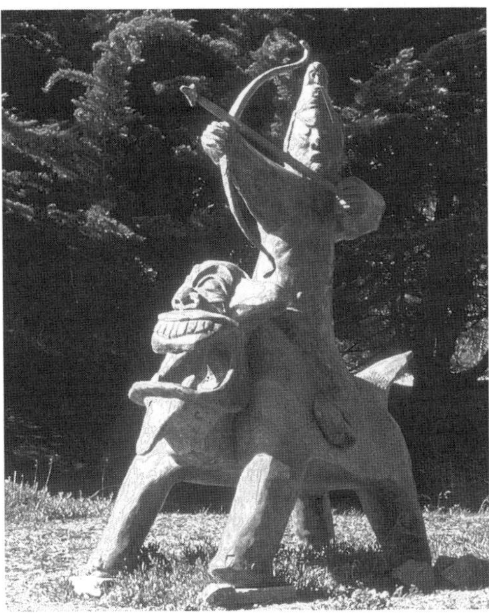

Figure 10–7: Get the "Point" of Centralizing?

NOTES

1 Bates used the phrase "central fixation" in many of his writings. This phrase has been changed to "centralization" or "centralizing" by many Natural Vision teachers, including myself, because the word "fixation" could be misunderstood by students to mean "staring" or "locking." "Centralizing" better describes the mental process of seeing one point at a time clearly and best. All references to "central fixation" have been changed accordingly in this book. The publisher of Bates' 1920 book *Perfect Sight Without Glasses* was Central Fixation Publishing Co.

2 Mary Dudderidge, "New Light Upon Our Eyes: An Investigation Which May Result in Normal Vision for All, Without Glasses," in *Scientific American.* (January 12, 1918), p. 61.

3 W. H. Bates, "The Reversal of Errors of Refraction by Education Without Glasses" in the *New York Medical Journal,* May 8, 1915.

4 Mary Dudderidge, "New Light Upon Our Eyes," p. 61.

5 Fritz Kahn, "The Eye," *Man in Structure and Function* (New York: Alfred A. Knopf, 1943), p. 665.

6 Margaret D. Corbett, *Help Yourself to Better Sight* (North Hollywood, CA: Wilshire Book Co., 1949), p. 203.

7 Steve Richards, "How to Extend Your Sight," *Invisibility* (Wellingborough, Northamptonshire, England: The Aquarian Press, 1982), p. 52.

CHAPTER ELEVEN

The Third Principle—Relaxation

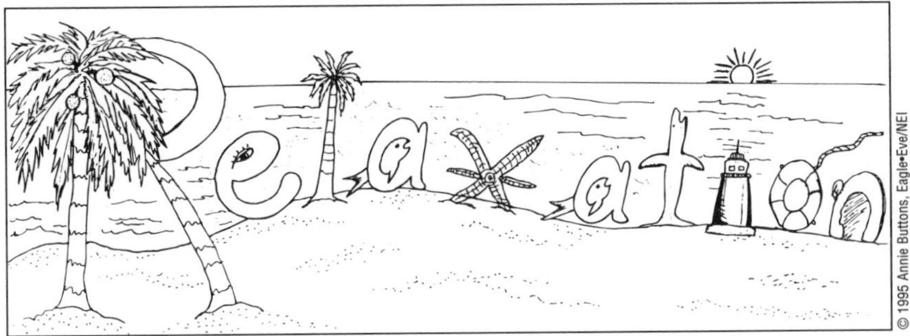

Figure 11–1: "Relaxation." Reprinted with permission from Annie Buttons.

Vision can be improved by natural methods. Tension causes eye strain. Relaxation relieves this tension. Normal eyes are always relaxed. Vision should come to the eye effortlessly as scent to the nostrils, music to the ears, touch of velvet to the finger tips.[1]

—Margaret Y. Ferguson, D.C., 1945

The reflection of the moon in the lake is clear only when the water is calm.

—Chinese proverb

RELAXATION

Relaxation is the third, and most important, principle of natural vision. The two principles discussed in the two previous chapters—movement and centralization—and the three habits of natural seeing are based on relaxation, especially of the mind.

The initial tendency is for many natural vision students to strain to see better. Bates stated that most vision problems are due to strain. Poor vision habits create excessive strain, and lower sight.

Everything Bates discovered and taught regarding natural vision is based on relaxation. Children and animals never strain to see. Natural, clear vision occurs automatically and subconsciously.

BATES ON RELAXATION

In the beginning of *Perfect Sight Without Glasses,* Bates emphasizes the importance of the principle of relaxation to normal vision.

> THE FUNDAMENTAL PRINCIPLE
>
> ... Do you observe also that the harder you try to see the worse you see? Now close your eyes and rest them ... If you have been able to relax ... you will have ... improved or clear vision ...

Bates not only taught relaxation as the key to natural, clear vision, he discovered that many situations people avoid—because of popular misconceptions about what is harmful or beneficial to sight—are, in fact, opportunities to master greater levels of relaxation. Examples include reading fine print, reading in dim light, and reading while commuting. How these situations, commonly thought to be a strain to sight, can be used to *improve* sight, is discussed in Chapter 22, "Reading—For All Ages."

From *Perfect Sight Without Glasses:*

> Fortunately, all persons are able to relax under certain conditions at will. In all uncomplicated errors of refraction the strain to see can be relieved, temporarily, by having the student look at a blank wall without trying to see. To secure permanent relaxation sometimes requires considerable time ... The ways in which people strain to see are infinite, and the methods used to relieve the strain must be almost equally varied. Whatever the method that brings most relief, however, the end is always the same, namely relaxation. By constant repetition and frequent demonstration and by all means possible, the fact must be impressed upon the student that *perfect sight can be obtained only by relaxation. Nothing else matters.* [TQ emphasis.]
>
> Most people, when told that rest, or relaxation, will reverse their eye troubles, ask why sleep does not do so. The answer to this question was given in Chapter VII [of *Perfect Sight Without Glasses*]. The eyes are rarely, if ever, completely relaxed in sleep, and if they are under a strain when the subject is awake, that strain will certainly be continued during sleep, to a greater or less degree, just as a strain of other parts of the body is continued.
>
> The idea that it rests the eyes not to use them is also erroneous. The eyes were made to see with, and if when they are open they do not see, it is because they are under such a strain and have such a great error of refraction that they cannot see. Near vision, although accomplished by a muscular act, is no more a strain on them than is distant vision, although accomplished without the intervention of the muscles. The use of the muscles does not necessarily produce fatigue. [The eye muscles are much more powerful than they need to be to perform their normal functions.] Some men can run for hours without becoming tired. Many birds support themselves upon one foot during sleep, the toes tightly clasping the swaying bough and the muscles remaining unfatigued by the apparent strain. Fabre tells of an insect which hung back downward for ten months from the roof of its wire cage, and in that position performed all the functions of life, even to mating and laying its eggs. Those who fear the effect of civilization, with its numerous demands for near vision, upon the eye may take courage

> from the example of this marvelous little animal which, in a state of nature, hangs by its feet only at intervals, but in captivity can do it for ten months on end, the whole of its life's span, apparently without inconvenience or fatigue.[a]
>
> The fact is that when the mind is at rest nothing can tire the eyes, and when the mind is under a strain nothing can rest them. Anything that rests the mind will benefit the eyes. Almost everyone has observed that the eyes tire less quickly when reading an interesting book than when perusing something tiresome or difficult to comprehend. A schoolboy can sit up all night reading a novel without even thinking of his eyes, but if he tried to sit up all night studying his lessons he would soon find his eyes getting very tired. A child whose vision was ordinarily so acute that she could see the moons of Jupiter with the naked eye became myopic when asked to do a sum in mental arithmetic, mathematics being a subject which was extremely distasteful to her....
>
> [a] The Wonders of Instinct, English translation by de Mattos and Miall, 1918, pp. 36–38.

Better Eyesight magazine, June 1923:

> When a person has normal sight the eye is at rest, and when the eye is at rest, strange to say, it is always moving to avoid the stare.

Better Eyesight magazine, October 1923 (some of this material is repeated from the previous chapter):

> Most people with imperfect sight when they look at the Snellen Card at twenty feet believe that they see imperfectly without any effort or staring. Some people feel that to have perfect sight requires something of an effort. It is interesting to demonstrate that these two beliefs are very far from the truth. As a matter of fact it requires an effort to fail to see and it requires no effort to have normal sight.
>
> In every case of imperfect sight whether due to nearsightedness or to any injury it can always be demonstrated that the nerves of the whole body are under a strain and in every case of perfect vision it can be demonstrated that no effort whatever is made ... When you have imperfect sight and look at the first letter of a line of letters on the Snellen Card which you cannot read you can always note that you do not see the first letter or any other letter better than the rest. Usually the whole line looks pretty much the same shade of gray. Why is it? Because you are trying to see the whole line at once ... if you try to do the impossible, try to see the whole line of letters at once [clearly] you will always fail, because you will have to make an effort. It is not an easy thing at all to fail, it is difficult, you have to try, or you make an effort to do the impossible in order to fail. To prove that imperfect sight is more difficult and requires hard work, a great deal of trouble, and much effort, is a great benefit.

Better Eyesight magazine, January 1924: "The normal eye is only at rest when it is moving.... "

Better Eyesight magazine, March 1924:

> 1. Imperfect sight is the result of hard work; effort produces strain; perfect sight is attained with ease; lack of effort produces relaxation.
> 2. Tension indicates imperfect relaxation; stare, effort, trying to see—these interfere with perfect vision.
> 3. Under strain one cannot imagine, remember, nor see perfectly.

Better Eyesight magazine, December 1925 (notice how Bates combines the three principles of normal vision—movement, centralization, and relaxation):

> SHIFTING
>
> ...All persons with normal eyes and normal sight do not concentrate or try to see by any effort. Their eyes are at rest, and when the eyes are at rest, they are constantly moving. When the eyes move, one is able to imagine stationary objects, in turn, to be moving in the direction opposite of the head and eyes. It is impossible to imagine, with equal clearness, a number of objects to be moving at the same time, and an effort to do so is a strain which impairs the vision, the memory, or the imagination. To try to do the impossible is a strain which always lowers the mental efficiency. This fact should be emphasized. Many students have difficulty in imagining stationary objects to be moving opposite to the movements of the eyes or head ... When pain, fatigue or other symptoms are present, it always means that the individual is consciously or unconsciously trying to imagine stationary objects are not moving. The effect is a strain ... The right way to shift is to move the eyes [and head] from one point to another slowly, regularly, continuously, restfully or easily without effort or without trying to see ... When the vision is imperfect, objects not observed may be seen better, or an effort is made to see them better than those directly observed. In fact, it is always true, that in all cases of imperfect sight, the eyes do not see best where they are looking and centralization is lost. To shift properly requires relaxation or rest. To shift improperly and lower the vision requires an effort. When one stares at a point without blinking or shifting, fatigue, distress or pain is felt. To continue to stare without shifting is hard work. To see imperfectly is difficult ... Imperfect sight or a failure to see requires much trouble and hard work. This fact should be demonstrated repeatedly by the student until thoroughly convinced that rest of the eyes, mind or body can only be obtained by shifting easily, continuously, and without effort.

Better Eyesight magazine, January 1926 (repeated from the Movement chapter): "SWINGING.... make no effort to imagine stationary objects to be moving."

Better Eyesight magazine, October 1927: "... relaxation is always a benefit, not only to the eyes, but to all the nerves of the body."

Better Eyesight magazine, December 1927:

> *Question:* Trying to make things move gives me a headache ... Why?
>
> *Answer:* Making an effort to do a thing will not help you. When you are walking along the street, the street should appear to go in the opposite direction without effort on your part ...
>
> *Question:* Why do "movies" hurt my eyes when they should benefit them?
>
> *Answer:* Unconscious strain. Do not stare at the pictures, but allow the eyes [and head] to roam over the whole picture, seeing one part best. Also keep things swinging.

Better Eyesight magazine, March 1928:

> When the period [or any other small object of interest] has a slow, short, easy swing, the eye is at rest and when it is at rest it is always moving to prevent concentration, trying to see and other efforts to improve the vision.
>
> It has been demonstrated that when the vision is good, any effort, no matter how

> slight, always impairs or lowers it. When this truth is demonstrated, it follows that normal vision cannot be obtained when an effort is employed.
>
> ... With perfect sight, no blur is seen, and the eyes are at rest.

MORE ON RELAXATION

Ophthalmologist R. S. Agarwal writes:

> Preservation of good eyesight is almost impossible without proper eye education and mental relaxation. The quieter the mind, the better is the eyesight preserved[2]. . . . I found this view card of Tåj Mahal more charming and beautiful, very relaxing to the mind. Anything which relaxes the mind is a benefit to the eyesight.[3]

Jacob Liberman, Ph.D., O.D., writes in *Light: Medicine of the Future,* "... our eyes are meant to see for us, if we let them. In other words, *vision is meant to be effortless*."[4]

Aldous Huxley writes, "Learn to combine relaxation with activity; learn to do what you have to do without strain; work hard, but never under tension."[5]

A mother rocks her baby to sleep. Movement is relaxing.

Vision is primarily a receptive activity.

THE PROBLEM IS ABNORMAL STRAIN

From Chapter X, "Strain," in *Perfect Sight Without Glasses:*

> Temporary conditions may contribute to the strain to see which results in the production of errors of refraction; but its foundation lies in wrong habits of thought. In attempting to relieve it the physician has continually to struggle against the idea that to do anything well requires effort. This idea is drilled into us from our cradles. The whole educational system is based upon it; and in spite of the wonderful results attained by Montessori through the total elimination of every species of compulsion in the educational process, educators who call themselves modern still cling to the club, under various disguises, as a necessary auxiliary to the process of imparting knowledge.
>
> It is as natural for the eye to see as it is for the mind to acquire knowledge, and any effort in either case is not only useless, but defeats the end in view. You may force a few facts into a child's mind by various kinds of compulsion, but you cannot make it learn anything. The facts remain, if they remain at all, as dead lumber in the brain. They contribute nothing to the vital processes of thought; and because they were not acquired naturally and not assimilated, they destroy the natural impulse of the mind toward the acquisition of knowledge, and by the time the child leaves school or college, as the case may be, it not only knows nothing but is, in the majority of cases, no longer capable of learning.
>
> In the same way you may temporarily improve the sight by effort, but you cannot improve it to normal, and if the effort is allowed to become continuous, the sight will steadily deteriorate and may eventually be destroyed. Very seldom is the impairment or destruction of vision due to any fault in the construction of the eye. Of two equally good pairs of eyes one will retain perfect sight to the end of life, and the other will lose it in the kindergarten, simply because one looks at things without effort and the other does not.
>
> The eye with normal sight never tries to see. If for any reason, such as the dimness of the light, or the distance of the object, it

cannot see a particular point, it shifts to another. It never tries to bring out the point by staring at it, as the eye with imperfect sight is constantly doing.

Whenever the eye tries to see, it at once ceases to have normal vision. A person may look at the stars with normal vision; but if he tries to count the stars in any particular constellation, he will probably become myopic, because the attempt to do these things usually results in an effort to see. One person was able to look at the letter K on the Snellen card with normal vision, but when asked to count its twenty-seven corners he lost it completely.

It obviously requires a strain to fail to see at the distance, because the eye at rest is adjusted for distant vision. If one does anything when one wants to see at the distance, one must do the wrong thing. The shape of the eyeball cannot be altered during distant vision without strain. It is equally a strain to fail to see at the near point, because when the muscles respond to the mind's desire they do it without strain. Only by an effort can one prevent the eye from elongating at the near point.

The eye possesses perfect vision only when it is absolutely at rest....

Things are seen, just as they are felt, or heard, or tasted, without effort or volition on the part of the subject. When sight is perfect the letters on the Snellen card are waiting, perfectly black and perfectly distinct, to be recognized. They do not have to be sought; they are there. In imperfect sight they are sought and chased. The eye goes after them. An effort is made to see them.

The muscles of the body are supposed never to be at rest. The blood-vessels, with their muscular coats, are never at rest. Even in sleep thought does not cease. But the normal condition of the nerves of sense—of hearing, sight, taste, smell and touch—is one of rest. They can be acted upon; they cannot act. The optic nerve, the retina and the visual centers of the brain are as passive as the finger-nail. They have nothing whatever in their structure that makes it possible for them to do anything, and when they are the subject of effort from outside sources their efficiency is always impaired.

The mind is the source of all such efforts from outside sources brought to bear upon the eye. Every thought of effort in the mind, of whatever sort, transmits a motor impulse to the eye; and every such impulse causes a deviation from the normal in the shape of the eyeball and lessens the sensitiveness of the center of sight. *If one wants to have perfect sight, therefore, one must have no thought of effort in the mind.* [TQ emphasis.] Mental strain of any kind always produces a conscious or unconscious eyestrain and if the strain takes the form of an effort to see, an error of refraction is always produced.... Unfamiliar objects produce eyestrain and a consequent error of refraction, because they first produce mental strain. A person may have good vision when he is telling the truth; but if he states what is not true, even with no intent to deceive, or if he imagines what is not true, an error of refraction will be produced....

Mental strain may produce many different kinds of eyestrain. According to the statement of most authorities there is only one kind of eyestrain, an indefinite thing resulting from so-called overuse of the eyes, or an effort to overcome a wrong shape of the eyeball. It can be demonstrated, however, that there is not only a different strain for each different error of refraction, but a different strain for most abnormal conditions of the eye....

The health of the eye depends upon the blood, and circulation is very largely influ-

> enced by thought. When thought is normal—that is, not attended by any excitement or strain—the circulation in the brain is normal, the supply of blood to the optic nerve and the visual centers is normal, and the vision is perfect. When thought is abnormal the circulation is disturbed, the supply of blood to the optic nerve and visual centers is altered, and the vision lowered. We can consciously think thoughts which disturb the circulation and lower the visual power; we can also consciously think thoughts that will restore normal circulation, and thereby reverse, not only all errors of refraction, but many other abnormal conditions of the eyes. We cannot by any amount of effort make ourselves see, but by learning to control our thoughts we can accomplish that end indirectly.
>
> You can teach people how to produce any error of refraction, how to produce a squint [strabismus], how to see two images of an object, one above another, or side by side, or at any desired angle from one another, simply by teaching them how to think in a particular way. When the disturbing thought is replaced by one that relaxes, the squint disappears, the double vision and the errors of refraction are corrected; and this is as true of abnormalities of long standing as of those produced voluntarily. No matter what their degree or their duration their reversal is accomplished just as soon as the person is able to secure mental control. The cause of any error of refraction, of a squint, or of any other functional disturbance of the eye, is simply a thought—a wrong thought—and the reversal is as quick as the thought that relaxes. In a fraction of a second the highest degrees of refractive error may be corrected, a squint may disappear, or the blindness of amblyopia may be relieved. If the relaxation is only momentary, the correction is momentary. When it becomes permanent, the correction is permanent.
>
> This relaxation cannot, however, be obtained by any sort of effort. It is fundamental that students should understand this; for so long as they think, consciously or unconsciously, that relief from strain may be obtained by another strain their reversal will be delayed.

From Bates' writing above, it is clear that strain is the cause of most vision problems. The individual with blurred vision is interfering with the normal, relaxed way of using the mind and body.

Better Eyesight magazine, September 1920:

> SLEEPINESS AND EYESTRAIN
>
> ... eyestrain has always been demonstrated when fatigue was present, and that fatigue has always been relieved when eyestrain was relieved. Perfect sight is perfect rest, and cannot coexist with fatigue.... Sleepiness is a common symptom of habitual eyestrain, and when the sight improves the need for sleep is often markedly reduced.

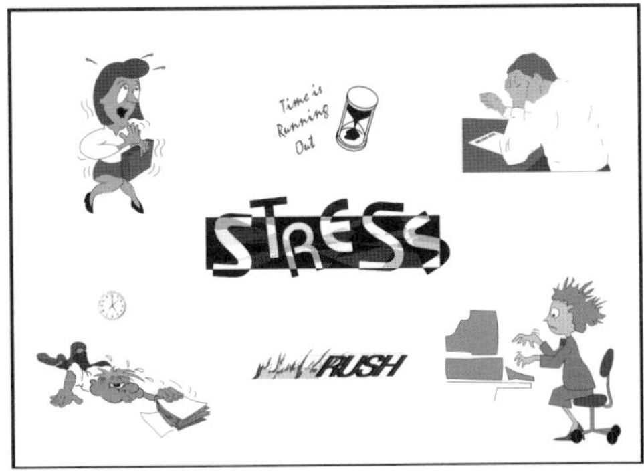

Figure 11–2: Stress.

Optometrist Bruce May states: "Essentially, myopia appears to be the response of the total person to some form of stress."[6]

An optician told one of my students, "The only time I need my bifocals is when I have a lot of stress."

RELAXATION—THE HEARING CONNECTION

See *Figure 9–7: The Vestibulo-Ocular Connection*.

Margaret Corbett writes in her book *Help Yourself to Better Sight:*

> All the special senses work together—seeing, hearing, smelling, tasting, and touching. If the nerves governing one of these special senses are tense, all are tense—if relaxed, all are relaxed. We who teach eye relaxation always notice that, as we build vision, the hearing becomes more acute.[7]

From *Better Eyesight* magazine, March 1920:

> Along with the improvement in her eyes has been a considerable improvement in her hearing. Noises in her ears which she describes as a "ringing and a singing" are promptly relieved by palming, and she says that the relief, which at first was only temporary, is now becoming constant. She also says that she hears conversation better than she used to.

THE SOLUTION IS RELAXATION

Relaxation is the basis of natural, clear vision. Whatever a student does to secure a greater relaxation automatically supports better vision.

Many students have changed their ways of living to improve their vision. Several of my students have quit stressful jobs they felt were not only interfering with relaxed vision habits, but were interfering with their overall health and happiness.

Some students have started massage therapy or other forms of natural healing to accelerate the release of tension created by many years of strained vision habits.

Most people would agree that stress is a major problem in our society today. Some researchers have shown that stress levels have risen exponentially in the last several decades.

Vision improves automatically by eliminating the incorrect, strained vision habits we acquired which lowered the vision in the first place. Clarity is automatic.

A balloon floats on the top of the water automatically. But, if enough weights are

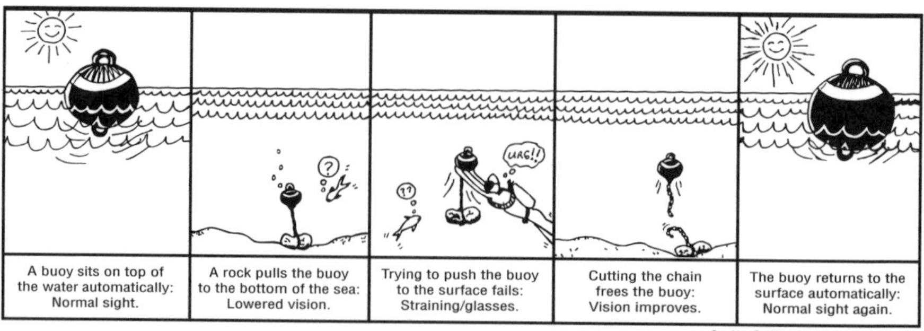

UAG!!
A buoy sits on top of the water automatically: Normal sight.
A rock pulls the buoy to the bottom of the sea: Lowered vision.
Trying to push the buoy to the surface fails: Straining/glasses.
Cutting the chain frees the buoy: Vision improves.
The buoy returns to the surface automatically: Normal sight again.
Graphics © 1995 Annie Buttons, Eagle•Eye/NEI

Figure 11–3: "A Buoy." Reprinted with permission from Annie Buttons.

attached to the balloon, it will sink to the bottom of the sea. Straining to push the balloon to the surface again will only fail. It will keep falling to the bottom of the sea over and over again. The solution is to simply remove the weights from the balloon. It then automatically floats to the surface again. No effort is needed.

MOVEMENT = CENTRALIZATION = RELAXATION = CLARITY

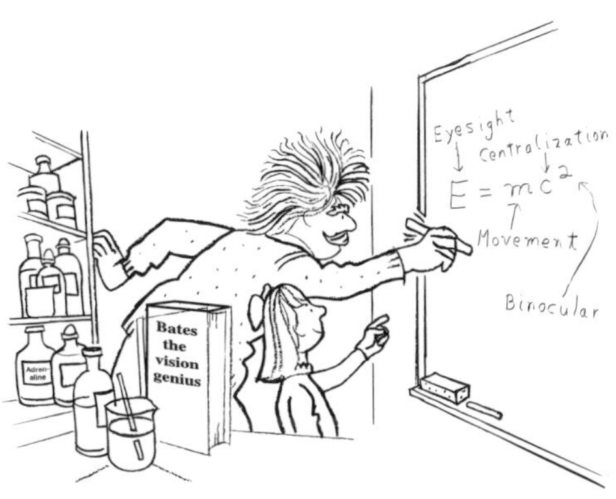

Figure 11–4: E=mc².

Bates wrote in the May 8, 1915, issue of the *New York Medical Journal:*

> The sole cause of all uncomplicated or functional errors of refraction is a conscious or an unconscious effort or strain to see. The only solution to this strain is relaxation. Relaxation or rest of the eyes is accomplished only by centralization.[8]

In the beginning, students often think that the three principles of natural vision are separate from each other. But as they re-integrate these three principles more each day, they realize that movement goes with centralization which goes with relaxation.

If the student of natural vision accepts the idea that the re-establishment of visual relaxation is the key to normal vision, the question then becomes, "What is visual relaxation?" The answer is found in the three habits of natural seeing—Sketch (Shift), Breathe, and Blink, discussed next.

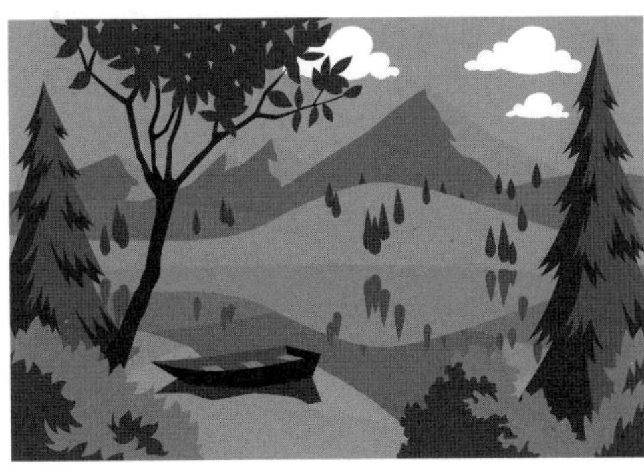

Notes

1 Margaret Y. Ferguson, "The Dr. Bates Method of Eye Training" in the *Journal of the California Chiropractic Association,* December 1945, p. 13.

2 R. S. Agarwal, *Mind and Vision* (Pondicherry, India: Sri Aurobindo Ashram Press, 1983), p. 1.

3 Ibid., p. 146.

4 Jacob Liberman, *Light: Medicine of the Future* (Santa Fe: Bear & Co., 1991), p. xx.

5 Aldous Huxley, *The Art of Seeing* (New York: Harper & Brothers Publishers, 1942), p. 37.

6 Bruce May, *Rx for Nearsightedness: Stress-Relieving Lenses,* Optometric Extension Program Foundation pamphlet (1981).

7 Margaret D. Corbett, *Help Yourself to Better Sight* (North Hollywood, CA: Wilshire Book Co., 1949), p. 201.

8 William H. Bates, "The Reversal of Errors of Refraction by Education Without Glasses" in the *New York Medical Journal,* May 8, 1915.

PART FOUR

The Three Habits of Natural Vision

The three habits of natural seeing are Sketching (Shifting), Breathing, and Blinking.

CHAPTER TWELVE

The First Habit—Sketching (Shifting)

SKETCH

Sketching, or "shifting" as Bates called it, is the first habit of natural vision. Sketching teaches the student two of the three principles of normal sight—movement and centralization. Movement and centralization were discussed extensively in previous chapters.

BATES ON SHIFTING

Better Eyesight magazine, September 1927:

> Shift your glance constantly from one point to another, seeing the part regarded best and other parts not so clearly. That is, when you look at a chair, do not try to see the whole object at once; look first at the back of it, seeing that part best and other parts worse.... This is centralizing.... Your head and eyes are moving all day long.

One might think that in order to see an object clearly, one must lock the sight rigidly onto the object of interest. The opposite is

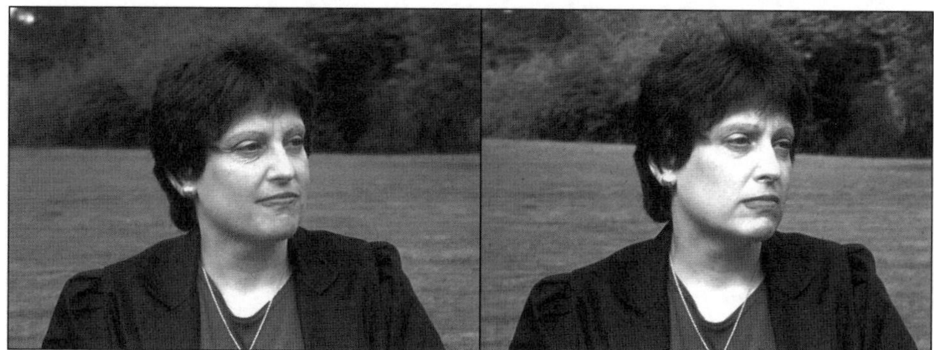

Figure 12–1: Sketching vs. Staring.

the case. Never lock your vision; sketch or shift to different objects all day long.

Better Eyesight magazine, December 1927:

> The importance of practicing certain parts of the routine habits at all times, such as blinking, centralizing . . . , and imagining stationary objects to be moving opposite to the movement of the head and eyes, is stressed.

In the last two quotes from Bates, in using the phrases "all day long" and "at all times," it is clear that the Bates method is not about "eye exercises." Natural vision habits are the keys to normal sight. As I like to remind my students frequently, the three habits of natural vision are not necessary more than twenty-four hours per day!

From *Perfect Sight Without Glasses:*

> Shifting may be done slowly or rapidly, according to the state of the vision. At the beginning the person will be likely to strain if he shifts too rapidly; and then the point shifted from will not be seen worse, and there will be no swing. As improvement is made, the speed can be increased. It is usually impossible, however, to realize the swing if the shifting is more rapid than two or three times a second.

"To realize the swing" means to notice the illusion of oppositional movement, discussed in the Chapter 9, "The First Principle—Movement," and Chapter 10, "The Second Principle—Centralization."

THE NOSE-HELPERS

See *Plate 11: The Nose-Helpers.*

Bates referred to first habit of natural vision in various ways—shifting, swinging, swaying, and dodging (the stare).

Many modern Bates teachers have utilized the idea of a nose-helper to teach shifting. The nose-helpers include the nose-pencil for "sketching" objects, the nose-feather for "brushing," the nose-paintbrush for "painting," the nose-crayon for "drawing," and/or the nose-laser beam for "beaming."

Natural vision students can use one, some, all, or none of the nose-helpers.

Sketching, shifting, swinging, swaying, dodging, brushing, painting, drawing, and beaming all refer to the same habit. These words can be used interchangeably. They all teach the student to move and centralize.

SKETCHING WITH THE NOSE-PENCIL

Sketching involves an imaginary nose-pencil. The student pretends the erasure end of the pencil is attached to the tip of the nose using imaginary super-glue. The student can then "sketch" the world all day long.

Characteristics of the imaginary nose-pencil are:

1. It is thin and weightless; sketching is easy and effortless;
2. It becomes longer and shorter as you sketch far objects, then midrange objects, then near objects and back again; it changes its length instantaneously and automatically; and
3. The point of the pencil touches the object you are sketching at all times. The nose-pencil is a way of visually "reconnecting" to the world. (Blurry, diffused vision is a "disconnection" from objects in the world.)

In the beginning, the simplest and easiest form of sketching is "edging" or "outlining." Simply trace the shape of a tree, house, flower, door, and so on. In art, students are taught to first draw the outline of an object, and then to fill in the details. So it is with the sketching habit. For example, after sketching the outline of a house, sketch the windows, doors, curtains, chimney, shutters, walkway, and so on. Interest, curiosity, and discovery are key characteristics of normal sight. Similarly, after sketching the outline of a tree, sketch the branches and leaves.

Vision Functions by Edges

Cover the middle vertical edge of *Plate 12: The Edge* with your finger, a ruler, or pencil. Does the right half now look the same as the left half?! What is happening?

Sight functions primarily by detecting edges. *The Edge* is composed of two identical gradients. Both gradients are lighter on the right, and gradually become darker toward the left. The edge in the middle appears where the darker edge of the right gradient meets with the lighter edge of the left gradient! However, when this edge is covered, the eyes no longer have a "clue" as to the change between the two gradients.

Show this page to a friend with the middle edge covered with a ruler. Ask your friend if there is any difference between the left side of the right half and the right side of the left half. Then take away the ruler. Surprise!

Move the Head, Not Just the Eyes

The nose-pencil is attached to the nose to remind us to move the head—not just the eyes. By moving the head while keeping our primary interest where the nose-pencil is touching, it is impossible to stare.

The purpose of sketching is to eliminate the habit of staring. This is of greatest importance. Bates and many other researchers have proven it is impossible to see clearly while staring. Ultimately, staring must be eliminated to have normal vision.

If it seems to the reader I am belaboring the issue of not staring—I am doing so on purpose. The staring habit is deeply ingrained in many students, and the importance of relearning natural movement and centralization cannot be overemphasized. Repetition is an important part of teaching students how to improve their sight.

The Picture is *Inside,* not Outside

The *picture* we see is not out in the world. Objects are out in the world, and light rays from those objects enter our eyes. Light rays land on the retina, and then, stimulated light receptors send messages along the optic nerve to the brain. The picture we see is formed in the brain.

So, in reality, we are sketching the picture created in and by the brain. You might think about sketching as if you were a one-inch-tall person sitting inside of your brain and sketching the picture formed inside your brain.

This is one reason straining to see does not make any sense. If the picture were out in the world, it might make sense to strain to see it *out there.* But the picture is *not* out there; it is in the brain. A person who is straining to see is straining to see the picture inside the brain. I call this "brain strain." This makes no sense, because there are no muscles in the brain! Perfect, normal sight requires no effort, and Bates frequently stated that any effort to see lowers vision.

The nose-pencil reconnects the student to herself inside the brain. Blur is not caused by external stimuli so much as how a person *responds* internally to the external stimuli. The return to clarity is a reflection of an individual's return to a normal, healthy state of *internal* relaxation—a return to a balance with nature.

Artificial Improvement Is Not Sufficient

Any form of artificial eyesight "correction" will never address the real cause of blurred vision. The original strain remains until it is released by the individual. Natural clarity *and blur* are in the hands of the individual—and no one else. The purpose of natural vision classes is to educate an individual how he can re-establish his own normal vision.

Some people subconsciously and "spontaneously" re-establish their own natural, clear sight. Since returning to clarity can be accomplished *without even knowing what to do,* a student can return to clarity *by knowing what to do*.

SHIFTING VS. SKETCHING

Sometimes Bates' term "shifting" will feel more natural than "sketching" or "brushing." For example, if you are interested in pebbles on a beach (re: The Pebble Game), you might "shift" from one to another. But, if you are watching a bird flying over a field, following it with a smooth nose-feather motion might feel more natural. As long as the principles of movement and centralization are incorporated, and you are not straining to see, you are practicing the first habit of natural vision correctly.

Movement + Centralization = Sketching or Shifting.

VARIATIONS ON NOSE-PENCIL SKETCHING

Four variations on the nose-pencil are the Nose-Feather, the Nose-Paintbrush, the Nose-Crayon, and the Nose-Laser Beam.

The Nose-Feather

The nose-feather image is especially valuable in learning the *ease* of natural seeing. It is also helpful in improving texture awareness. The nose-feather is not wide, like a fluffy plume (sorry), because a wide feather could encourage diffusion. A thin feather reminds the student to centralize.

One elderly woman I taught kept complaining every week that she just could not "get" the nose-feather image on her nose. In the last class, she said she had good news and bad news. "I finally 'got' the nose-feather—but now I can't get rid of it! It is there on my nose everywhere I go!"

The Nose-Paintbrush

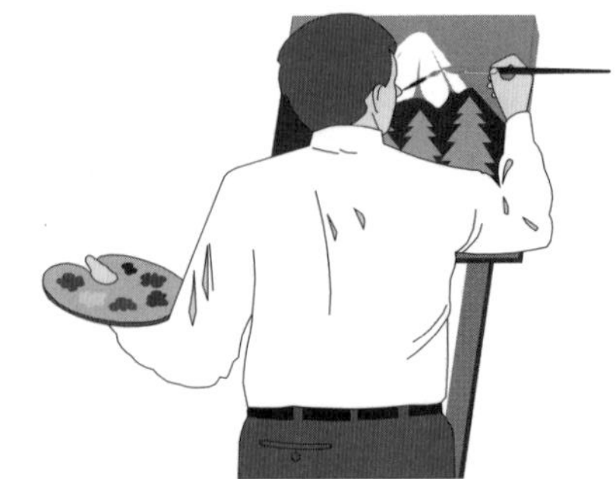

The nose-paintbrush is excellent for that artist inside all of us. Aldous Huxley's natural vision improvement book is appropriately entitled *The Art of Seeing.* Fortunately, there is an infinite supply of imaginary paint to paint the world for your entire lifetime!

The Nose-Crayon

Children enjoy "nose-doodling" with the nose-crayon. Teach your children to nose-doodle, breathe, and blink all day long!

The Nose-Laser Beam, the "High-Tech" Nose-Helper

The nose-laser beam is the "high-tech" vision improvement helper. Pretend the nose-laser beam illuminates the small point where you are centralizing. Everything around that point is less clear. This is a powerful image for many students.

I began using the nose-laser beam after observing a student tilting his head down much of the time in the first few classes. When I asked him if he was using his nose-feather, which he obviously wasn't, he answered, "No. It is too heavy!" He had excellent progress after switching to the nose-laser beam.

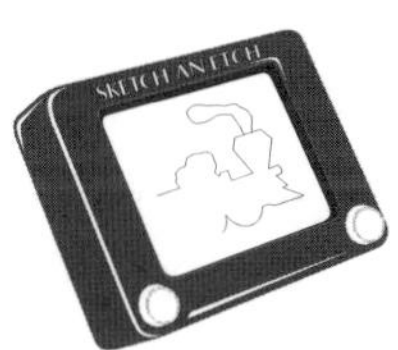

Yes, You Can Imagine, or Pretend!

Some students tell me they cannot "imagine." This is not true. Everyone can imagine. I have not had one student in thirteen years of teaching who told me they could not imagine painting a large pink elephant when their eyelids were closed!

Some students prefer the word "pretend" instead of imagine. Everyone can pretend. Children frequently pretend while playing games.

I do not teach "visualizing" to my students. Visualizing means you can actually "see" the object you are creating in your mind—as if it were actually in front of you. Visualizing is not necessary for improving vision.

Nose-Helper Not Essential; Movement and Centralization Are

Some students say they do not like any of the nose-helpers. This is fine as long as the student relearns movement and centralization. Bates did not use any nose-helpers while teaching his students to improve their vision. The nose-helpers are simply a playful way to help re-integrate two of the three key principles—movement and centralization.

Bates taught his students to "shift." Shifting includes both movement and centralization. Specific activities Bates created—for example, the Long Swing and the Sway—were designed to teach students to move and centralize all day long. If the student relearns the principles and habits of natural vision without a nose-helper, there will be no disadvantage in the long run.

Remember, people with normal sight usually are not aware of the correct habits they are using all day long.

Sketching (Shifting) Is Not an Exercise; It Is a Habit!

Sketching, or shifting, is the correct way of seeing the world—all day long. It is *not* an eye exercise. It is the first of the three key vision *habits*.

The key to Bates' work was not "eye exercises"—as many people mistakenly believe. People who talk about "Bates eye exercises" often do not understand Bates' work. Many people fail with the eye-exercise approach because the habits of natural seeing are not relearned. Exercises are practiced for a short time each day; vision habits are for twenty-four hours per day.

It is not due to not doing "eye exercises" the vision became blurred—it is due to the formation of strained vision habits. Therefore, eye exercises are not the solution to blur.

Bates discovered how we are meant to see all day long. He taught his students to relearn the correct *habits* of natural vision—permanently.

BUT IT DOESN'T FEEL NATURAL (AT FIRST)

For many students, sketching feels unnatural in the beginning. This reaction occurs for three main reasons:

1. Sketching is somewhat exaggerated in the beginning. Larger sketching is best in the beginning to be sure the head is released and mobile. Ultimately the head movement can be very small, barely perceptible by other people, but the head and neck are still relaxed and mobile;
2. Blurred vision is slow, or "frozen," vision; normal vision is "swift" vision. It takes time to relearn swift, constantly shifting sight;
3. Sketching and shifting *consciously* is unnatural.

The three habits of natural vision are meant to be subconscious. As long as the habits students are practicing are conscious, they are not normal or natural. Of course, they become subconscious, normal, and natural by practicing them more and better each day.

THE MIND IS PRIMARY

What we see is conscious; but *how* we see is meant to be subconscious. I believe this is one of the reasons people have so many problems with their vision. Too much conscious attention is directed to the eyes. People use eyeglasses, contact lenses, unnecessary eye drugs, and eye surgeries—it is all about the eyes. This was not nature's plan for the visual system.

It is interesting when potential students talk to me about their sight, how many people say to me, "I use my eyes a lot!"—as if they are *consciously* trying to see all day. Babies and animals do not know they have eyes. They have pictures which are created in their minds, and they move their body and *interest* through these pictures all day long. The eyes are not consciously involved. This is important. Students are interested in improving their *sight.* Awareness of eyes is not necessary. The sooner a student forgets the eyes exist, the faster will be the improvement of sight.

As students practice sketching, many find they are doing well at moving the head, but they are not centralizing—their attention is not at the tip of the nose-pencil. Centralization is a more subtle concept than movement, and generally takes longer to relearn. After a while, the student realizes it does not make any sense to move the head unless he is shifting his *attention* from one point to another. *The mind is primary; the eyes are secondary.*

MORE WHAT WE ARE UNLEARNING THAN LEARNING

From *Better Eyesight* magazine, December 1925:

> The [key to the] reversal of imperfect sight then, is to stop all effort. It is not accomplished by doing things. It can only come by the things that one stops doing.

The purpose of sketching is to eliminate the staring habit. It isn't so much what a student is *doing* that improves vision as much as what the student is *not doing.* Staring and straining to see lower vision; *not* staring and *not* straining improves vision—automatically.

It may be helpful to remember most people have clarity early in life. Correct vision habits are present whenever a person has normal, clear vision; and when vision is normal, it is completely natural, automatic, subconscious, and effortless.

Basically, a Natural Vision teacher reminds students of exactly the same vision habits they used to have when their vision was clear.

Chapter Thirteen

The Second Habit—Breathing

The second habit of natural vision is breathing. Natural, abdominal breathing is basic, fundamental, and essential for normal health and normal sight.

ANATOMY OF BREATHING

See *Figure 13–1: The Respiratory System.*

The respiratory system is composed primarily of the nasal passages, trachea (windpipe), two lungs, and the diaphragm.

The lungs are large, pink-gray, highly elastic, cone-shaped organs. The lung on the right side of the body has three lobes, while the lung on the left side has two lobes. The absence of a third left lobe allows room for the heart.

The inside surface area of the lungs, where oxygen and carbon dioxide are exchanged, is about thirty times the surface area of the skin—nearly 600 square feet! The lungs themselves do not actually "breathe." Breathing is performed primarily by the diaphragm.

The diaphragm is a large, powerful, tough, dome-shaped muscle which lies below the two lungs and the heart. The diaphragm is not attached to the lungs. The digestive organs lie below the diaphragm—the liver below the right side of the diaphragm, and the stomach, spleen, and left kidney below the left side.

NATURAL, ABDOMINAL BREATHING

Abdominal Breathing

See *Plate 13: Abdominal Breathing.*

The lungs do not expand and contract by themselves. The diaphragm and intercostal muscles expand and contract the ribcage, and their combined motions create an expansion and contraction of the lungs.

When we inhale, the diaphragm tenses (contracts) and moves downward into a flatter, shorter shape. The lungs then expand and fill with oxygen.

When we exhale, the diaphragm relaxes (expands) and moves upward into a more curved, longer shape. The lungs then contract and expel carbon dioxide and other gases. The majority of air inhaled and exhaled is effected by the action of the diaphragm. The movement of the diaphragm up and down is about two or three inches. The diaphragm is the largest internal moving part of the human body.

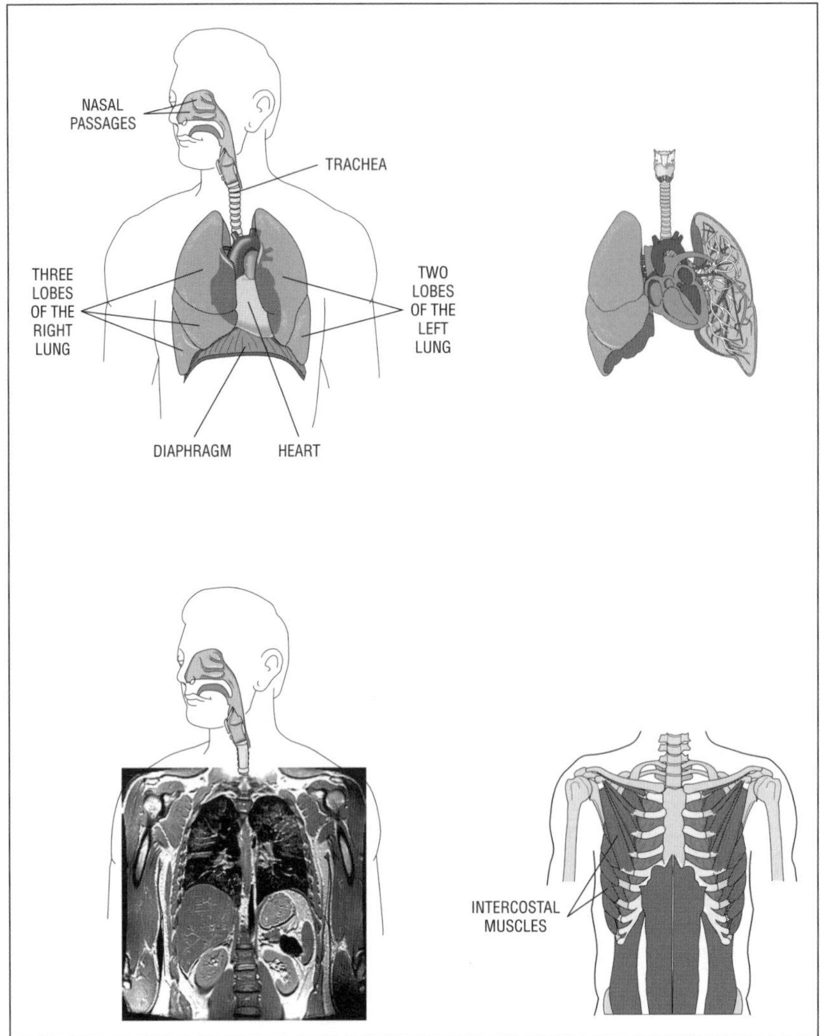

Figure 13–1: The Respiratory System.

In addition to the diaphragm, the intercostal muscles expand and contract the ribcage (chest), aiding inhalation and exhalation. The diaphragm and ribcage movements aid the circulation of blood and other fluids in the body.

Natural breathing is primarily diaphragmatic, abdominal, or "tummy" breathing. Although breathing can be controlled consciously to some extent, breathing is usually an automatic, subconscious activity. The normal breathing rate is approximately sixteen breaths per minute.

During inhalation the downward movement of the diaphragm pushes down on the digestive organs in the abdomen, which then expands outward. (Air does not fill the abdomen!) During the second half of inhalation the chest expands slightly outward and upward. There is also a small expansion on the right and left sides of the abdomen and ribcage and the back.

It is important not to pull the abdomen inward while inhaling; similarly, do not use the neck and shoulder muscles to lift the shoulders. Many people have formed these two incorrect patterns of breathing.

During exhalation the diaphragm returns upward, releasing pressure on the digestive organs, which then move back to their original positions. During the first half of exhalation the chest, abdominal sides, and back return to their original contracted positions.

Breathing through the Nose

Breathe through the nose, not the mouth. Nasal passages, mucus, and cilia in the nose help filter out dust and bacteria from the air. Cilia are little hairs that beat in the opposite direction of the incoming air. The nasal passages also help warm the air to body temperature before the incoming air reaches the capillaries in the lungs.

SHALLOW/CHEST BREATHING

Many natural vision students have discovered that they do not breathe naturally. They have shallow, "chest" or thoracic breathing. Oftentimes the breathing pattern consists of short gasps of air. Shallow breathing is not only an incorrect vision habit, it is an incorrect living habit. Restrictive breathing is a result of stress. And it can become a vicious cycle—shallow breathing reduces the amount of oxygen to the heart, which creates more tension in the muscles and nerves of the body, which constricts the breathing further. The abdominal muscles are contracted chronically tight when the tummy is pulled continually inward. This allows the lungs to expand only in the chest area, and therefore, breathing is very limited.

One of my students said, "I'm surprised I'm alive because I found out this week that I never breathe!"

Emotional, mental, or spiritual distress, repressed feelings, birth trauma, accidents, illness, incorrect diet, and polluted and/or stagnant air can lead to shallow chest breathing.

June Biermann and Barbara Toohey write in their book *The Woman's Holistic Headache Relief Book:*

> BODY SIGNALS
>
> Besides monitoring your life changes for stress, you can also watch your body patterns. Our bodies give off signals when they're tense. Learn these signals and you'll know when you'd better start doing something about the tightness, tension, and anxiety you're exhibiting.
>
> Breathing. The best indicator of what's going on inside you. Often the very first sign. Short and shallow means tension; holding your breath means extreme tension.[1]

Tip: If a truck or car passes by you with a lot of toxic fumes, take a deep breath of air before the fumes reach you, and then slowly exhale until the fumes are gone.

Some students feel discouraged when they discover they have incorrect breathing habits. I was at first, but I was also happy to discover them because I could start relearning natural breathing again.

Tip: If you find a moment when you are

not breathing, exhale whatever air is in your lungs, then inhale. It is easier to exhale first than inhale from a non-breathing state.

Some singing teachers teach their students abdominal breathing by having them lie on the floor on their back and placing a book on their abdomen. The teacher says, "Now, let's move the book upward and downward by abdominal breathing." A person who attempts to sing using shallow chest breathing will soon become exhausted.

EXPERIENCE ABDOMINAL BREATHING

If you become light-headed or dizzy while experiencing abdominal breathing activities, stop and come back to the activities later. These symptoms may be a temporary reaction to the incorrect habit of shallow breathing.

1. One of the best ways to study abdominal breathing is to lie comfortably on your back on a firm surface. Take off your shoes, watch, glasses/contact lenses. Wear loose clothing and place a small pillow or cushion under your knees. The mouth is closed and the jaw relaxed.

Close your eyelids. Place one hand on your abdomen and the other on your chest. The placement of your hands on the abdomen and chest helps you feel which area is rising and falling and when.

Exhale all of the air from your lungs. As you begin to slowly inhale, the abdomen and the hand on it should begin to rise. The chest

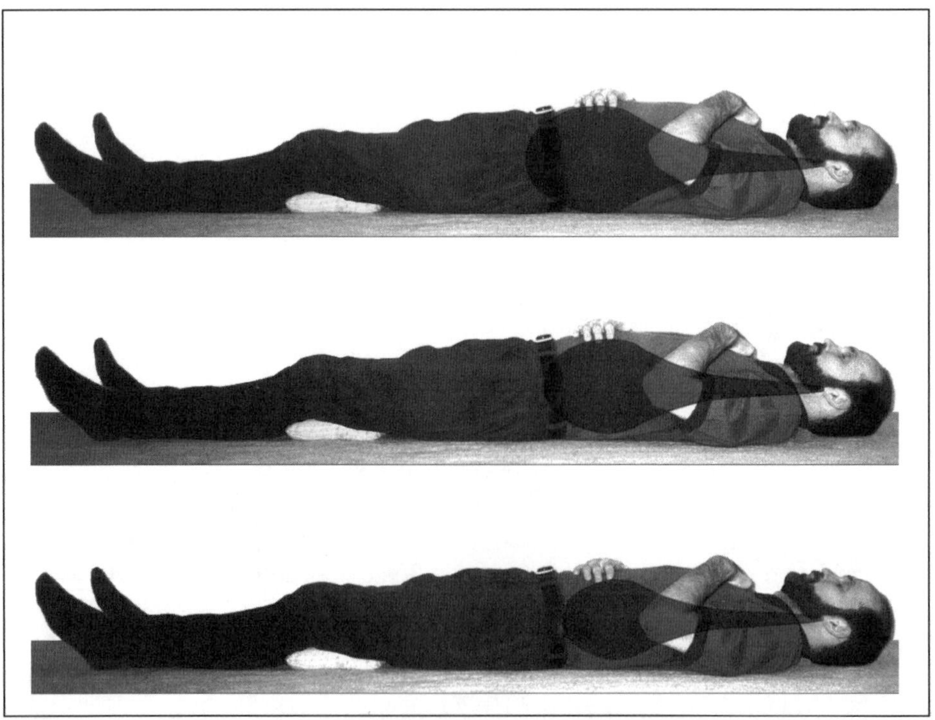

Figure 13–2: Experience Abdominal Breathing (1).

should rise slightly near the end of the inhale.

If the chest rises first, you probably do not have normal, abdominal breathing. Some students discover that the abdomen does not rise at all—only the chest.

As you begin to slowly exhale, the chest should lower slightly, followed by the lowering of the abdomen.

2. The above study of abdominal breathing can also be done sitting in a chair or even standing. One hand can be placed on the abdomen. Optionally, the other hand can be placed on the chest.

Many students have found an eyedropper image helpful to breathing properly. The idea is to study your breathing patterns so you can become aware of them. You can then practice better breathing habits a little more each day. Like sketching, abdominal breathing is not an exercise. The idea is to relearn abdominal breathing as a normal, natural habit.

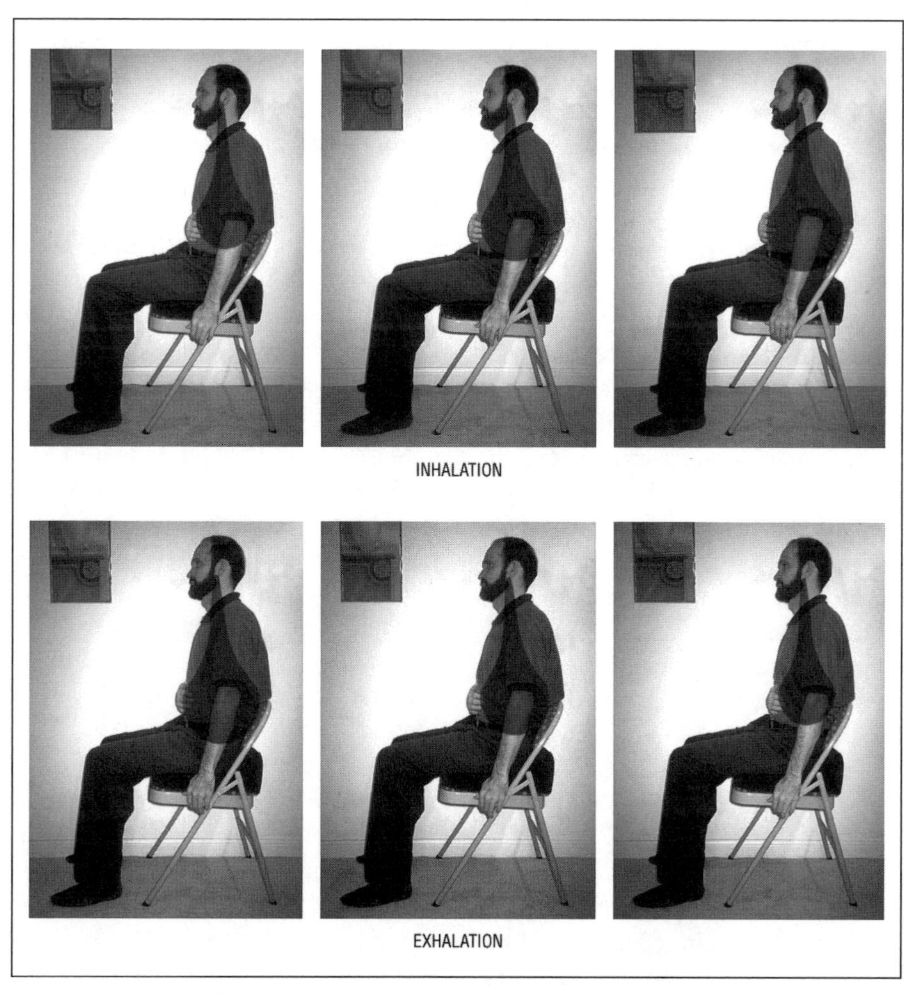

Figure 13–3: Experience Abdominal Breathing (2).

THE EMOTIONAL CONNECTION

It is not a coincidence that the diaphragm lies just below the heart. Abdominal breathing is literally an "opening" of the heart. Alexander Lowen discusses the relationship between the diaphragm and feelings connected with the heart in his book *Bioenergetics*.[2]

Breathing can dramatically affect our moods. If we have a lot of stress, breathing can help calm and center us. Slower breathing can slow down the rate of heartbeats.

Wilhelm Reich's work with character analysis led him to the therapeutic discovery of "muscular armoring" and his famous "Reichian body work." Repressed emotions can be frozen, or locked, in chronic muscle spasms. According to Reich, each emotion has an *impulse to action.* If the individual under stress does not release the emotional tension physically, by crying for example, muscles associated with the stress can become contracted. If this suppressive behavior becomes habitual, the person can acquire chronic spastic contractions. "Fight or flight," adrenaline-pumping stress can become the status quo. Normal breathing is interfered with, and the person forms a habit of shallow "chest" breathing.

Reich developed breathing techniques to reestablish a connection to the original crisis, and provided an opportunity for healing. The question is—if breathing shuts down due to a crisis, will the crisis be resolved when the breathing returns to normal? Many healers have concluded the answer is "Yes" in many cases.

Tom's Personal Log: During a stress-reduction workshop I took in 1980, many of the facilitators kept telling me that I was not breathing, and suggested I breathe more.

I knew I was good at not breathing for long periods. I was even proud of how long I could go without breathing.

The Monday morning following this workshop, my shoulders, chest, and abdomen dropped down into their normal positions. But it had been so long since they were in the normal positions, it hurt! I had to tighten my abdominal muscles to stop the pain. I began to realize how much tension I had been holding for many years.

After nine years of healing, my breathing had finally started to become normal.

I reached a breakthrough in 1990. During a particularly high period of stress, I checked my breathing pattern when preparing to go to sleep. I was sure my breathing would not be normal—but it was! I have come a long way in relearning normal, natural breathing.

One of my students said that she realized she had stopped her normal breathing long ago when, as a child, a big gust of wind blowing through a tunnel frightened her.

Many people hold their breath when they are "concentrating hard." The real problem starts when non-breathing and shallow breathing become habits. Then a person may not breathe correctly during activities in which he is not "concentrating hard."

Someone who sighs a lot is likely not breathing normally. The body is gasping for oxygen.

BREATHING AND STARING

Staring almost always accompanies shallow breathing or holding the breath. Many parts of the body can become tense and locked, especially the neck and shoulders. If incorrect breathing habits make a person stare, vision will lower.

BREATHING AND POSTURE

Correct posture is important to allow space for abdominal breathing. Incorrect posture, discussed in Chapter 9, "The First Principle—Movement," often accompanies staring.

TOM'S PERSONAL LOG: A short time after I began chiropractic healing, I discovered I slept in the fetal position: on my side, with my head, shoulders, and chest curled forward toward my bent knees. This incorrect posture constricts the lungs and prevents normal abdominal breathing. It took me more than a year to unlearn this fetal sleeping position.

SMOKING IS OUT

Toxins inhaled while smoking congest the capillaries in the lungs. These toxins reduce as much as 60% of oxygen that can be assimilated into the bloodstream, and reduce the elimination of carbon dioxide and other gases from the body.

Additionally, many people who smoke have poor night vision. Healthy rods in the retina can pick up extremely low levels of light at night. The ability is interfered with by toxins inhaled while smoking.

It is interesting to note that certain groups of human beings are the only creatures on this planet that do not run from smoke. Animals know better. Fortunately, it seems that many people are quitting this harmful habit.

EXERCISE, YOGA, AND BREATHING

Exercise is important for maintaining normal, abdominal breathing—especially in this modern age of sedentary occupations and lifestyles. Striding (brisk, energetic walking) and swimming are excellent for breathing and overall health. Walking, running (on appropriate surfaces), and bicycling are also very good.

Yoga is another excellent method of improving breathing and posture. Many yoga teachers emphasize maintaining regular, continuous breathing while performing various postures.

I do not teach students "deep" breathing, or controlled breathing. For vision, it is important to study the correct, natural pattern of abdominal breathing, and to integrate this habit back into our lives.

THE MOVEMENT CONNECTION

Breathing is a natural form of movement—an "internal massage"—essential for stimulation of and circulation in all of the organs and tissues of the body. Normal, diaphragmatic breathing directly and rhythmically stimulates the liver, stomach, colon, kidneys, pancreas, spleen, and other abdominal organs.

Important nerves and muscles pass through the diaphragm. A chronically tight diaphragm can interfere with digestion, elimination, the lower limbs, and sexual functions.

Acupuncture is concerned with the balanced movement of energy through the body. Shallow, constricted breathing blocks and imbalances the flow of energy. Proper breathing is a natural "energy pump," stimulating and balancing energy flow throughout the body.

TOM'S PERSONAL LOG: After years of massage therapy, chiropractic, and osteopathic work, I realized that in order for me to be healthy, my breathing needs to return to normal. I can have all the external bodywork done I want, but if I hold my diaphragm tight, I will never be completely relaxed and healthy.

THE CENTRALIZATION-RELAXATION CONNECTION

Many students discover a sense of "centeredness" as they relearn abdominal breathing. Natural breathing throughout the day helps one be calmer and more peaceful. Many yoga and meditation techniques use breathing as a method of concentration. Some breathing teachers emphasize the close relationship between breathing, relaxation, and concentration to release chronic tension.

BATES ON BREATHING

Bates makes only one reference to breathing in *Perfect Sight Without Glasses:* "Palming was successful in half an hour ... the nose opened, and the breathing [of a girl with a cold] ... became normal."

Although there is little reference to breathing in Bates' *Better Eyesight* magazines, many modern Bates teachers have taught abdominal breathing as a key natural vision habit. Normal breathing is connected to correct vision habits.

Better Eyesight magazine, January 1923:

> BREATHING
>
> Many people with imperfect sight are benefited by breathing. One of the best methods is to separate the teeth while keeping the lips closed, breathe deeply as if one were yawning. When done properly one can feel the air cold as it passes through the nose and down the throat. This method of breathing secures a great amount of relaxation of the nose, throat, the body generally, including the eyes and ears.
>
> A man aged sixty-five had imperfect sight for distance and was unable to read fine print without the aid of strong glasses. After practicing deep breathing in the manner described, he became able at once to read diamond type quite perfectly, as close as six inches from the eyes. The improvement was temporary but by repetition the improvement became more permanent.
>
> At one time I experimented with a number of students, first having them hold their breath and test their vision, which was usually lower when they did not breathe. They became able to demonstrate that holding their breath was a strain and caused imperfect sight, double vision, dizziness and fatigue, while the deep breathing at once gave them relief.
>
> There is a wrong way of breathing in which when the air is drawn into the lungs the nostrils contract. This is quite conspicuous among many cases of tuberculosis.
>
> Some teachers of physical culture in their classes while encouraging deep breathing close their nostrils when drawing in a long breath. This is wrong because it produces a strain and imperfect sight. By consciously doing the wrong thing, breathing with a strain, one becomes better able to practice the right way and obtain relaxation and better sight.
>
> By the habit of practicing frequently deep breathing, one obtains a more permanent relaxation of the eyes with more constant good vision.

Once again, I do not teach "deep" breathing. Normal abdominal breathing is sufficient for normal sight.

Many holistic practitioners find it necessary to teach students and clients to breathe normally again. This is a reflection of how much stress and tension many people live under today.

YAWNING

Yawning is natural, normal, and essential for normal health. Yawning helps maintain a proper pH level in the bloodstream. It also pumps cerebral spinal fluid.

Many people in this country have been trained to not yawn: "Don't yawn in public. It is rude." (Hmmm. Sounds like not pointing and not moving.) I once had a guest from Africa attend one of my introductory lectures, in which I included yawning. After the lecture he shared with me how strange it is that children in the United States are told to not yawn in public.

Yawning in this society is considered to be a sign of boredom. This is incorrect. Yawning is a sign of being tired or relaxed. It does not indicate the level of interest.

As I like to remind my students, "Babies yawn, cats and dogs yawn, and people in Italy yawn!" It is time for adults in the United States to relearn natural yawning.

Yawning is contagious! If you practice a few, the "real" ones will start!

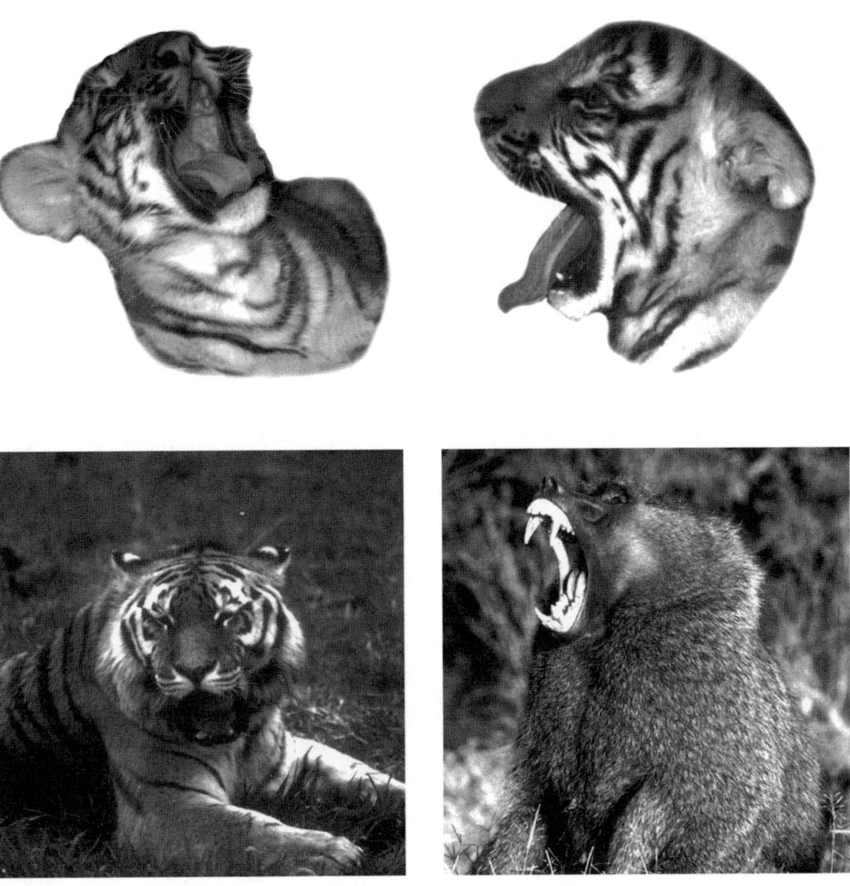

Figure 13–4: Yawning.

Even by thinking of the word "yawn" you may start yawning!

Ever notice how thinking stops during a yawn?!

Yawning is a habit that has been suppressed in this society. Yawn when you are not with other people. You can be more subtle when other people are present. I frequently compliment my students for yawning!

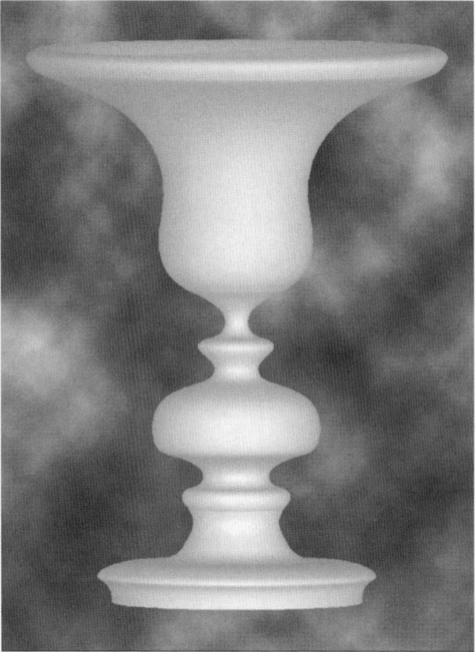

Figure 13–5: The Yawning Vase.

MORE ON BREATHING

Oxygen supplied to the eye by breathing is especially important because the retina consumes more oxygen by weight than any other part of the human body. The extraordinary lengths to which nature goes to supply oxygen to the retina is described in Chapter 17, "The Retina."

The study of breathing helps natural vision students to further appreciate the interrelationship among the three principles of natural vision—Movement, Centralization, and Relaxation. Each principle supports the other two. It is all one way of living in balance with nature.

The most important point of this chapter is for the student to relearn natural abdominal breathing as a continuous, automatic, and subconscious habit. We are meant to breathe as easily and automatically as a newborn baby for our entire lifetime. It is not supposed to be interfered with for long periods of time.

NATURAL BREATHING IS RELAXING

Frederick Léboyér writes in his excellent book about breathing and childbirth, *The Art of Breathing:*

> —We are told to relax.
> —To relax? Excellent. How?
> —I don't know. They don't tell us anything....
> —Your teachers, probably, do not know. As for the secret, as I'm sure you suspect, it's breathing.[3]

Natural abdominal breathing is relaxing, and relaxation is the most important principle of normal sight.

NOTES

1. June Biermann and Barbara Toohey, *The Woman's Holistic Headache Relief Book* (Los Angeles: J. P. Tarcher, Inc., 1979), p. 74.
2. Alexander Lowen, *Bioenergetics* (New York: Penguin Books, Inc., 1976).
3. Frederick Léboyér, *The Art of Breathing* (Longmead, England: Element Books Ltd., 1985), p. 32.

Chapter Fourteen

The Third Habit—Blinking

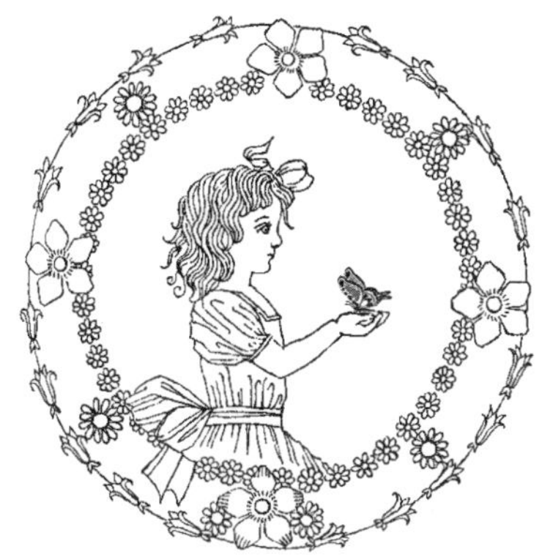

When most I wink, then do mine eyes best see.

—William Shakespeare, Sonnet No. 43

The third habit of natural vision is blinking.

ANATOMY AND PHYSIOLOGY

See *Plate 14: Eyelids, Eyelashes, and Eyebrows.*

The *eyelids,* our "natural windshield wipers," sweep away particles that enter the eye and protect the eye from external injury and excessive light. Each eyelid has two or three rows of *eyelashes,* which help prevent dust particles from entering the eye. The *eyebrows* divert perspiration, rain, and other particles from the forehead out toward the temples away from the eyes.

The Eyelid Muscles and Blinking

See *Plate 15: The Orbicularis Eyelid Muscle (Side View),* and *Plate 16: The Orbicularis Eyelid Muscle (Front View).* The upper eyelid closes by the contraction of the *orbicularis palpebrae muscle,* which encircles the front of the eye, and by the relaxation and lengthening of the levator palpebrae superioris muscle. The upper eyelid opens by the opposite actions.

The lower eyelid, which has a smaller range of movement than the upper eyelid, closes by the contraction of the orbicularis palpebrae muscle; it opens by the opposite action.

The orbicularis palpebrae muscle is shown in dark red; the eyelids are closed in these two illustrations.

See *Plate 17: The Levator Palpebrae Superioris Muscle (Side View)* and *Plate 19: The Levator Palpebrae Superioris Muscle (Top View).* The upper eyelid is opened by the contraction of the levator palpebrae superioris muscle (from the Latin *levator,* meaning "to raise," and *palpebra,* meaning "eyelid"). The levator palpebrae superioris muscle is located above the superior oblique and superior rectus muscles. The front part inserts into the upper eyelid, and the rear part attaches to the back of the eye orbit.

Blinking is the action of quickly and easily lowering and raising the eyelids. Like sketching and breathing, blinking is normally done unconsciously but can also be done consciously.

Ptosis, A Drooping of the Eyelid

Ptosis is a drooping of the upper eyelid. Ptosis can be caused by deficient development, or paralysis, of the levator palpebrae superioris muscle. In both cases, this muscle is unable to contract sufficiently to raise the upper eyelid to its normal position.

Secretion Portion of the Lacrimal (Tear) System

See *Plate 20: The Lacrimal (Tear) System.* The *lacrimal gland* (from the Latin *lachrima,* meaning "tear") is located above the eye, toward the temple, underneath the eyebrow ridge, and between the eyeball and the eye socket. This almond-size, sponge-like gland is controlled by the parasympathetic part of the autonomic nervous system and continually produces aqueous (watery) *lacrimal tears.* Tears are delivered to the front of the eye by the six to twelve lacrimal ducts.

Lacrimal tears are slightly alkaline, containing sodium chloride (salt) and proteins. Tears provide moisture to the eyes and remove dust and particles of dirt. They also contain oxygen and other nutrients for the cornea.

In addition to cleansing the eye, tears contain antibacterial protein called *lysozyme.* This powerful enzyme protects the eye from infections by dissolving the protective outer coats of harmful bacteria. Without lysozyme in the tears, micro-organisms would grow on the cornea and infections could occur on the eye.

Located inside the eyelids are about thirty *sebaceous glands* (Meibomian and Zeis glands), which secrete an oily lubrication, called *sebum.* Sebum coats the eye and the eyelids, providing lubrication between them, and prevents the watery lacrimal tears from running over the edges of the eyelids onto the cheeks.

Together, the lacrimal and sebaceous glands create three different layers of tears over the eye:

1. The layer of tears closest to the cornea, sclera, and eyelid is composed of mucous proteins. It coats the eye evenly and allows the second, watery layer of tears to easily adhere to the eye.
2. The middle watery layer, provided by the lacrimal glands, is the cleansing and nutrient layer. It washes away foreign particles and supplies the cornea with proteins, salt, and moisture.
3. The third outer layer is oily. It helps prevent the middle watery layer from evaporating too rapidly and provides lubrication between the eye and the eyelids.

These three layers of tears also help keep the front of the eye warm in cold weather.

The Conjunctiva

See *Plate 21: The Conjunctiva.* A thin transparent membrane called the *conjunctiva* (shown in green) extends along the inner surfaces of both eyelids, over the front portion of the sclera, and over the cornea. The conjunctiva forms a barrier, called the *fornix conjunctiva,* which prevents tears and particles from traveling into the back of the eye orbit. Without the conjunctiva, water could flow into the back of the eye socket when you are swimming!

The conjunctiva is extremely sensitive to pain, and one learns quickly never to allow an object to touch the eye—our most important sensory organ. A grain of sand in the eye is immediately flooded with copious tears and expelled out and over the lower eyelid onto the cheek.

Conjunctivitis is an inflammation of the conjunctiva.

The Irrigation System

During blinking, the eyelids pump tears out of the lacrimal glands via the lacrimal ducts into the upper outer corner (fornix) of the conjunctiva. The tears cleanse, moisten, and disinfect the cornea, sclera, and conjunctiva as they travel toward the lower, inner corner of the eye. Some tears evaporate during this process.

The Drainage Portion of the Lacrimal System

Excess tears drain from the eye through two small orifices at the inner corners of both eyelids. These two minute openings, called *lacrimal puncta,* can often be seen by close inspection in a mirror. The lacrimal puncta glide along the sclera collecting tears into the lacrimal sac. By means of pumping action during blinking and a suction action by the nose, excess tears drain from the lacrimal sac down through the nasolacrimal duct into the nasal cavity, where they evaporate due to respiration.

A Third Eyelid?!

The small, round, pinkish fold of tissue at the inner corner of the human eye is called the *lacrimal caruncle.* Some consider this to be the remainder of an old *nictitans,* a third eyelid. Many nocturnal birds and some reptiles have a nictitans, which is discussed further in Chapter 17, "The Retina."

Dry Eye Syndrome

Insufficient tearing from the lacrimal glands, overly rapid evaporation due to wind, or excessive heat can create dryness in eyes. This can result in a burning sensation, oversensitivity to light (photophobia), mucous discharge, corneal changes, and impairment of vision.

Many people have dry eyes due to not blinking frequently enough. Some estimate over six million Americans have chronically dry eyes. Many natural vision students have eliminated dry eyes by simply relearning correct blinking. Many have also lowered their sensitivity to bright light, and have been able to discard their sunglasses completely. They now feel relaxed in sunlight by simply blinking softly and frequently.

In strong wind or dry weather situations, it is important to blink more frequently to prevent the eyes from drying out due to rapid evaporation of tears.

Dry eyes can also be caused by undesirable effects[1] from medication or diseases. Consult with your eye doctor if you have serious eye problems.

Artificial Tears—Helpful or Harmful?

Moist, protective tear layers are essential for the health of the eyes. However, one might question whether artificial tears are a help or detriment if used on a long-term basis. Does the continuous use of artificial tears suppress the normal production of natural tears, thus creating more of a dependence on the artificial tears? Are the artificial tears truly an adequate replacement for natural tears?

Artificial tears may be needed for a short time in acute problems. Again, consult with your eye doctor for any serious eye problems.

Irritant vs. Emotional Tears

The tears live in an onion that should water this sorrow.

—William Shakespeare

Lael Wertenbaker, in *The Eye: Window to the World,* writes:

> While all animals that live in air produce tears to keep the eyes moist, man is the only animal that weeps. In 1957, intrigued by the dual purpose of crying, chemist Robert Brunish analyzed the ingredients of emotional and irritant tears. Tears induced by onion fumes and strong wind, he discovered, contained a lower concentration of the protein albumin. In the 1970s, biochemist William Frey began investigations whether this protein was related to the chemical changes in our blood stream caused by stress. Tears might well play a role in filtering out the body's stressful chemicals. The machismo ethic of suppressing tears, Frey thinks, might irritate peptic ulcers and other stress-related diseases. By not allowing himself to weep, the strong, silent male might not take advantage of natural relief.[2]

Fritz Kahn, in *Man in Structure and Function,* writes about crying:

> All higher animals produce tear fluid to irrigate the cornea, but only man cries as an expression of emotional disturbance. Only a thinking and emotionally sensitive person cries. An infant yells, but it does not cry. Children cry when they learn to think and to feel. Crying is a process connected with speech; it is a substitute for speech, a protective mechanism whereby a speaking individual can still express his feelings even though he may be prevented from speaking. People ... cry when they are unable to make themselves heard or to obtain justice with the weapons of speech and thought. When it has achieved nothing by means of logic, a speaking creature appeals to sympathy by crying. Crying is a reflex which has extended its field of action from the physiological to the moral realm—it is a new phenomenon in the developmental history of life.[3]

Bates on Blinking

From Bates' "Fundamentals" card:

> The normal eye blinks, or closes and opens very frequently.
>
> ... By moving the head and eyes a short distance from side to side, being sure to blink, one can imagine stationary objects to be moving.[4]

Better Eyesight magazine, April 1922: "Rest your eyes continually by blinking, which means to open and close them so rapidly that one appears to see things continuously."

Blinking is a rest for the eyes. Normal sight is based on relaxation.

Better Eyesight magazine, September 1923:

> BLINKING
>
> ... Usually unconsciously the normal eye closes and opens quite frequently and at irregular intervals and for very short spaces of time. Most people can demonstrate that when they regard a letter that they are able to see quite clearly it is possible for them to consciously close their eyes and open them quick enough and see the letter continuously. This is called Blinking and it is only another name for dodging. Dodging what? Dodging the [harmful] tendency to look steadily at things all the time. All the methods which have been recommended for the improvement of the vision, ... centralizing, palming, swinging, blinking, can all be grouped under the one word—dodging.

As with many other aspects of natural health, natural vision is based on continuous, easy movements. Here Bates refers to this constant movement as dodging.

When relearning normal blinking, some students think that during the blink, they will not be able to see an object of interest continuously. This is not true. The period of time for a normal blink is very short.

Better Eyesight magazine, November 1923:

> BLINKING
>
> The normal eye when it has normal sight blinks quite frequently. By blinking is meant closing the eyelids and opening them so quickly that neither the student nor his observers notice the fact ... Blinking is necessary in order to maintain normal vision continuously, because if one consciously prevents blinking, the vision for the distance or the ability to read fine print are modified. It is interesting to me how blinking, which is so necessary for good vision, has been so universally ignored by the writers of books on diseases of the eyes. Blinking is a rest, it prevents fatigue, and very important, it improves the sight in myopia, and helps to maintain good vision more continuously.

Blinking, when done properly, is so quick and easy, people with normal sight do not usually notice they are blinking.

Better Eyesight magazine, January 1924: In a remarkable article entitled "My Young Assistant," Emily C. Lierman (who later married Dr. Bates) writes about a three-year-old girl named Ethel, who was giving a man vision lessons.

> Ethel complained, "You are staring. You shouldn't stare; that is bad ... You must blink your eyes. Just let me show you how." Ethel has perfect sight. Her eyes are never still and she blinks unconsciously all day long.

Better Eyesight magazine, February 1924:

> *Question:* What one method of improving sight is best?
> *Answer:* Swinging and blinking.

Better Eyesight magazine, March 1924:

> By blinking is meant frequent closing of the eyes. It is usually done so rapidly that it is not conspicuous. Many persons with normal sight have the illusion that they do not blink. They believe their eyes are always at rest and that their eyes are continually open all the time.... One person was able to distinguish a small letter on the bottom line at twenty feet, 20/10. He was positive that he saw the letter continuously.

> It was found ... [that] he closed and opened his eyes frequently, without being conscious of the fact....
>
> [While studying people as they looked at moving pictures:] In all cases where the sight was normal, blinking occurred almost every second....
>
> When light is good ... blinking occurs at less frequent intervals.

Better Eyesight magazine, June 1924. Article by Emily C. Lierman:

> Although weary and tired, after I had worked with Lewis over two hours, I was repaid a thousandfold when he read every letter of the 70 line and 50 line as he moved the ... [reading] card slowly from side to side ... blinking all the time. He was instructed to stand and swing his body from side to side to lessen the tension of his body; also to blink his eyes all the time to stop staring ... On his second visit he read the smallest letters on the card, the 10 line....

Better Eyesight magazine, July 1924. Article submitted by Natural Vision teacher Dr. Edith T. Fisher, M.D., referring to one of her students:

> I explained to him that by making an effort to relax he was increasing the strain. While he was talking I noticed that he had not blinked. His forehead was deeply wrinkled and there was a constant twitching of the facial muscles ... First I explained about blinking, but when he tried this he contracted all the facial muscles ... [After palming] I reminded him to blink, and though he did not contract all his facial muscles it was still a great effort for him. He said, "I don't think I ever blinked before" ... Three days later ... his vision had improved ... He blinked easily now, but still stared at times.

> Tom's Personal Log: I had so much tightness in my eyelids that it was impossible for me to blink easily and naturally in the beginning. I was only able to blink hard. It has taken me many years to re-establish soft eyelids and blinking.

Better Eyesight magazine, August 1924. Emily Lierman writes about one of her students:

> As Frederick answered my questions he looked directly at me and ... I noticed he listened without blinking, for more than two minutes or longer. As the normal eye blinks unconsciously every few seconds, I soon realized what his trouble was....

The habits of poor vision are usually never thought about by persons with poor sight. Both the correct and incorrect habits of vision are primarily subconscious. It takes time to form poor blinking habits. It also takes time to re-establish proper blinking habits.

Better Eyesight magazine, August 1924: "BLINKING. Normal eyes blink constantly."

Better Eyesight magazine, January 1925. Article by Emily Lierman:

> At one time a young man ... came to us suffering from severe mental strain. His large staring eyes would make anyone uncomfortable ... His eyes protruded and he stared without blinking....

Better Eyesight magazine, March 1925:

> Blinking is done quickly, and not slowly like a wink ... Blink consciously, whenever possible, especially when reading.

In spite of Shakespeare's words quoted at the beginning of this chapter, winking is not the same as blinking. Winking is usually done consciously with one eyelid. It is not a natural vision habit and should not be confused with normal blinking, which is (usually) subconscious and relaxed.

Better Eyesight magazine, December 1925:

> Blinking is necessary to maintain normal vision in the normal eye. When blinking is prevented the eyes become tired, and the vision very soon becomes worse. Some persons, without knowing it, will blink five times in one second, as demonstrated by the [motion] camera ... When blinking they may fail to obtain relaxation, because they too often blink with an effort ... blinking is done easily without effort. Blinking is very important. It is not the brief periods of rest from closing the eyes which helps the sight so much, as the shifting or movements of the eyes. It should be repeatedly demonstrated that the eyes are only at rest when they are shifting.

Here Bates emphasizes the connection between the important principle of movement and the habit of blinking. A student might at first guess that the less movement one has, the less tired he will become. In regards to vision, the opposite is true. The eyes are designed for movements. Rigid staring lowers sight. Staring is almost always associated with infrequent blinking and shallow breathing.

When a student begins to understand how the principles and habits of normal sight all support each other, he is well on the path of success.

In beginning lessons, blinking is often done with an effort by many students. The eyelid muscles are relatively tense due to locking the eyelids open for long periods of time and due to the harmful habit of squinting. With practice, proper blinking becomes easy and automatic once again.

Better Eyesight magazine, August 1927:

> The normal eye with normal sight blinks frequently, easily and rapidly, without effort or strain. If children do not blink frequently, but stare and try to see things with the eyes open continuously, the vision is always impaired. At first the child should be reminded to blink consciously but it soon becomes an unconscious habit and the vision is improved.

Here Bates links blinking to the principle of relaxation. The three vision habits are to be practiced easily—without any effort.

Better Eyesight magazine, August 1927:

> *Question:* I have found blinking and shifting to be of great benefit to me but, although I have been practicing both for six months, it has not become a habit. I still have to practice both consciously. What means can I use to blink and shift normally?
> *Answer:* Continue to consciously practice blinking and shifting until you acquire the unconscious habit. It is merely a substitution of a good habit for a bad one.

Better Eyesight magazine, September 1927: "To use your eyes correctly all day long, it is necessary that you: 1. Blink frequently. ..."

It is interesting that in his later years, Bates' summaries of proper vision habits place the blinking habit first. Perhaps this is because blinking is the simplest habit.

Better Eyesight magazine, October 1927: "The normal eye blinks quickly, easily and frequently."

In *Better Eyesight* magazine, December 1927, Bates connects the habit of blinking to the health of the whole person:

> It can always be demonstrated that when a student with imperfect sight looks intently at one point, keeping the eyes open constantly, or trying to do so, that a strain of the eyes and all the nerves of the body is usually felt, and the vision becomes imperfect. It is impossible to keep the eyes open continuously without blinking. Each time the eyes blink, a certain amount of rest is obtained and the vision is benefited. For this reason, the student is instructed to blink frequently while swaying . . . and at all other times . . . The importance of practicing certain parts of the routine habits at all times, such as blinking . . . is stressed.

Better Eyesight magazine, February 1928. Article by Emily Lierman:

> To begin with, he blinked too fast, which is as [incorrect] as not blinking at all. When . . . students acquire the habit of blinking too fast, they are very apt to stare while they blink . . . I had emphasized that he must not snap his eyes shut nor open them too quickly . . . This new way of teaching him to blink without blinking too fast helped him . . . to blink one blink at a time, instead of blinking rapidly with a nervous twitch. . . .

Better Eyesight magazine, April 1928:

> *Question:* I notice that my [strabismic] eye does straighten after palming, but reverts when I stop. How can I tell when and how I strain?
>
> *Answer:* Avoid staring after palming, and blink all the time. You can demonstrate that staring is a strain by consciously doing it for a few seconds. . . .
>
> *Question:* How can one overcome the stare if it is unconscious?
>
> *Answer:* Blink consciously, whenever possible, especially when reading. Never look at an object for more than a few seconds at a time. Shift . . .
>
> *Question:* By blinking do you mean shutting and opening the eyes quickly, or is it done slowly like a wink?
>
> *Answer:* Blinking is done quickly, and not slowly like a wink. Watch someone with perfect sight do this unconsciously, and follow his example.

Practicing frequent blinking helps to break the staring habit.

THE FREQUENCY AND DURATION OF NATURAL BLINKING

Normal, natural blinking occurs approximately every two to four seconds (fifteen to thirty blinks per minute) on the average.

The duration of a blink, i.e., the time between closing and opening the eyelids, is very short—about 1⁄40 of a second.

And, of course, blinking should be done very softly.

NOTES ON BLINKING

- Natural blinking is automatic, rhythmical, soft, casual, easy and light—like the wings of a butterfly, i.e., without effort. See *Plate 18: Blinking.* The upper eyelid should come down completely and touch the lower eyelid during blinking. Watch the blinking habits of people who have normal sight.
- Blink as you shift your attention from one object to another, and from one part of an object to another part. Blink when you shift your attention from near to far, and again from far to near.
- Frequent, soft blinking is meant to be a subconscious habit. Therefore it must be practiced consciously until it is a

subconscious habit again. People with normal vision do not know they blink frequently—it is automatic. As one of my students said, "Practice makes *permanent.*"

- Remember the staring contest in grade school, where we challenged our classmate to "Make me blink!"? Those with the strongest corrective lenses usually win the contest. Besides, "Tough guys don't blink."
- As mentioned above, blinking encourages shifting of our attention from one point to another. The theme of one of the earlier Bates teachers was "shift and blink." Blinking aids in the mobility of the eyes, and helps prevent staring.
- Gesell, in his book *Vision: Its Development in Infant and Child,* referring to a twenty-week-old infant, states, "Intent fixation dissolves with a flash release, often accompanied by blinking. . . ."[5]
- Blinking is a free "massage" for the eyes all day long. Blinking also encourages important micro-movements of the extrinsic eye muscles.
- Lymphatic fluid around the eyes increases its circulation by blinking.
- Proper blinking helps prevent strain and fatigue.
- It is important to have correct blinking habits during computer work. Blinking is far less frequent for those who experience eyestrain during computer work.
- Many people do not blink enough while reading books.
- Humans are the only creatures on this planet who squint and strain with effort to see. Animals do not squint, even in the brightest sunlight.
- When you are thinking about a problem, and seeing objects around you is not essential, close your eyelids. Do not lock your eyelids open for long periods of time as this creates a strain.
- Ever see a fish blink? No, because fish have no eyelids! The water automatically cleanses their eyes. The eyes of fish are open when they sleep.
- Some programs incorrectly teach students exercises in which they are instructed to hold their eyelids open for long periods of time. This is harmful. Blinking frequently is normal and essential for natural clear vision. In one program, the student is repeatedly told to keep his head still. While performing five different eye exercises he did not blink for 39, 82, 41, 40, and 41 seconds.
- A student of mine, a yoga teacher, read in a book to first practice not blinking for thirty seconds, and then to "build up" to thirty minutes! She had serious vision problems.
- Nearsights tend not to blink for long periods of time when their attention is in the far distance.
- Farsights tend not to blink for long periods of time while reading or doing other activities up close.
- A person who does not blink looks *blank!*
- Sometimes students see more clearly during or just after yawning. Yawning can create excess tears on the cornea and create a pseudo-contact lens effect. The same effect is often experienced when taking a shower. Usually this clearer vision will disappear within one or two more blinks because the excess tears or water are swept away.

Improved sight can also be due to the relaxation provided by yawning.

- Oftentimes, a person will have infrequent or no blinking when staring, fatigued, or breathing shallowly. The eyelids become tense and locked. Everything becomes immobile. Immobility is the problem; circulation is the solution.
- Contact lenses can interfere with normal blinking due to irritation of the eyelids while passing over the edges of the contact lense. Some contact lense wearers blink much less than normal.
- Some meditation techniques confuse the stilling of the mind with rigidly stilling the body—including the eyes and eyelids. Some yoga books suggest staring fixedly at the flame of a candle—without moving the eyes and without blinking. This is very harmful to eyesight. One of my students who followed such instructions could not understand why his vision was not improving.

One yoga book states "Vision has to be fixed at the tip of the nose without winking the eyelids." This is a strain, as is turning the eyes upward and/or inward in a fixed position. These are all contrary to Bates' principles and habits of normal vision.

TV AND MOVIES—BLINKING ALLOWED

In regards to someone who is giving a speech on TV, one study suggests that a relatively high blinking rate (48–67 blinks per minute) indicates the speaker is more nervous, edgy, anxious, or stressed. This study also suggests that a relatively low blinking rate (7–11 blinks per minute) indicates the speaker is enjoying pleasant feelings, feels "in control" or "extraordinarily confident," and has a higher comfort level. This is contrary to Bates' findings on blinking also.

Many actors and actresses on TV have very low rates of blinking. Many actors and actresses in the US are trained not to blink while performing on television. A normal (not average!) rate is associated with higher anxiety. Even some TV news broadcasters are told not to blink too frequently when reporting the news.

There is a popular space travel series on TV in which many of the actors do not blink for extremely long periods of time. With the high number of hours Americans watch TV, one may be concerned about the harmful influence of infrequent blinking habits on the viewers, especially children.

A BUTTERFLY BLINKING STORY

An excellent way to enjoy this story is to have someone read it to you while palming with closed eyelids.

👁 Pretend you are sitting in a comfortable chair in a beautiful meadow, while the sunshine gently warms your skin. A beautiful iridescent-winged butterfly floats softly over your shoulder and out in front of you. This

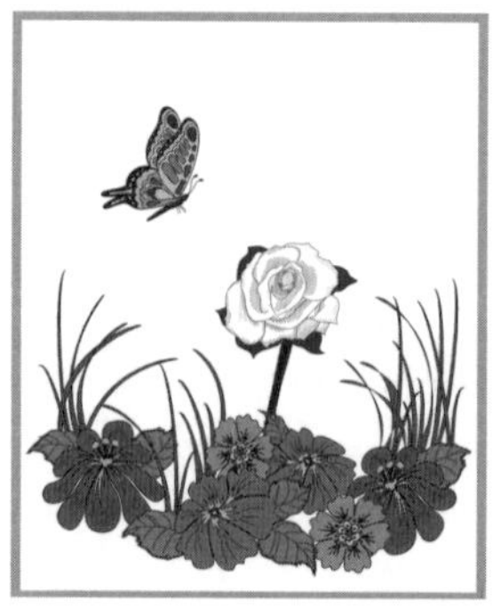

magnificent butterfly is so light, it seems as if it is part of the air itself. The butterfly wings sparkle from the sunshine as it floats to the right, and then to the left. Returning to the center, our butterfly puts down one toe and spins around in the air like a ballerina.

The butterfly then floats slowly out into the distance, over an ocean of flowers. Five feet out it floats; ten feet; and fifteen feet. Notice how the wind creates waves over all of the colorful flowers. At about twenty feet, the butterfly notices a single, large, snow-white rose in the center of the field of flowers.

As the butterfly floats around the rose, it becomes intoxicated by its wonderful fragrance. Finally, the butterfly lands softly in the center of the white rose. As we brush the butterfly's soft wings, they remind us of how soft the eyelids are as we blink frequently all day long.

The wings open and close every two or three seconds. This reminds us of the frequency of natural blinking.

After this story, stop palming and open your eyelids. Practice "butterfly blinking" while using your nose-feather to brush objects around you. Remember abdominal breathing. Brush, Breathe, and Butterfly Blink!

SQUINTING—A HARMFUL HABIT

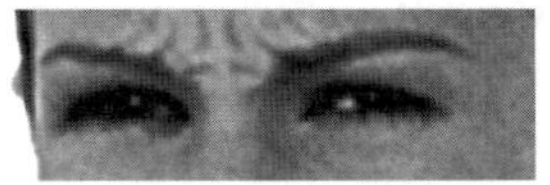

Figure 14–1: No Squinting.

Squinting is a conscious narrowing of the eyelids, forming a small horizontal slit. This narrowing of the eyelids blocks part of the peripheral light rays entering through the pupil. Although a person can often see better artificially, squinting is a harmful habit. One Bates teacher refused to continue lessons with a student who kept using this type of "trick vision." A Natural Vision teacher never teaches squinting.

By the way, the word "squint" used here does not refer to the "squint" used by Bates and others in reference to strabismus. There is no connection between these two different usages of this word.

Better Eyesight magazine, July 1927:

> Partly closing your eyes brings on a strain which increases your imperfect sight ... it injures your eyes.

Better Eyesight magazine, December 1927:

> *Question:* Why do some people see better by partly closing their eyes?
>
> *Answer:* People with poor sight can see better [artificially] by partly closing their eyes, but when they have perfect sight, squinting makes it worse.

Squinting, in *all* its variations, always involves an effort, and therefore has nothing to do with seeing clearly naturally. Since effort to see always lowers natural sight, vision is worse after squinting.

WHY SQUINTING CREATES AN ARTIFICIAL, SHARPER IMAGE—THE PINHOLE EFFECT

Many people have discovered it is possible to see more clearly without their corrective lenses by squinting or by looking through a tiny hole. How is this possible?

The eyeball allows light rays to pass through the pupil at many different angles. When the eye is in the normal shape (for clear vision), the light rays entering the eye refract, i.e., they curve or bend as they pass through the cornea and the lens and finally land on the retina. None of these light rays interfere with each other. They all land at the proper locations. Each light ray is properly "focused" on the retina.

However, not all the light rays are refracted. The single light ray coming from directly in front of the eye (along the visual axis) does *not* refract or bend. This single, central light ray passes perpendicularly through the cornea and lens and does not curve or bend. It continues in its original direction, in a straight line back to the fovea centralis, located in the center of the back of the eye. This fact might now make a nearsight, whose eyeball is too long, and a farsight, whose eyeball is too short, wonder why they do not see clearly in the center of the field of vision at all distances without corrective lenses.

Now we must examine the role of the peripheral light rays. Peripheral light rays that pass non-perpendicularly through the cornea and lens refract. When the eyeball is in the normal shape, none of the peripheral light rays fall in the fovea centralis.

When the eyeball is chronically squeezed out of shape, as in nearsightedness and farsightedness, the peripheral light rays do not fall in focus on the retina. They spread out and interfere with each other, landing incorrectly on top of each other. Some of these peripheral light rays fall into the fovea, where they are not supposed to go, creating blurred central vision.

For nearsights and farsights, peripheral light rays also interfere with each other in the peripheral parts of the field of vision. But because the rods, which pick up our peripheral vision, are incapable of seeing better than 20/400, peripheral interference is somewhat irrelevant. This is because the "out of focus" peripheral light rays only result in nearsights and farsights seeing less clearly than 20/400 vision in the *peripheral* vision. For nearsights and farsights, the peripheral vision is simply *less* clear than the *unclear* peripheral vision of the person who has perfect eyesight.

With the creation of a pinhole "tunnel," the majority of the peripheral light rays are eliminated. You are now letting only the "central," non-refracted light rays through. When a nearsight forms a small "pinhole" with the forefinger (very close to the head, but not touching the eye), a distant object is usually seen more clearly, without any corrective lenses. Similarly, when a farsight looks at something close, the close object is usually seen more clearly. The smaller the pinhole, the sharper the object (but it is also dimmer). The peripheral light rays no longer interfere with the cones in the fovea.

Theoretically, if the fovea and the pinhole were sufficiently small, we would be able to see perfectly clearly, but only light rays from one atom from the object straight ahead!

The pinhole effect shows your minimum potential eyesight without glasses.

Those people with astigmatism usually see more clearly with the pinhole experience. But, because the astigmatic cornea has angular distortions (a wavy surface), the clearer vision might not be as clear as someone who has only nearsightedness or farsightedness. In astigmatism, the single light ray from straight ahead might not continue in a straight line back to the fovea.

Using the forefinger to see better is not recommended, as it is still artificial vision. Besides, vision functions best when both eyes are used together.

The Pinhole Camera

A pinhole camera works by focusing light rays without a lens. An advantage of the pinhole is that objects are clear at all distances. The biggest disadvantage of the pinhole is the image is usually very dim.

A larger aperture on a pinhole camera would allow more light through to create a brighter image, but without a lens or cornea, the image would become blurred. And, of course, with a larger aperture, it would no longer be a "pinhole" camera.

The nautilus, a mollusk, sees using a pinhole eye. Its eye has no lens or cornea to focus light.

"But I Do Not See Clearly, or More Clearly"

The image seen through the pinhole may not be perfectly clear for all nearsights and farsights, because it is not possible to eliminate all the peripheral light rays passing through the pinhole.

Additionally, diffraction may occur on the edges of the finger, distorting to some degree the light rays entering the eyes. As Bates pointed out above, a person with normal sight who squints will not see better. This is due to the diffraction of light rays passing through the pinhole.

The pinhole experience may be diminished if a person has certain pathologies, including problems with the cornea, aqueous humor, lens, vitreous humor, retina, and other parts of the eye and visual system.

More on the Harm of Squinting

Squinting is harmful to vision because it always involves an effort. The eyes, eyelids, face, head, neck, and shoulders become tight, and the breathing usually stops or becomes shallow. Usually a person is very rigid when squinting. Squinting is a very "unsightly" habit.

Even if the eyelids are lowered relatively softly to create better vision with the pinhole effect, it is still harmful. The author of one Bates method book teaches his students this harmful "trick" of slightly lowering the upper eyelids, stating, "Keep the upper lids down ... as if they were half-open eyes." Students of natural vision are cautioned never to do this.

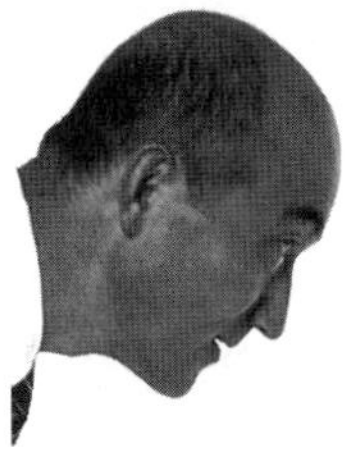

Figure 14-2: No "Trick" Vision.

It is also possible to see more clearly, again artificially, by bending the head forward and downward, while raising the eyes. The narrow angle of light along the eyebrows, or eyebrow ridge, creates a partial pinhole effect. This is not only a harmful vision habit but creates a strain on the neck. Additionally, the eyes would be looking in the opposite direction (up) of the head direction (down). Do not do this.

According to Fritz Kahn, " ... myopia is derived from the Greek words μυω, 'to close,' and ωψ, 'the eye,' and refers to the habit nearsighted people develop of half-closing the lids in order to see more clearly."[6] (In *Perfect Sight Without Glasses,* Bates translated the same Greek words to mean "closes the eye, or blinks.")

Worse than the tension created in the eyelids, face, and neck by any type of squinting is the mental harm. Vision is primarily a right-hemisphere activity and is based on trust. People who squint do not trust their sight to be clear automatically and easily. Straining to see is a distrust of natural vision.

BLINKING—THE SOCIAL CONNECTION

Many people with poor vision think it is impolite to blink when they talk with someone. Notice the similarity to believing it is impolite to move when talking with someone, discussed in Chapter 9, "The First Principle—Movement."

One of my recent students stated that, in the past, when she had normal sight, she felt self-conscious blinking frequently (normally) when talking with people who did not blink frequently. As a result, she practiced blinking less, and her vision became blurred.

BLINKING—THE EMOTIONAL CONNECTION

Similar to the poor vision habit of staring, many people with poor vision think that if they close their eyelids—even for a fraction of a second—they will not be protected from potential danger. Ironically, a person is *less* protected by *not* blinking frequently, since vision lowers with infrequently blinking.

BLINKING AND FLASHES

Better Eyesight magazine, May 1923:

> *Question:* I am practicing the methods in your book to reverse myopia and astigmatism. Sometimes, for short periods, I see perfectly, then things fade away. Can you explain this?
>
> *Answer:* This is what we call getting flashes of perfect sight. With continued practice these flashes will come more frequently and eventually will be permanent.

Many students have flashes while improving their vision. In the beginning, flashes are usually brief moments of dramatically improved or even perfect sight. This can be quite startling—so startling that many students return immediately to incorrect vision habits—staring with non-movement and diffusion, stopping breathing, and stopping blinking. The student thinks that if he remains still enough, she can keep, or "lock onto," this clearer vision. The student should continue normal blinking when she has a flash.

Students are very happy when they have a long flash, and it remains clearer even while blinking.

Squeezing the eyelids very tight can also create a flash for some students, but it is an incorrect habit. A student should never associate any type of effort with his vision.

Not all students have flashes; for some, the external eye muscles let go slowly while improving vision.

FINAL NOTES ON BLINKING

Blinking is one of the keys to normal, clear vision. It should be apparent from this chapter that the simple habit of blinking is of great importance. Blink frequently and softly all day long. Practice correct blinking until it becomes a subconscious habit—again.

NOTES

1 This author does not prefer the term "side effects," commonly used in conjunction with unwanted reactions caused by many drugs. I believe that in many cases the so-called "side effects" are actually the "primary effects," and

that the supposed primary benefits of the drugs are actually the "side effects." The reader is referred to George Vithoulkas' *The Science of Homeopathy,* the most important book I have read on health and disease, and *A New Model for Health and Disease,* both listed in the bibliography.

[2] Lael Wertenbaker and the Editors of U.S. News Books, *The Eye: Window to the World* (Washington, D.C.: U.S. News Books, 1981), p. 28.

[3] Fritz Kahn, "The Eye," *Man in Structure and Function* (New York: Alfred A. Knopf, 1943), p. 645.

[4] A small card made by Bates with a summary of his teachings; date unknown.

[5] Arnold Gesell, Francis L. Ilg, and Glenna E. Bullis, *Vision: Its Development in Infant and Child* (New York: Paul B. Hoeber, Inc., 1949), p. 90.

[6] Fritz Kahn, "The Eye," *Man in Structure and Function,* p. 656.

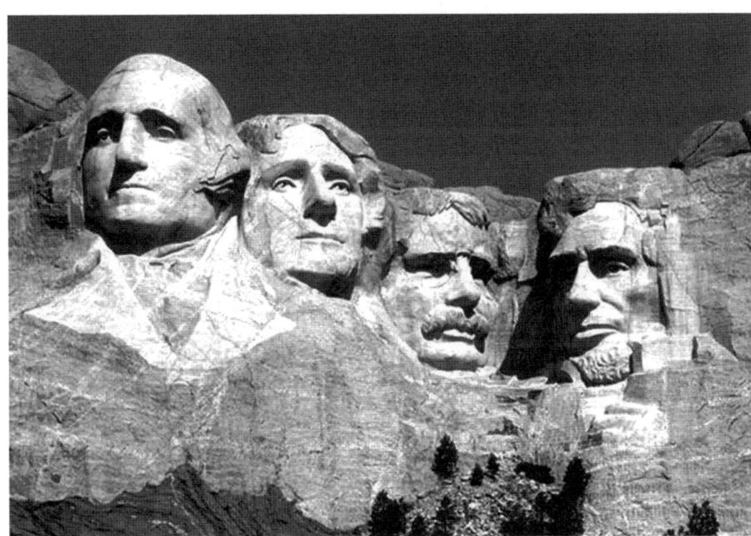

Figure 14–3: . . . and Blink, by George!

Chapter Fifteen

Sketch, Breathe, and Blink Summary

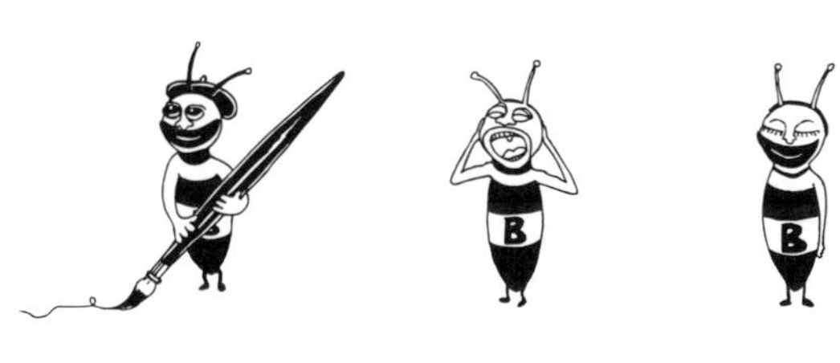

Figure 15–1: "The Three B's" (or "The B-Attitudes"). Reprinted with permission from Annie Buttons.

BRINGING THE THREE VISION HABITS TOGETHER

Initially the vision habits may feel separate from one another. This is because the student usually emphasizes one habit at a time in the beginning. This feeling of separation lessens as the habits are re-integrated more each day. With practice, the student will discover that the Sketching habit *goes with* the Breathing habit, which *goes with* the Blinking habit. When a person has normal vision, each habit supports and cooperates with the other. The same is true of the principles of Relaxation, Movement, and Centralization.

Not only do the habits and principles of natural vision blend together in time, the student begins to create a "rhythm of sight."

"IN THE BEGINNING ..."

Some students, especially during the first few classes, have told me the habits I am teaching them are incorrect. Yet with practice these students begin to realize that they *are* correct, and how harmful are the ingrained, incorrect vision habits they have practiced for many years. A Natural Vision teacher only *reminds* students of exactly how they used to see the world when they saw clearly and naturally. The natural vision habits are not new. From one perspective, natural vision classes are only history lessons.

Some students think these vision habits are incorrect because so few people in our society have correct vision habits. If a person copies the habits of the majority in our society, he will not see clearly. Bates talked about poor vision habits being "contagious." Students must not copy the "average" habits.

Initial objections, if not resistance, to the

correct habits of natural vision are not only common, they are expected. After all, how many years has the student had incorrect vision habits? One of my students who was 69 years old wore glasses for 64 years.

One of my students was describing the correct vision habits to her mother, who had perfect eyesight. Her mother's response was, "You mean you *haven't* been doing those things?!"

THE EYES ARE LISTENING

I frequently hear new students say, "I have bad eyes." Since vision is primarily a mental function, many Bates teachers consider it harmful to refer to the eyes as "bad." Since natural vision habits are not a moral issue, I teach students to substitute the word "incorrect" for the word "bad."

As one Bates teacher said, "The eyes hear what you say and think about them." Notice that you never hear people say they have "bad" ears.

IT IS SO SIMPLE, BUT ...

One of the peculiar aspects of relearning to see correctly is that the principles and habits are so simple.

I once took a college graduate course in Quantum Chemistry. The subject was so complex and difficult that the average grade on the final exam was 21 out of 100 points! The subject matter was nearly incomprehensible to me, and, apparently, many other students.

Unlike this chemistry course, the habits and principles of natural vision are simple. But if they are so simple, why do they seem so difficult to relearn? Because the incorrect vision habits have become ingrained in our body and mind. The state of our sight is largely a reflection of how we are living. And many people in this society live with excessive stress.

PLATEAUS ARE A TIME TO COAST

In any learning process there are plateaus. Plateaus are periods of time when, no matter how much the student practices correct vision habits, the vision improvement seems to level off.

It takes time for the mind and body to adjust to the vision habits you have practiced. Once the level of vision skills you have practiced is solid, a foundation is created for further progress. Simply continue to practice better vision habits each day, and when your vision is ready to progress further, it will.

KEEPING THE PERSPECTIVE

It is important to keep a reasonable perspective while improving vision, otherwise some students might become too frustrated with their rate of progress.

If the student has had incorrect vision habits for many years, these habits probably will not change completely in only a few weeks. Bates told one of his student simply to continue doing exactly what she had been doing which has given her such "great benefit."

Two or three years to rid oneself of the need for corrective lenses—which many natural vision students have done—may seem like a long time. But compared to twenty or thirty years of incorrect, strained vision habits and wearing strong corrective lenses, this is a relatively short time.

One student, who wore glasses for twenty-five years, asked me after two classes if a 5% improvement, as measured by her eye doctor, was a good improvement. I asked her, "How many *years* did it take for you to *lose* 5% of your vision?!"

Once explained and demonstrated thoroughly, the principles and habits of natural vision are easy to understand. This does not mean, however, that it is always easy to re-establish them quickly.

The visual system evolved over millions of years, and clarity is not lost for trivial reasons. Bates stated that it took time and hard work to establish blurred vision. Fortunately, the body and mind know how to heal and are generous in accelerating healing when given the opportunity. It takes time, patience, commitment, and dedication to relearn any correct habit. Happily, the rewards of improving vision naturally are incalculable.

"POSITIVITY" ESSENTIAL FOR SUCCESS

One way to deal with frustration is to keep your attention on the progress and benefits you have received by practicing the correct vision habits thus far. There are many forms of progress, including:

1. Endurance, which is the ability to practice the correct vision habits for a longer period each day;
2. Faster speed of sight; blurred vision is relatively slow;
3. Brighter colors and contrast;
4. A looser neck;
5. Better centralization skill;
6. Improved movement awareness in the peripheral vision;
7. Greater depth perception, which indicates the right hemisphere is reactivating for normal vision;
8. Better clarity; even brief moments of improved vision are a very positive sign. How many years ago did you have the sight you experienced in that flash?!

Students must keep at least a 51% positive attitude to succeed!

Pilot Baron Manfred von Richthofen, the famous WW1 "Red Baron" flying ace, stated, "Success flourishes only in perseverance."

FAILURES

Better Eyesight magazine, December 1922, in a article entitled "Failures":

> People who found no help were always people who fought me for all they were worth. I remember a physician who came to me for nine months, every day, and devoted from one to two hours trying to prove that I was wrong.... I advised him to try and prove that I was right. In a very short time he was reversed [of his vision problem].
>
> The people who find no help are the people who do the wrong thing against my advice.

Blurred vision is due to excessive strain learned by an individual. Failures are due to individuals not releasing this excessive strain from their eyes and lives. There are many reasons why this occurs. We live in a society that carries much tension. It may require a significant amount of time and energy to re-establish a healthy balance in our visual system.

The more tension there is in a society, the more important the relaxed vision habits become. Perhaps the many forms of natural healing are no longer optional, but mandatory if we are to remain healthy under society's present conditions.

One of my students arrived at the third class of the course and shared with us her realization that this process required commitment. She said she was not committed to her work, relationship, or anything else for

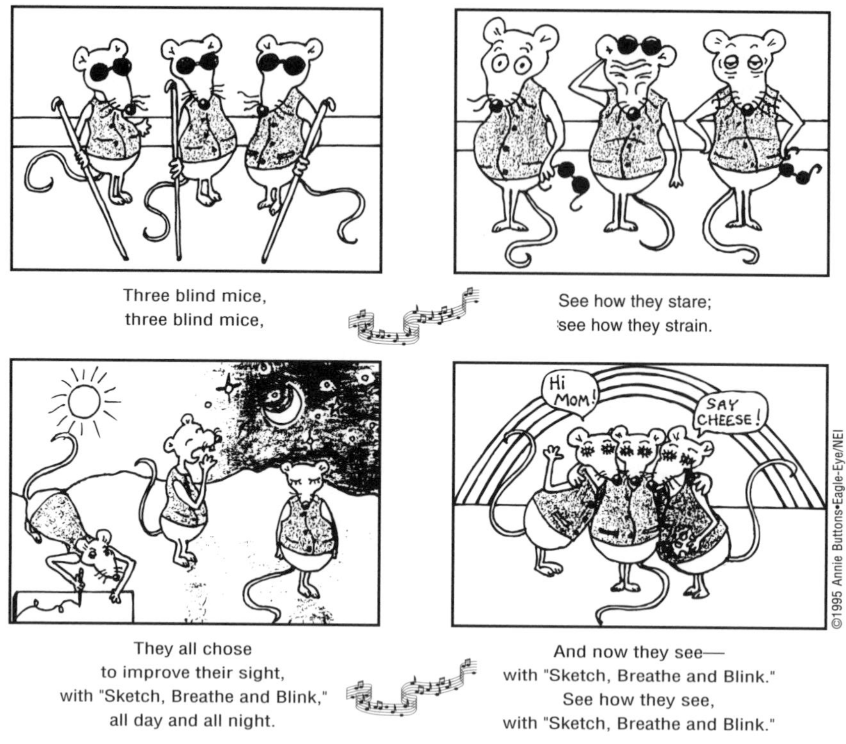
Three blind mice,
three blind mice,
See how they stare;
'see how they strain.
They all chose
to improve their sight,
with "Sketch, Breathe and Blink,"
all day and all night.
Hi MOM!
SAY CHEESE!
And now they see—
with "Sketch, Breathe and Blink."
See how they see,
with "Sketch, Breathe and Blink."
©1995 Annie Buttons•Eagle-Eye/NEI

Figure 15–2: "The Three Seeing Mice." Reprinted with permission from Annie Buttons.

that matter, and she certainly was not going to be committed to improving her vision. I never saw her again.

MOTIVATION

At a health convention, I once remarked to a woman, "If I can improve my sight, so can you." She thought about my statement for a few moments and replied, "Even if you couldn't do it, I can!"

Motivation to change incorrect vision habits is essential for success. Students of natural vision improvement are motivated for many different reasons.

Some find glasses and contact lenses inconvenient. Some like the idea of improving their overall health by improving their sight. Some are motivated to improve their vision to avoid more serious vision problems later on. (See Chapter 27, "Serious Vision Problems.") Some want to avoid risky surgeries, which still may not remove the true, underlying cause of their blurred vision. Others want to avoid moving into glasses in the first place.

Closely connected to motivation is ingenuity. One of my students placed a small, plastic flower on her fingernail to remind her of the three vision habits to practice throughout the day. She had one of the fastest improvements of all my students. Another student, in realizing relaxation is the key and that self-healing requires extra energy, decided to go to sleep one-half hour earlier at night.

One Bates teacher talked about two boys who had read a book on eyesight improvement and knew that the less they wore their glasses, the faster would be their improvement. So, on the way to their first lesson, they walked along the streets of New York to the teacher's classroom without their glasses on. Since both boys were very nearsighted, one would need to lift the other up onto his shoulders to read the street signs!

Some students have even chosen to stop driving a car until they improved their vision sufficiently to pass their driver's exam without glasses.

BATES SUMMARIZES THE KEY HABITS AND PRINCIPLES OF NORMAL SIGHT

Only a few years before his death, Bates summarized the keys habits of normal sight in his *Better Eyesight* magazines. It seems as if, even for Bates himself, the habits and principles of natural vision had finally become perfectly clear and concise. Perhaps these two summaries are Bates' greatest, final gift to humanity.

Regardless of the facts and theories of the eyes discussed in the early chapters of this book, it is possible to see clearly and naturally only by utilizing the correct vision habits and principles created by nature.

From *Better Eyesight* magazine, September 1927:

> PERFECT SIGHT
>
> If you learn the fundamental principles of perfect sight and will consciously keep them in mind your defective vision will disappear....
>
> ...All errors of refraction are functional, therefore are reversible.
>
> ...All defective vision is due to strain in some form.
>
> You can demonstrate to your own satisfaction that strain lowers vision. When you stare you strain. Look fixedly at one object for five seconds or longer. What happens? The object blurs and finally disappears. Also, your eyes are made uncomfortable by this experiment. When you rest your eyes for a few moments the vision is improved and the discomfort relieved.
>
> ...Strain is relieved by relaxation.
>
> To use your eyes correctly all day long, it is necessary that you:
>
> 1. Blink frequently. Staring is a strain and always lowers the vision.
> 2. Shift your glance constantly from one point to another, seeing the part regarded best and other parts not so clearly. That is, when you look at a chair, do not try to see the whole object at once; look first at the back of it, seeing that part best and other parts worse. Remember to blink as you quickly shift your glance from the back to the seat and legs, seeing each part best, in turn. This is centralization.
> 3. Your head and eyes are moving all day long. Imagine that stationary objects are moving in the direction opposite to the movement of your head and eyes. When you walk about the room or on the street, notice that the floor or pavement seems to come toward you, while objects on either side appear to move in the direction opposite to the movement of your body.

Better Eyesight magazine, December 1927:

> The importance of practicing certain parts of the routine habits and principles at all times, such as blinking, centralizing, and imagining stationary objects to be moving

> opposite to the movement of one's head and eyes, is stressed. The normal eye does these things unconsciously and the imperfect eye must at first practice them consciously until it becomes an unconscious habit.

These are quite possibly the two most important sentences ever written about natural, clear vision.

In the first sentence Bates identifies the key vision habits and principles to practice. In the second, he tells students they must practice them consciously until they are unconscious habits—exactly like they used to be when they used to have normal eyesight.

In essence, vision students are simply relearning to see—naturally.

See *Plate 60: The Land of Sketch, Breathe, and Blink.*

PART FIVE

Light, the Retina, and Stereoscopic Vision

Chapter Sixteen

Light

And God said, "Let there be light," and there was light. And God saw the light, that it was good ...

—Scriptures

This chapter covers many aspects of light, including sunlight, closed-eyelids sunning, artificial light and lighting hardware, ultraviolet light, and sunglasses.

THE EYES ARE ORGANS OF LIGHT

The eyes are organs of light. Our eyes have evolved over millions of years under the influence of sunlight. To remain healthy, the visual system needs to receive the full spectrum of sunlight. The sun's light impacts the retina, where it is converted to electro-chemical energy and transmitted to the brain and body.

SUNLIGHT

Sunlight, a Primary Source of Energy

See *Plate 22: The Electromagnetic and Visible Spectrums*.

The sun radiates energy toward the Earth in the form of electromagnetic waves. The higher-energy electromagnetic waves consist of cosmic, gamma, x-ray, and far-ultraviolet (UV) waves. Medium-energy waves consist of the mid- and near-UV, "visible," and short infrared waves. The lower-energy waves consist of long infrared, micro, TV, radio, and electric waves.

All electromagnetic waves travel at 186,000 miles per second. Since light travels at one billion feet per second, I remind students there is no need to strain to see!

Each type of electromagnetic wave has a *frequency* associated with it.

Thanks to Einstein, we know that higher-energy waves, like x-rays, have higher frequencies or oscillations, i.e., they vibrate up and down more times per second than medium- or lower-energy waves. Frequency is measured in cycles per second, or Hertz (Hz).

For example, high-energy x-rays have a frequency of approximately one quintillion (10^{18}) cycles per second; visible light has a medium frequency of approximately one quadrillion (10^{15}) cycles per second; low-energy radio waves have a frequency of only 1000 (10^{3}) cycles per second.

Each type of wave also has a *wavelength*

associated with it. Wavelengths of electromagnetic radiation are commonly measured in nanometers (nm)—billionths (10^{-9}) of a meter—from crest to crest.

X-rays have a wavelength of approximately one nanometer. Visible lightwaves have wavelengths in the range of 400 to 700 nm. Long radio waves have a wavelength of approximately one billion nanometers, or one meter.

As you can see, the higher the frequency or energy, the shorter the wavelength of a particular wave; the lower the frequency, the longer the wavelength.

Sunlight, the Atmosphere, and the Earth

See *Plate 23: Sunlight, the Atmosphere, and the Earth.*

The Earth's surface does not receive all of the rays from the sun.

Higher-energy cosmic, gamma, x-ray, most of the far-UV waves, and the lower-energy medium- and far-infrared, micro, radio and electric waves are absorbed or reflected by the atmosphere.

The medium-energy mid- and near-UV, the "visible" spectrum, and the near-infrared (heat) waves are the main rays that penetrate the Earth's atmosphere and reach the planet's surface. These light rays are essential to the health of all living creatures.

The Visible Spectrum = Colors!

Everything in life strives for color.

—Goethe

Light is the first of painters.

—Ralph Waldo Emerson, *Nature*

The cones and rods "see" less than 1% of the sun's electromagnetic spectrum, the "visible" spectrum. Visible light comprises four-fifths of the sun's energy penetrating the atmosphere.

Invisible *ultra*violet light has *higher* energy than violet light.

The colors of the visible spectrum with their associated range of wavelengths are:

- Violet 400–450 nm
- Blue 450–500 nm
- Green 500–550 nm
- Yellow 550–600 nm
- Orange 600–650 nm
- Red 650–700 nm

Invisible *infra*red light has *lower* energy than red light. Infrared light is heat, like the warmth we feel from a room heater. The warmth we feel on our skin from the sun is also infrared light.

In bright light, the human retina is most sensitive to yellow-green light, at ~555 nm, and least sensitive to violet and red light. In darkness, humans are most sensitive to "green" light at ~496 nm. ("Green" light is actually seen as "white" or "gray" in "true" nighttime vision. This is explained further in the next chapter.)

Sunlight, an Essential Nutrient

It has recently been determined that sunlight has many surprising health benefits to humans.

—Research scientist

Go outside and play in the sun, it's good for you.

—Mom

See *Plate 24: Go Outside and Play in the Sun.*

Douglas Kiang, reviewer for *Inside Mac Games,* writes:

> As a reviewer for *Inside Mac Games,* I am lucky enough to see many, many games come across my desktop on a regular basis. Every so often, perhaps once a year, a new title comes along that impels me to throw off my staid reviewer's necktie and dance a little dance around my office, at which point my wife usually comes along, unplugs my Macintosh, and shoves me outside, [saying], "See that? That's called the sun."[1]

Living beings have evolved over many tens of thousands, if not millions, of years under the influence of light from the sun. Life on Earth depends on sunlight. Sunlight warms the oceans. By the process of evaporation, clouds are created, which then move over the land and bring rain. Photosynthesis is responsible for creating the food we eat.

The discoverer of Vitamin C, Nobel Prize winner Albert Szent-Gyorgyi, states that the energy which we take into our bodies ultimately comes from the sun.[2]

Research by John Ott, author of *Health and Light* and *Light, Radiation of You,* and other scientists have shown that for plants, animals, and humans to be healthy, they must have not only the proper quantity of light, but the proper *quality.* The best quality of light comes from the sun, which provides a natural "full spectrum" of both visible and invisible light.

Richard J. Wurtman, a researcher at the Massachusetts Institute of Technology, has shown a connection between light and the rhythmical secretion of hormones in the body.[3]

Inadequate quantity and quality of light can lead to hypertension, headaches, insomnia, arthritis, and other physical, emotional, and mental interferences to our health.

Light for Sight and Health

See *Plate 25: Light for Sight and Health.*

Light entering the eyes is utilized by the body in two ways:

1. Light energy travels to the visual cortex, where a picture of the world is created; and
2. Light energy travels to the hypothalamus, which sends messages to the pineal and pituitary glands. Together, these organs and glands regulate many functions of our mind and body.

The hypothalamus appears to be the master organ of the body, and its functions are highly dependent upon quantity and quality of light received from the eyes.

The hypothalamus regulates the pineal gland, which secretes melatonin—a sedative-like hormone—at night to prepare our body for sleep. Bright light inhibits the pineal gland's secretion of melatonin. Some reports indicate that standard indoor lighting is not sufficient to suppress the secretion of melatonin during the daytime.

The diurnal (day/night) and seasonal changes we experience bodily are largely due to the changes in light via the pineal gland. The pineal gland regulates our internal "body clock" and sends messages back to the hypothalamus to regulate body functions.

The hypothalamus also sends messages to the pituitary gland. The hypothalamus, in conjunction with the pituitary and pineal glands, influences our sleeping and eating patterns, activity levels, the thyroid gland, the adrenal glands, reproductive organs, growth, body temperature, and blood pressure. Metabolic processes are also synchronized by the pineal gland.

The "spark" that initiates these internal processes is light.

The sea lamprey, a species dating back 300 million years, has a "third eye" on top of its head. Not used for seeing, this eye sends light directly to the brain to regulate the fish's metabolism. The skull of some animals is so thin that light from the sun directly influences their pineal gland.

In her book *How Animals See,* Sandra Sinclair describes the tuatara lizard and other animals which have a third eye:

> Presumably the third eye has no great importance in image formation but rather functions more as light-gatherer that activates the body's hormonal clock . . . Most of [a tuatara lizard's] lifetime is spent hibernating, but the third eye never shuts, perhaps monitoring changes in light that tell this lizard when it's time to wake up.[4]

Edith Raskin writes in her book *Watchers, Pursuers and Masqueraders—Animals and Their Vision:*

> How does that seasonal masquerader, the snowshoe hare, know when to change its coat from brown to white and back again? In an attempt to solve this mystery, scientists placed masks over the eyes of snowshoe hares. A curious thing happened—the blindfolded hares did not change. Those blindfolded in the winter remained white in summertime, while those blindfolded in the summer stayed brown in winter.
>
> Evidently if the hares' eyes were covered they did not respond to the seasons. Although they were able to feel daily temperature changes, the summer warmth and the winter cold were no guide for them.
>
> . . . How, precisely, do scientists explain seasonal changes in animals such as the deer and the snowshoe hare? As the seasons change, the hours of daylight change. The eyes of these animals receive the daylight and this light stimulates the optic nerve to transmit nerve impulses to the brain. At the base of the brain is a gland called the pituitary, which is no bigger than a peanut. The brain sends on the nerve impulses to this gland. Receiving these signals, the gland releases its own messengers into the blood. These messengers are chemical substances called hormones.
>
> The pituitary hormones are carried by the blood to different parts of the animal's body. The length of time the eyes receive light determines the extent of hormone messengers sent into the blood. The hormones, in turn, regulate seasonal changes in the deer or snowshoe hare. For instance, in the snowshoe hare, the more light the more hormone, and so its coat is brown; the less light there is, the less hormone, and so its coat is white.[5]

Many relationships have been established between the light that enters our eyes and the brain stem, the cerebral cortex, and the limbic system.

Disturbances in the quality (full spectrum), quantity (photocurrent), intensity (brightness), and timing of light (diurnal cycles from bright daylight to dark night) can lead to health problems. Research has shown that many people who suffer from "Seasonally Affected Disorders" (SAD) have remarkable improvements in the areas of depression, moodiness, and fatigue by simply rebalancing and resynchronizing their body and mind with full-spectrum light.

The Melatonin Controversy

Melatonin is now being produced synthetically and sold as a drug to regulate the body's

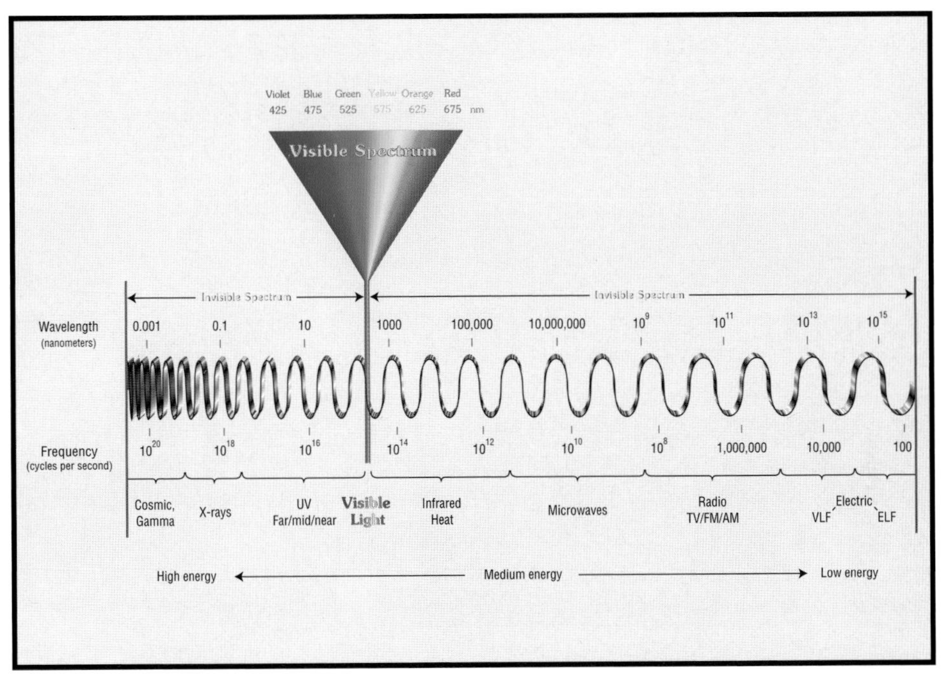

Plate 22. The Electromagnetic and Visible Spectrums.

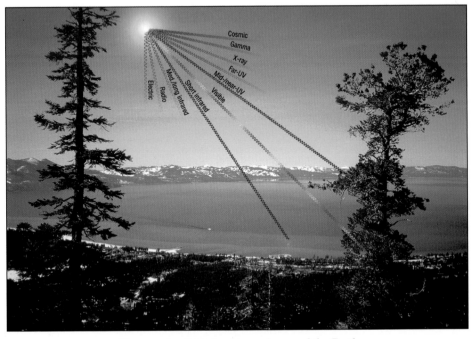

Plate 23. Sunlight, the Atmosphere, and the Earth.

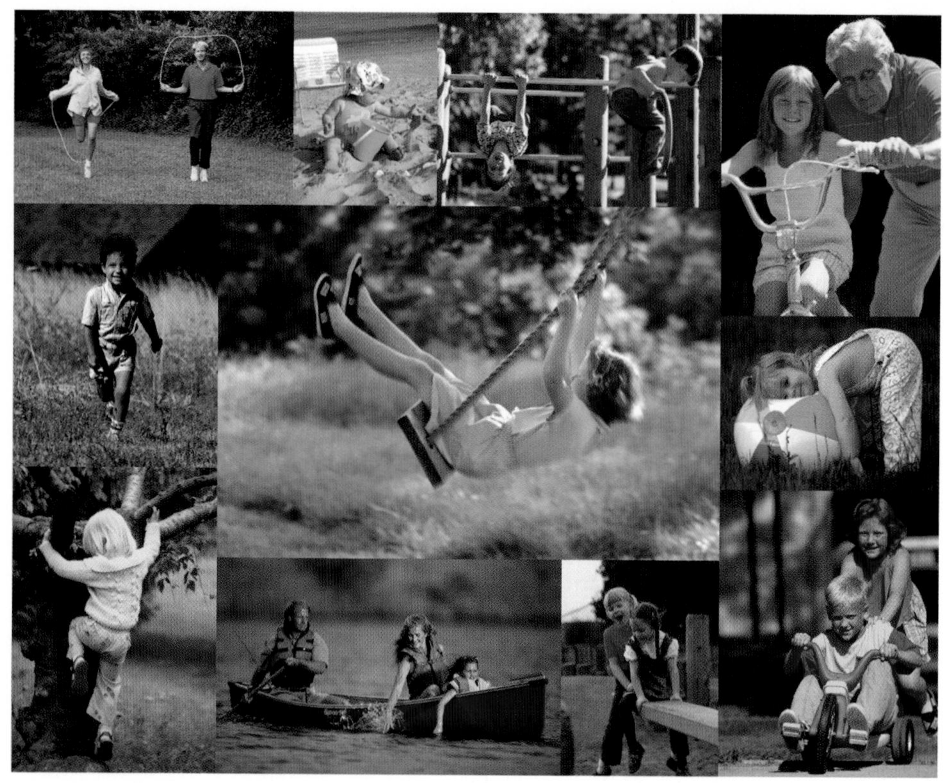

Plate 24. Go Outside and Play in the Sun.

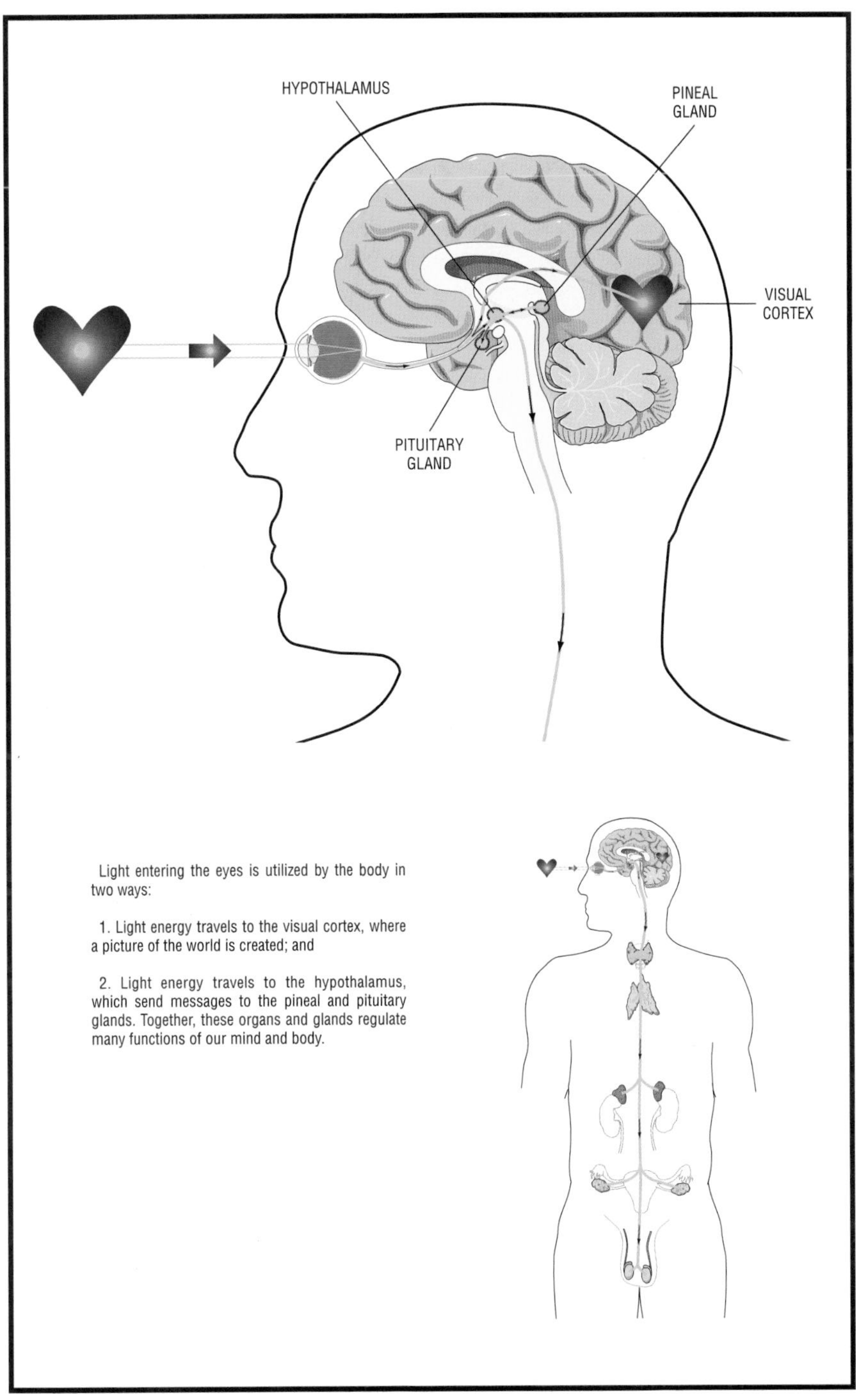
HYPOTHALAMUS
PINEAL GLAND
VISUAL CORTEX
PITUITARY GLAND
Light entering the eyes is utilized by the body in two ways:
1. Light energy travels to the visual cortex, where a picture of the world is created; and
2. Light energy travels to the hypothalamus, which send messages to the pineal and pituitary glands. Together, these organs and glands regulate many functions of our mind and body.

Plate 25. Light for Sight and Health.

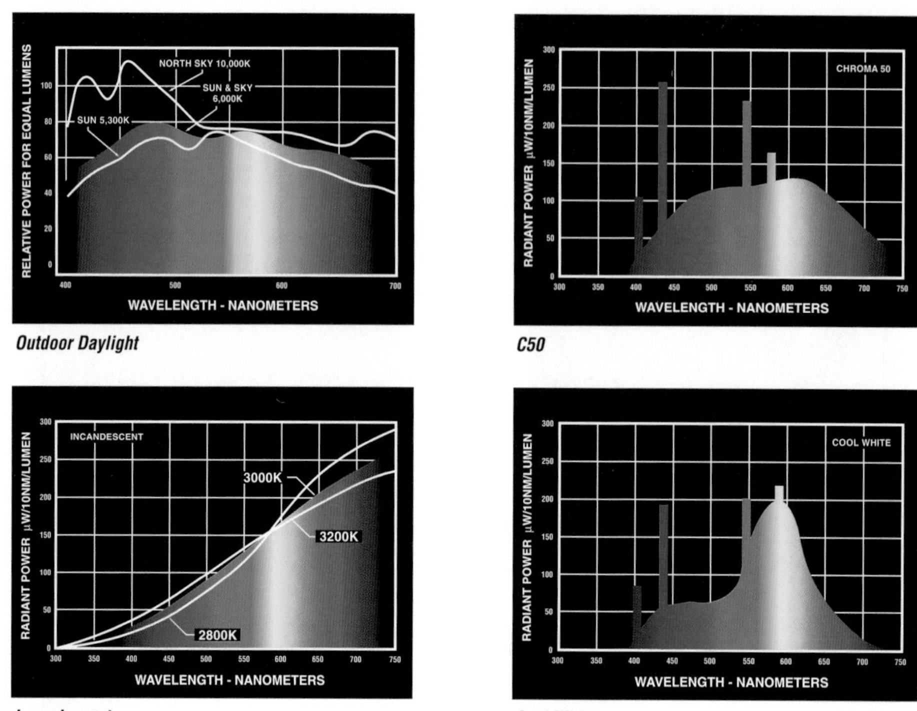

Plate 26. Spectral Power Distribution Curves.
Reprinted with permission from GE Lighting, a division of General Electric Company.

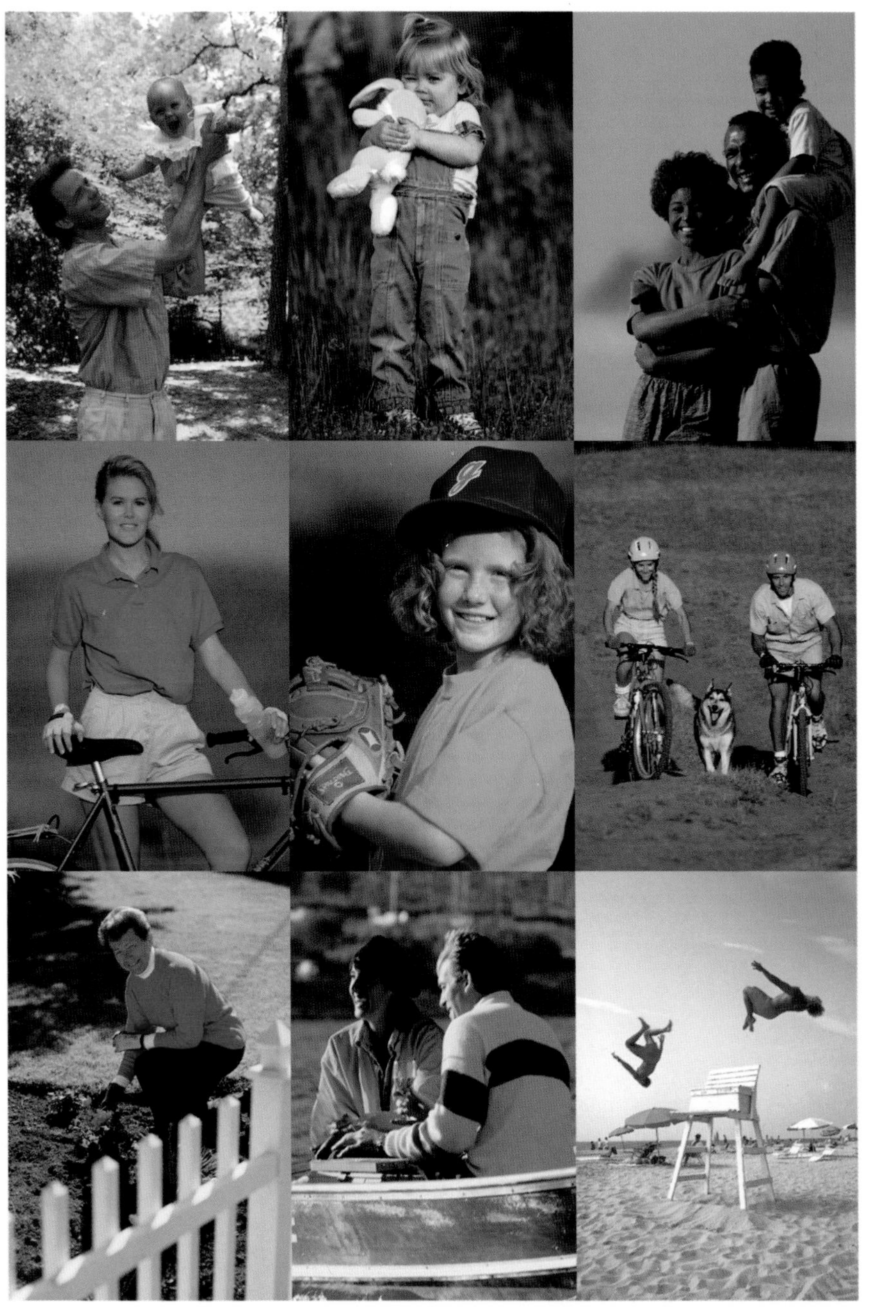

Plate 27. Living in Natural Light.

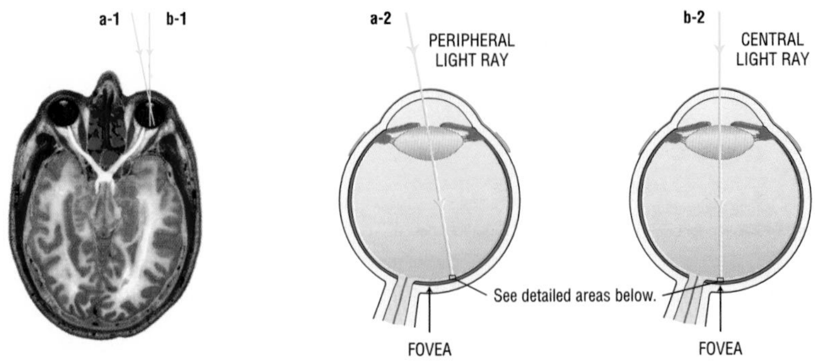

THE TEN LAYERS OF THE PERIPHERAL PART OF THE RETINA

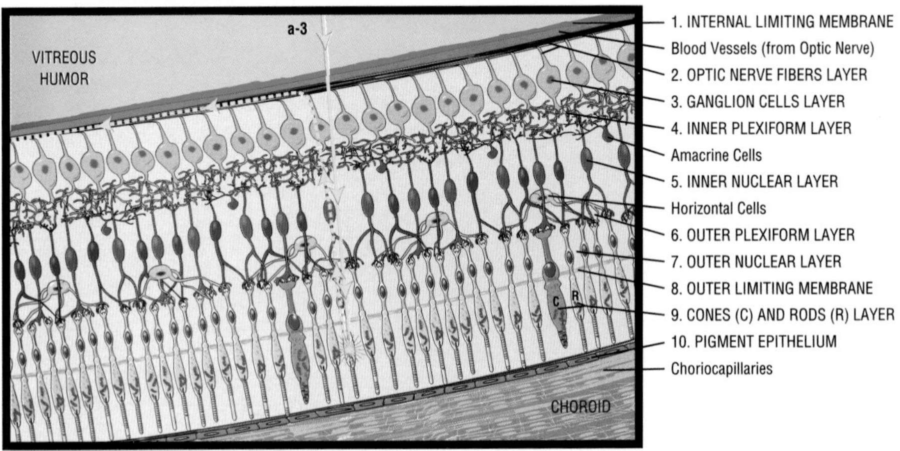

THE FOVEA CENTRALIS

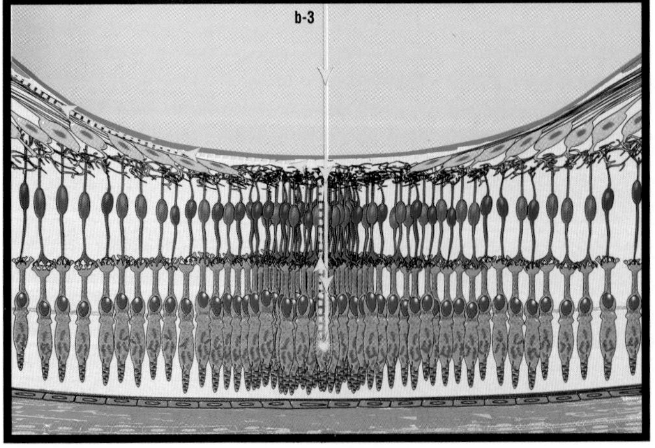

The fovea centralis is a "pit" in the center of the retina. While there are few cones in the peripheral parts of the retina, as shown above, there is a very high concentration of cones in the fovea. There are no rods in the center of the fovea.

At the fovea, the upper layers of the retina are compressed and moved off to the side. This allows the central light rays to reach the cones with less interference.

The absence of blood vessels above the foveal cones is partially compensated by the increased vascularization of the choriocapillaries underneath the fovea.

This structure results in our finest acuity and color perception being in the center of our visual field, and is the physical basis for the principle of centralization.

Plate 28. Retina Cross-Sections.

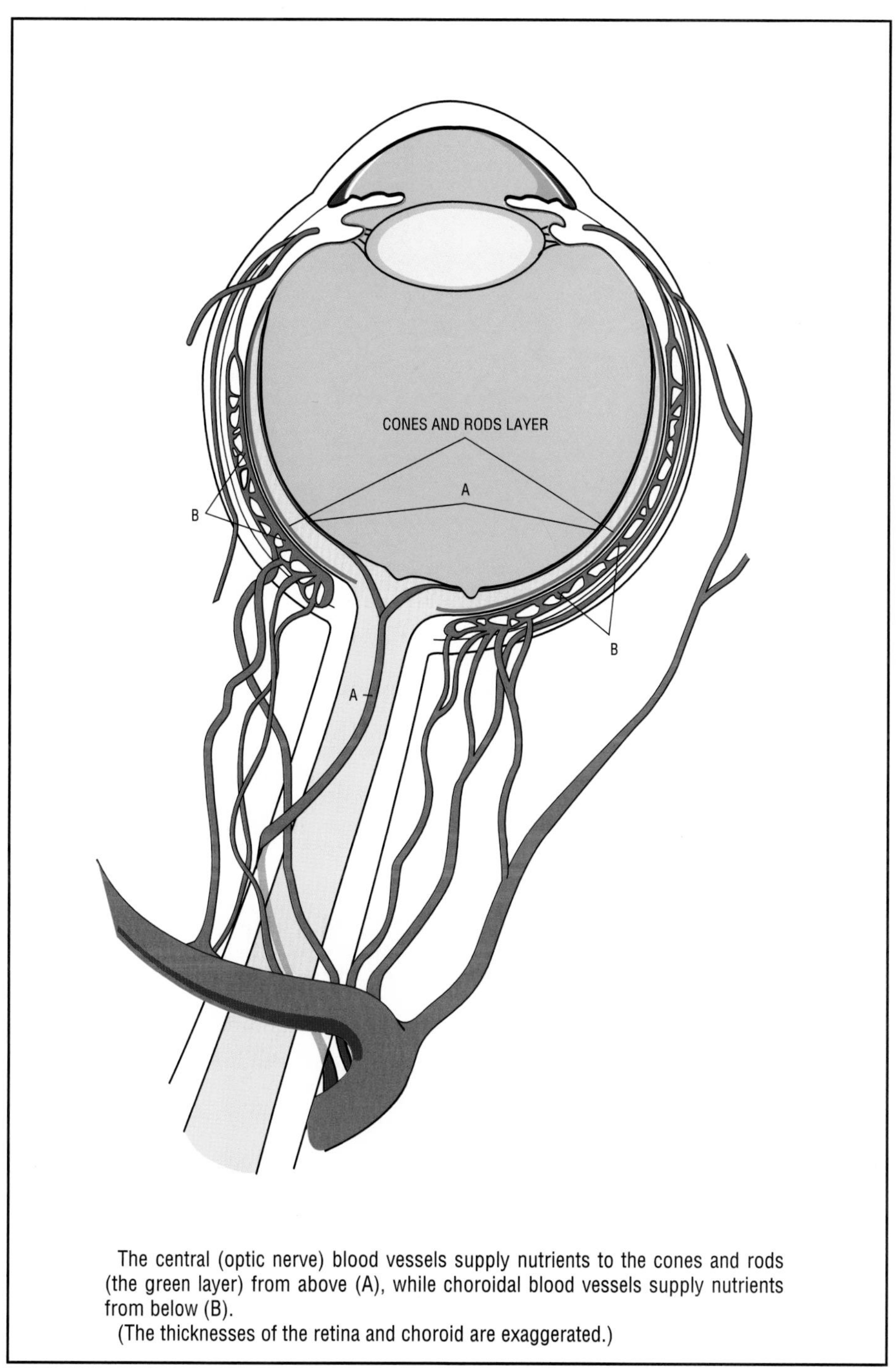

The central (optic nerve) blood vessels supply nutrients to the cones and rods (the green layer) from above (A), while choroidal blood vessels supply nutrients from below (B).
(The thicknesses of the retina and choroid are exaggerated.)

Plate 29. Blood Vessel Sandwich for the Cones and Rods.

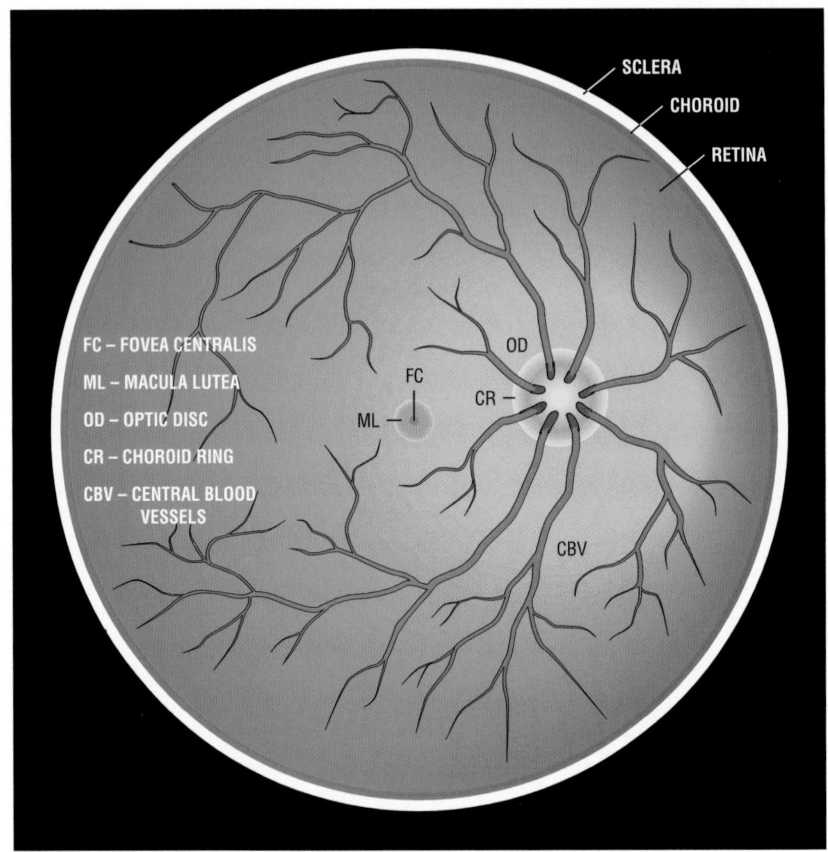

Plate 30. Retina (1).

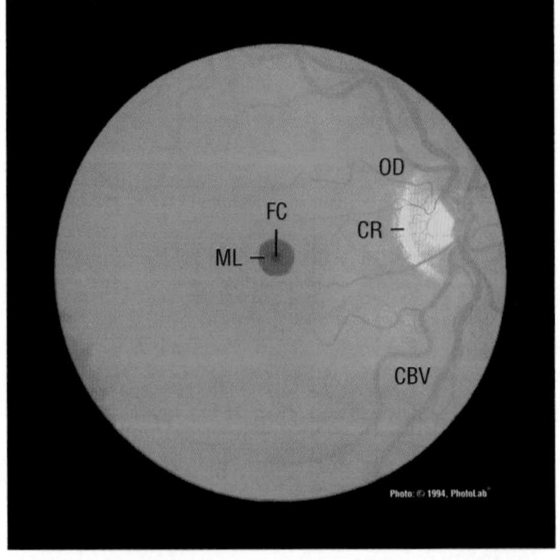

Plate 31. Retina (2).

metabolism. As with many types of drug use, this could be dangerous, especially if used on a long-term basis.

Could long-term use of artificial melatonin lead to the suppression of natural melatonin from the pineal gland? Has the real cause of the pineal gland imbalance been corrected by using an artificial melatonin? Are pineal functions interfered with by wearing sunglasses and by being indoors too much?

Syntonics—Healing with Light

Syntonics (from Greek *syn-*, meaning "together," and *tonos*, meaning "tone"—thus "harmony") is a field of natural health that uses color lights to open up constricted pathways of light energy traveling from the eyes to the brain. Even when two individuals have the same amount of light entering their eyes, the amount of light energy *reaching their brains* can be vastly different. Many people in this society have restricted energy flow (photocurrent) from the eyes to the brain.

Many individuals have reactions or aversions to specific colors, especially when viewing them in a dark room. It appears that certain life stresses can shut down the flow of specific colors from the eyes to the brain. When individuals view certain colors, especially colors associated with their sub-dominant hemisphere, many types of healing can occur. Reversal processes, discussed later in Chapter 20, "The Two Sides of Health and Healing," are typically experienced during syntonic light sessions.

Syntonic sessions tend to improve metabolism, increase life force energy, and put a person back into "sync" with nature. Jacob Liberman's book *Light: Medicine of the Future* contains a list of syntonic practitioners.

Sunning with Closed Eyelids

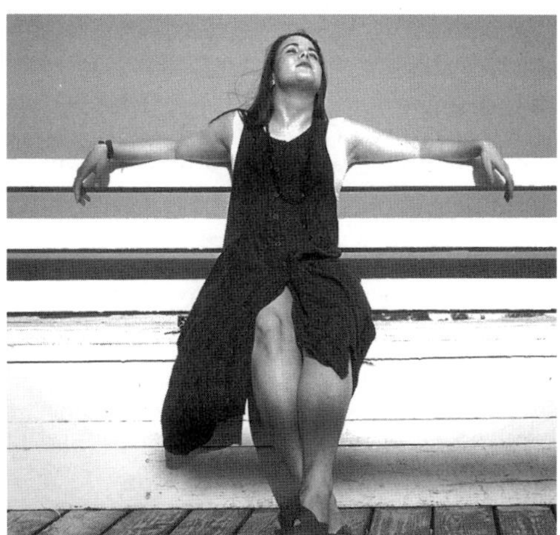

Closed-eyelids *sunning* is one of the best ways to regain light tolerance. The eyes are organs of light; they are designed for, and need, natural light. People who are over-sensitive to light *need light,* not sunglasses and darkness.

Bates researched various forms of self-healing, including sunning. After Bates wrote *Perfect Sight Without Glasses,* he concluded *closed-eyelids* sunning was the only form of sunning a student should practice.

From *Better Eyesight* magazine, December 1927:

> An important part of the routine activities is the use of the direct sunlight. The student is told to sit in the sun with his eyes closed, moving his head a short distance from side to side, and allowing the sun to shine directly on his closed eyelids. He is instructed to forget about his eyes, to think of something pleasant and let his mind drift from one pleasant thought to another. Before opening his eyes, he palms for a few minutes. When the sun is not shining, a

> strong electric light ... is substituted ... allowing it to shine on his closed eyelids as in the sun....

In *Better Eyesight* magazine, July 1927, Mr. Ian Jardine, a Natural Vision teacher, tells of his own introduction to closed-eyelid sunning:

> ...Then I was shown how to sun my eyes by letting the rays of the sun fall on the closed eyelids, while moving the head gently from side to side. This seemed a strange thing to do, as previously I had worn blue glasses to shield the eyes from strong light.

Closed-Eyelid Sunning

Closed-eyelid sunning is a natural, healthy activity. Animals "sun" naturally. Sunning is not an "exercise"; it is a self-healing activity. Remember to keep the eyelids *closed* while sunning.

TO SUN:

Sit in a comfortable chair facing the sun. A reclining chair is especially relaxing. Close your eyelids. Depending upon the relationship of your head to the sun, tilt your head slightly toward the sun. Then, swing your nose-feather gently to the right, then to the left, then to the right, and continue alternating back and forth slowly across the sun.

Even though the eyelids are closed, notice how the sun appears to move in the opposite direction of your head movement.

The infinity sign/figure-8 shape is an excellent pattern while sunning. Remember to move the nose-feather up through the center and down on the outsides of the loops, i.e., counterclockwise on the left and clockwise on the right.

Even a few minutes of sunning can be very beneficial. Do not sun for so long a period that you get a sunburn. Five to ten minutes at a time is fine for most people. If at first the light is too bright, you can sun while sitting under a shady tree.

If the sun is not available, you can "sun" indoors by using a regular 100-watt light bulb. Of course, the sun is always the best.

Another wonderful way to sun is to do the Long Swing at sunrise or sunset. Remember to keep the eyelids closed while sunning.

Tom's Personal Log: I was sitting on a bench with a friend at a park one day. I noticed she had closed her eyelids and was moving her

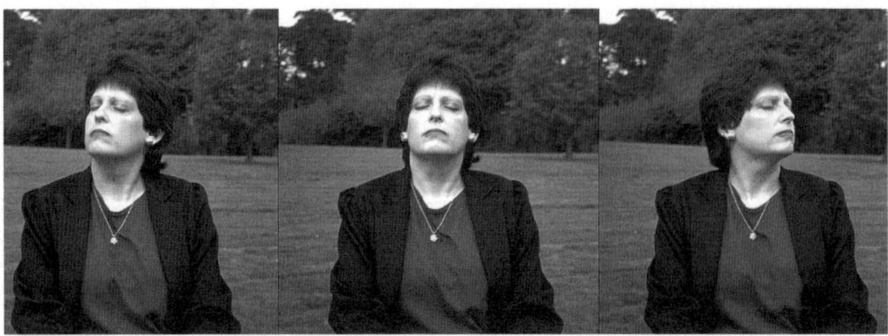

Figure 16–2: Sunning.

slightly uplifted head gently to the right and left, across the sun.

She did not know about "sunning" by reading or hearing about it. This was simply natural for her to do. She has normal sight.

The Sunning Sandwich

One way to develop better brightness-to-darkness and darkness-to-brightness adaptation is to alternate sunning with palming. You can enjoy closed-eyelid sunning for three minutes, followed by three minutes of palming. Then do three minutes of sunning again, three minutes of palming, and so forth. Palming is described in Chapter 21, "Palming and Acupressure."

Strobing (or Flashing) While Sunning

Do not do this activity if you are prone to photo-convulsive seizures.

Another variation on sunning is to flicker your fingers in front of your closed eyelids. This creates a stroboscopic or flashing effect, which stimulates micro-movements in the eyes.

BATES ON LIGHT

From *Perfect Sight Without Glasses:*

> It is not light but darkness that is dangerous to the eye. Prolonged exclusion from the light always lowers the vision, and may produce serious inflammatory conditions. Among young children living in tenements this is a somewhat frequent cause of ulcers upon the cornea, which ultimately destroy the sight. The children, finding their eyes sensitive to light, bury them in the pillows and thus shut out the light entirely.
>
> The universal fear of reading or doing fine work in a dim light is, however, unfounded. So long as the light is sufficient so that one can see without discomfort, this practice is not only harmless, but may be beneficial.
>
> Sudden contrasts of light are supposed to be particularly harmful to the eye.... There is no evidence whatever to support these statements.... Such practices as reading alternately in a bright and a dim light, or going from a dark room to a well-lighted one, and vice versa, are to be recommended. Even such rapid ... fluctuations of light as those involved in the production of the moving picture are, in the long run, beneficial to all eyes. I always advise students to go to the movies frequently and practice centralizing. They soon become accustomed to the flickering light, and afterward other light and reflections cause less annoyance.

ARTIFICIAL LIGHTING

Until man duplicates a blade of grass, Nature can laugh at his so-called scientific achievements.

—Thomas A. Edison

Ever since Thomas Edison invented the electric light bulb in 1879, we have been participating in an experiment with artificial light. Due to modern technology the amount and quality of light many people are exposed to has been radically altered.

Quantitatively, many people in our society are outdoors only 10% of the time, compared to 80% before the invention of the electric light bulb. When outdoors, many people wear dark sunglasses, which reduces even further their reception of natural sunlight—an essential nutrient.

Qualitatively, the spectrum of light we are under when indoors differs significantly from the natural light our visual system has evolved under. Many studies have shown that common types of artificial light can be harmful to our health.

For example, studies have shown that biological stress and learning difficulties increase when individuals are under standard "cool-white" fluorescent tubes. Based partly on research by Dr. Fritz Hollwich[6] in 1980, Germany placed a ban on cool-white fluorescent lights in medical facilities.

Conventional lighting, including standard incandescent light bulbs and cool-white fluorescent tubes, are very poor substitutes for natural sunlight. If a person is going to spend a great portion of the day indoors, it is important to weigh the benefits and drawbacks of various types of artificial lighting.

Since there are disadvantages with each type of artificial light, *no* artificial light is an adequate substitute for natural sunlight. What type of lighting is best for homes and workplaces? The answer is complicated.

See the *Light Comparison Table* in Appendix D.

Natural, "Full-Spectrum" Sunlight

See *Plate 26: Spectral Power Distribution Curves.*

"Outdoor Daylight" shows the sun providing a fairly even distribution of the visible spectrum. Notice how the "Outdoor Daylight" spectrum changes depending upon the location and time of day.

Outdoor sunlight also provides a small amount of mid- and near-UV light in about a 1:10 ratio.

Note that the vertical and horizontal axes are different between "Outdoor Daylight" and the other three graphs. Spikes in fluorescent spectrums are characteristics of the phosphor coating used inside the tubes.

The CCTs and CRIs of Light

Changes in a light's spectrum are, in part, due to the source's temperature, known as chromaticity, or Correlated Color Temperature (CCT). CCT is a measure of a light source's apparent "whiteness," yellowness (warmth), or blueness (coolness), and is measured in units of degrees Kelvin (K). CCT is a measure of the light source's direct appearance to our eyes. CCT measurements do not include the mid- and near-UV spectrum.

A candle flame has a very warm, orange/yellow CCT of approximately 1600K; the sun and sky at sunrise are 1800K (yellow/warm); one hour after sunrise, the sun has a CCT of approximately 3600K (warm); at noon 4870K (slightly warm; almost white); an overcast sky is approximately 7100K (bluer/cooler); the Northwest sky is 25,000K (very blue/cool). Near 5500K, the sunlight is "white."

Notice the inverse relationship with CCTs—a "warmer" light source has a lower CCT, and a "cooler" light has a higher CCT. The terms "warmer" (yellow/orange/red) and "cooler" (blue/indigo/violet) refer to the psychological effects of the light source, not its temperature.

Another indicator of a light's "naturalness" is the Color Rendering Index (CRI), which ranges from 1 to 100. CRI indicates how well the colors of objects are rendered (reflected), using a light source at a specific CCT. Outdoor sunlight has a "perfect, natural" CRI rating of 100. Unlike CCT, CRI measurements include visible spectrum and mid- and near-UV factors.

The CRIs of lights that have different CCTs cannot be compared. This is because even though two light sources may have the same CRIs, they may render colors very differently if they have different CCTs.

An incandescent bulb with a high CRI of 95, but a low CCT of 2700K, is yellow/red intense and blue-deficient. See *Plate 26, "Incandescent."* It would not be valid to compare this incandescent bulb's light quality to another light with a CRI of 95, but a higher CCT of 5000K. It is valid to compare the CRIs only of lights that have the same CCTs.

Generally, a light source with a CCT of 5000K and a CRI of 80–89 will give a good color rendering. A CCT of 5000 and a CRI of 90–100 will give excellent color rendering.

The Quest for Artificial, Full-Spectrum Lighting

In recent years light manufacturers have become aware of the many benefits of full-spectrum lighting. They have attempted to improve on the poor (and many say *unhealthy*) light spectrums provided by standard incandescent and cool-white fluorescent lights. Much research and development has gone into creating an artificial light (or combination of lights) that attempts to emulate, as closely as possible, the natural full-spectrum light provided by the sun.

In evaluating artificial light sources, both CCT and CRI need to be taken into consideration. Generally, light that has a CCT between 5000K and 7500K *and* a CRI of 90 or more is considered to be "full-spectrum" light. At least one company says that the proper ratio of mid- and near-UV light must be included in the light to be considered "truly" full spectrum.

Some modern fluorescent tubes or fixtures have these characteristics. Most standard incandescent and halogen bulbs have very high CRIs, but low CCTs. So, they do not "qualify" as full-spectrum lights.

An additional consideration is how efficiently the light is produced. Efficiency, also known as efficacy, is measured in lumens per watt. Lumens refers to the amount of light produced; wattage is the power consumed. A very high-wattage light bulb or tube may produce a small amount of light, and therefore, would be relatively inefficient. A more efficient light bulb or tube may produce a large amount of light with the same or even fewer watts.

Let's review the pros and cons of various types of artificial lights.

"Regular," Incandescent, Tungsten Lightbulbs

Regular incandescent lightbulbs were invented by Thomas Edison in 1879. Incandescent bulbs use a tungsten filament (wire) that glows when electricity passes through it.

Advantages of regular, incandescent bulbs:

1. Initial cost is low.
2. Easy to replace.
3. Provide good contrast and shadow—contrast is important to sight.
4. Variable brightness, by changing wattage.
5. Very high CRI of 95–98.
6. Can be used with dimmer (variable) switches, although dimming produces an even more distorted spectrum. If a

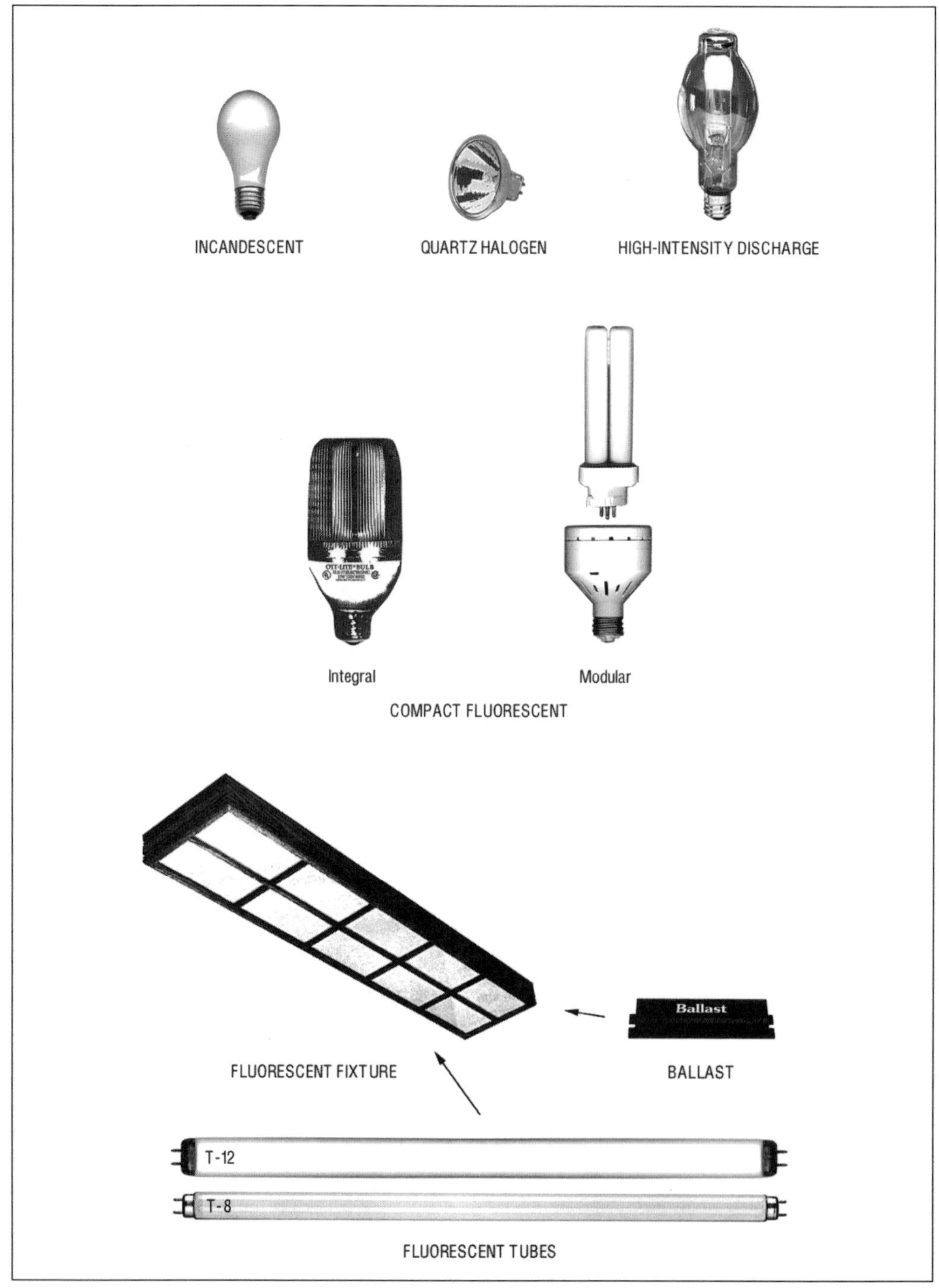

Figure 16–3: Lighting.

low level of light is desired, it is better to use a lower-wattage bulb than a "dimmer" switch. The lower-wattage bulb produces a better spectrum than a higher-wattage bulb lowered in wattage by a dimmer.

Disadvantages of regular, incandescent bulbs:

1. Expensive in the long term due to frequent replacements—much shorter lifetime than fluorescent tubes.
2. Inconvenience of frequent replacement.
3. Minimal mid- and near-UV light is emitted.
4. A very low CCT of 3000K. As can be seen in the *Plate 26, "Incandescent"* graph, incandescent bulbs provide a very poor balance of colors, being very yellow-red intense, and violet-blue deficient. Note that natural sunlight *peaks* in the blue region.
5. As can also be seen from *Plate 26,* incandescent bulbs are very energy-inefficient in regards to the production of light. Ninety percent of the energy from an incandescent bulb is given off not in the form of light, but as infrared heat; essentially, an incandescent bulb is an expensive space heater.
6. Approximately 22% of light output is lost during lifetime.
7. Many bulbs fail when switched-on or jarred.
8. Much less efficient than advanced fluorescent tubes.
9. Sixty-cycle flicker.

The incandescent bulb has a relatively high "visual efficiency" because the human visual system has a greater sensitivity to yellow than blue. In other words, an incandescent bulb emits a high amount of energy in the yellow region, and we see yellow better than the other colors. Even though it has a high CRI of 95–98, the total spectrum is very imbalanced, and objects illuminated by this light render colors very "warm."

There are some incandescent bulbs that claim to be "full-spectrum." One such popular bulb has no CCT or CRI ratings on its package. The intensity of light from a 150-watt bulb seems like the light from a standard 75-watt incandescent bulb. The color of light appeared unnatural (dull purple) to some people. Some students say the spectrum looks more natural, and therefore feels better, than a regular incandescent bulb. One product claims an average life of 3500 hours, compared to a typical 750-hour, standard incandescent bulb.

"Quartz" Halogen Lightbulbs

Halogen lightbulbs contain a tungsten filament and halogen gas (typically iodine), which results in a "whiter" spectrum than most incandescent bulbs and higher lumens per watt (greater efficacy). Halogen lightbulbs are often used in automobile headlights.

Because halogen bulbs operate at a higher temperature, they require the use of quartz glass instead of regular glass. Halogen bulbs are usually more expensive than regular incandescent bulbs.

Advantages of halogen bulbs:

1. Very bright and can be precisely focused.
2. High CRI, 95 typical.
3. Last longer than incandescent bulbs.

4. Approximately 12% more energy-efficient than incandescent bulbs.
5. Can be used with dimmer (variable) switches.
6. Lose less light over its lifetime than incandescent bulbs; 10% light loss versus the incandescent's 22%.

Disadvantages of halogen bulbs:

1. Low CCT.
2. Initial cost higher than incandescent bulbs.
3. High heat output, sometimes requiring a special fixture.
4. Much less efficient than advanced fluorescent tubes.
5. Much shorter lifetime than fluorescent tubes.
6. Sixty-cycle flicker.

One report recently warned of supposed harm of UV from halogen light. Unlike regular glass used for regular incandescent and most fluorescent lights, UV light created in the halogen bulb is transmitted through the quartz glass. One government agency is recommending people not use halogen lights unless manufacturers add "regular glass" to prevent the UV from escaping.

The reader will need to decide whether different sources of UV light are harmful or *beneficial.*

High-Intensity Discharge (HID) Lights

High-Intensity Discharge (HID) lights are made in three types: mercury, sodium, and metal halide.

Mercury HIDs are the older type. They have a high CCT but a very low CRI. Mercury HIDs are not as efficient as the newer HIDs, and are becoming obsolete.

Sodium HIDs have higher CRIs, but lower CCTs.

Metal halide HIDs have CCTs ranging up to 3800K, and CRIs up to 75.

Because of their very high efficiencies, modern HIDs are used primarily outdoors to light large areas at night, like streets and parking lots. HIDs cannot be used with a dimmer.

"Compact" Fluorescent (CF) Lights

"Compact fluorescent" (CF) lights fit in standard "screw-in" light fixtures and can, therefore, replace many standard incandescent bulbs. Because some CFs are taller and wider than regular incandescent bulbs, they may not fit into some lamps or lighting fixtures unless a taller lampshade harp or a socket extender is used.

The lower-wattage CFs are rated to be equivalent to much higher-wattage incandescent bulbs. For example, an 18-watt CF is often stated to be the equivalent of a 75-watt incandescent bulb.

However, CFs seem to put out less light than the "equivalent" incandescent bulb. This is partly due to the high visual sensitivity to yellow and the yellow-intense incandescent bulb factors discussed above. There can be a period of adjustment when switching to CFs. CFs are more economical in the long run because they last much longer than incandescent bulbs.

Many of the newer CFs use the much improved *electronic* ballast discussed below.

I am not aware of any CFs that provide mid- and near-UV spectrum. Also, many CFs do not produce as much contrast as incandescent bulbs. Contrast is important to eyesight.

Current CFs cannot be used with dimmer switches.

One-piece (integral) CFs use a built-in ballast, which can be either electronic or magnetic. Integral CFs have the disadvantage of having to throw away the entire unit when it burns out.

Two-piece (modular) CFs incorporate a reusable magnetic ballast contained in the screw-in base, and a replaceable fluorescent tube that attaches to the base. The tube is typically rated at 10,000 hours, while the base/ballast is rated at approximately 50,000 hours.

Modular CFs currently use only magnetic ballasts—a disadvantage. The magnetic ballast in a CF base can be much heavier than the light incandescent bulb it is replacing. As a consequence, replacement in some fixtures may not be practical. The wattages of both the tube and the ballast need to be added to get the total wattage of a modular CF.

Never use any type of fluorescent light with a dimmer switch, even if it is set at full power. Doing so could cause premature burn-out, and could create a fire hazard.

Fluorescent Lights

Standard fluorescent tubes, invented in 1938, are much more energy-efficient than incandescent bulbs. In contrast to the 10% efficiency of incandescent bulbs, approximately 30% of the energy used to power fluorescent tubes is converted to light.

Many "full-spectrum" fluorescent tubes are not only energy-efficient, but have a much longer lifetime than typical cool-white fluorescent tubes. So, even though the full-spectrum tubes have a higher initial cost, their long-term cost can be much less than the equivalent light from standard fluorescent tubes. The longer lifetime also eliminates inconvenient, frequent replacements of tubes. I have found this to be major advantage.

As seen in *Plate 26: Spectral Power Distribution Curves,* the typical "Cool White" fluorescent tube provides an imbalanced spectrum compared to "Outdoor Daylight." The phosphor composition in the "Cool White" maximizes the yellow-green region, where our eyes are most sensitive to colors. The "Cool White," which has a low CRI of 68 and a CCT of only 4200K, is deficient in the green, blue, violet, and UV parts of the spectrum. Like incandescent bulbs, cool-white fluorescents are deficient in the blue region, where sunlight has its maximum intensity.

There are many types of fluorescent tubes, ranging from cool-white to the advanced full-spectrum tubes.

Fluorescent Tube Types

For many years, most four- and eight-foot fluorescent tubes had a diameter of one and a half inch, known as "T-12" tubes.

Some manufacturers now produce more efficient, one-inch-diameter "T-8" fluorescent tubes. T-8s are rated at 32 watts, while the larger T-12s typically operate at 40 watts. The smaller surface area inside the T-8s allows the use of more expensive and efficient phosphor combinations. T-8s can produce more lumens (light) per watt and can result in higher CRI ratings (at CCTs of 5000–5500K). However, the total lumen output is usually less than that from T-10s and T-12s.

Even though T-8s have a smaller diameter, the bipin width is the same as the standard T-12s. This means T-8s can be used in standard fluorescent fixtures. T-10s have an intermediate diameter of a 1¼", and have the same bipin width as the T-12s and T-8s. T-5s are miniature, low-wattage (typically 6W) tubes, with a small bipin width.

Advanced Full-Spectrum Fluorescent Tubes

As can be seen in *Plate 26,* "C50" (Chroma 50) produces a more balanced spectrum than the "Incandescent" bulb and the "Cool White" fluorescent tube. The Chroma 50's spectrum is closer to the spectrum of "Outdoor Daylight." The Chroma 50 has a CCT of 5000K, and a CRI of 90.

"Diffusion is Still Confusion"

"Full-spectrum" fluorescent tubes do not, by themselves, provide adequate lighting.

Due to the design of fluorescent tubes, and the way fluorescent tubes use phosphors to produce light, fluorescent light is more diffused than incandescent (point) light sources. Diffused light gives a relative dullness to objects, i.e., less contrast.

A CF is slightly less diffused than a standard four-foot fluorescent tube because of the CF's smaller size.

Contrast is very important to sight. Sight functions largely by the detection of edges and shadows. Contrast indoors can be obtained by using incandescent or halogen bulbs, or by allowing natural sunlight to enter through windows or skylights.

Fluorescent Hardware Considerations

The fluorescent tubes mentioned above will fit in most fluorescent fixtures. However, fluorescent lights cannot be used with dimmer switches—at least not yet.

Some fluorescent tubes emit the mid- and near-UV spectrum. The glass or plastic used with some fluorescent tubes is specially designed to let the UV light out of the tube.

Many fluorescent fixtures have plastic coverings, called diffusers. Since UV light is absorbed by conventional diffusers, it is important that the UV light produced by special fluorescent tubes not be absorbed by the diffuser.

There are three solutions to this problem:

1. Use a special UV-transmitting diffuser.
2. Use an "egg-crate" diffuser, which has large, square holes through which the light passes—a practical solution; egg-crate diffusers are available at many hardware and lighting stores.
3. Do not use a diffuser; however, aesthetics may not make this a practical solution.

Ballasts for Fluorescent Lights

Unlike regular incandescent bulbs, fluorescent tubes require a transformer, or ballast, to regulate the electricity delivered to the tubes. Ballasts come in two types: the older magnetic type, also known as "core-coil," and the newer electronic type. Usually, either type will power two four-foot, 40-watt (or less) fluorescent tubes.

Advantages of magnetic ballasts:

1. Initially less expensive than the newer electronic ballasts.
2. Already installed in many fluorescent fixtures.

Disadvantages of magnetic ballasts:

1. Many have an annoying hum or buzz. Magnetic ballasts have sound ratings, which are usually indicated on the label on the ballast. A ballast with sound rating "C" can be annoying—especially if listened to for a long time. If you are going to use a fluorescent fixture containing a magnetic ballast, be sure to

get the quieter type with sound rating "A." Unfortunately, the sound level can increase over time with either type.

2. Physical vibration, which can cause the entire fixture, especially the metal parts, to vibrate, producing additional irritating noise.
3. Less energy-efficient than electronic ballasts, which makes them more expensive to operate in the long run.
4. Subtle but "unnerving" flicker, or strobe-like, effect. Magnetic ballasts alternate off and on at 60 cycles per second. This flicker can be eliminated by converting the source of power from alternating current (AC) to direct current (DC), but this would be impractical for many people.
5. Generation of more heat than electronic ballasts.
6. Delay, accompanied by flickering, when starting.
7. Heavier than electronic ballasts.

Advantages of electronic ballasts:

1. Silent; no noise; no vibration.
2. Thirteen to twenty-five percent more energy-efficient than magnetic ballasts, which makes them less expensive to operate in the long run.
3. Operate at 20,000–25,000 cycles (on/off) per second; no noticeable flicker or stroboscopic effect.
4. Start more quickly (nearly instantaneously) than magnetic ballasts.
5. Operate cooler than magnetic ballasts.
6. Weigh less than magnetic ballasts.

Disadvantages of electronic ballasts:

1. Higher initial cost.
2. May need to replace magnetic ballasts in current fixtures.

Ballast issues can become very complex. Ballasts come in different grades, or qualities. Also, some manufacturers recommend "matching" a specific ballast with a specific fluorescent tube. These issues are beyond the scope of this book.

Considering the advantages of electronic ballasts, they are highly recommended.

"*Investigate* Before You *Invest*"

Since new technology in lighting is often expensive, it is worthwhile comparing prices of lights and hardware. Consult with lighting manufacturers, and lighting and hardware stores in your area.

Since advanced types of fluorescent lights have a very long lifetime, and since you probably will not replace these lights until they burn out, it may be worthwhile spending some time to research which ones are best for you.

As advanced lighting products are produced in greater quantities, and as more companies enter this market, prices should come down. For example, the cost of some electronic ballasts has dropped from $59 to $39 in the last four years.

There is a myriad of features in the new lights and fixtures. So, as a financial advisor once cautioned his students, "*Investigate* before you *invest.*"

Helping the environment is another reason for using energy-efficient full-spectrum fluorescent tubes, CFs and electronic ballasts.

X-rays, and Other Radiation

At least one light researcher has expressed concern about, and has gone to lengths to eliminate, low-level x-rays coming from cathodes of fluorescent tubes.

When concerned about any form of radiation, it is helpful to consider that radiation diminishes in intensity exponentially with the distance from the source. For example, if a point light source puts out *x* units of radiation at one foot, only 25% of that radiation will be received at two feet; only 11% of the radiation at three feet, and *only 1% of the radiation at ten feet.* So, what may be a concern at one foot may be of negligible or no concern at ten feet.

If you are concerned about x-ray, or any other kind of radiation from any device, increase the distance between yourself and the device. As just discussed, a small increase in distance results in a large reduction in radiation exposure.

Alternatively, lead-impregnated tape can be wrapped around the ends of the fluorescent tubes where the cathodes are located, to reduce or eliminate x-ray emissions.

LIGHT "JET-LAG"

The technological advances in lighting have made artificial light available at all hours of the day *and night.* As a result, many people are now suffering from over a century of full-spectrum light "jet lag." Many people have become desynchronized with the daily and seasonal influences of light. The darkness of night is just as important as the bright full-spectrum light of day. This timing distortion is a direct consequence of modern technology.

DAYTIME FULL-SPECTRUM LIGHT—ALL DAY AND ALL NIGHT?

Many of the advanced full-spectrum lights attempt to simulate natural, *noon-time* sunlight. This means that a person is under a static, "noon-time" light during the entire time spent under these lights. But the spectrum of natural sunlight changes throughout the day. We have all observed the changing colors of sunrise, noon-time, and sunset. Perhaps the next development in full-spectrum lighting will be a light that adjusts its spectrum based on the time of day.

Of course, at nighttime sunlight is absent. Does the use of advanced full-spectrum *daylight* lights *at night* throw us even more out of balance with nature?

When researching artificial light sources, the quality of light is an important issue, but so is the *change* in the characteristics of light throughout the 24-hour day—an issue that has been largely ignored.

MORE ON ULTRAVIOLET

Three Types of UV Light

In discussing UV light, it is important to distinguish between the lower-energy mid- and near-UV light discussed above, and the higher-energy far-UV. Many articles have been written about the supposed "harm" of UV light, especially in respect to sunglasses, cataracts, and skin cancer. Unfortunately, oftentimes no distinction is made between higher- and lower-energy UV light.

The sun radiates three types of UV light:

1. High-energy, far-UV (100–290 nm), also called UV-C. Far-UV is naturally absorbed by the ozone layer in the atmosphere. Any far-UV that reaches the Earth's surface and enters the eye is absorbed by the cornea.
2. Medium-energy, mid-UV (290–320 nm), also called UV-B. Mid-UV naturally penetrates the atmosphere and reaches the Earth's surface. Of the mid-UV light that reaches the eye, the

cornea absorbs some of the mid-UV, while the lens absorbs any mid-UV light not absorbed by the cornea.

3. Low-energy, near-UV (320–380 nm), also called UV-A. Near-UV also naturally reaches the Earth's surface. The lens absorbs all near-UV light that enters the eyes.

Apparently, *no* type of UV light reaches the retina.

Most UV light is absorbed by whatever it strikes on the Earth's surface. It is not reflected. Therefore, the great majority of UV light that passes through the atmosphere does not enter our eyes.

Natural and Essential Mid- and Near-UV Light

The Earth's surface receives a small but significant amount of mid- and near-UV light. These two types of UV light are essential to human, animal, and plant life, and for this reason are included in some advanced fluorescent lights.

Bees and some other insects and animals can "see" ultraviolet light. Ultraviolet patterns on a flower guide the bee to its nectar. Vitamin D, necessary for calcium assimilation, is produced in the skin by UV light.

Some have considered the health benefits of mid- and near-UV light important enough to install special UV-transmitting plastic in the windows of homes and buildings.

The lenses used in conventional glasses and contact lenses absorb about 90% of the UV light. One optometrist provides his clients with special, UV-*transmitting* lenses. According to this optometrist, it is important to verify that lenses *claiming* to be UV-transmitting *actually do* transmit the UV light.

Standard non-UV transmitting contact lenses cause a pupil to be larger than its normal size. John Ott, in his book *Health and Light,* writes of an experiment conducted in 1969 by Philip Salvatori, chairman of the Board of Directors of Obrig Laboratories:

> The experiment consisted of fitting a [person] with an ultraviolet transmitting contact lens for one eye and a non-ultraviolet transmitting lens over the other eye.
>
> Indoors, under artificial light containing no ultraviolet, the size of both pupils appeared the same, but outdoors, under natural sunlight, there was a marked difference. The pupil covered with the ultraviolet transmitting lens was considerably smaller. This would seem to indicate that the photoreceptor mechanism that controls the opening and closing of the iris responds to ultraviolet wavelengths as well as visible light.[7]

Sunlight and Nutrition

Research has shown that there can be harm from sunlight if a person has poor nutrition. See Dr. Zane R. Kime's book, *Sunlight Could Save Your Life,* listed in the Bibliography.

Mid-UV Causes Cataracts?

Some have "suggested" that mid-UV light "may" be a cause of cataracts. One study was based on a sample of 838 fishermen who did not wear eye protection. The fishermen who had greater exposure to mid-UV had a higher rate of cataracts. Admittedly, there could have been a completely different reason these fishermen had more cataracts. Although no claim is made that this study "proved" mid-UV causes cataracts, much attention has been directed to recommending UV-absorbing sunglasses be worn as a precaution.

One national agency has stated that the research connecting long-term exposure to sunlight to cataracts is inconclusive, and even flawed.

Bates said cataracts can be caused by mental strain. See Chapter 27, "Serious Vision Problems."

Bates on UV

Quoting from *Perfect Sight Without Glasses:*

> As for the ultra violet part of the spectrum, to which exaggerated importance has been attached by many recent writers, the situation was found to be much the same as with respect to the rest of the spectrum; that is, "while under conceivable or realizable conditions of overexposure injury may be done to the external eye, yet under all practicable conditions found in actual use of artificial sources of light for illumination the ultra violet part of the spectrum may be left out as a possible source of injury."[8]

SUNGLASSES—LEARNING TO LIVE IN DARKNESS

See *Plate 27: Living in Natural Light.*

From *Better Eyesight* magazine, December 1922:

> *Question:* Does Dr. Bates approve of dark glasses to protect the eyes from the glare of the sun at the seashore?
>
> *Answer:* No. Dark glasses are injurious to the eyes. The strong light is beneficial to the eye....

The Harmful Consequences of Wearing Sunglasses

One consequence of wearing dark sunglasses is that the pupil dilates unnaturally. The pupil is not supposed to dilate unless there is low light in the environment. Doesn't the use of sunglasses confuse the visual system?

The person who goes out into the bright sunlight after buying their first pair of contact lenses often experiences discomfort in the bright light. In addition to the abnormally enlarged pupil (due to the non-UV transmitting lense), the contact lense scatters light abnormally into the extreme peripheral parts of the retina. Is this one reason many people become over-sensitive to normal light (photophobia) and then buy dark sunglasses, which then cause the pupil to dilate even larger while in natural daylight?

Are not these artificial devices confusing and harmful to the visual system?

Tom's Personal Log: When I was given my first pair of contact lenses, bright sunlight was very painful when leaving the store. I immediately returned to the store and bought the darkest sunglasses I could find. Now I had two unnatural devices in front of my eyes, and when driving a car, there was a third, the UV-absorbing, tinted windshield.

Over the next few years, I became more and more sensitive to and uncomfortable in the sunlight. I began to dread the coming of summer.

Many sunglasses advertisements warn us never to be in the sunlight without "protection" from the UV. As mentioned above, there is rarely a distinction between the essential mid- and near-UV light, and the far-UV light, which is absorbed by the ozone layer.

Diversity of opinion could hardly be greater on this topic, as light pioneers like John Ott, Jacob Liberman, some holistic-oriented eye doctors, and many others are warning us of the harmful effects of the full spectrum of light *not* entering the eyes!

Dark sunglasses are artificial. They did not exist for the masses 100 years ago. People used to wear hats. Modern sunglasses were developed primarily for pilots flying at very high altitudes, where protection is needed from solar glare. They became popular to the masses soon after.

Military studies have shown that *anything* that lowers the levels of light entering the eyes decreases visual performance.

TOM'S PERSONAL LOG: As a result of studying the relationship between light and health, I have not worn sunglasses since 1982. If I have not adapted to bright light, I use a hat.

In a newspaper article regarding sunglasses for babies and children, a famous toy store manager suggests babies should be given sunglasses right after birth—as soon as they come out of a hospital. An optometrist states that sunglasses should be put on children "as young as is practical." For those interested in natural vision and health, this is not a good idea.

Glamour is a motivation for some people to wear glasses. Sometimes parents tell me their children, who do not need prescription glasses, want to wear glasses to look fashionable. This fashion will be at the cost of interfering with the visual system and health.

ADDICTED TO DARKNESS

One of the greatest dangers in wearing sunglasses as a habit is that the individual can become addicted to darkness. By not allowing the eyes to experience normal sunlight, a person can become more sensitive to the bright outdoor light. One then becomes dependent upon the dark sunglasses as a necessary crutch.

This scenario is quite similar to becoming more dependent upon prescription glasses—the more you use them, the more you will *need* to use them.

With "shades" and sunscreen lotions being a billion-dollar-a-year industry, it appears that many Americans are becoming both UV- and visible-light-deficient.

Are some modern health problems related to "malillumination," as John Ott describes it? Just how have animals and people gotten by, for millennia, without sunglasses? I have concluded that *not* receiving the full spectrum of natural sunlight is harmful to health, and using the best possible lighting indoors is important.

I regularly watch vision students become *less* sensitive to sunlight. Most vision students eliminate their contact lenses and wear glasses less and less while improving their sight. Many of my students have completely discarded sunglasses within eight weeks—and they now feel relaxed in bright sunlight.

All people who have blurry vision have strain on their visual system. How much of this chronic strain causes over-sensitivity to normal sunlight? How much of the application of the relaxation principle during vision improvement allows the student to become less sensitive to normal sunlight? As mentioned in Chapter 14, "The Third Habit—Blinking," the re-establishment of normal tearing by returning to normal blinking can also lower abnormal over-sensitivity to light.

FINAL NOTES ON LIGHT

Books, Articles, and Resources

I recommend students read the following outstanding books and articles discussing the relationship between light and health:

- Jacob Liberman's *Light: Medicine of the Future.*
- John N. Ott's *Light and Health,* and *Light, Radiation and You.*
- Richard J. Wurtman's "The Effects of Light on the Human Body," in *Scientific American,* July 1975.
- Dr. Zane R. Kime's *Sunlight Could Save Your Life.*

These books and articles are listed in the Bibliography. There is a list of lighting resources in Appendix B, "Resources—Lighting."

Practical Suggestions

- Natural, full-spectrum light from the sun is essential to our health. Be outdoors in natural lighting at least one hour per day. Even indirect sunlight on cloudy days is beneficial.
- If you are over-sensitive to bright light, do closed-eyelid sunning to rebuild your light tolerance.
- If you have been indoors for a long time, and then go outside into the bright light, wait a few moments to adapt to the bright light. Sunning with closed eyelids, even for a few seconds, can help you adapt quickly to bright light.
- If the sunlight is still too bright, wear a hat, not sunglasses. Notice that most professional tennis players, and many other athletes do not wear sunglasses, even when looking into the bright sky.
- If you feel you must use sunglasses, wear ones that are "neutral-gray" and with the least tint you can comfortably get by with. If possible, use *maximum* UV-transmitting sunglasses. (See Appendix B, Resources—Lighting.) Wear sunglasses only if you consider them necessary for certain situations. Worn for short periods of time, sunglasses are not harmful. Do not become addicted to sunglasses!
- People who live in a location where there is bright light have naturally adapted to that light. For example, people who live in areas where there is a lot of snow do not need sunglasses on a regular basis—they have adapted to the brightness of the snow. Due to the speed of modern transportation, people can travel quickly to a new location with very different light. For example, if you live in San Francisco and drive to the mountains to go skiing, suddenly there is bright glare from the snow, to which you are not accustomed. You may want to wear sunglasses for a short time. When returning to San Francisco, do not continue to wear the sunglasses as a habit.
- When indoors, use the best full-spectrum lighting possible. Lights that provide continuous mid- and near-UV light are preferred. Natural vision students who have installed full-spectrum lights have been very happy with them. They really *do* make a difference to your health.
- In addition to full-spectrum fluorescent lights, use incandescent or halogen

bulbs to provide the important contrast and shadows.

- Replace magnetic ballasts with electronic ballasts.
- If possible, arrange your lifestyle to awaken at sunrise, and retire soon after sunset.
- Since the eyes are organs of light, the more natural, full-spectrum light you give your eyes, the more healthy your eyes and *you* will be.

Notes

1 Douglas Kiang, reviewer, Tuncer Deniz, editor. Reprinted with permission. "Buried in Time," *Inside Mac Games* (Glenview, Illinois: Inside Mac Games, July/August 1995), p. 102.

2 A. Szent-Gyorgyi, *Introduction to a Submolecular Biology* (New York: Academic Press, 1960).

3 Richard J. Wurtman, "The Effects of Light on the Human Body," *Scientific American*, Vol. 233, No. 1 (July 1975), pp. 68–77. An excellent report.

4 Sandra Sinclair, *How Animals See* (New York: Facts on File Publications, 1985), p. 87.

5 Edith Raskin, *Watchers, Pursuers and Masqueraders: Animals and Their Vision* (New York: McGraw-Hill Book Company, 1964), pp. 23–25.

6 Fritz Hollwich, *The Influence of Ocular Light Perception on Metabolism in Man and in Animals* (New York: Springer-Verlag, 1980).

7 John N. Ott, *Health and Light* (New York: Simon & Schuster, 1973), p. 109.

8 No reference given by Bates for this quote.

Chapter Seventeen

The Retina

Studying the structure and functions of the retina can help the student to better understand the principles and habits of natural vision.

See *Plate 28: Retina Cross-Sections.*

Light passes through the cornea, aqueous humor, pupil, lens, and the vitreous humor before finally reaching the retina. The *retina* (from the Latin *rete,* meaning "net") "nets" the light entering the eye. The retina attaches to the choroid with a single row of pigment epithelium cells.

The human retina is paper-thin, ~1/100", or 0.25 mm, in thickness. This semi-transparent membrane consists of nerve cells, fibers, supporting structures, blood vessels, and most importantly, the specialized photoreceptor cells called cones and rods. The entire eye is designed for the cones and rods. The 137 million light receptors (7 million cones and 130 million rods) in each eye are among the smallest cells in the human body. A TV pales in comparison, with only 400,000 points of light creating its picture.

Light entering the retina does not immediately strike the cones and rods on the top layer of the retina, as one might guess. Light must travel through eight retinal layers before reaching the light receptors (see *Plate 28, a-3),* which lie in the ninth layer. There is one exception to this—at the fovea centralis (see *b-3*).

When light rays strike cones and rods, chemicals in these light receptors transform light energy into electrical impulses. These signals travel through the various "brain" cells in the middle and upper layers of the retina, along nerve fibers to the optic disc. Light signals then travel faster than 400 feet per second through the optic nerve to the brain where, finally, a "picture" is created.

In humans, light rays that miss the cones and rods strike the light-absorbing pigment epithelium and choroid. The internal pressure of vitreous humor helps keep the retina attached to the choroid.

TEN RETINAL LAYERS

The ten layers of the retina from the top, internal layer to the bottom, external layer are:

1. Internal limiting membrane, which is adjacent to the vitreous humor.
2. Optic nerve fibers layer—axons of ganglion cells travel to the optic disc, and

then along the optic nerve to the brain; this layer also contains the main branches of the central arteries and veins from the optic nerve.

3. Ganglion nerve cells layer.
4. Inner plexiform (molecular) layer—includes amacrine cells.
5. Inner nuclear layer—containing bipolar neuron cells; amacrine cells lie near the inner plexiform layer, and horizontal cells lie near the outer plexiform layer.
6. Outer plexiform (molecular) layer.
7. Outer nuclear layer—contains the nuclei of the cones and rods.
8. Outer limiting membrane.
9. Cones and rods layer.
10. Pigment epithelium—a single-cell layer that attaches to the choroid.

There are also long columnar cells, called Müller cells (not shown in *Plate 28*), which extend from the internal limiting membrane to the cones and rods layer. These cells provide support for the entire retina.

TWO BLOOD SUPPLIES

See *Plate 29: Blood Vessel Sandwich for the Cones and Rods.*

Blood is transported to the eye via the ophthalmic artery, and returns via the ophthalmic vein.

The retina and nerve fiber portion of the optic nerve are shown in yellow. The cones and rods layer is shown in green. Notice how the blood vessels supply both sides of the retina, while passing through the retina only at the optic disc.

The thickness of the choroid layer and its blood vessels are exaggerated in *Plate 29.* In reality, the choroid is thinner than the sclera.

The Central, Retinal Blood Vessels

Approximately one-half inch from the back of the eye, two blood vessels—one from the ophthalmic artery and the other from the ophthalmic vein—enter the optic nerve. These two blood vessels, called the central retinal artery and vein, travel forward through the center of the optic nerve toward the eye. They enter the eye at the optic disc.

Plate 30: Retina (1) and *Plate 31: Retina (2)* show a portion of the back of the retina of the right eye. The central blood vessels can be seen fanning out from the optic disc (OD) into the retina. The optic disc is located ~15° to the right of, and slightly above, the center of the back of the eye. The central arteries and veins travel through the top layers of the retina, above the cones and rods layer.

Plate 30: Retina (1) shows an angular distance of ~70° from one edge to the other. The entire visual portion of the retina encompasses ~200°.

Plate 31: Retina (2) is a photograph of a smaller portion of the retina. As the retina at the fovea is extremely thin, the dark choroid can be seen underneath it. Part of the choroidal ring (CR) can be seen as a bright yellow arc at the outer border of the optic disc. This is where the choroid meets the optic nerve. This image shows ~35° from one edge to the other.

See *Plate 29: Blood Vessel Sandwich for the Cones and Rods, Plate 30: Retina (1)* and *Plate 31: Retina (2).*

The macula lutea (ML) is located in the center of the retina, and the fovea centralis (FC) is located in the center of the macula. Notice how none of the central blood vessels pass through the fovea. To do so would interfere with the ability of the cones to pick up sharp detail and colors in our central vision. Since the rods are incapable of picking up sharp detail and color, blood vessels in peripheral parts of the retina are of lesser importance.

WATCHING RETINAL CORPUSCLES

When viewing a field of deep bluish-purple light, like the sky at certain times of the day (never looking directly into the sun, of course), one might notice tiny particles traveling along specific paths. These are images of corpuscles traveling through tiny retinal capillaries located in front of the cones and rods layer. Light entering the eye casts a shadow of these corpuscles mainly onto the rod light receptors, and you can watch them move! In fact, if you check your pulse, you can watch the corpuscles surge rhythmically with your heartbeat! Corpuscles are not seen exactly in the center because no capillaries pass over the cones in the fovea.

Seeing the corpuscles can be a little tricky, because the lighting needs to be just right.

Note: These corpuscles are not "floating specks," which are discussed in Chapter 30, "Questions and Answers."

The Choroidal Blood Vessels

In addition to the central artery and vein, other blood vessels from the ophthalmic artery and vein enter the back of the eye. These blood vessels pass through the sclera into the choroid, the eye's "vascular layer." Choroidal blood vessels supply nutrients to the bottom (outer) side of the retina by means of capillaries. This "choriocapillaris" layer lies parallel to, and comes in contact with, the pigment epithelium. The cones and rods layer lies just on the other side of the single-cell-layer pigment epithelium.

Since the fovea has few blood vessels supplying it from above, the choriocapillaris is thickened below the fovea to supply it additional nutrients.

Choroidal blood vessels also supply nutrients to the front of the eye.

See *Plate 29: Blood Vessel Sandwich for the Cones and Rods.*

The two sources of blood vessels (central and choroidal) create a "blood vessel sandwich" above and below the layer of cones and rods in the retina. The cones and rods are given a maximum supply of nutrients with minimum interference—an extraordinary design of nature.

IN THE BEGINNING, THERE WERE RODS ...

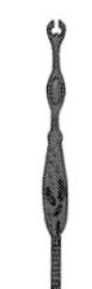

The first eyes could detect only light and dark.[1]

—Sandra Sinclair

One Type of Rod

Millions of years ago, creatures in the deep, dark oceans evolved a primitive visual system composed of rods. Rods allowed these creatures to pick up indistinct and colorless objects moving in very low levels of light. Rods also helped determine relative levels of heat and cold based on brighter and darker environments. There is only one type of rod.

The 130 million rods in the human retina are not designed for sharp detail. In fact, rods are incapable of "seeing" objects better than

20/400. This is only 1/20th of normal, "20/20," sight. This means you cannot see the 20/200, "big E" line on the eye chart with your peripheral vision. Rods register all of the lightwaves in the visible spectrum only as shades of grays or white. They are incapable of sending messages of color to the brain.

Rods are Very Sensitive—In Darkness

See *Plate 32: Darkness-Adapted Rods Sensitivity Chart.*

While the quality of light is measured in terms of CRI and CCT (as discussed in the previous chapter), the quantity of light is measured in foot-candles. One foot-candle (called a candela) is the amount of light illuminating an area of one square foot at a distance of one foot from a candle.

Note in *Plate 32* that the Radiance vertical axis is logarithmic (not linear).

The sensitivity of rods depends on the intensity of light in the environment. In very low levels of light—for example, at nighttime—the rods have their highest sensitivity.

The rods function in the bright light (like in the daytime) but they are not as sensitive to light at that time. The curve in *Plate 32* would be much lower (less sensitive) in the daytime.

Rods are most sensitive to the wavelengths in the blue-green region, from 450 to 550 nm. This means that a *dim* green object might be seen as bright as a *bright* violet object. In other words, both objects would be seen with the same intensity of grayness. At night, "green" leaves on a tree lit by moonlight appear to be a brighter gray than "orange" leaves.

As can be seen from *Plate 32,* rods are incapable of picking up wavelengths of red light. Ever notice how dark a red fire truck seems to be at night? It appears nearly black. Some firetrucks are painted yellow because they are easier to see at night.

Plate 35: Daytime Cones/Darkness-Adapted Rods Sensitivity Chart, compares the sensitivity of darkness-adapted rods to bright light-adapted cones. In nighttime, we can take advantage of the fact that cones are red-sensitive, while the rods are not, by using a red flashlight. The cones are activated to provide sharp detail (and the color red), while the rods are unaffected by the red light. When you turn off the red flashlight, the rods are still adapted to the darkness. Some stores even sell "night vision lights." When I was in the service, we used red flashlights at night.

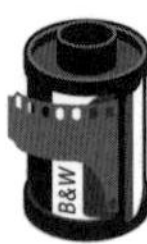

In photography, there are different types of film. There is "black and white" film and there is color film.

There are also different "speeds" of film. The speed of the film is determined by the film's "graininess," or clumping, of silver in the negative. High-speed film, like ISO/ASA 1000, has a coarser grain than low-speed film. High-speed film is more sensitive to low levels of light but has less definition (sharpness) than low-speed film.

Rods function similar to high-speed black and white film (or should we say this film functions like the rods!).

Rod Night Adaptation

When night or darkness arrives, the rods go through a remarkable change.

When the retina is examined immediately after being in darkness, it has a reddish-purple color. This "visual purple" is due to a pigment produced inside the rods called *rhodopsin* (from the Greek *rhodon,* meaning "rose," and *opsis,* meaning "sight").

Rhodopsin is produced continually by the reaction of the yellow-orange aldehyde *retinal* with one type of a colorless protein called *opsin.* Retinal is a modified form of Vitamin A, found in carrots and many other vegetables.

When bright light is absent, rhodopsin increases its concentration in the rods, giving the rods the ability to pick up extremely low levels of light. The higher the concentration of rhodopsin, the greater a rod's sensitivity to light.

When light hits a highly "rhodopsin-energized" rod, an electrical signal is sent through the retinal cells to the brain. But now the rhodopsin pigment is disassociated; the visual purple is "bleached out." This rod can no longer pick up low levels of light—at least temporarily. As long as the level of light remains low, rhodopsin is reformed at a greater rate than it is depleted, and the rod quickly regains its sensitivity to low levels of light.

Bright light, like daytime light, causes the rate of depletion of rhodopsin to be greater than the rate of formation. As a result, the rods lose their sensitivity to low levels of light.

So, the rods are like rechargeable batteries. In darkness, they become fully "charged"; but in bright light they become relatively "discharged."

Smoking often reduces nighttime vision. The rods need to be healthy to pick up low levels of light. Fortunately, much of nighttime vision can be restored when smoking is stopped.

Excellent Night Vision

Due to the high concentration of rhodopsin at night, rods can pick up extremely low levels of light. When fully adapted to darkness, the rods are up to 30,000 times more sensitive to light than the cones are in daytime. (Cones have *no* sensitivity to extremely low levels of light.) A highly-sensitized rod can be "triggered" by a single photon—the smallest unit of light energy.

Steve Richards writes, "The normal human eye in good health is capable of detecting the light of a match on a clear, dark night at a distance of thirty miles!"[2]

From Brightness to Darkness, and Back

When a person goes from bright light into sudden darkness, the rods reach ~80% of their low-level light sensitivity in fifteen minutes. Rods reach complete night adaptation in one hour.

When you wake up in the middle of the night, the rods have adapted to very low levels of light. You can see the objects in your room. But when you turn on a bright light (Ouch! The visual purple does not like bright light!), the visual purple is quickly lost, and along with it, low-light sensitivity. When the light is turned off, almost no objects can be seen in the room, and the process of night adaptation starts again.

Going to the movie theater in the daytime, when the movie has already begun, is an education in darkness adaptation. When the door to the theater closes behind you, you can see the movie screen and the aisle lights, but little else. The pupil enlarges and the rods begin adapting to the darkness. Gradually, you see better and better, and soon enough, you can walk down the aisle. "No one is sitting in this chair. Oops! I guess I haven't adapted to darkness as much as I thought!"

By the end of the movie, before the lights are turned on, the theater seems brighter than when you first entered. You adapted to the darkness during the movie. If it is still daytime when you leave, bright light hits the rhodopsin-sensitized rods and the visual purple is bleached away once again.

Nighttime Tip #1. If you have adapted to very low levels of light, look away from any sudden bright light. If you look toward the light, you will not be able to see as well, if at all, for a short period of time.

Nighttime Tip #2. If you are leaving a room in which you have adapted to the darkness, but plan to return very soon, before entering the bright room, cover one eye. In this way, the eye you cover will still be darkness-adapted when you return to the dark room.

Rods—Our "Movement Detectors"

The rods are excellent "movement detectors." Rods allow animals to detect and catch *moving* prey, and to escape *moving* predators. As discussed in Chapter 9, "The First Principle—Movement," the rods (and cones) are not designed to be stimulated with a constant, steady source of light. Light rays need to change their positions on the retina. As long as we are moving, light rays from stationary objects change their positions on the retina.

While working with some older computer monitors, a "flicker" can be seen in the peripheral vision. This is due to the rods picking up the slower "refresh" rate of the screen. Since the cones do not pick up movement as well as the rods, the point at which you are centralizing seems steady. Monitor flicker is discussed more in the Chapter 24, "Computers, TVs, and Movies."

Some people have retinas in which there are rods but no cones—a condition known as *rod monochromacy.*[3] For this 0.003% of the population, the picture of the world has no detail and is completely colorless.

... AND THEN THERE WERE CONES

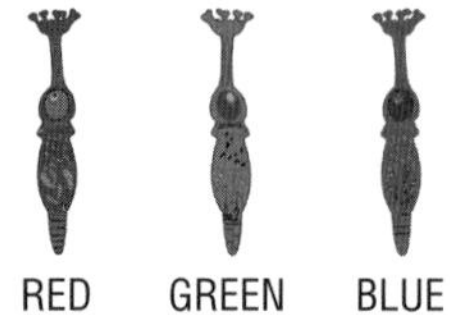

As animals evolved from the deep dark oceans to bright land, some of the rods evolved into cones. The high intensity of surface light is utilized by the cones to pick up sharp detail and colors. Cones are found primarily in diurnal (daytime) animals and humans. The majority of the seven million cones in the human retina are located in the fovea centralis.

Three Types of Cones

See *Plate 33: Daytime Cones Sensitivity Chart.*

There are three types of cones in the retina:

1. "Blue" cones are most sensitive to violet and blue light.
2. "Green" cones are most sensitive to green and yellow light.
3. "Red" cones are most sensitive to green, yellow, and red light.

These three types of cones result from retinal combining with three different types of opsins inside the cones. "Blue" cones have a higher concentration of "blue-opsins"; "green" cones have higher concentration of "green-opsins"; and "red" cones have a higher concentration of "red-opsins."

By combining the sensitivities of the three cones in *Plate 33,* we can see that the greatest sensitivity is in the yellow-green region. Note the logarithmic vertical scale.

Tri-Chromatic Vision—Our Natural RGB Monitor

See *Plate 34: The Eye—Our Natural RGB Monitor.*

Most computer displays (CRTs, VDTs) and TVs are "RGB" monitors. By combining red, green, and blue lights on a screen in different amounts, all colors can be created.

The full range of colors perceived by the brain is a result of different amounts of the blue, green, and red cones being stimulated by a particular object.

For example, light waves from an "orange" ball would stimulate more "red" cones than "green" cones, and none of the "blue" cones. The brain interprets this mixture of red and green signals as orange. Similarly, a blue object would stimulate more "blue" cones than "green" cones, and none of the "red" cones.

The three different types of cones—red, green, and blue—allow us to see all the colors of a rainbow. This is known as tri-chromatic vision. Cones can also pick up white, which is the combination of all colors.

Cones Need Medium-Bright Intensity

Plate 33 shows the sensitivity of the three types of cones in bright light. When darkness approaches, the cones begin losing their sensitivity to light. In "true" nighttime vision, where the intensity of light is very low, the cones have *no* sensitivity. The cones need at least a medium intensity of light to be activated.

Artificial lights—for example, a flashlight—used at nighttime are designed with enough intensity to activate the cones. We can then see detail and colors.

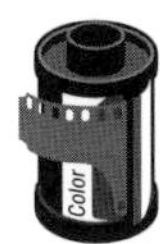

Returning to the film analogy, the cones function somewhat like low-speed color film, like ISO/ASA 100. Low-speed film has a finer grain than high-speed film. It produces good definition (sharpness), higher contrast, and strong color saturation. However, low-speed film is less sensitive to light than high-speed film.

Most Colorblind People See Colors

Many people think that people who are "colorblind" cannot see colors. However, most colorblind people have lost only part of their color vision. Usually, only one or two types of cones are either absent or not functioning normally. If the green cones are not functioning normally, a person will be deficient picking up green. However, red and blue and combinations of red and blue can still be seen.

Five to eight percent of men and 0.3–0.5% of women are colorblind. Although color blindness is considered to be hereditary, some natural vision students have improved their color blindness using the Bates method.

Clara Hackett, in her natural vision book *Relax and See,* presents some excellent activities for people who have color blindness. She writes:

> The absence of all appreciation of colours is very rare. In most cases, there is a lack of perception of red, green, and/or blue. Many colour-blind people can develop their colour sense.
>
> ... The techniques [described] are practical for self-instruction. If you are colour-blind, there is a good chance that you can benefit from them. Essentially, they add up to a double learning process. You will learn basic facts about colours and practice identifying, matching, making and sorting colours. You will also practice some of the basic elements of good vision and these will help to simplify and speed the colour learning process.
>
> A first essential is to achieve relaxation. Tension affects your mind and memory and may interfere, too, with "sighting" of colour. If previous attempts to learn colour were futile, tension may have been a factor.[4]

Syntonics, mentioned in the previous chapter, has also benefited some people who have color blindness.

A DIFFERENCE BETWEEN DAY AND NIGHT

According to historians, early Muslims determined the beginning of day when natural sunlight allowed them to see the colors of threads in a pile of mixed fibers. When the colors were not distinguishable anymore, it was the beginning of night.

See *Plate 36: Cones and Rods Sensitivity—Day and Night Cycle.*

In the daytime, cones have good sensitivity to colors and detail. Rods are not as sensitive to light in the daytime because visual purple is absent. In true nighttime vision, the rods become extremely sensitive to low levels of light, and the cones drop to zero sensitivity—in other words, the cones do not function.

Of course, if a light source has enough intensity in the night, it can activate the cones, and therefore, color and detail are seen. Notice that detail can be seen on the moon at night. There is sufficient intensity of light from the moon to activate the cones. Still, true nighttime vision is primarily rod vision.

DIFFERENT DENSITY DISTRIBUTIONS

Understanding of density (concentration) distribution of cones and rods in the retina helps us use our central and peripheral vision correctly.

See *Plate 37: Measuring Density Distributions of Cones and Rods.*

The Vertical Density Graphs (discussed below) are based on measurements taken along, and above and below, the vertical line V1-V2. These graphs show the typical density distribution of the cones and rods along lines passing through the fovea, without the "distraction" of the optic disc.

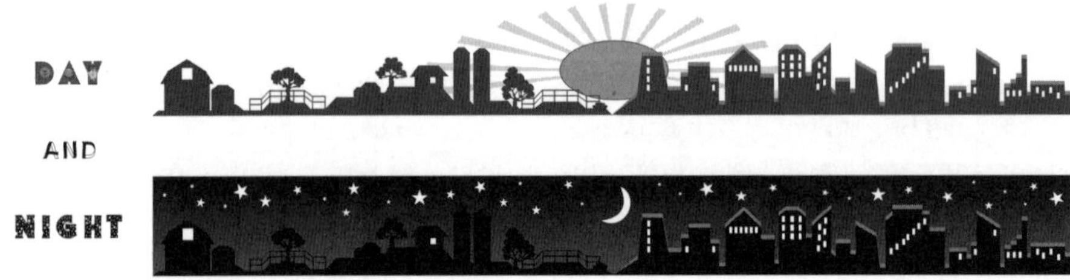

The Horizontal Density Graphs (discussed below in the section "The Blind Spot—No Cones or Rods") are based on measurements taken along, and to the left and right of, the line H1-H2. Notice how this line passes through the optic disc (OD), where there are no cones or rods.

Cone Density Distribution

Maximum Cone Density at the Fovea Centralis

See *Plate 28: Retina Cross-Sections, b-3, Plate 30: Retina (1),* and *Plate 37: Measuring Density Distributions of Cones and Rods.* See also *Plate 38: Cones Vertical Density Graph (V1-V2)* and *Plate 39: Cones 3-D Density Model (Side View).*

The *macula lutea* (from the Latin *macula,* meaning "spot," and *lutea,* meaning "yellow"—literally, "yellow spot") is ~1.25 mm (5°) in diameter and contains a very high concentration of cones.

The *fovea centralis* (from the Latin *fovea,* meaning "pit," and *centralis,* meaning "central"—literally, "the central pit") is a very small depression located in the center of the macula. The fovea is about ⅕ the size of the macula, or ~0.25 mm (1°) in diameter. The fovea consists almost exclusively of cones. There are only cones exactly in the center of the fovea—no rods.

Plate 38 shows the density of cones as measured vertically along the retina.

Density, in this case, refers to the number of light receptors per square millimeter (mm^2). 1 mm ≈ 1⁄25". Density can also be considered the concentration of light receptors. Generally, the higher the density, the better we can see.

Moving from the peripheral part of the retina into the macula, the density of cones increases exponentially. Cone density increases to a maximum of ~150,000/mm^2 exactly in the center of the fovea.

The fovea is literally a pit in the retina. As mentioned at the beginning of this chapter, there is an exception to the light rays needing to penetrate eight retinal layers to reach the cones and rods. At the fovea, some of the top retinal layers, particularly the ganglion and bipolar cells, are compressed and moved off to the side. Additionally, the cones "reach" slightly upward toward the top of the retina. With less distance to travel, light rays can hit the foveal cones without scattering the light as much.

These facts result in our sharpest vision—by far—being at a pinpoint in the center of the visual field. The area of peak concentration of cones in the center of the fovea is so small, the eyes need to shift from one dot of a colon (:) to the other in order to see each dot distinctly!

Charles H. May, in *Diseases of the Eyes,* writes:

> Cones are concerned with visual acuity and color discrimination at high intensities of illumination (photoptic vision); rods are responsible for vision at low degrees of illumination (scotoptic vision) when sight is more effective in the periphery of the retina and is colorless. When the image of an object falls upon the macula, there is distinct vision; when it falls upon any other part of the retina, there is indistinct vision. Two points give rise to *separate visual impressions* when their images are at least 0.002 mm. apart, since this represents the diameter of the cones at the fovea. In other words, to be seen distinctly, two objects must subtend a visual angle of one minute or more.[5]

One minute of an arc is one-sixtieth of 1°, or 0.016°. (A circle is 360°; 90° forms a right angle.) As you can see, so-to-speak, the area of sharpest vision is extremely small.

One way to remember the relationship of cones to other aspects of our central vision is to think of all the "C" words: "Cones see Clearly and Colorfully only in the Center at the fovea Centralis; Chickens have all Cones!"

Minimal Cone Density in the Periphery

The density of cones, along with clarity and color perception, decreases dramatically moving away from the fovea. The density of cones drops to only 3% of their maximum, at a distance of only 7° from the center of the fovea. The density of cones is even lower outside the macula, and drops to zero in the far peripheral parts of the retina.

Not only does the cone density drop dramatically in the peripheral parts of the retina, the eight upper layers of the retina lie above those few peripheral cones. As a consequence, peripheral cone perception ranges from very poor to none. At a distance of 70° into the peripheral retina, acuity is only 1% of the central vision; this is ~20/2000 vision. Color is imperceptible in the far parts of the peripheral vision.

In *Plate 39,* the (minimal) peripheral cones are darkened to indicate they are "buried," like the rods, under eight retinal layers.

The cones *do* pick up some color in the peripheral vision, especially close to the central vision, but it is "diluted" compared to color in the central vision.

Zoologist John Downer, in his book *Supersense: Perception in the Animal World,* writes:

> The cones are concentrated in the fovea, and the rest of the retina has a higher proportion of rods which only provide monochrome [black and white] vision. The illusion of full colour outside the central image is provided by the brain. This can be demonstrated by moving a previously unseen object into a person's field of view. The person is unable to identify the colour until the object is close to their main image area.[6]

Experience Cone Density Distribution

As discussed in Chapter 10, "The Second Principle—Centralization," it is impossible to see clearly except in the center. People who have blurry vision attempt, usually subconsciously, to see everything clearly at the same moment. This is called diffusion. The attempt to do the impossible, Bates said, is a strain, and lowers sight.

In order to see clearly, a person needs to have his visual attention at the place within the picture where it is clear, and the only place the picture is clear is exactly in the center.

EXPERIENCE CONE DENSITY DISTRIBUTION

See *Plate 8: Centralizing—The Two Pencils.*

Take two different colored pencils, for example, yellow and green. Hold the bottoms of the pencils, with the eraser ends positioned on top. Hold the pencils vertically out in front of you about one foot away. Separate them horizontally about 16" away from each other.

Sketch the yellow pencil while wiggling the peripheral green pencil. The cones in fovea pick up sharp detail and bright color on the yellow pencil. The green pencil, if held far enough out in the periphery, will appear gray and "unclear." No peeking at the green pencil!

There are so few, "buried" cones in the peripheral part of the retina, they are of no value in picking up the detail and color of the "green" pencil. In fact, if you had not known beforehand the second pencil was green, you most likely would not be able to identify its color. On the other hand, the movement of the peripheral "gray" pencil is picked up well by the rods.

Now sketch the green pencil. A very different experience! Now the cones in the fovea pick up the sharp detail and bright green color of the green pencil—right where you centralize. The "yellow" pencil is now "colorless" and indistinct. Wiggle the yellow pencil. Once again, the rods pick up the peripheral "gray" pencil's movement very well.

Rod Density Distribution

Maximum Rod Density in the Periphery

See *Plate 28: Retina Cross-Sections, a-3, Plate 30: Retina (1),* and *Plate 37: Measuring Density Distributions of Cones and Rods.* See also *Plate 40: Rods Vertical Density Graph (V1-V2),* and *Plate 41: Rods 3-D Density Model (Side View).*

The rods are not distributed evenly on the retina. The maximum density of rods is ~160,000/mm^2, and they are located in a 360° circle around, and ~18° away from the fovea. The density of rods being "maximized" around the fovea allows us to have our best nighttime vision (only 20/400 at best) close to the center of our visual field. This is important, because in very low levels of light, we have *no* vision exactly in the center of our visual field. This is yet another remarkable design of nature—giving us our best night vision close to where we have no (central) vision.

Note: The loss of central vision described here is not the same as the "blind spot" caused by the optic nerve. This is discussed further below.

Moving toward the far periphery (from the circle of maximum density), the density of rods slowly diminishes to about one-quarter of its maximum. The furthest parts of the visual portion of the retina contain only rods, no cones.

Zero Central Rods

Moving toward the fovea (from the circle of maximum density), the density of rods quickly drops to zero. There are no rods located exactly in the center of the fovea, only cones. In fact, by the rods dropping to zero density, the cones can rise to their maximum "pure" density in the center of the fovea.

Since there are no rods in the center of the fovea centralis, and since the cones do not function in very low levels of light, all humans are correctly "blind" in the center of the visual field in true nighttime vision. *True nighttime vision* is any situation in which the intensity of light is sufficient to activate the rods, but not the cones.

Fortunately for our nighttime vision, the area of zero rods in the fovea is very small. This means the point of interest must be very small (and dim) for it to disappear. The corollary to this is—if the tiny central point is seen at *any* time, that point must be cone vision, and detail and color can be seen at that point.

If an object is very dim, but also large, the *center* of that object will disappear, but the peripheral parts of that object will be picked up by the rods.

EXPERIENCE ROD DENSITY DISTRIBUTION

Part A: At nighttime, sketch a star in the sky. Notice there seems to be a "ring" of bright stars ~18° away from that star, all the way around it in a circle. This effect is due to the "ring" of high-density rods located ~18° around the fovea.

If the star you are interested in is dim enough, and if you are centralizing on it, it will disappear! This is because the cones cannot pick up very low levels of light and there are no rods in the center of the fovea.

Part B: In the dark, find a watch or other object which has small, dim, fluorescent dots. If you sketch one dot directly, it will "disappear." When you shift away from the dot, it "lights up" in your peripheral vision.

These are excellent ways to study rod vision. The student can determine how well she is centralizing by watching the tiny dim spot disappear.

The "disappearing act" of the tiny, dim star is experienced in darkness in one of the natural vision classes. This is one of the students' favorite classes.

If you were an astronomer, how would you ever see a tiny dim star? One possibility would be to use a powerful telescope, so that a dim star appears brighter. The star might then have enough intensity of light to activate the cones, and could then be picked up with the central vision. What if the star was still too dim, even in the telescope? You could locate the star in the peripheral vision, and then take a picture of the star. The film will register the star's light, but only if the film's "light receptors" are sensitive enough. After the picture is developed, you still need to put enough light on it to finally see the star clearly.

Many telescopes used for night viewing are a combination of two telescopes. The smaller, low-power telescope, called the finder, attaches to the side of the large telescope. The finder, analogous to our peripheral rods, picks up a larger but less detailed area in the night sky to "find" planets and stars.

R.L. Gregory writes in *Eye and Brain—The Psychology of Seeing:*

> Astronomers "look off" the fovea when they wish to detect very faint stars so that the image falls on a region of the retina rich in rods.[7]

Do not diffuse, even in true nighttime vision. Centralizing is an important mental function and should be practiced at all times. In true nighttime vision, with only 20/400 vision, continue to centralize and shift your attention. Pick up your peripheral vision similar to the way you do in the daytime—"peripherally."

Being diurnal creatures, the human visual system is not designed primarily for night vision. If you are in very low-level light situations and need to see clearly, use a flashlight to activate the cones.

DIFFERENT NETWORKING

A close look at the middle layers in *Plate 28: Retina Cross-Sections,* reveals a difference in how the cone and rod signals are processed.

Each cone is connected to its own bipolar cell in the inner nuclear layer. This one-to-one connection between the cones and the bipolar cells is one reason we pick up a sharper image with the cones. This one-to-one cone connection is not maintained all the way to the brain, however. There is some mixing of cone signals in the inner plexiform layer, where several cones can connect to one ganglion cell.

Unlike the cones, several rods are connected to one bipolar cell, Additionally, the rods are connected by horizontal cells, located just above the outer plexiform layer. This grouped arrangement is called association cells and allows for better sensitivity to light at night and better movement perception by the rods; a disadvantage of association cells is a less distinct image.

This "tree branch" arrangement of rods and bipolar cells is one reason objects appear larger at nighttime compared to daytime. If only one rod is struck by a light ray, the brain interprets it as if an entire group of rods has been struck.

There are 137 million cones and rods, but only one million nerve fibers travel from the retina to the brain.

PUTTING IT ALL TOGETHER

In medium to high levels of light, the cones pick up sharp detail and colors, but only in the central vision. The rods are capable of picking up very low levels of grays in darkness, and are excellent at movement perception in the peripheral vision.

Plate 42: Cones and Rods Vertical Density Graph (V1-V2) is simply a combination of *Plate 38* and *Plate 40*. *Plate 43: Cones and Rods 3-D Density Model (Side View)* is simply a combination of *Plate 39* and *Plate 41*.

Plate 35: Daytime Cones/Darkness-Adapted Rods Sensitivity Chart is a combination of *Plate 32* and *Plate 33*. *Plate 35: Daytime Cones/Darkness-Adapted Rods Sensitivity Chart* shows how darkness-adapted rods pick up light much better than the bright light-adapted cones. (Of course both of these sensitivity charts cannot occur simultaneously, since both darkness and brightness cannot occur simultaneously.) The shift in maximum sensitivity from ~496 nm in darkness with the rods to ~555 nm in bright light with the cones is known as the Purkinje shift. (Do you remember the images of Purkinje?)

See *Plate 44: How We See*.

a. In the daytime, we think we see like a camera. We think every part of the picture is equally sharp and colorful.
b. In daytime, humans only see clearly and most colorfully in the center due to the high density of cones in the fovea. The peripheral parts of the picture are much less clear and colorful. Also, the area of human vision is not a rectangle shape, but more an irregular, oval shape.
c. In true nighttime vision, humans are incapable of seeing a very small and dimly lit central area. This is because there are no rods in the center of the fovea, and the cones are incapable of picking up very low levels of light. We are "blind" in the center. Notice how the rods have their greatest sensitivity in a circle ~18° from the central point of interest.

The iris constricts in bright light, forming a small pupil, and expands in dim light, forming a large pupil. Not only does a large pupil size let in more light, but the size of the picture we see is larger by about 10%. For the right eye, most of this increase is toward the temple and slightly below eye level. For the left eye, the visual field increases to the left and slightly below eye level. Notice in *Plate 44: How We See, c*, the size of the picture on the lower left, left, and upper left side does not increase in nighttime. Why? Just cover your left eye to find out!

Notice the blind spot due to the optic nerve.

See also *Plate 45: A Difference Between Day and Night*.

THE BLIND SPOT—NO CONES OR RODS

See *Plate 30: Retina (1)*, *Plate 31: Retina (2)*, and *Plate 37: Measuring Density Distributions of Cones and Rods*.

The optic disc is a depressed, light-pink area located inside the eye where the optic nerve joins the eyeball. The optic disc is ~2 mm in diameter and located ~15° from the fovea, toward the middle of the head and slightly above the horizon. It has a slightly vertical oval shape.

See *Plate 46: Cones 3-D Density Model (Top View)* and *Plate 47: Rods 3-D Density Model (Top View)*. These illustrations show the blind spot at the optic disc, indicated by the small white oval located ~15° to the right of the fovea centralis. These models are of the right eye as if you were looking into the eyeball at the retina. The right side of the models are toward the nose and the left side of the models are toward the temple.

The white point in the center of *Plate 47* indicates there are no rods in the center of the fovea. Notice the "ring" of high-density rods ~18° away from and around the fovea. In *Plate 46* the high density of cones in the macula is indicated by the many brightly colored, concentric circles in the center.

Plate 48: Cones and Rods Horizontal Density Graph (H1-H2) shows the cones (colored) and rods (black and white) densities along and beyond the (nearly) horizontal line H1-H2 in *Plate 37*. Notice in *Plate 48* how both the cone and rod density curves drop to zero density at the optic disc.

See *Plate 49: The Blind Spots* and *Plate 51: Binocular Vision*. There are no cones or rods in the optic disc—only nerve fibers and the central retinal blood vessels. This area creates one "blind spot" for each eye. When seeing with only the right eye, there is an area located ~15° to the right of and slightly below the point of centralization where there is no vision. The left eye's blind spot is located ~15° to the left of and slightly below the point of centralization.

The area not seen with the blind spot increases the greater the distance an object is located from you. At a distance of ten inches from the eye, the area of the blind spot is about the size of a quarter; at one meter it is the size of an apple; and at three meters, it is about the size of a basketball; and at twenty meters, the size of a horse!

Usually, a person is not aware of the blind spots because the area not seen by the right eye is picked up by the left eye, and vice versa. See *Plate 49* and *Plate 51*. Another excellent design by nature, for if the optic disc were in the middle of the back of both eyes, we would have no central vision—night or day.

The brain tends to fill in the blind spot area to some extent. This can create a false sense of security for a person with sight in only one eye. It is especially important for people with diminished or lost sight in one eye to continue moving so that the area of the blind spot does not remain constant. Some people with sight in only one eye have been struck by an object coming toward them along the angle of the blind spot because they were not moving.

EXPERIENCE THE BLIND SPOT

Part A:

Cover your right eye. Hold this page with the words "*Fovea Centralis*" out in front of the left eye approximately eight inches away. While sketching the letter "*v*" in the word "*Fovea*" with your nose-pencil, slowly move this page closer to and farther away from your head. At a certain distance, the words

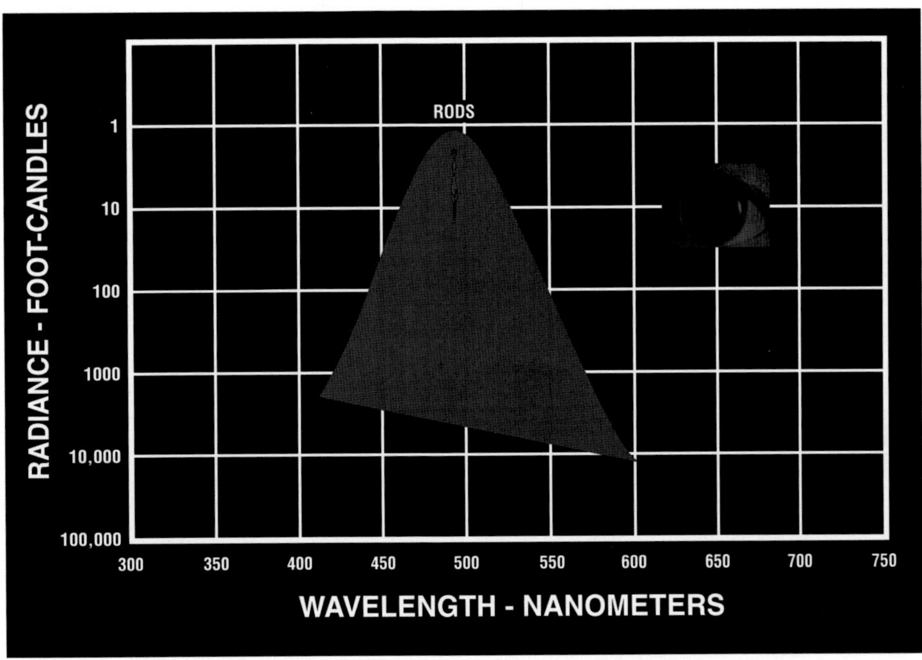

Plate 32. Darkness-Adapted Rods Sensitivity Chart.

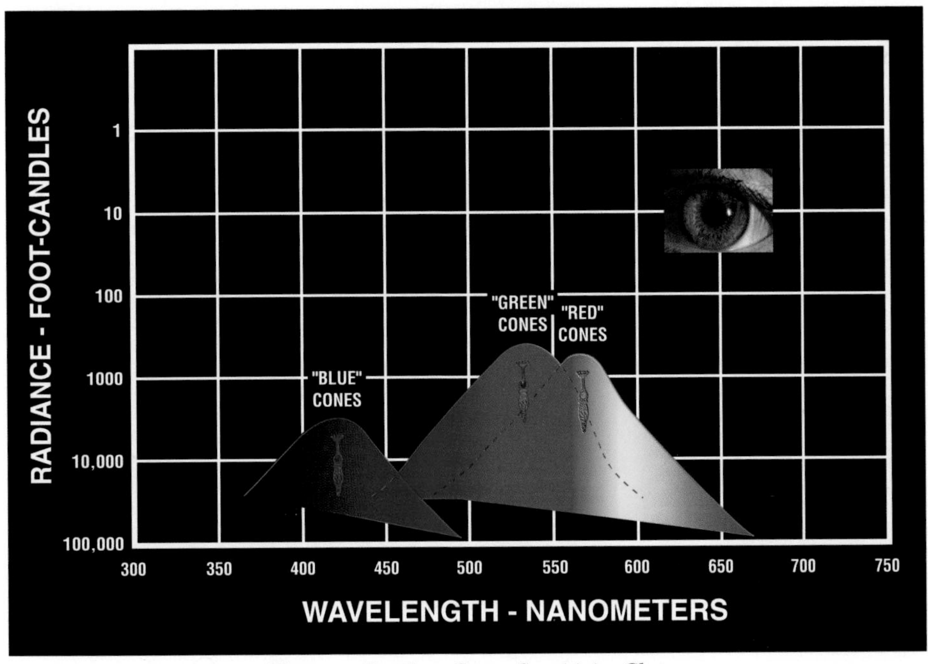

Plate 33. Daytime Cones Sensitivity Chart.

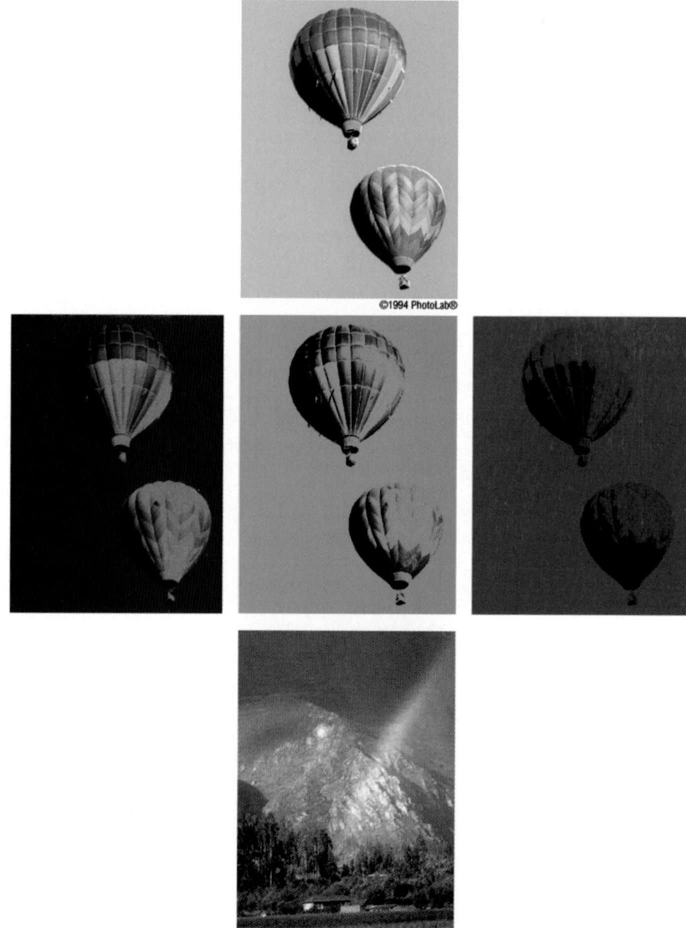

Plate 34. The Eye—Our Natural RGB Monitor.

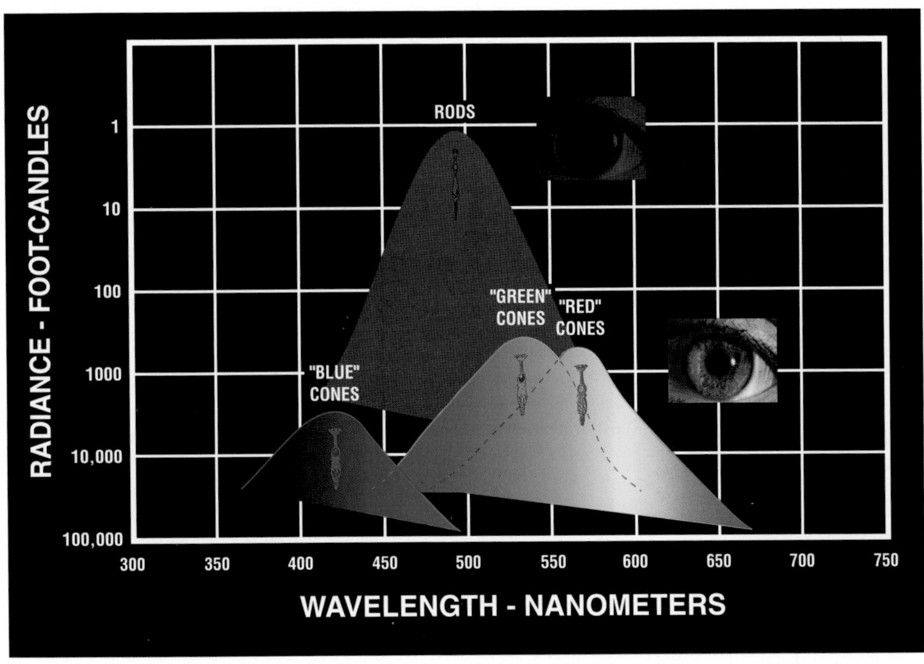

Plate 35. Daytime Cones/Darkness-Adapted Rods Sensitivity Chart.

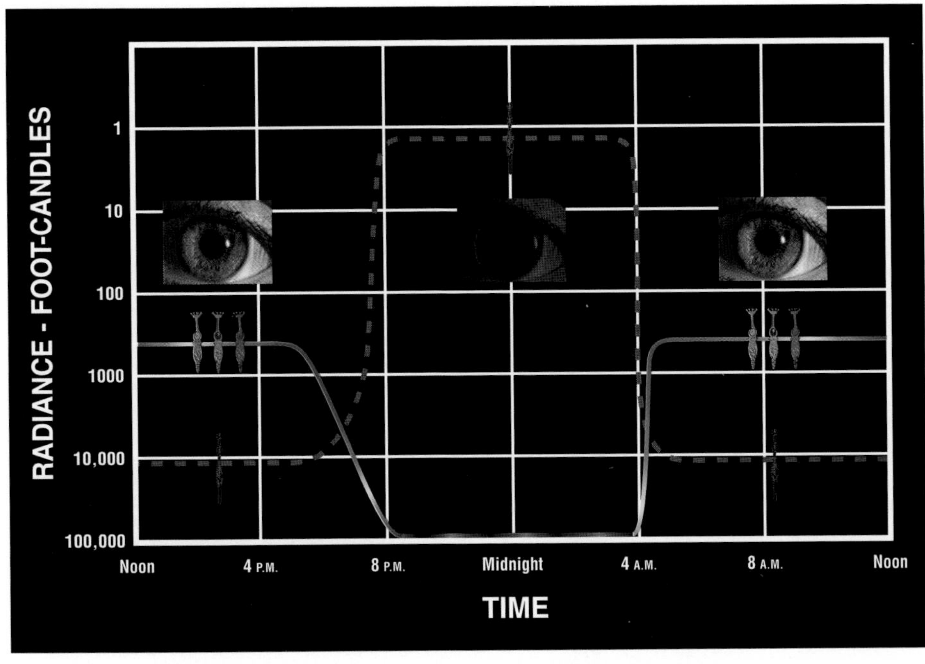

Plate 36. Cones and Rods Sensitivity—Day and Night Cycle.

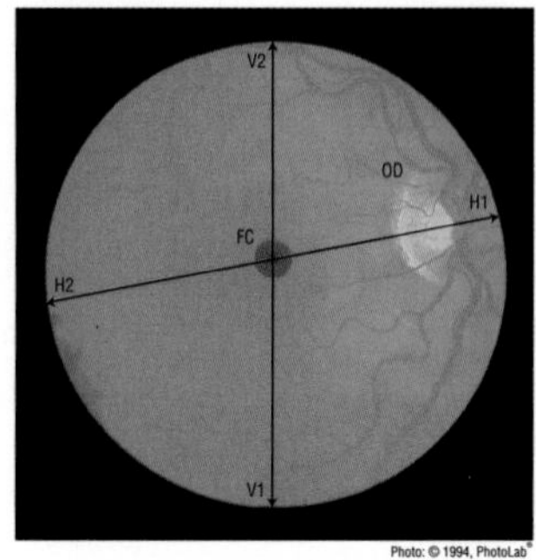

Plate 37. Measuring Density Distributions of Cones and Rods.

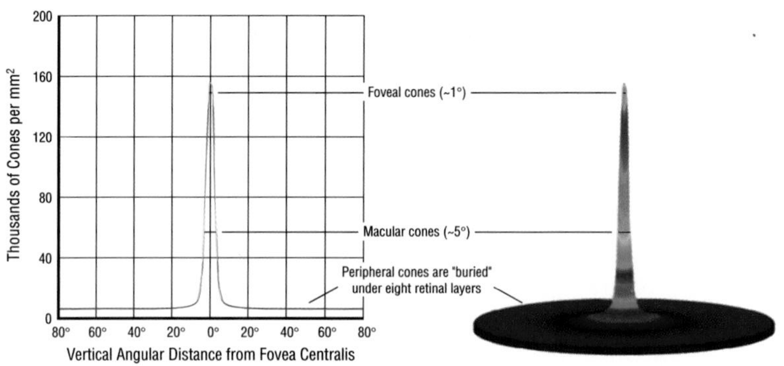

Plate 38. Cones Vertical Density Graph (V1-V2).

Plate 39. Cones 3-D Density Model (Side View).

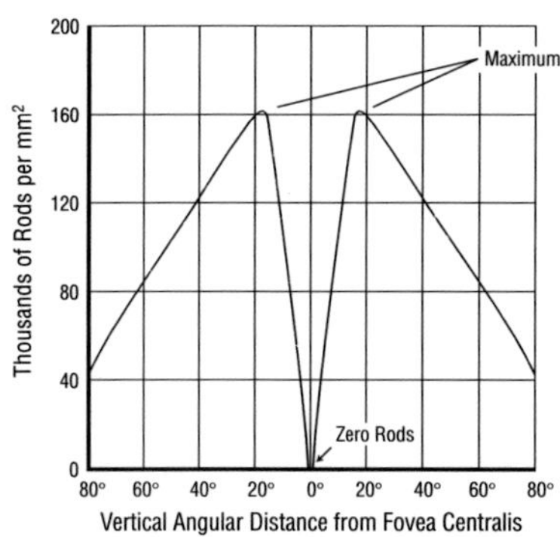

Plate 40. Rods Vertical Density Graph (V1-V2).

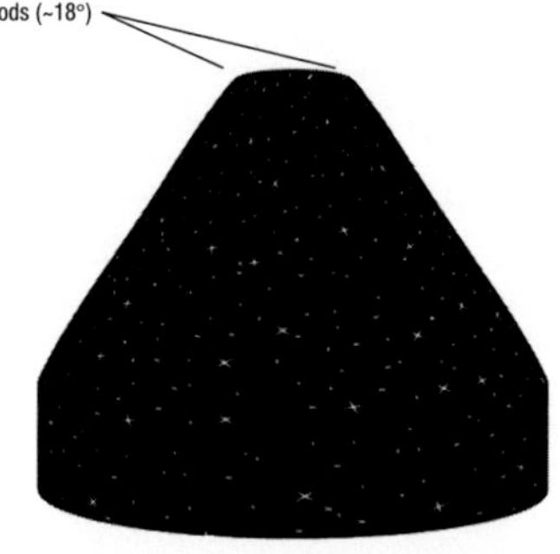

Plate 41. Rods 3-D Density Model (Side View).

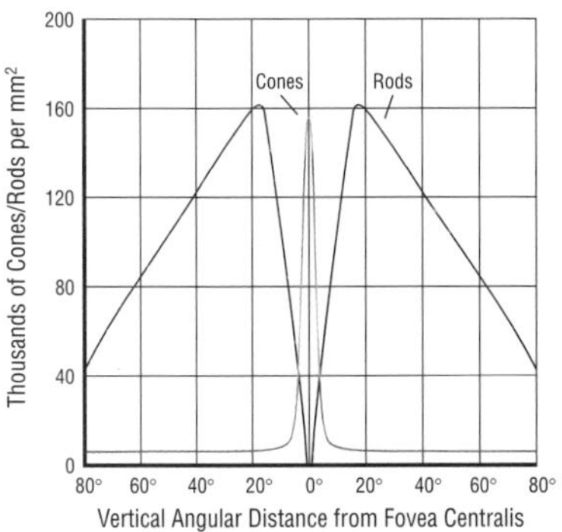

Plate 42. Cones and Rods Vertical Density Graph (V1-V2).

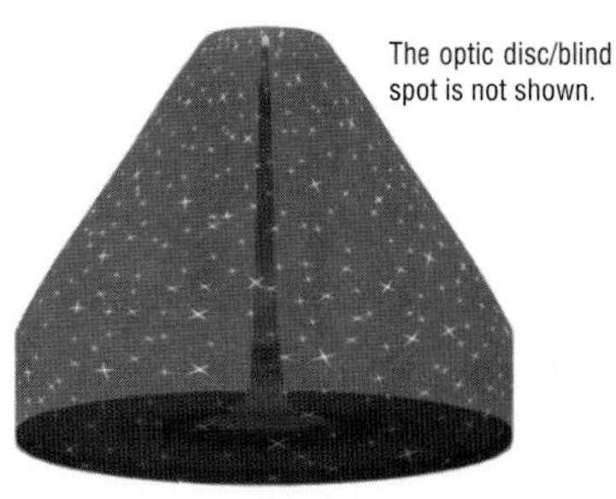

The optic disc/blind spot is not shown.

Plate 43. Cones and Rods 3-D Density Model (Side View).

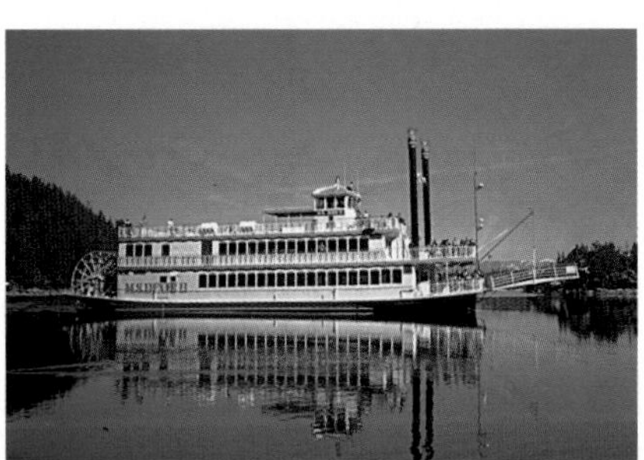

a

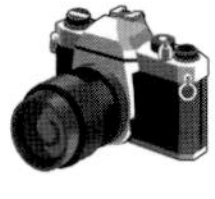

We think we see the world like a camera "sees" it. A camera's picture contains sharp detail and even colors throughout a rectangular image. Any attempt to see the world in this manner is a strain to the human visual system.

b

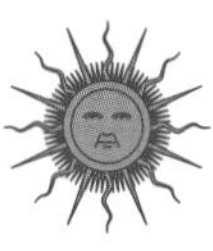

For humans in the daytime, only the center of the image is clear and contains the best color. Sharp detail and colors diminish in the peripheral vision. Compare the clarity and colors of the man in the center of the boat—the point of centralization in the image at left—with the people at the front of the boat. Also, the picture seen with one eye is not rectangular; rather, it is a distorted oval shape. The shape of right eye's daytime visual field is shown at left. The blind spot due to the optic nerve is not shown.

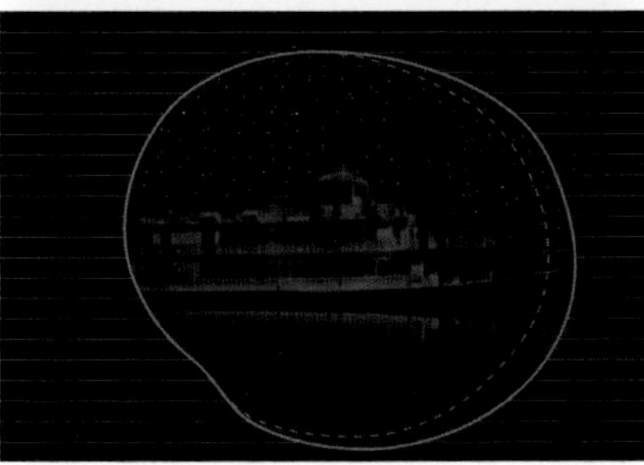

c

In true nighttime vision, a small dim object (man in the center of the boat) cannot be seen with our central vision. We are "correctly blind" where we centralize. The best nighttime vision is located in a circle ~18° around the point of centralization. This is indicated by the faint halo around the vanished central man. This is due to the maximum density of rods located around the fovea centralis by ~18°. Additionally, our visual field is ~10% larger at nighttime due to the larger pupil size. The blind spot due to the optic nerve is not shown.

Plate 44. How We See.

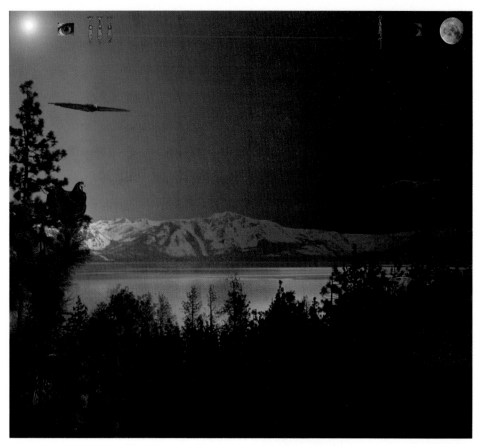

Plate 45. A Difference Between Day and Night.

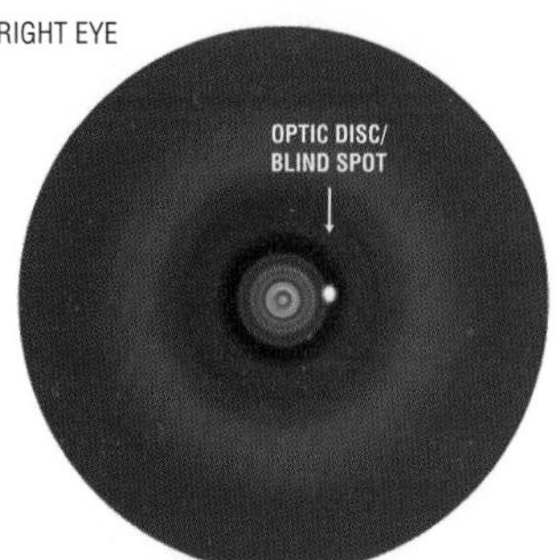

Plate 46. Cones 3-D Density Model (Top View).

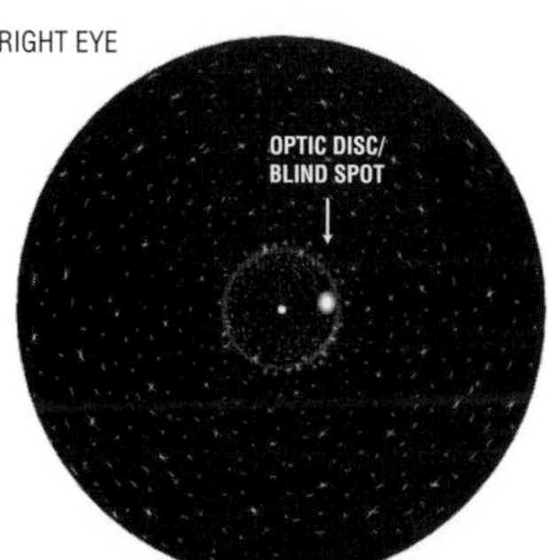

Plate 47. Rods 3-D Density Model (Top View).

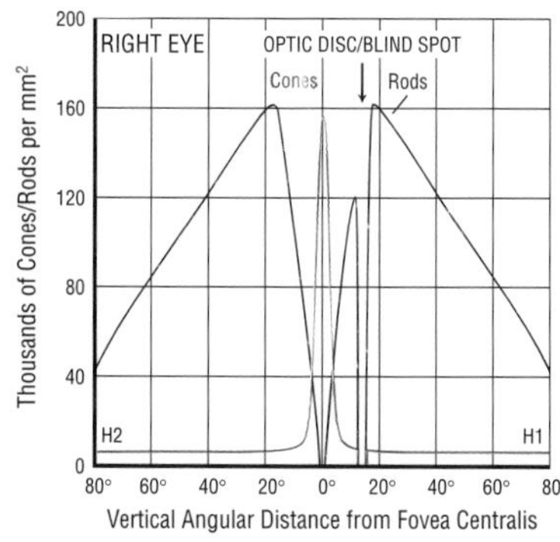

Plate 48. Cones and Rods Horizontal Density Graph (H1-H2).

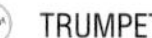

While centralizing on the trumpet, the peripheral object LBS cannot be seen by the left eye due to the left eye's optic disc. This is indicated by the left black ray.

LBS can be seen by the right eye. This is indicated by the blue ray.

While centralizing on the trumpet, the peripheral object RBS cannot be seen by the right eye due to the right eye's optic disc. This is indicated by the right black ray.

RBS can be seen by the left eye. This is indicated by the red ray.

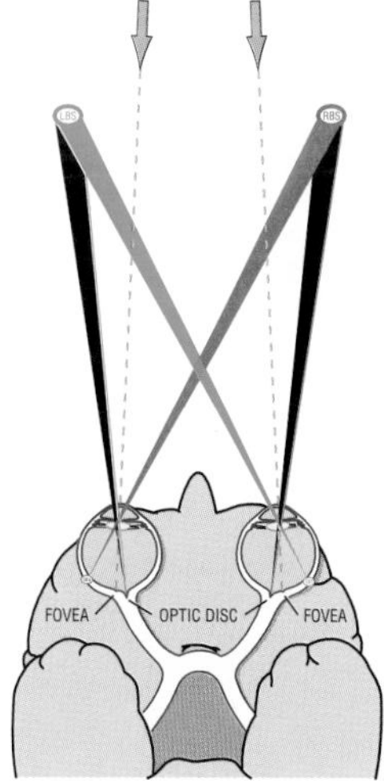

Plate 49. The Blind Spots.

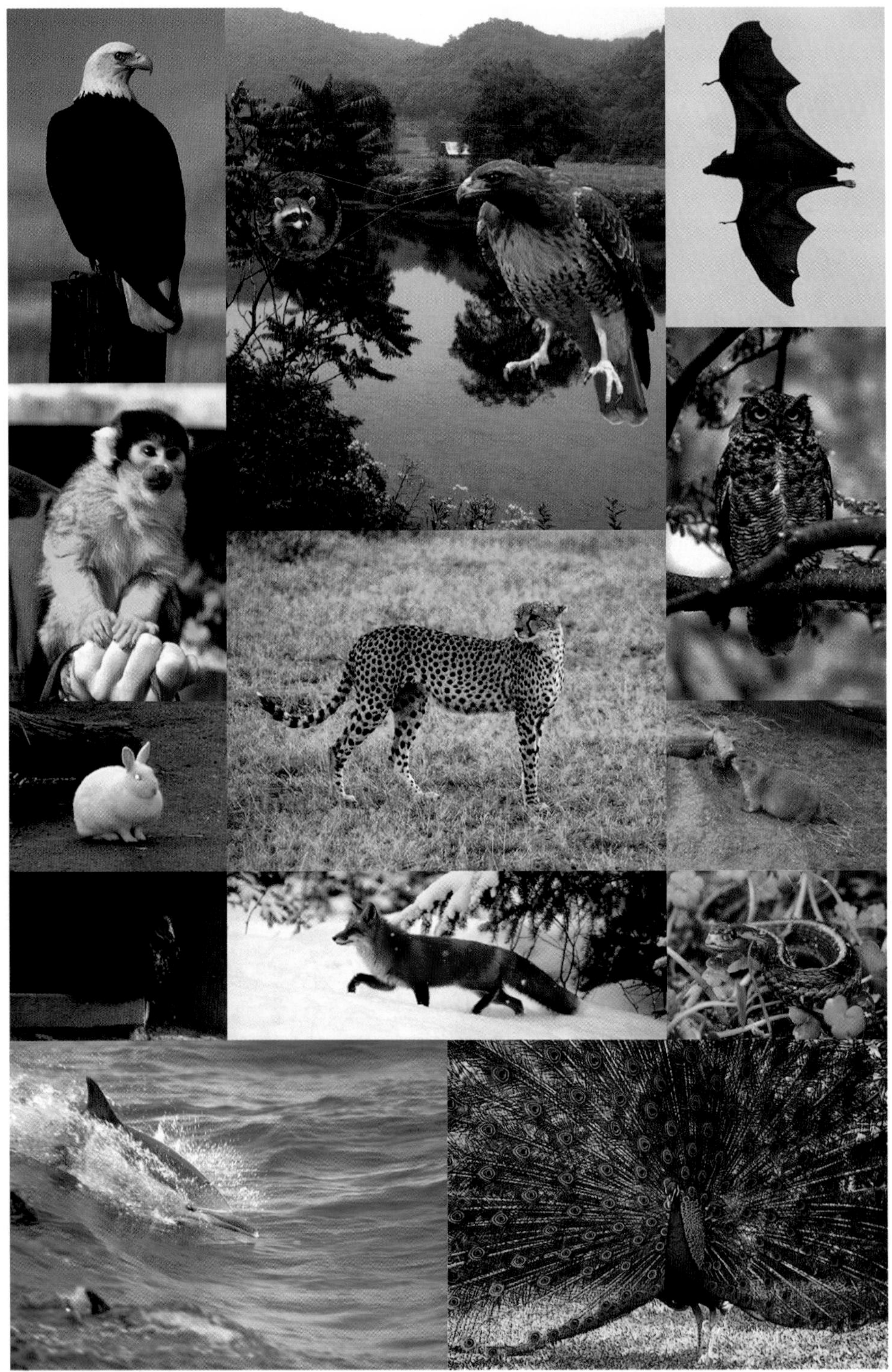

Plate 50. Animal Vision.

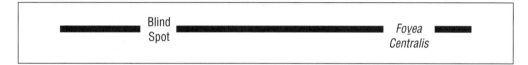

"Blind Spot" will disappear. No peeking! The light rays from the words "Blind Spot" land in the optic disc, where there are no light receptors. When the page is moved closer to or farther away from your eye, the light rays from the words "Blind Spot" fall onto the rods (and cones) outside the optic disc.

Part B:

Sketch the letter "v" in the word "*Fovea*" in *Part A*. When you have found the distance at which the words "Blind Spot" disappear the best, then sketch the letter "t" in the sentence "*Fill it in, Brain!*" Magic! The brain fills in the empty space in the line to the left with what logically should be there—a "continuous" line. Moving this page closer and farther away reveals the empty space once again.

If you would like to experience the blind spot with your right eye, turn this page upside-down, and repeat the same instructions.

If you have difficulty with these experiences, rotate this page a couple of degrees counterclockwise (clockwise when using the right eye.) Since the optic disc is a couple of degrees above the horizon relative to the fovea, this may help "Blind Spot" disappear. (Most students do not need to do this.)

The brain filling in the empty space, when it is at the blind spot, is an indication of how mental the process of seeing is. How much of the picture we see all day long is "filled in" between the spaces of the cones and rods in the retina?

THE BIRDS' AND THE BEES' VISION

See *Plate 50: Animal Vision.*

Most animals are either diurnal (daytime) or nocturnal (nighttime) creatures. As such, each has developed a visual system that best suits its purposes.

The eyes of land and air predators are placed forward in the head for excellent depth perception. (Predator fish must move their heads left and right to spot prey that is straight ahead.)

Along with humans, some primates, reptiles (including alligators, crocodiles, lizards), and almost all diurnal birds have at least one fovea in each eye.

Among animals that have cones, not all have all three types of cones. Many have only one or two types, which means their color vision is limited. Among mammals, only apes and most monkeys have color vision close to humans.

NICTITANS, THE THIRD EYELID

Most nocturnal birds and some reptiles, like lizards, crocodiles and alligators, and camels, have a functioning third membrane called a *nictitans* (from the Latin *nictatus,* meaning "to wink"). This special thin, transparent membrane is located near the inner angle of the eye or beneath the lower eyelid.

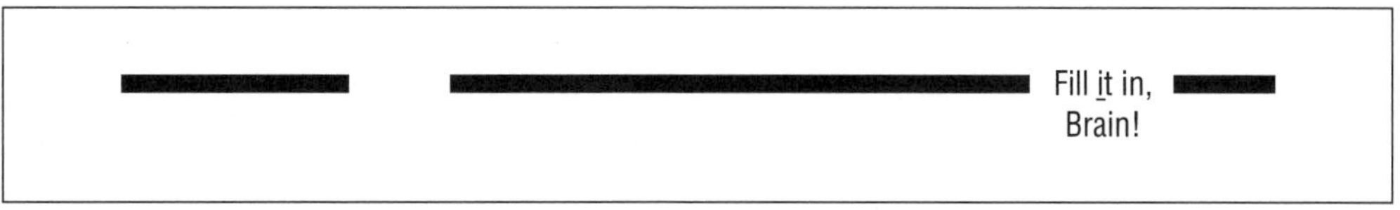

Even when closed, the transparent nictitans allows the animal to continue seeing—a decided advantage. The nictitans helps protect animals from dirt and debris. By closing the nictitans, birds can protect their eyes while in flight. Nocturnal birds, like the owl, can use the nictitans to protect their eyes from bright sunlight during the day.

Birds

Birds have very large eyes relative to the size of their head and body. Some eyes are so large, they touch each other inside the bird's head! (Thus, the phrase "bird brain.") A larger eye has more cones, which provides sharper vision. Birds have the highest quantity and density of light receptors of all animals. A sparrow has a cone density of 400,000 mm^2, which is more than twice that in the human eye.

As mentioned above, nearly all birds have a fovea. About half of all birds have two foveas in each eye.

For all birds, the lower eyelid moves upward for protection from dirt and other particles and to close the eyes during sleep; the owl is the only bird that can lower its upper eyelid.

Daytime Birds

Some daytime birds, including eagles, hawks, chickens and canaries, have all cones, but no rods. Unlike humans, these animals see everything sharp and colorful simultaneously, similar to the picture from the camera in *Plate 44: How We See, a.* Unfortunately, "pure" cone vision makes a daytime bird unable to see in true nighttime.

Raptor (predatory) birds such as eagles, hawks, and falcons have the best distance vision of all creatures on Earth. The buteo hawk has the highest density of cones at 1,000,000 mm^2. This is more than five times that of humans. An eagle can spot a mouse on the ground from high in the sky, while a vulture can spot a carcass from nearly two and a half miles away.

All raptors have two deeply pitted foveas in each eye. These specialized foveas produce magnified "telescopic" sight both straight ahead and to the sides. One fovea picks up a point of clarity straight ahead, and the other picks up a point of clarity in the peripheral vision.

Due to its very high concentration of cones and specialized foveas, the red-tailed hawk can see the raccoon across the river with greater clarity than humans. (See *Plate 50.*)

A chicken has all cones. The entire visual field is equally sharp and colorful in the daytime. However, because it lacks rods, the chicken is essentially "blind" at night and needs to hide from the rod-equipped fox. The eyes of chickens and ducks are placed on the sides of their heads, typical of prey animals.

Nighttime Birds

Pronounced nighttime birds, like night owls and some bats, have only rods and no cones. Owls see only indistinct, gray shapes. (Some diurnal owls have some cones, and therefore some color vision.) Nocturnal owls have more rods than humans. For example, the barn owl has four times as many rods as humans.

Additionally, the rods in owls are in larger groups (association cells), resulting in even greater sensitivity to light at night—up to 100 times more sensitive than the darkness-adapted vision of humans.

One advantage of not having a fovea centralis is that a tiny, dim object does not disappear from the central vision at night. The central object will be "grainy" and colorless, but at least it can be seen.

Most nocturnal birds are not able to accommodate. Even if they could, the best vision would still be much less than 20/20, since the rods do not pick up sharp detail. Movement and very low-level light perception are more important for nocturnal birds.

The owl compensates somewhat for its immobile eyes by having twice as many vertebrae in its neck. With the extra vertebrae, an owl can turn its head almost 180° in each direction. This gives some children the impression the owl can rotate its head all the way around, 360°! The owl can also bend its head all the way back.

Contrary to their reputation, bats do use their eyes to see at night. In fact, the fruit bat has excellent night vision. Many bats (but not fruit bats) also use a form of sonar, sending out chirps that echo off of insects and other prey. The time it takes for the echo to return helps the bat gauge the prey's distance.

Other Animals

The color vision of many mammals is limited to faded yellows and blues. Red colors appear dark brown, while greens appear white or gray.

Other Daytime Animals

Within the large, wild cat families, only the cheetah is a diurnal predator. Notice in *Plate 50* the black stripe extending from the eye to the mouth. This helps prevent reflection from the bright sunlight. Football players have copied the cheetah's ways! Some lizards have a black circle around their eyes which serves the same purpose.

Although their retinas contain mostly rods, cheetahs, leopards, and seabirds have a thin, horizontal band of concentrated cones in the middle of their retinas—a semi-fovea. This gives cheetahs sharper vision to spot gazelles and antelope along the flat plains of Africa. But gazelles and antelopes also have horizontal foveas to spot their predators.

Notice the forward position of the cheetah's eyes, typical of land predators. This provides excellent depth perception. The cheetah is the world's fastest land mammal, accelerating from a stand-still to over 70 miles per hour within a few seconds. Only the three birds, the golden eagle, peregrine falcon, and Indian swift, can travel faster. Cheetahs are currently an endangered species.

The native black tail prairie dog (actually a squirrel that sounds like a small dog!), squirrels, and turtles have nearly all cones. They have no night vision. Note the location of the eye on the side of its head, allowing excellent peripheral vision, like chickens and rabbits. This is typical of prey animals.

The vision of the mandrill monkey is very similar to human trichromatic (RGB) vision, whereas some other monkeys have more limited color vision.

The South American squirrel monkey has very good cone vision, but is slightly deficient in the red region.

The chameleon, a type of lizard, has an extremely high density of cones in its fovea—nearly 800,000 mm^2, almost matching that of the buteo hawk. Turtles have almost completely cone vision.

Other Nighttime Animals

Nocturnal animals have virtually all rods, with few or no cones. Since the rods are very poor at picking up red light, a red flashlight can be used at night to find night animals without frightening them away. At night, human eyes can detect red better than most night animals.

Cats have both rods and cones; however, the rods far outnumber the cones. The density of cones in cats is only 24,000 mm^2, about ⅙ that of humans. Cats do not have a fovea. The night vision of a cat is about eight times better than human night vision. Part of this better night vision is due to the tapetum which is described below.

Cats, including lions, are primarily nighttime animals. A cat's pupil is round when large but becomes a narrow vertical slit when closed. This helps protect their night-adapted rods from sudden bright light.

Research on the vision of dogs is conflicting. About half of the studies suggest dogs do not see color, and the other half suggest they do. Some think dogs have very limited color vision in the blue region. In any case, the majority of seeing by dogs is with the rods, and therefore the picture is gray. The fovea is absent in dogs.

Other nocturnal animals include rats, mice, lemurs, flying squirrels, raccoons, rabbits, crocodiles, dolphins, alligators, raccoons, skunks, and badgers. These animals have essentially all rods.

Dolphins, being nighttime hunters, have 7,000 times more rod association cells than humans; cats have 2,000 times more.

Deep-sea fish have the most light-sensitive retinas of all creatures. Their retinas are particularly designed to pick up blue wavelengths of light, as most red light is absorbed near the surface of the water.

Rabbits have "wide-angle" eyes at the sides of their head, typical of land prey animals. Rabbits have almost 360° wrap-around vision. With almost no defense from predators except freezing and running, their panoramic vision is important for survival. Since rods are movement detectors, "freezing" can be an effective method of avoiding detection. Rabbits have no cones.

The Tapetum—Doubling Sensitivity

Many animals including owls, cats, lions, cows, sheep, oxen, rabbits, raccoons, some dogs, elephants, bears, wolves, dolphins, whales, and some deep-water fish have eyes that glow at night. This is due to an extra highly reflective layer called the *tapetum lucidum.* The tapetum (from the Latin *tapete,* meaning "carpet," and *lucere,* meaning "to shine"; literally "the shining carpet"), which is not present in humans, lies in the choroid, just beyond the pigment epithelium in the retina.

In animals with tapetums, light that misses the light receptors passes through a relatively transparent epithelium layer and reflects from the mirror-like tapetum back into the rods (and cones, if any) layer. The tapetum gives the light ray a second chance of hitting a rod or cone, giving these animals better nighttime vision. Some of the light reflected from the tapetum exits the eyes again, creating a cat's "glowing" eyes at night.

Some animals even have a "super tapetum" made of guanine crystals. These crystals reflect light even better than the common tapetum.

Notice in *Plate 50* how the eyes of the rabbit "glow" from the camera flash. This is due to the rabbit's tapetum. The pupils are large because the rabbit is in the shade at sunset.

Ultraviolet and Infrared Vision

Bees, butterflies, deer, and many lizards can see UV light. UV light patterns on flowers and insects are important for feeding on nectar and for mating.

Some snakes, e.g. the green tree python, pit vipers, and rattlesnakes, some owls, and some bats can see in the infrared region. At night, a mouse is not as protected as it thinks, as the viper snake can see the mouse's "heat" image.

Special "thermographic" camera technology now allows us to take infrared "heat" pictures. For example, a heat picture can be taken of a hand-print on a wall just after the hand has moved away.

Goldfish can see both infrared and UV light.

There are several books listed in the Bibliography that describe the vision of animals. *How Animals See,* by Sandra Sinclair, is a standout.

CHAPTER SUMMARY

I once asked a group of students how they would design the light receptors in the retina. One student said, "The retina should have all cones during the day, and then transform into all rods at night."

There are many types of visual systems, only a few of which have been discussed in this chapter. For humans the cones are maximized in the center of the visual field, for excellent acuity and color. Rods pick up indistinct gray images, motion, and very low levels of light in the periphery.

In the movie *Tombstone* an observer of the famous Wild West lawman Wyatt Earp states, "He's got the eyes of both predator and prey." Basically, nature has given us "eagle-eyes" in the center of the visual field, and "night-owl" vision in the periphery.

Notes

1 Sandra Sinclair, *How Animals See* (New York: Facts on File Publications, 1985), p. xv.

2 Steve Richards, "How to Extend Your Sight," *Invisibility* (Wellingborough, Northamptonshire, England: The Aquarian Press, 1982), p. 52.

3 Natalie Angier, "New Clues to Vision: People Whose Glasses Must Be Rose-Colored; When the retina has no cones, scientists can see the rods at work," *The New York Times* (November 17, 1992), p. B6.

4 Clara A. Hackett and Lawrence Galton, *Relax and See* (London: Faber and Faber, Limited, 1957), pp. 196–97.

5 Charles H. May, *Diseases of the Eye* (Baltimore, Maryland: William Wood and Company, 1943), p. 294.

6 John Downer, *Supersense: Perception in the Animal World* (New York: Henry Holt and Company, 1988), p. 52.

7 R. L. Gregory, *Eye and Brain: The Psychology of Seeing* (New York: McGraw-Hill Co., 1966), p. 48.

Chapter Eighteen

Stereoscopic Vision

BINOCULAR VISION

Horizontal Fields

See *Plate 51: Binocular Vision.*

In *Horizontal Visual Fields,* object *a* is the point of centralization. Notice in *Left Eye Horizontal Visual Field, b,* and *Right Eye Horizontal Visual Field, c,* both visual fields are equal in size, but opposite to each other. Each eye sees a horizontal angle of field of 145° (85° from the point of centralization, *a,* toward the temples, plus 55° from *a* to the nose).

See *Combined Horizontal Visual Fields, e.* The two visual fields overlap almost completely in the middle area with an angle of 120°, *d.* This large area of overlapping, binocular vision is possible because both eyes are located in front of the head and are facing forward.

The total horizontal visual field is 170°, *e* (85° for the right eye + 85° for the left). However, there are two small areas, one to the far left (*b*', 25°), and the other to the far right (*c*', 25°), which are still monocular. This is due to the nose blocking the far right side of the left eye's field of vision and the far left side of the right eye's field of vision.

Binocular vision is especially important for humans and animals that have a fovea centralis. Light from the object of interest, *a,* enters the fovea of each eye. Information reaching the brain is doubled at this point of centralization—the only part of the visual field where we see clearly.

For most of the peripheral vision (green area *d,* minus the foveal vision), the rods are also activated twice. This gives us better movement perception and depth perception. A disadvantage of maximum, forward binocular vision is the loss of some side and all rear vision. Since forward vision is primarily found in predators, this is rarely a problem.

Full Visual Fields

In *Plate 51: Binocular Vision, Full Visual Fields,* "Dixie Man" is the man located exactly in the center of the picture (between two columns on the second deck) and is the object of centralization.

Combined Visual Fields shows the total visual fields, *b* + *c*. *d* is the area of overlapping, binocular vision, while *b*' and *c*' are monocular.

The angle upward from the center of the visual field to the eyebrow is 45°; downward from the center to the cheek is 65°. The total central vertical angle is 110°.

Blind spots are eliminated in the *Combined Visual Fields.* However, the two optic disc areas are monocular, because each area is only seen with one eye.

The Fused Finger

See *Plate 51: Binocular Vision, The Fused Finger.*

Examine your right forefinger carefully while holding it about eight inches in front of your head. When asked how many fingers there are, we say there is only one finger, and we think we see this finger like a camera sees it, as in *Camera Finger.*

A closer examination reveals there are actually two fingers that are "fused" into one. Up close, the right eye sees a significantly different view of the finger than the left eye does. Close or cover each eye alternately to discover this fact. Note the fingernail images seen with each eye separately.

The brain merges the two different images, the best it can, into "one" finger. The finger we see is actually a composite of the two separate images from each eye, as in *Fused Fingers.* This is not the same as a camera's view.

This demonstration is more dramatic if you hold your hand vertically about four inches in front of your head. Position the thumb so it is close to the head and the small finger is farther away. Alternate closing each eyelid. The two views of the hand are very different. The right eye can see the right sides of all the fingers, but not the left sides, and vice versa. With both eyes open, you see both sides simultaneously.

Now hold a finger or hand out at arm's length. Examine the finger or hand carefully again. Close each eye alternately to discover there is less difference between the two sides.

The closer an object is to a person, the greater the difference between the two pictures of that object. The brain uses the amount of difference between the two images, along with the size of the object, to determine its distance. The difference between the images in each eye changes the most from directly in front of the head out to a distance of about twenty feet.

Theoretically, a finger or hand positioned at infinity would be seen the same with each eye. With our visual system, however, objects at twenty feet and beyond are essentially at infinity as far as fusion and depth perception are concerned.

Binocular Vision for Depth Perception

The main advantage of having two eyes in the front of the head with overlapping visual fields is better depth perception. Binocular vision helps us determine an object's distance.

As discussed above, the difference between the two images is one way the brain gauges depth.

Another way the brain judges an object's distance is by its size. A rabbit one foot away appears much larger than the same rabbit twenty feet away. But what if the rabbit twenty feet away was so large it appeared to be the same size as the rabbit only one foot away? How can the brain tell the difference? This is where the difference in the images in the two eyes comes into play. The two images on the right and left retinas of a smaller rabbit one foot away would have a greater difference between them than the two images on the retina of a far-away, larger rabbit. Also, by experience, we know that rabbits are not huge!

Two other ways the brain can judge the distance of an object is by convergence and accommodation. Convergence, discussed more below, is alignment of the two eyes so that the object of interest (centralization) lands in the foveas for sharp acuity. The more the eyes turn inward, the greater the convergence, and the closer that image must be. The accommodation of the eye to see a near object is another clue the brain has to gauge the distance of an object. As mentioned in Chapter 3, "Understanding Lenses and Prescriptions," accommodation occurs basically within the first twenty feet.

Judging Relative Distances

Refer to *Plate 52: Judging Relative Distances.*

The model in *a-1* is the same model as in *a-2*; *b-1* is the same as *b-2*; and *c-1* is the same as *c-2*.

a-1, b-1, and *c-1* are views of the models from the top.

a-2, b-2, and *c-2* are views from behind the eyeballs, looking toward the letters L, C, and R. These models show the different images created on the retinas when two objects (L and R) are at different distances from the eyes.

The eyes in these models are directed toward the center of the letter C, as indicated by the gray lines extending from the fovea centralis of each eye out to and through the center of the letter C.

In examining these models, there are several discoveries we can make about how the retina "sees" multiple objects. The brain processes different retinal images and then draws conclusions regarding the relative distances of those objects.

First, notice how all letters on the retina are flipped upside-down and leftside-right. Next, notice that L is to the left of C, but on the retina the image of L is to the right of C. R is to the right of C, but on the retina the image of R is to the left of C. The image of the world is completely reversed on the retina.

In *a-1/a-2,* L, C, and R are the same distance from the eyes. Also, L is the same distance to line AB as R is to line CD. AB and CD represent the lines of sight from the fovea to letter C. In *a-2,* the images of L, C, and R on the retina are the same size, and the images of L and R are the same distance to the image of C.

In *b-1/b-2,* L has been moved closer to the eyes, while R has been moved farther away. In *b-1,* notice how the letters L and R are now closer to line AB, while they are farther away from line CD. This may be easier to see if you rotate the illustration counterclockwise so that AB is vertical; then, rotate the page clockwise to make CD vertical.

In *b-2,* in the left eye, the images of L and R are now closer to C, while in the right eye they are farther away. The positions of the letters on the two retinas are now quite different from each other, and from the images on the retina in *a-2.* In *b-2,* how does the brain fuse these two different pictures from the retinas?

The image of C does not change its location or size on the retina because C has not been moved from its original location and the eyes are still centralizing on C.

In *c-1/c-2,* L has been moved farther away from the eyes, and R closer. Compare all of the images on the six retinas. There are only two that are identical. Which ones are they?

Along with the other methods described above, the brain uses the difference in distances between images of L and R on the two retinas to make judgments about the relative and absolute distances of these letters. The main differences occur when the two objects are within the first twenty feet.

If the distances between the images of L and R on the retinas are the same, as in *a-2*, the brain may assume L and R are at the same distance from us. If the distance between the images of L and R is smaller on the retina of the left eye than on the right eye, as in *b-2*, the brain may conclude L is closer than R. Finally, if the distance between images of L and R is greater on the retina of the left eye than on the right eye, as in *c-2*, the brain may conclude L is farther away than R.

Notice in *b-2* that the images of L are larger on the retinas because L is closer to the eyes; the image of R is smaller because it is farther away. In these models, the brain may assume a larger letter is closer, and a smaller letter is farther away.

These letters are the same size. If they were different sizes, the brain might need more information to judge their distances. Learning the size of objects by experience, like the rabbit example above, is an important part of learning to gauge distances of objects.

The images in the above models are relatively large, and close to the eyes. If these same three letters were placed 100 feet away, and the letters L and R were moved the same distances closer and farther away, the differences between their images on the two retinas would be much less. This is one reason it is easier to gauge the relative distances of objects within the first twenty feet.

A Topsy-Turvy World

Some studies have been conducted in which a person wears special goggles which make objects appear upside down, and the right side on the left. After a certain period of time, while still wearing these goggles with prisms, some objects are seen right-side up in their correct orientations![1]

3-D Vision, More Than Just Stereoscopic Vision

The sense of depth created by binocular vision is called stereoscopic vision. The brain merges both the two-dimensional images, one from the right eye and one from the left eye, into one three-dimensional image. Stereopsis (from Greek, meaning "solid sight") means the appearance of depth when both eyes are used.

In addition to stereoscopic vision, the right hemisphere of the brain creates an even *more* 3-D image.

In natural vision classes, students sketch scenic pictures with their imaginary nose-pencils. At the end of the second class, most vision students experience a marked feeling of depth in these scenic pictures—as if the student could actually walk into the scene, sensing the edges around objects.

This sense of 3-D depth perception is not the same depth perception experienced by stereoscopic vision, as this "extra sense" of 3-D can be experienced with only one eye. This 3-D experience is one of the *qualities* of vision that resurfaces when the visual system begins to relax and returns to a natural balance.

During his initial telephone call, one of my students told me he had perfect sight for 26½ years, and that he had been wearing glasses for only six months. He told me that as much as he wanted to improve his acuity, he also wanted his 3-D vision back. He said that the more he wore his glasses, the "flatter" the world seemed to get, especially while wearing the glasses. Unfortunately, most people who have worn glasses for many years do not remember natural 3-D vision. It can be startling to many students when it begins to return.

So, a person may have stereoscopic vision, due to the proper convergence of the two eyes, but he may not have right hemisphere, 3-D vision. Left-brain, mechanical glasses, the "machines of seeing," switch off many right-hemisphere qualities of vision. *Sight through glasses is not similar to the experiences of true natural vision.*

The ophthalmologist Dr. R. Agarwal, in his in book, *Mind and Vision,*[2] describes this extra sense of 3-D and some other aspects of natural vision:

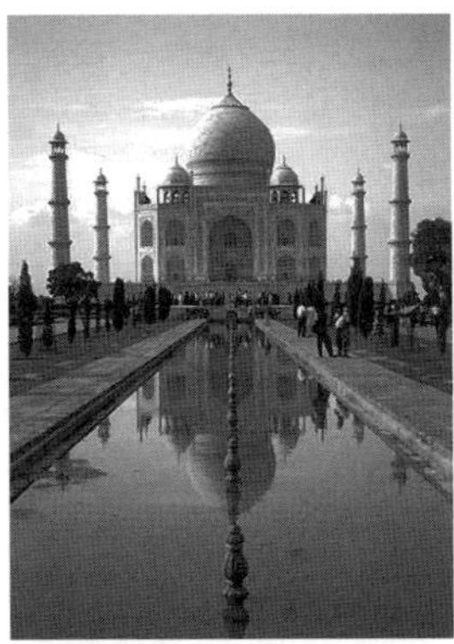

So I gave a picture of the Taj Mahal to this girl student. She was asked to look at the people right in front and at those who were on the floor of the Taj Mahal as if they were a mile away, very far. By alternate shifting of sight she could feel the distance between the people in front and the Taj Mahal. Taj Mahal appeared as if a real monument before her. Instantly the girl observed that the sun had also come there, as if from nowhere, and was shining brilliantly on the golden dresses of the girls in the photograph. Suddenly she cried out, "Ah, it is really beautiful." She saw the depth in the windows of the Taj Mahal. The shadows of the front walls of the Taj falling on the walls behind added to its three-dimensional appearance. The four minars, the conical trees, the water canal and the carpet of green grass, all appeared quite real to her. The mind [began] to see everything in its true perspective, as if Taj was visible with its length, breadth and height. The people in front seemed to be walking in reality... The coloured saree of the lady became hundred-fold beautiful and magnificent with all its sober designs. When the mind got completely relaxed, the visual cells of the retina began to function with their full capacity.[3]

Since the retina is part of the brain, the *brain* began to function with its full capacity.

Later he writes of another student:

... she was taught centralization and was given a picture of the Taj Mahal. At first glance the view-card appeared to be a flat coloured picture but by looking at it in a particular way without effort or strain she was able to enjoy it. The Taj appeared in all its glory in a bright light. The effect of the sun could be seen on the building, the shadows could be seen behind the persons walking in front of Taj. The three-dimensional effect could be produced easily with each eye separately.[4]

This story shows that this extra sense of three-dimensional vision is not dependent upon stereoscopic vision. There is a definite, extra quality of 3-D vision, difficult to describe or quantify, produced in the mind when a person has relaxed, natural vision habits.

The Stereoscopic Pictures Fad

Recently, images have been produced which, at first glance, seem like a group of meaningless, random dots. However, when a person centralizes at a certain distance in front of, or in back of, the image, a 3-D picture is formed in the brain. Though the 3-D effect is entertaining, the diffusion necessary to create the effect may be harmful. One computer software company even warns of getting a headache by viewing such images created by their software.

Natural, clear vision is based on relaxation of the mind. Creating more strain with these images is not recommended.

I believe that the 3-D effect experienced with these images may be more entertaining to people who wear glasses, because they have lost much of their natural, right-hemisphere 3-D vision.

BATES ON STRABISMUS (SQUINT) AND AMBLYOPIA

Before discussing the somewhat complex topics of fusion, amblyopia, convergence, and strabismus (the latter is also known as squint), let's read what Bates had to say on these topics. "Squint" was a term used (more in the past) to refer to strabismus; "squint" as used here does not refer to the harmful vision habit of narrowing the eyelids. The term "strabismus" has been substituted for the term "squint" in many of Bates' extracts.

Almost the entire chapter on strabismus and amblyopia from *Perfect Sight Without Glasses* is reprinted here:

CHAPTER XXI
STRABISMUS AND AMBLYOPIA:
THEIR CAUSE

Since we have two eyes, it is obvious that in the act of sight two pictures must be formed; and in order that these two pictures shall be fused into one by the mind, it is necessary that there shall be perfect harmony of action between the two organs of vision. In looking at a distant object the two visual axes must be parallel, and in looking at an object at a less distance than infinity, which for practical purposes is less than twenty feet, they must converge to exactly the same degree. The absence of this harmony of action is known as squint, or strabismus, and is one of the most distressing of eye defects, not only because of the lowering of vision involved, but because the want of symmetry in the most expressive feature of the face which results from it has a most unpleasant effect upon the personal appearance. The condition is one which has long baffled ophthalmological science. While the theories as to its cause advanced in the text-books seem to fit some cases, they leave others unexplained, and all methods of [improvement] are admitted to be very uncertain in their results.

The idea that a lack of harmony in the movements of the eye is due to a corresponding lack of harmony in the strength of the muscles that turn them in their sockets seems such a natural one that this theory was almost universally accepted at one time. Operations based upon it once had a great vogue; but today they are advised, by most authorities, only as a last resort. It is true that many persons have benefited by them; but at best the correction of the strabismus is only approximate, and in many cases the condition has been made worse, while a restoration of binocular vision—the power of fusing the two visual images into one—is scarcely even hoped for.[a]

The result of even the most successful strabismus operation, in long-standing strabismus, is merely cosmetic in the vast majority of cases.—Eversbusch: *The Diseases of Children,* edited by Pfaunder and Schlossman. English translation by Shaw and La Fetra, second edition, 1912–1914, vol. vii, p. 316.

The muscle theory fitted the facts so badly that when Donders advanced the idea that strabismus was a condition growing out of refractive errors—hypermetropia being held responsible for the production of convergent and myopia for divergent strabismus—it was universally accepted. This theory, too, proved unsatisfactory, and now medical opinion is divided between various theories. Hansen-Grut attributed the condition, in the great majority of cases, to a defect, not of the muscles, but of the nerve supply; and this idea has had many supporters. Worth and his disciples lay stress on the lack of a so-called fusion faculty, and have recommended the use of prisms, or other measures, to develop it. Stevens believes that the anomaly results from a wrong shape of the orbit, and as it is impossible to alter this condition, advocates operations for the purpose of neutralizing its influence.

In order to make any of these theories appear consistent it is necessary to explain away a great many troublesome facts. The uncertain result of operations upon the eye muscles is sufficient to cast suspicion on the theory that the condition is due to any abnormality of the muscles, and many cases of marked paralysis of one or more muscles have been observed in which there was no strabismus. Relief of paralysis, moreover, may not relieve the strabismus, nor the relief of the strabismus the paralysis. Worth found so many cases which were not benefited by training designed to improve the fusion faculty that he recommended operations on the muscles in such cases; while Donders, noting that the majority of hypermetropes did not [have] strabismus, was obliged to assume that hypermetropia did not cause this condition without the aid of co-operating circumstances.

That the state of the vision is not an important factor in the production of strabismus is attested by a multitude of facts. It is true, as Donders observed, that strabismus is usually associated with errors of refraction; but some people have strabismus with a very slight error of refraction. It is also true that many persons with convergent [inward] strabismus have hypermetropia; but many others have not. Some persons with convergent strabismus have myopia. A person may also have convergent strabismus with one eye normal and one hypermetropic or myopic, or with one eye blind. Usually the vision of the eye that turns in is less than that of the eye which is straight; yet there are cases in which the eye with the poorer vision is straight and the eye with the better vision turned in. With two blind eyes, both eyes may be straight, or one may turn in. With one good eye and one blind eye, both eyes may be straight. The blinder the eye, as a rule, the more marked the strabismus; but exceptions are frequent, and in rare cases an eye with nearly normal vision may turn in persistently. A strabismus may disappear and return again, while convergent strabismus will change into divergent [outward] strabismus and back again. With the same error

[a] The result obtained by the operation is, as a rule, simply cosmetic. The sight of the strabismic eye is not influenced by the operation, and in only a few instances is even binocular vision restored.—Fuchs: *Text-Book of Ophthalmology*, p. 795.

of refraction, one person will have strabismus and the other not. A third will have strabismus with a different eye. A fourth will have strabismus first with one eye and then with the other. In a fifth the amount of the strabismus will vary. One will get well without glasses, or other [solutions], and another with these things. These improvements may be temporary, or permanent, and the relapses may occur either with or without glasses.

However slight the error of refraction, the vision of many strabismic eyes is inferior to that of the straight eye, and for this condition [amblyopia], usually no apparent or sufficient cause can be found in the constitution of the eye. There is a difference of opinion as to whether this curious defect of vision is the result of the strabismus, or the strabismus the result of the defect of vision; but the predominating opinion that it is, at least, aggravated by the strabismus has been crystallized in the name given to the condition, namely, *amblyopia ex anopsia,* literally *dimsightedness from non-use*—for in order to avoid the annoyance of double vision the mind is believed to suppress the image of the deviating eye. There are, however, many strabismic eyes without amblyopia, while such a condition has been found in eyes that have never been strabismic.

The literature of the subject is full of the impossibility of reversing amblyopia, and in popular writings persons having the care of children are urged to have cases of strabismus [addressed] early, so that the vision of the strabismic eye may not be lost. According to Worth, not much improvement can ordinarily be obtained in amblyopic eyes after the age of six, while Fuchs says, "The function of the retina never again becomes perfectly normal, even if the cause of the visual disturbance is done away with."[a] Yet it is well known, as the translator of Fuchs points out in an editorial comment upon the above statement,[b] that if the sight of the good eye is lost at any period of life, the vision of the amblyopic eye will often become normal. Furthermore, an eye may be amblyopic at one time and not at another. When the good eye is covered, a strabismic eye may be so amblyopic that it can scarcely distinguish daylight from darkness; but when both eyes are open, the vision of the strabismic eye may be found to be as good as that of the straight eye, if not better. In many cases, too, the amblyopia will change from one eye to the other.

Double vision occurs very seldom in strabismus, and when it does it often assumes very curious forms. When the eyes turn in the image seen by the right eye should, according to all the laws of optics, be to the right, and the image seen by the left eye to the left. When the eyes turn out the opposite should be the case. But often the position of the images is reversed, the image of the right eye in convergent strabismus being seen to the left and that of the left eye to the right, while in divergent strabismus the opposite is the case. This condition is known as *paradoxical diplopia.* Furthermore, persons with almost normal vision and both eyes perfectly straight may have both kinds of double vision.

All the theories heretofore suggested fail to explain the foregoing facts; but it is a fact

[a] *Text-Book of Ophthalmology,* p. 633. [Although in the main body of Bates' text the reference number (^{1}) for the first footnote is missing, this footnote clearly refers to Fuchs' quote.]

[b] Cases have been reported, some surely authentic, in which an amblyopic strabismic eye has acquired good vision, either through correction of the refraction, or because loss of sight in the good eye has compelled the use of the amblyopic eye.—Ibid.

> that in all cases of strabismus a strain can be demonstrated, and that the relief of the strain is in all cases followed by the reversal of the strabismus, as well as of the amblyopia and the error of refraction. It is also a fact that all persons with normal eyes can produce strabismus by a strain to see. It is not a difficult thing to do, and many children derive much amusement from the practice, while it gives their elders unnecessary concern, for fear the temporary strabismus may become permanent. To produce convergent strabismus is comparatively easy. Children usually do it by straining to see the end of the nose. The production of divergent strabismus is more difficult, but with practice persons with normal eyes become able to turn out either eye, or both, at will. They also become able to turn either eye upward and inward, or upward and outward, at any desired angle. Any kind of strabismus can, in fact, be produced at will by the appropriate kind of strain. Some persons retain the power to produce voluntary strabismus more or less permanently. Others quickly lose it if they do not keep in practice. There is usually a lowering of the vision when voluntary strabismus is produced, and accepted methods of measuring the strength of the muscles seem to show deficiencies corresponding to the nature of the strabismus.

Since, as Bates points out, strabismus can result in an unpleasant effect on a person's appearance, many people with strabismus tend to be less social than people without strabismus. Children can make particularly cruel and painful comments to a child who has strabismus.

Oftentimes, people wonder why the person with strabismus is pointing one eye in various directions while talking with them. They usually think this is being done on purpose, but it is not. Rather, people with strabismus are usually self-conscious and embarrassed by their turning eye. People with strabismus are usually highly motivated vision students. These students want to have normal-looking eyes.

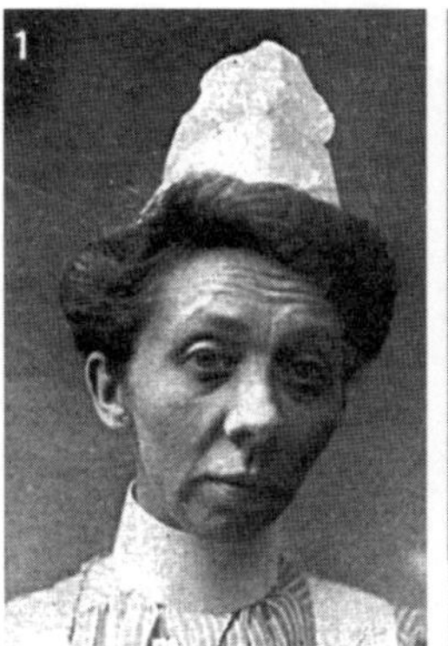

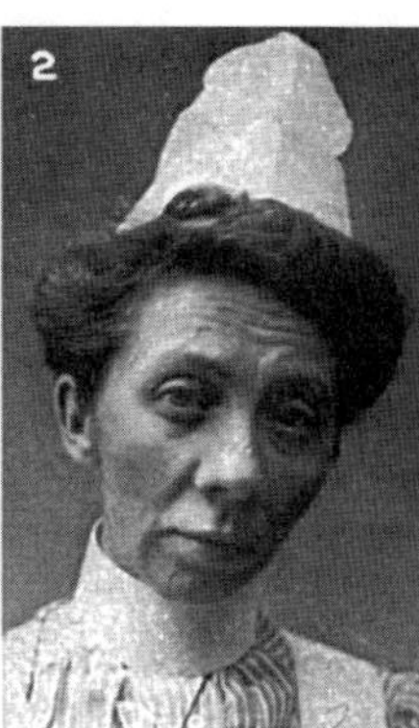

Figure 18–1: Voluntary Production of Strabismus.[5] No. 1—Reading the Snellen card with normal vision; visual axes parallel. No. 2—The same person making an effort to see the card; myopia and convergent strabismus of the left eye have been produced.

According to Bates, the "strength" of the muscles is not a factor in strabismus. Here he is actually referring to the common misconception that there is a "weakness" in one or more muscles. This is explained further below.

Most people who have strabismus have amblyopia. This is discussed more in section "Amblyopia—A 'Switched Off' Image," below.

Bates stated that strabismus was caused by strain, and in that respect, was no different than nearsightedness, farsightedness, and astigmatism. They are all caused by strain. Strabismus is usually grouped with nearsightedness, farsightedness, and astigmatism as a functional problem. This grouping helps separate these four vision problems from pathologies of the eyes.

The Story of Esther

From *Better Eyesight* magazine, August 1927:

SCHOOL CHILDREN
by Emily C. Lierman

... ESTHER

Esther, aged seven, first came to me in January 1927, to be relieved of strabismus. She had worn glasses since she was three years of age for the relief of strabismus in the right eye. Her parents noticed, after she had worn glasses a short time, that she was more nervous than before. Later, they were much concerned because she acquired bad habits, such as holding her head to one side instead of straight, especially while studying and reading her school lessons. Her glasses were then changed. It was thought that wrong glasses had been prescribed because she still kept her head to one side as before, and her nervousness became more pronounced. The parents were told that in time the strabismus would be corrected if Esther wore her glasses all the time.

The strabismus continued to get worse instead of better, so the parents brought her to me. The vision of her right eye was 10/15, but in order to read the letters of the ... card, she had to turn her head so that it almost rested on her right shoulder. Her left vision was 15/15 and she read the letters of the card in a normal position. I [checked] her right eye again, placing the card up close. She turned her head just as much to one side as she did when the card was placed ten feet away. I asked her mother to hold the child's head straight, and again told Esther to tell me what the letters were. I held the [reading] card two feet away while she covered her left eye. She said everything was all dark, and she could see nothing.

It did not take me long to find out that Esther was a bright child, and that she would willingly do anything for the benefit of her poor eye. She said to me, "It is too bad that my sister should have two good eyes and that I should have only one good one." I encouraged her to follow my directions closely and I told her if she continued to do so and practiced as often as she should at home, that we would then try to correct the vision of the poor eye.

I found her to be quite an artist. When her eyes were covered, I asked her if she could remember a drawing of some kind. "Oh, yes," she answered, "while my eyes are closed and covered I can imagine that I am drawing your picture."

I said, "All right, you keep on imagining that you are drawing my picture and later on I will let you sit at my desk and draw a picture of me." We talked about pleasant things for five or ten minutes while she had her eyes covered.

I then taught her to swing her body from left to right, glancing for only a second at the reading card, and then looking away to her left. I purposely avoided having her swing to the right, because she had the desire while reading or trying to see more clearly to always rest her head on the right shoulder. I drew her mother's attention to the fact that, as she swung, both eyes moved in the same direction as her body was moving. When she stopped blinking, which I had encouraged her to do rhythmically with the swing, her right eye turned in and her head also turned to one side.

After she had practiced swinging for a little while, I noticed that she gaped a few times, which meant that she was straining. It is good for parents to notice this, in helping the child practice for the relief of strabismus, and to stop all practice with the exception of closing the eyes to rest them.

Esther palmed again for a little while and then I showed her some celluloid toy animals and asked her to name each one of them. She named each one correctly with the exception of the buffalo, so I did not use that one for her case. If a child [who is given lessons] for strabismus is asked to tell things in detail, the child must be familiar with the objects. While she again covered her eyes to rest them, I placed the animals on the floor five feet away from where she was sitting. I told her mother to touch each animal and have Esther name them. Out of eight animals, she named three incorrectly. They were among the last ones she tried to see. We then noticed that her head turned to one side in order to see them. All this time her left eye was covered.

Then I had Esther sit at my desk and asked her to draw my picture. The drawing was quite well done for a little girl of her age. She kept her head straight while drawing. When strain is relieved, the symptoms of imperfect sight are relieved also. She enjoyed drawing, therefore it did not produce a strain. When she was asked to read the ... card letters, she strained in order to see them and the condition of her eyes became worse.

Esther was encouraged to do something that she liked at every lesson, such as writing figures from one to ten, or drawing a line without using a ruler. At the first attempt, the lines were very crooked and the figures not straight.

Swinging and palming, practiced several times daily, soon improved the right eye to normal. At the last visit, her head remained straight and the strabismus had entirely disappeared.

The vision of her right eye became better than normal, as far as reading the [letter] card was concerned. She read the bottom line at twelve feet and seven inches. This line is read by the normal eye at nine feet. She did equally as well with the left eye, which, of course, had normal vision in the beginning.

To be sure that the child was entirely relieved of strabismus, I told her to look at my right eye, then at my left eye, then to my chin and other parts of my face as I pointed with my finger to each part. She followed me with both eyes moving and her head perfectly straight and as yet she has had no relapse.

"Then, One Day I Broke My Glasses"

John Ott writes in his book *Health and Light:*

> ... then, one day I broke my glasses. While waiting for a new pair to be made, I wore my spares. The nose piece was a little tight and it bothered me, so I took them off most of the time.... It might be well-noted here that after six months of not wearing glasses, except for what little driving of the car was absolutely essential, and for focusing my projector when showing pictures, I began to notice that wearing my glasses even for these short periods seemed to strain my eyes more and more. Accordingly, an appointment with my oculist for a regular check-up seemed advisable. This time it was necessary to go back for a second examination which my doctor explained was customary in order to double check any such drastic change as was the case with the condition of my eyes. The principal difference in my new prescription was that the rather strong prisms previously needed to correct a muscular weakness were no longer needed.[6]

Prisms are used to compensate for strabismus. In strabismus, a muscle is not "weak," as is commonly believed and stated. It is chronically tight, pulling the eye out of its normal position.

The Mechanical Solution to Strabismus—Prisms

Figure 18–2: Prism Correction, a, shows an esophoric right eye. The left eye is centralizing correctly on the green bead. Accordingly, the green bead appears to be in the center of the left eye's visual field.

Since the right eye is turned inward too far, the green bead appears too far to the right side of the right eye's visual field (see *a,* dotted line).

b shows how a prism can be used to change the angle of light rays from the green bead into the right eye. Now, theoretically, the green bead should be in the center of the visual field of the esophoric right eye. A strabismic eye is often amblyopic, so the use of a prism may be of no visual benefit to the strabismic person. (The strabismic eye might appear straight to other people.)

One might guess that the alignment of the green beads in the center of both visual fields would encourage an amblyopic eye to "switch on," but this does not always occur.

As with nearsighted, farsighted, and astigmatic lenses, the prism lense solution supports the tension of the eye muscle(s), and, perhaps worse, the underlying mental strain. The underlying cause of the problem has not been addressed or removed.

I have had at least two people describe to me multiple, unsuccessful strabismus operations. After early failures, the eye muscles

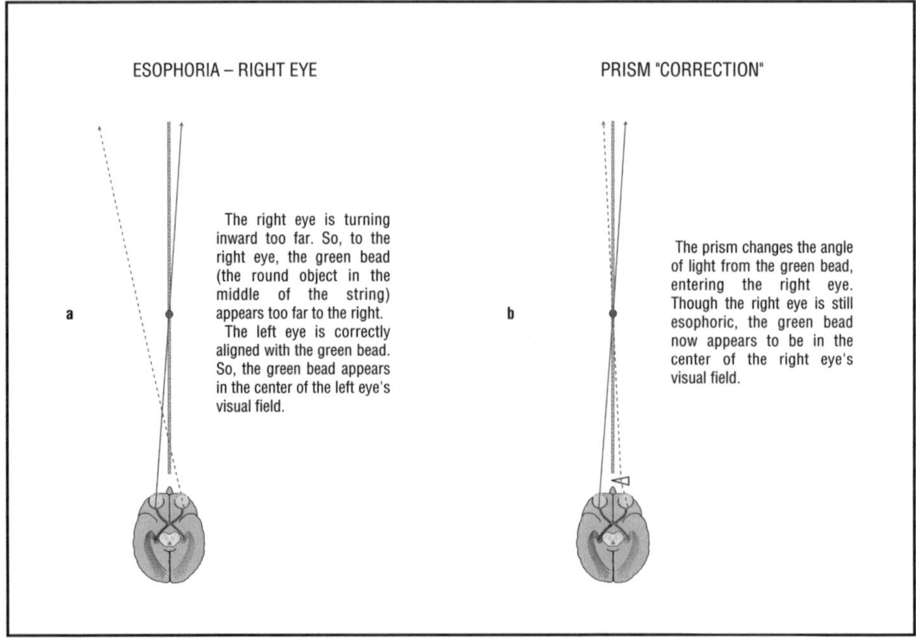

ESOPHORIA – RIGHT EYE
PRISM "CORRECTION"
a
The right eye is turning inward too far. So, to the right eye, the green bead (the round object in the middle of the string) appears too far to the right.
The left eye is correctly aligned with the green bead. So, the green bead appears in the center of the left eye's visual field.
b
The prism changes the angle of light from the green bead, entering the right eye. Though the right eye is still esophoric, the green bead now appears to be in the center of the right eye's visual field.

Figure 18–2: Prism Correction.

were intentionally cut much shorter, leaving the strabismic eye turning in the direction *opposite* to the original deviation. The theory is that, perhaps someday, the strabismic eye would look straight. This has not occurred yet for these two individuals.

Bates on Strabismus, Continued

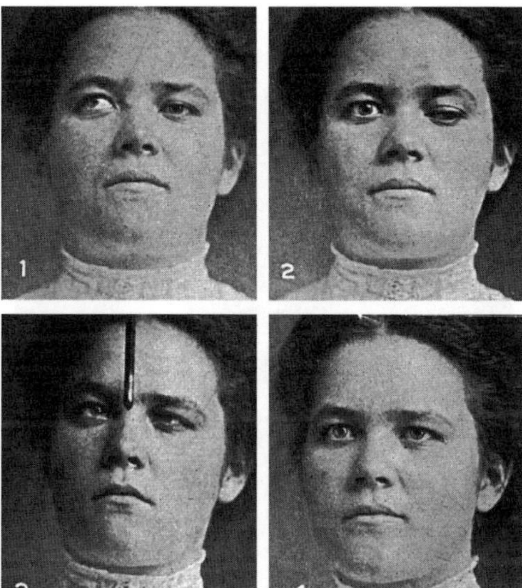

Figure 18–3: Case of Divergent Vertical Strabismus Eliminated by Eye Education.*[7] *No. 1—The right eye turns out and up, the left being straight. No. 2—Student learns to look down and out with the left eye while the right looks straight. No. 3—Student learns to turn both eyes in by looking at a pencil held over the bridge of the nose. No. 4—Student has permanently improved. All four pictures were taken within fifteen minutes of each other, the student having learned to reproduce the conditions represented at will.

A man at a health fair once demonstrated to me his ability to move his eyes, independently and simultaneously, in any directions he wanted.

In the following chapter in *Perfect Sight Without Glasses,* Bates discusses the reversal of strabismus and amblyopia:

> The evidence is conclusive that strabismus and amblyopia, like errors of refraction, are purely functional troubles; and since they are always relieved by the relief of the strain with which they are associated, it follows that any of the methods which promote relaxation and centralization may be employed for their reversal....
>
> In the case illustrated the student had divergent vertical strabismus in both eyes. When the left eye was straight the right eye turned out and up, and when the right eye was straight the left eye turned down and out. Both eyes were amblyopic and there was double vision, with the images sometimes on the same side and sometimes on opposite sides. She suffered from headaches, and having obtained no relief from glasses, or other methods ..., she made up her mind to an operation and consulted Dr. Gudmund J. Gislason, of Grand Forks, N. D., with a view to having one performed. Dr. Gislason, puzzled to find so many muscles apparently at fault, asked my opinion as to which of them should be operated upon. I showed her how to make her strabismus worse, and recommended that Dr. Gislason teach her by eye education without an operation. He did so, and in less than a month ... effected a complete and permanent reversal both of the strabismus and of the amblyopia. The same method has proved successful with other students.
>
> Some students do not know whether they are looking straight at an object or not. These may be helped by watching the deviating eye and directing them to look more nearly in the proper direction. When the deviating eye looks directly at an object the strain to see is less, and the vision is consequently improved.

> . . . The improvement resulting from eye education in cases of strabismus and amblyopia is sometimes so rapid as to be almost incredible. The following are a few of many other examples that might be quoted:
>
> A girl of eleven had convergent vertical strabismus of the left eye. The vision of this eye at the distance was 3/200, while at the near point it was so imperfect that she was unable to read. The vision of the right eye was normal both for the near point and the distance. She was wearing glasses when she came to the office—convex 4.00 D. S. combined with convex 0.50 D. C., axis 90, for the right eye; and convex 5.50 D. S. for the left eye—but had obtained no benefit from them. [Bates then teaches her movement and centralization, and] in less than ten days her vision was normal in both eyes, and in less than two weeks it had improved to 20/10, while diamond type was read with each eye at from three inches to twenty inches. In less than three weeks her vision for the distance was 20/5, by artificial light, and she read photographic type reductions at two inches . . . and at the end of three years [no relapse] had occurred. . . .
>
> A very remarkable case was that of a girl of fourteen who had strabismus from childhood. . . . [She followed] my instructions, and in less than a week the strabismus was corrected and she had perfect vision in both eyes. At the beginning . . . she could not count her fingers at three feet with the poorer eye, and in three weeks . . . she had perfect sight. . . .
>
> A girl of eight had had amblyopia and strabismus since childhood. The vision of the right eye was 10/40, while that of the left was 20/30. Glasses did not improve either eye . . . She was told that the cause of her defective sight was her habit of looking at objects with a part of the retina to one side of the true center of sight. She was advised to see by looking straight at the Snellen card. In less than half an hour the vision of the left eye became normal, while the right improved from 10/40 to 10/10. The improvement was complete in two weeks.

FUSION 1

EXPERIENCING FUSION 1: 1+1 = 1!

You may want to have someone read these directions to you, and to check your alignments (which are very important) as you do these activities. Be sure there is plenty of light, and that the lighting is as equal as possible on the left and right sides.

These activities can be a bit complicated at first. Once they are understood, they are fairly simple to do. You may want to consult with a vision teacher.

If you become tired doing these activities, take a break. Come back to them later when you are rested.

You can substitute two different colored pencils for your fingers in the following activity. Two different colored pencils, like yellow and green, are a bit easier to use than the fingers, because it is easier to distinguish between them when shifting your attention near and far.

If you use pencils, use a yellow pencil in place of the near finger, and a green pencil in place of the far finger. Place the eraser end up, holding the other end at the bottom with your fingers. Position any lettering or details on the pencil so they are facing toward you.

Part A—Experiencing *Fusion 1, The Far Finger (or Green Pencil):*

Refer to *Plate 53: Fusion 1, Far Finger, a-1,* and *Fusion/Far Finger, a-2.*

Locate an object far into the distance; in

the Fusion 1 images, the distant object is Dixie Man. Dixie Man is located exactly in the center of the boat; see *c-2*. Hold your left forefinger (or green pencil) at arm's length straight out in front of you, in line with the distant object. Hold your forefinger vertical, pointing upward, and at eye level.

Sketching (SB&B!) the left forefinger, touch your nose with the base of your right forefinger, holding it vertical and at eye level also. The top of your right forefinger should now be near the forehead. Move your right forefinger straight out 5–6 inches from your head exactly in line with the left forefinger and the distant object. Do not put your attention on the near forefinger.

Continuing to sketch the center of the far finger (indicated by the black circle in *a-1* and *a-2*) you may notice one, solid far finger, as expected, but two semi-transparent near fingers. (It is OK if the two near fingers seem to be solid instead of semi-transparent.) One of the near fingers should appear to be to the right of the far finger; it is seen by the left eye. The second near finger should appear to be to the left of far finger; it is seen by the right eye. Of course there is only one near finger, but we should notice two near fingers.

Remember to take a break if you get tired from these activities.

"What if I have only one near finger, not two?" If you do not experience two near fingers yet, let's at least prove to ourselves that there could be two near fingers when our attention is on the far finger, and both pictures are "switched on" in the brain.

Continuing to sketch the far finger, simply alternate closing one eyelid at a time. Alternatively, you can cover one eye at a time using an eye patch. Eye patches are available at many drug stores.

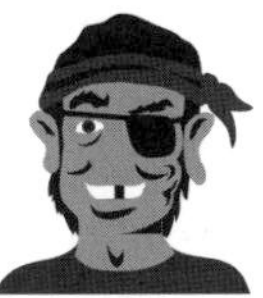

When the right eyelid is closed or covered—being sure to keep your attention on the far finger—the left eye sees the *solid* near finger to the right of the far finger. This is what we would expect, and is shown in *Plate 54: Amblyopia, d-1.* Conversely, when the left eyelid is closed, the right eye sees a solid near finger to the left, as shown in *d-2*. This is why there could be, or already are, two near fingers when both eyes are open and the attention is on the far finger.

See *a-2*. In summary, if the pictures from both eyes are "switched on" in the brain, and if normal convergence and fusion are occurring, you should see two near fingers when sketching the far finger—one to the right seen by the left eye, and one to the left seen by the right eye.

If you only have one finger up close (to the right or to the left) when sketching the far finger, at least you now know how there could be two near fingers. Continue to study the following, since the *idea* of what you should be experiencing can be beneficial later.

If you are seeing two near fingers, and if both the near and the far fingers are *perfectly* aligned straight out in front of your nose and head, the far finger will be seen exactly in the middle of the two near fingers. If it is not, move either the near finger or far finger to the right or left, so the far finger is seen exactly in the center of the two near fingers. Again, both the near and far fingers must aligned exactly straight in front of the nose and head.

This can be a little tricky for some students in the beginning. Many students mistakenly align one *eye* with the near finger and the far finger. Also, some students mistakenly bring their attention to the near finger, instead of keeping the attention on the far finger. In fact, oftentimes the surprise of the two near fingers causes some students to "jump" with their attention to the near finger. Of course, then there will only be one near finger, not two.

Although many students do not see the two near fingers initially, many see two near fingers in a very short time. Once the brain knows logically there can, and should, be two near fingers, both pictures are encouraged to "switch on." Note, however, the two near fingers will most likely not be seen unless the directions, especially the alignments of the head, near finger, and far finger, are followed precisely. Ask someone to assist you with this if you are having difficulty.

The two near fingers form a "window" or "gate." Continuing to sketch the far finger, move the near finger straight out a few inches, and then back in to the original position. Notice that when the near finger moves out, the window becomes narrower; when the near finger moves closer, the window becomes wider. Return the near finger to the original 5–6 inches distance from the nose.

Continuing to sketch the far finger, notice there are two distant objects. In *a-2,* when sketching the far finger, one Dixie Man is seen slightly to right of the far finger (seen by the right eye), while a second Dixie Man is seen slightly to the left (seen by the left eye).

With two near fingers and two Dixie Men, we experience the fact that fusion only occurs at one distance, in this case, at the far finger. Two images of the far finger are being processed by the brain into one, fused far finger, as in "The Fused Finger," discussed at the beginning of this chapter.

The *conscious* experience of two fingers and two distant objects can be tiring. The mind knows there is only one near finger and one distant object in reality, yet sees two of each. Is seeing believing? The process of *how* we see the world is meant to be a subconscious activity. Usually, the brain ignores the fact that there are two images of an object at a distance other than where you are centralizing. You may want to rest before continuing.

Part B—Experiencing *Fusion 1, The Near Finger (or Yellow Pencil):*

Refer to *Plate 53: Fusion 1, Near Finger, b-1,* and *Fusion/Near Finger, b-2.*

Aligning the head, fingers, and distant object as in Part A, now sketch the near finger. The area of centralizing is indicated by the small circle. There should be one solid near finger and two semi-transparent far fingers, and two distant objects. The two images of the near finger are now fused into one near finger.

If the head, near finger and far finger are correctly aligned, the near finger will be exactly in the middle of the two far fingers. (The two far fingers should also be in the middle of the two distant Dixie Men.) Notice again how fusion only occurs at one distance, in this case, at the near finger.

Unlike the experience in Part A, the left far finger is now seen by the left eye, and the right far finger is seen by the right eye. You can check this fact by alternately closing or covering one eye at a time. Remember to continue sketching the near finger.

Part C—Experiencing *Fusion 1, The Distant Dixie Man:*

Refer to *Plate 53: Fusion 1, Dixie Man, c-1,* and *Fusion/Dixie Man, c-2.*

Aligning the head, fingers, and distant object as in Parts A and B, sketch an object straight ahead, far into the distance (Dixie Man).

There should now be four fingers. The near finger creates a wide window (or gate), and the far finger creates a narrow window (in the center of the wide window). One Dixie Man should appear exactly in the center of both the wide and narrow "finger" windows. The two images of Dixie Man received by the eyes are now being fused into one image by the brain. Unlike *a-2* and *b-2,* notice how there is now only one boat.

Parts A, B, and C—Experiencing *Fusion 1:*

Now, shift between the distant object, the far finger, and the near finger, spending a few moments sketching each one. Notice again how fusion only occurs at one distance at a time—at the point of centralizing. The other two objects not being sketched are double.

Notice also how there is a "time delay" between shifting your attention from one finger to the other finger to the distant object. First, the mind chooses to shift to a different object. Then the messages are sent from the brain to the eyes. Finally the eye muscles converge and accommodate to the new object of interest. The mind is primary and the physical is secondary.

You may be able to feel the convergence of the eye muscles by repeating this experience, imagining shifting back and forth between the distant object and your finger with your eyelids closed.

Vision is primarily a mental function. Bates discovered that mental strain sends messages of imperfect sight to the eyes, while mental relaxation sends messages of normal sight to the eyes.

Fusion and Double Images Explained Further

Fusion is the merging, or combining, of the two pictures seen by the two eyes into one image. Fusion occurs in the brain, and at only one distance. There is one "fused" object at our point of interest, i.e., where we centralize. Fusion is possible only when there is binocular vision.

Convergence is the alignment of both eyes to a single point of interest (centralization). This alignment extends from the point of interest, through the eyeball, and into the fovea of each eye. The eyes are said to be converging, or intersecting, at that particular point of interest.

In most cases, fusion occurs automatically as a result of normal convergence.

In *Plate 53: Fusion 1, Far Finger, a-1,* and *Fusion/Far Finger, a-2,* the eyes are correctly intersecting on the far finger, creating one "fused" far finger. From the right eye's point of view, the near finger appears to be located to the left of the far finger; from the left eye's viewpoint, the near finger appears to be located to the right of the far finger. If both pictures remain "on," the brain has no option but to produce two images of the near finger while sketching the far finger.

For the right eye, Dixie Man appears to the right of the far finger; for the left eye, Dixie Man appears to the left of the far finger. Again, the brain has no option but to produce two images of Dixie Man while sketching the far finger.

The *correct* experience of double images observed in these experiences is not "double vision." Double vision refers to the experience of seeing two objects *where you are centralizing.* There is supposed to be only one fused object at the point of centralization. At least initially, double vision is frequently a consequence of strabismus, discussed more below.

To better understand fusion, and why there is a doubling of objects at other distances, refer to *Figure 18–4: Near Finger Supplement.*

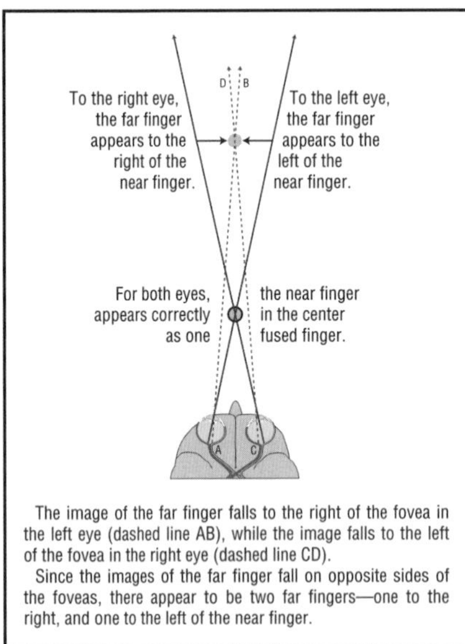

The image of the far finger falls to the right of the fovea in the left eye (dashed line AB), while the image falls to the left of the fovea in the right eye (dashed line CD).

Since the images of the far finger fall on opposite sides of the foveas, there appear to be two far fingers—one to the right, and one to the left of the near finger.

Figure 18–4: Near Finger Supplement.

The attention is on, and both eyes are correctly converging to, the near finger. The center of the image of the near finger falls in the fovea of each eye. The finger is in the center of the picture for each eye. The brain merges the two fingers into one "fused" near finger.

By following the line of sight from the left eye out to the near finger and beyond, we can see how the far finger is located to the left of the near finger. The far finger is to the left of the center of the picture for the left eye, while the far finger's image falls to the right of the fovea; see dashed line AB.

By following the line of sight from the right eye out to the near finger and beyond, the far finger is located to the right of the near finger. The far finger is to the right of the center of the picture, while the far finger's image falls to the left of the fovea; see dashed line CD.

Since the brain is seeing far fingers to both the right and left of the near finger (both to the left and to the right of the foveas), two far fingers are seen, not one. In the final analysis, the brain has no other option regarding the quantity and locations of the far finger.

Centralization and Fusion

When you notice a tree through your kitchen window, there are two ladybugs walking on the window, not one. If your attention goes to the ladybug, there are now two trees in the distance, not one.

Usually, the mind disregards the illusion of two images where we are not centralizing. The rods pick up the movements of objects not falling in the foveas. If a peripheral object is of interest or concern to us, the mind and eyes shift to centralize on the new object.

Also, the objects at other distances will be less clear than the object the eyes are centralizing and accommodating on.

When the pictures from both eyes are switched on in the brain, there are usually *two* images of objects in front of, and in back of, the object we are centralizing on. However, if the object we are interested in is more than twenty feet away, objects farther away usually do not appear to be double images.

The concepts of binocular vision and fusion help reinforce the importance of centralizing. The object of interest is meant to enter the fovea of each eye. In combination with the mechanism of accommodation, one can now appreciate that there is only one point in all the universe where we have sharp, colorful, and fused vision—at the point of centralization.

EXPERIENCING HEAD BALANCE

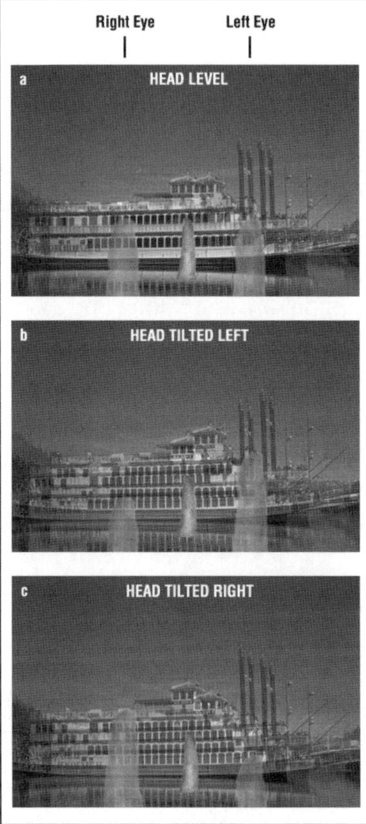

Figure 18–5: Head Balancing.

Repeat the initial alignments in *Part A, The Far Finger (or Green Pencil),* above.

Refer to *Figure 18–5: Head Balancing, a, b,* and *c*.

Keeping your attention on the far finger, move the (two) near fingers and the far finger downward until the tops of all fingers are at eye level. Notice the height of the two near fingers. Are the tops of the left and right near fingers at the same height, as in *a?* When the tops of the two near fingers are level, the head is balanced, at least from the right and left perspective.

Now, keeping the attention on the far finger, tilt your head very slightly to the left and then to the right. Be sure to only *tilt* your head, like the Leaning Tower of Pisa. Do not turn or rotate your head, or else the two near fingers may be lost. When you tilt your head to the left, the left near finger should move downward, and the right near finger should move upward, as in *b.* Conversely, when you tilt your head to the right, the right near finger should move downward, and the left near finger should move upward, as in *c.* (The doubled distant objects also move upward and downward.)

Optionally, an object far in the distance can be used instead of the far finger. With a very small head movement, sketch a far object while tilting your head. Again, notice the heights of the two near fingers.

If the two near fingers are not at the same height, tilt your head in the appropriate direction until they are at the same height.

This is a simple way of checking left/right head posture. Some people tilt the head to one side as a chronic habit—many without even knowing they do so. This is a strain on the neck, spinal column, and the visual system. Tilting the head to one side can lead to lack of normal fusion.

It is possible to experience the tops of the fingers being uneven, even though the head is level. This could be the case if a person has vertical strabismus. One eye may be looking up too high, while the other eye is looking straight ahead, normally, at the far finger. This is discussed more below.

Just for fun: Notice in a mirror that when

you tilt your head a small amount from left to right, the eyes rotate to retain their horizontal alignment! This action is created by the oblique muscles.

THE VISION HALO

For many students, the Vision Halo is an outstanding teacher of centralization, movement, and head balance.

Creating a Vision Halo

Refer to *Figure 18–6: The Vision Halo*.

1. Obtain a piece of strong but flexible wire. Plastic-coated, solid aluminum fencing wire, available at or through many hardware stores, works great. One and three-quarters loops from a 9"-diameter spool yields about 2½ feet of wire. This is longer than the final length needed to form the halo, but the extra length at the end makes it easier to shape the last portion of the halo.
2. Unwind the first ¾ part of the wire into a straight line as shown. Bend the last inch of the end of the wire (small arrow) outward a small amount so that the tip of the wire will not touch the head; file the end smooth.
3. Shape the circular part into an oval to fit around the head. Form a long, straight portion that points forward, away from the head. Make this part as straight as possible.
4. Bend the long forward part upward about 45° at the point shown. At approximately five inches out along this angled part, bend the remaining part straight downward at the point shown. Cut the excess wire so the vertical part is about eleven inches long. File the end smooth.
5. Side view of the Vision Halo.
6. Side view of Vision Halo on the head.
7. Front view of Vision Halo on the head.

Aligning the Vision Halo

It is important to place the vertical bar exactly in front of the nose, and vertical. The window formed by the two vertical bars may seem to have a slight "V" shape. This is normal.

Do not look at the vertical bar for more than a moment—only long enough to align it properly.

Just as there were two near fingers when sketching Dixie Man in *Part C,* The Distant Dixie Man, above, you should now have "two" vertical bars, forming a "window" or "gate," when sketching distant objects.

Learning about Vision Habits with the Vision Halo

- Since the halo moves when the student's head moves, there is a continuous biofeedback occurring. A locked head and neck makes the window freeze.
- If a student only moves the eyes to the left or right, the window will be lost—another reminder that the head is not moving.
- If the window is angled to the right or left, the student's head is tilting to the right or left, respectively.
- The tendency to want to see objects outside the window as clearly as objects inside the window is called diffusion. Vision is best within the window; this is called centralizing. This is especially

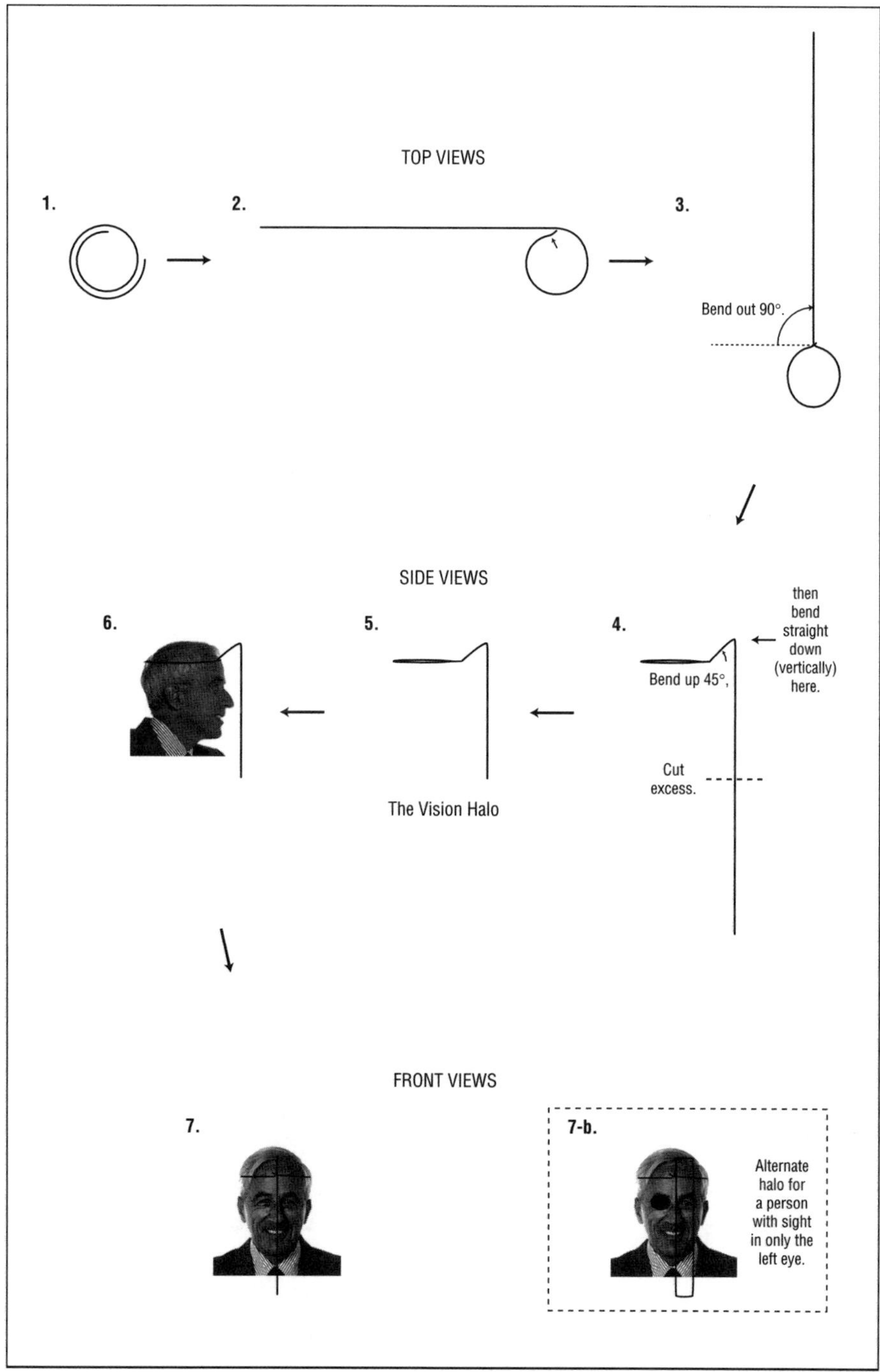

Figure 18–6: The Vision Halo.

valuable to students, as centralization is a somewhat subtle concept.

- Some students, who do not see two fingers in the Fusion 1 activities above, see two vertical bars while wearing the halo.

Important: *Never* wear the Vision Halo while driving a car, or any other activity in which it could be a distraction or unsafe.

Vision Halo for People with Sight in Only One Eye

Refer to *Figure 18–6: The Vision Halo, Step 7-b.*

For those with sight in only one eye, a variation on the Vision Halo can be made.

Instead of using 1¾ loops of wire, use 2½ loops of wire. The long straight part in *Step 2* and *Step 3* will then be much longer than shown.

Do not cut the wire in *Step 4*. Instead, bend the wire horizontally (at the point where it would normally be cut) one inch toward either the left or right. If the right eye has sight, bend the wire to the right; if the left eye has sight, bend the wire to the left. Bend the next part of the wire upward; then bend the last part horizontally toward the topmost part of the vertical bar, and attach it to (i.e., wrap it around) the top part. The "window" in this modified halo will not be exactly in the center of the head but is positioned slightly toward the side of the eye that has sight.

With this modification, a person with sight in only one eye can practice centralizing, movement, and head balance.

Tom's Personal Log: When I first took vision lessons, the Vision Halo helped me discover how much I was holding my head rigid. The window kept freezing, which meant I was not moving my head.

I also discovered how much I diffused into the areas outside the window. I found I seldom centralized.

After a few months of using the halo, I was able to practice better vision habits more each day when I was not wearing it. The benefits I received from the halo were very high. It helped me more quickly identify and begin to eliminate the incorrect vision habits I had for many years.

AMBLYOPIA—A "SWITCHED OFF" IMAGE

Fusion vs. Amblyopia

A common interference to fusion is amblyopia. It is estimated that 2% of Americans are amblyopic. As mentioned by Bates above, the more technical term for amblyopia is *amblyopia ex anopsia,* which means "dim-sightedness from non-use."

Amblyopia is the condition in which the image from one eye is not being processed correctly in the brain, even though both eyelids are open. The light rays are triggering the light receptors in the amblyopic eye, but the brain is not processing that image. In effect, the person is using only one image from one "switched on" eye to see. Amblyopia can occur even though each eye has perfect sight when used alone, i.e., when one eye is closed, or covered. Essentially, the sight from one eye is being suppressed, or partially suppressed.

Many conventional books refer to the amblyopic condition as, "The eye doctor looks into the amblyopic eye and sees nothing wrong, while the amblyopic eye looks out and sees nothing right."

In the Fusion 1 activities presented above, some students do not see two fingers; they only see one. We want to have two fingers; this tells us both pictures are switched on in the brain.

If you correctly experience all of the Fusion 1 activities shown in *Plate 53*, you can skip ahead to *Fusion 2—The Bead Game*, below.

Refer to *Plate 54: Amblyopia* and *Plate 53: Fusion 1*. The point of centralization is indicated by a small circle in all diagrams and images.

Compare *Right Eye Amblyopia/Far Finger, d-1*, to *Fusion/Far Finger, a-2*. In both of these images the attention is on the far finger. However, in *d-1*, the image for the right eye has "switched off." Only the image from the left eye is being processed by the brain, resulting in monocular vision. All objects—the near finger, the far finger, and Dixie Man—are one and solid. There are no doubled or semi-transparent images. The far finger is not a "fused" image since the right eye's image is not being combined in the brain with the left eye's image. The left eye sees the near finger to the right of the far finger, and Dixie Man is seen to the left of the far finger—the same positions as in *a-2*.

Left Eye Amblyopia/Far Finger, d-2, shows the picture seen when the left eye is amblyopic. Compare to *d-1* and *a-2*.

The other figures, *e-1* through *f-2*, show the pictures seen when viewing the near finger and Dixie Man, and when the right and left eyes are amblyopic.

It is fairly easy to understand all of the images in *Plate 54: Amblyopia* by repeating the activities in Fusion 1 and simply closing, or covering, one eye at a time. When you close one eye, you are simulating amblyopia. Then compare *d-1* and *d-2* to *a-2*, *e-1* and *e-2* to *b-2*, and *f-1* and *f-2* to *c-2*.

Variations on Amblyopia

Some students have one and a half fingers (or pencils). A "half" finger means that one of the two semi-transparent fingers (or Dixie Men) is more faint, or "ghostly," than the other semi-transparent finger. For example, when sketching the far finger, the right near finger may be seen relatively strongly, but the left near finger is very faint.

Or, there could be two strong near fingers at some times, and only one near finger at other times. These tell us one eye is switched on and the other is switching on and off.

Other variations include alternating amblyopia, where the picture from one eye turns off, and then the picture from the other eye turns off.

Amblyopia can be present only during certain activities.

Amblyopia can also be a function of the distance at which a person is centralizing. A student may have two near fingers while sketching the far finger, but only one far finger when sketching the near finger. Or, a student may have two fingers in the distance while sketching the near finger, but only one near finger while sketching the far finger.

As Bates mentioned above, there are many variations possible with amblyopia.

"Lazy Eye" or "Tense Eye"?

It is unfortunate the term "lazy eye" has been used to refer to amblyopia, for the amblyopic eye is not "lazy"; it is tense. (Another example of left-brain, "Puritan work ethic" language inappropriately applied to the primarily right-hemisphere, relaxed functions of the visual system.)

When people are told they have a "bad," "poor," or "lazy eye," the assumption is made that the problem is occurring because the eyes are not working hard enough. In truth, the opposite is the case—there is too much strain on the visual system.

Bates said that many types of amblyopia are caused by strain.

Strabismic Amblyopia

Since a person with strabismus would likely experience double vision if both pictures stayed on, the brain most often turns one of them off. It is stressful to see two images everywhere, so the mind simply switches off one of the pictures. The mind usually turns off the eye that has strabismus. Again, there are many variations possible.

Refractive Amblyopia

Amblyopia is often found in people who have a large difference in acuity between the two eyes. This is called refractive amblyopia.

For example, if the brain is receiving a 20/40 image from one eye and a 20/400 image from the other, it would be difficult to merge these two images into one. In fact, to do so would likely result in a poorer image than the 20/40 image alone. By switching off the 20/400 image, the person can have "full" 20/40 with the other eye.

By using corrective lenses that bring the eye with 20/400 back up to 20/40, the amblyopic eye may be encouraged to switch back on.

Some students have nearsightedness in one eye, and farsightedness in the other. Oftentimes, the nearsighted eye is amblyopic when the attention is in the distance, and the farsighted eye is amblyopic when the attention is up close.

Other Types of Amblyopia

Amblyopia can also be caused by trauma, toxicity, nutritional deficiencies, ptosis (drooping of an eyelid), cataracts, corneal problems, macular degeneration, and other problems. Your eye doctor may be able to provide more information on these conditions.

ACTIVITIES FOR AMBLYOPIA

There are several activities a student can use to encourage the amblyopic eye to switch back on. Before doing these activities, the student may want to read the following section on convergence and strabismus. As mentioned above, amblyopia is often connected to problems of strabismus.

ACTIVITIES FOR AMBLYOPIA

Part A: This activity is for amblyopes and students with a large difference in acuity between the two eyes.

1. Do the cross-crawl and/or the figure-8 pattern (up in the center) with the nose-pencil (or feather) for one or two minutes. This helps balance the right and left sides of the body and connects the right and left brains.
2. Check for two fingers, both near and far, as described in "Fusion vs. Amblyopia," above. If there is only one finger where there should be two, or if you have a large difference in acuity between your two eyes, continue.
3. Cover (patch) the "switched-on" eye, or the eye that has better acuity.
4. Sketch a picture, nose-feather an object, toss a ball, do the Long Swing, or sun (with closed eyelids), etc., for three minutes. This activates the amblyopic or less clear eye and encourages it

to switch on and see simultaneously, or to see better, with the other eye.

5. Cover the "switched-off" eye, and do the same activity as in #4 above, for one minute. It is important to activate both eyes, not just one.
6. Remove the patch, and do the same activity as in #4 with both eyes for three minutes. This teaches the two eyes to see together equally.
7. If amblyopic, check for two fingers again. We want to have two, steady fingers.
8. Palm for a few minutes.

If a student is nearsighted in one eye and farsighted in the other, do near-to-far swings with the nearsighted eye, spending more time sketching in the distance. Then do far-to-near swings with the farsighted eye, spending more time in the near area. Then do both eyes together near-to-far-to-near-to-far, etc.

The purpose of these activities is to "activate" and relax (not work) the eye with the greater strain. Effort should never be applied to any activities for improving vision. The three habits of natural vision, and the self-healing activities such as palming and sunning, bring relaxation to the visual system. Relaxation is the key to normal sight.

Part B: For amblyopes. (You may want to have someone assist you with this activity.)

1. Do the cross-crawl and/or the figure-8 pattern with the nose-pencil for one or two minutes.
2. Cover the "switched-on" eye.
3. Hold, or place, two pencils in front of you, vertically about four inches from your nose and about two inches away from each other horizontally. Now, position one pencil in front of your nose, and the other slightly to the side of the uncovered eye. You should now have a two-pencil "window" through which the amblyopic eye is looking. Sketch a distant object through this window.

The purpose of this activity is to experience the two-pencil window and to place the picture of the distant object, located between the two pencils, into your mind. This gives the brain an idea of what you want to see when holding only one pencil—without covering one eye.

4. Close both eyes, and remove the patch.
5. Keeping your eyes closed, remove the pencil in front of the amblyopic eye.
6. Pretend both eyes are open and you are seeing the distant object within the two-pencil window.
7. Being sure keep your attention on the object in the distance at all times, open both eyes and sketch the object in the distance. You may notice "two" pencils. The two pencils may appear only for a brief moment in the beginning. Also, they may not be equally strong. One may appear dim or "ghostly."

If you get the two-pencil window—even for a moment—congratulations! Both eyes were switched on at that moment! The eyes know how to see normally, and you have just given them the opportunity to improve!

If you did not get the window, continue to practice the above activities for amblyopia, and practice better vision habits each day. Palm and sun frequently.

This activity should be repeated until "two" pencils are seen consistently, while holding one pencil.

As in Part A, the purpose of this activity is to activate and relax (not work) the eye that is under more strain. Effort should never be applied to the visual system.

Important: If the student feels discomfort or gets tired, he should stop and rest. Palming is one of the best ways to rest the eyes after using the patch.

Some children who have amblyopia are given a patch to wear for long periods of time, even all day long. This can create more stress than the stress producing the amblyopia. Oftentimes, the child refuses to wear the patch.

If a patch is used, the approach should be one of teaching the amblyopic eye to relax. Therefore, any time a patch is used, games and activities that are enjoyable to the child should be employed. Implementing the principles and habits of natural vision are important when using a patch.

FUSION 2: THE BEAD GAME

THE BEAD GAME: CONVERGENCE

The Bead Game is one way of determining how well the eyes are converging and fusing.

In order to experience the Bead Game, two strings need to be seen, which means both eyes need to be switched on. Though a person with amblyopia may not experience two near fingers, two far fingers, or two Dixie Men in the Fusion 1 activities above, she may experience two strings in the Bead Game.

As Bates pointed out, a person may have proper convergence, yet still have amblyopia. In this case only one string would be seen. This, however, is not very common. Most students who have normal convergence have proper fusion.

A student will recognize the Bead Game as being an "infinite" fingers activity. If you were able to hold up many fingers out in front of you in a row, you would have a continuous "string" of fingers. The Fusion 1 activities with the near finger, far finger, and Dixie Man are a prelude to the Bead Game.

The Bead Game should *never* be approached as a near-to-far *exercise* or *drill,* as presented in several books, tapes, and "kits" on eyesight. The Bead Game is only used to observe convergence, or lack of convergence, of the two eyes.

ALIGNING THE STRING FOR THE BEAD GAME

Refer to *Plate 55: Fusion 2—The Bead Game.*

As with the finger alignments in Fusion 1, the alignment of the string is very important. You may want to have a second person do the Bead Game with you, holding the other end of the string. In this way you can check each other's alignment.

Obtain a string about three feet long. Place three different colored beads, or buttons, ⅜–½ inch in diameter, along the string. In the following examples, red, green, and blue beads are used. The red bead is the close bead, green is the middle bead, and blue is the far bead. If another person is not holding the other end of the string, you can tie it to a doorknob or other steady fixture.

While sitting in a chair, rest your elbows comfortably on a cushion or table. Hold one end of the string between the thumb and forefinger of one hand, such that the string goes over the forefinger out into the distance. The forefinger and string should be held one inch from, and at the same height as, the nose. The string held in your hand must be positioned exactly in front of the nose, and the head must be exactly straight. The correct alignment is

HORIZONTAL VISUAL FIELDS

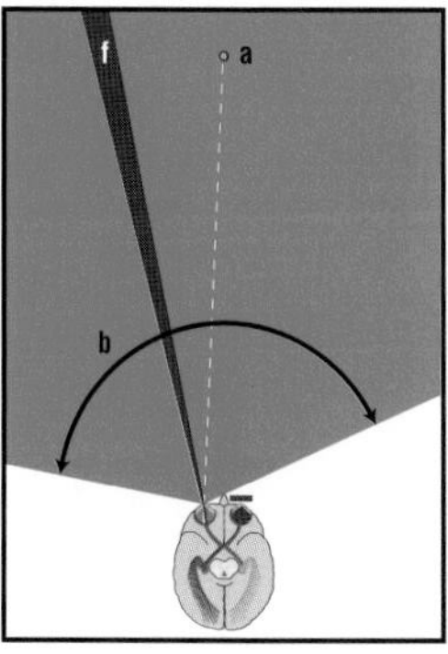

Left Eye Horizontal Visual Field, **b**
Monocular Vision

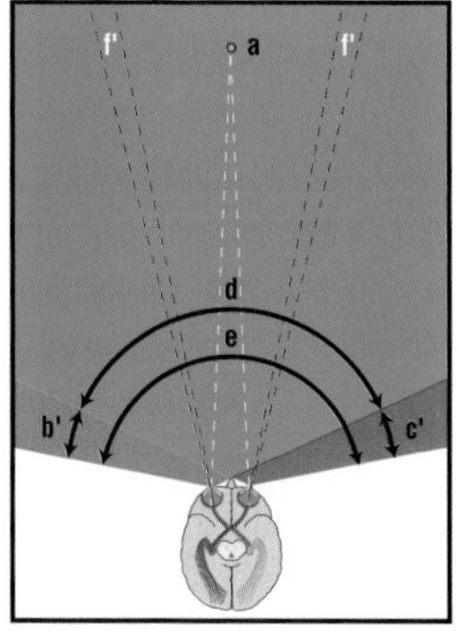

Combined Horizontal Visual Fields, **e**
Binocular Vision, **d**

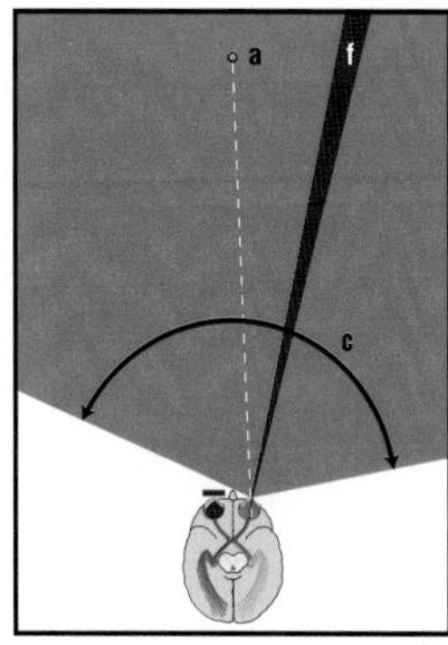

Right Eye Horizontal Visual Field, **c**
Monocular Vision

a. Centralization object.
b. Horizontal visual field of left eye; monocular vision; blue area.
c. Horizontal visual field of right eye; monocular vision; red area.
d. Binocular vision, **d**, is the intersection of **b** and **c**; green area. **b'** is left monocular vision. **c'** is right monocular vision.
e. Combined horizontal visual fields, **e**, is the union of **b** and **c**.
f. The blind spots, **f**, are eliminated with binocular vision. However, the two optic disc areas, **f'**, remain monocular.

FULL VISUAL FIELDS

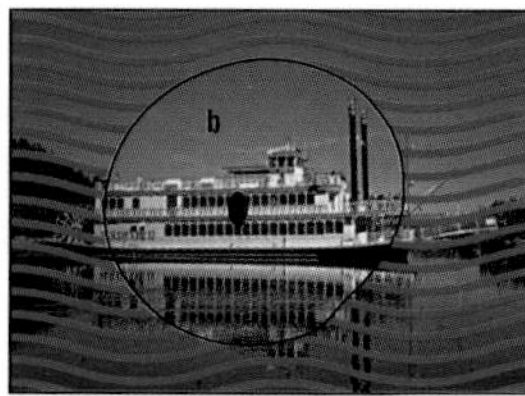

Left Eye Visual Field
Monocular Vision, **b**

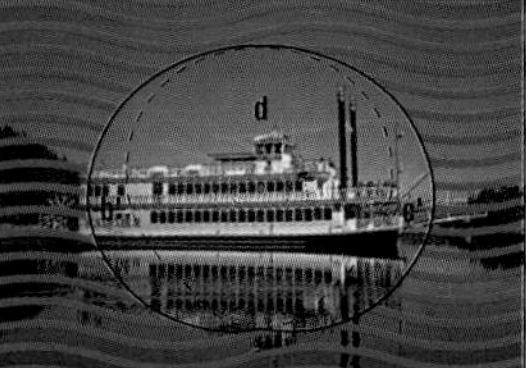

Combined Visual Fields
Binocular Vision, **d**

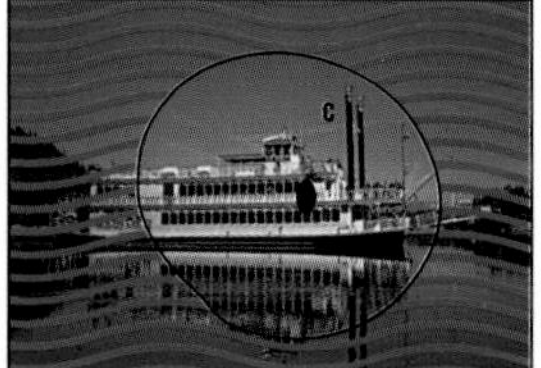

Right Eye Visual Field
Monocular Vision, **c**

"Dixie Man," the man located in the center of the boat, is the object of centralization. Binocular vision is area **d**, inside the black dashed-line area. The two blind spots are eliminated (gray dashed-line ovals) with binocular vision; these two optic disc areas remain monocular.

THE FUSED FINGER

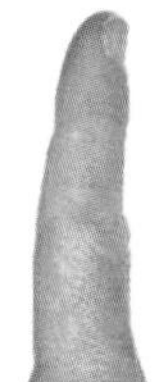

Finger As Seen
By Right Eye

+

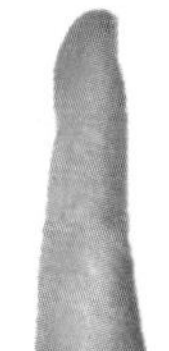

Finger As Seen
By Left Eye

=

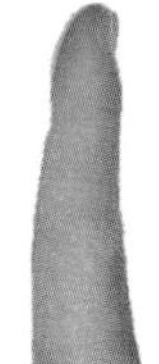

Fused Fingers

≠

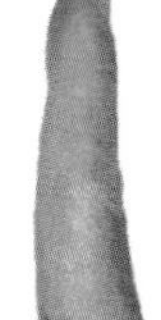

Camera Finger

Hold your right forefinger straight out in front of you approximately eight inches from your nose. The forefinger you see is a fusion of two images; it is not identical to a camera's picture. For example, notice the difference between the fingernails of the fused and camera fingers. Fusion is possible because of binocular vision.

Plate 51. Binocular Vision.

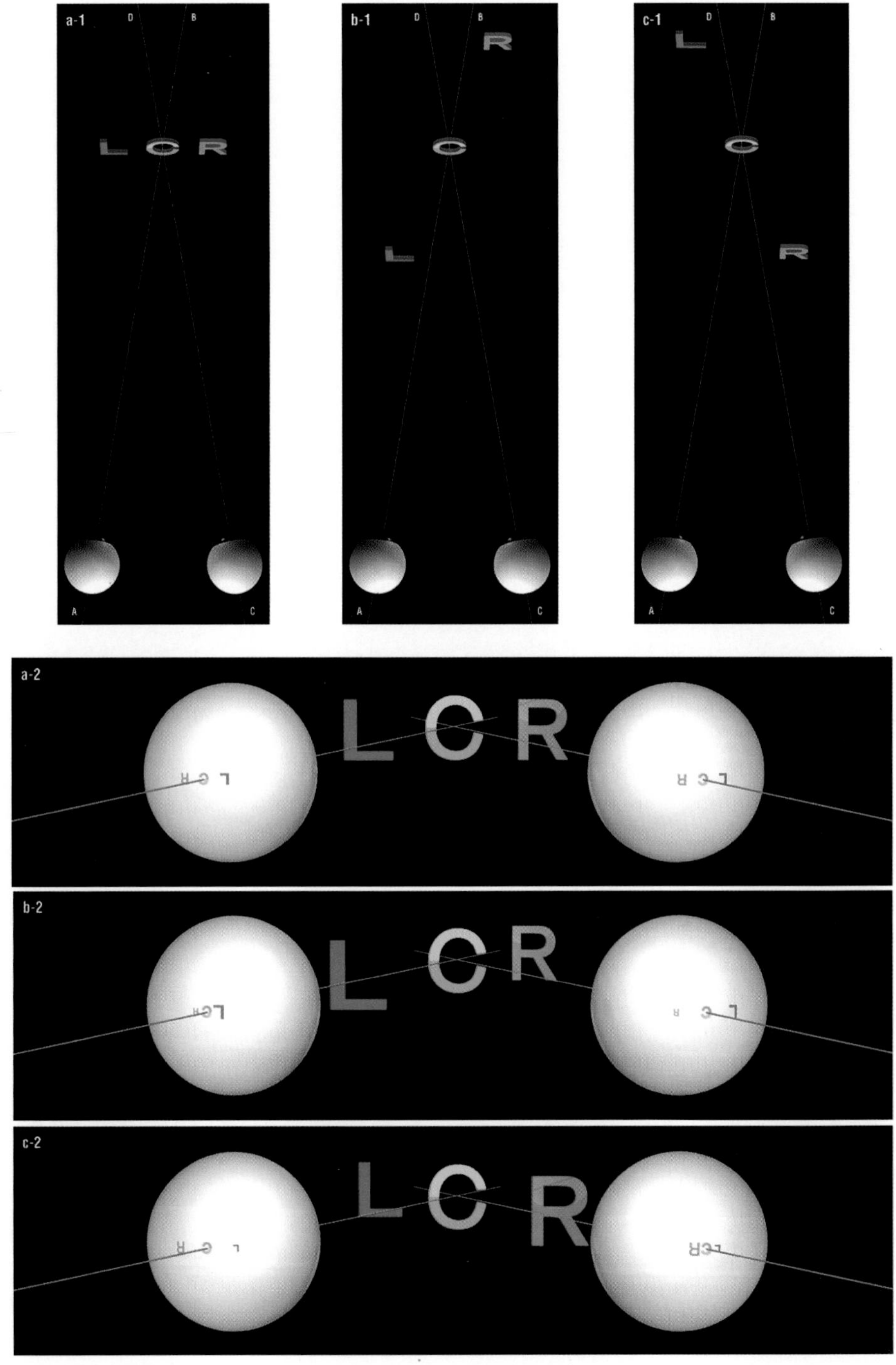

Plate 52. Judging Relative Distances.

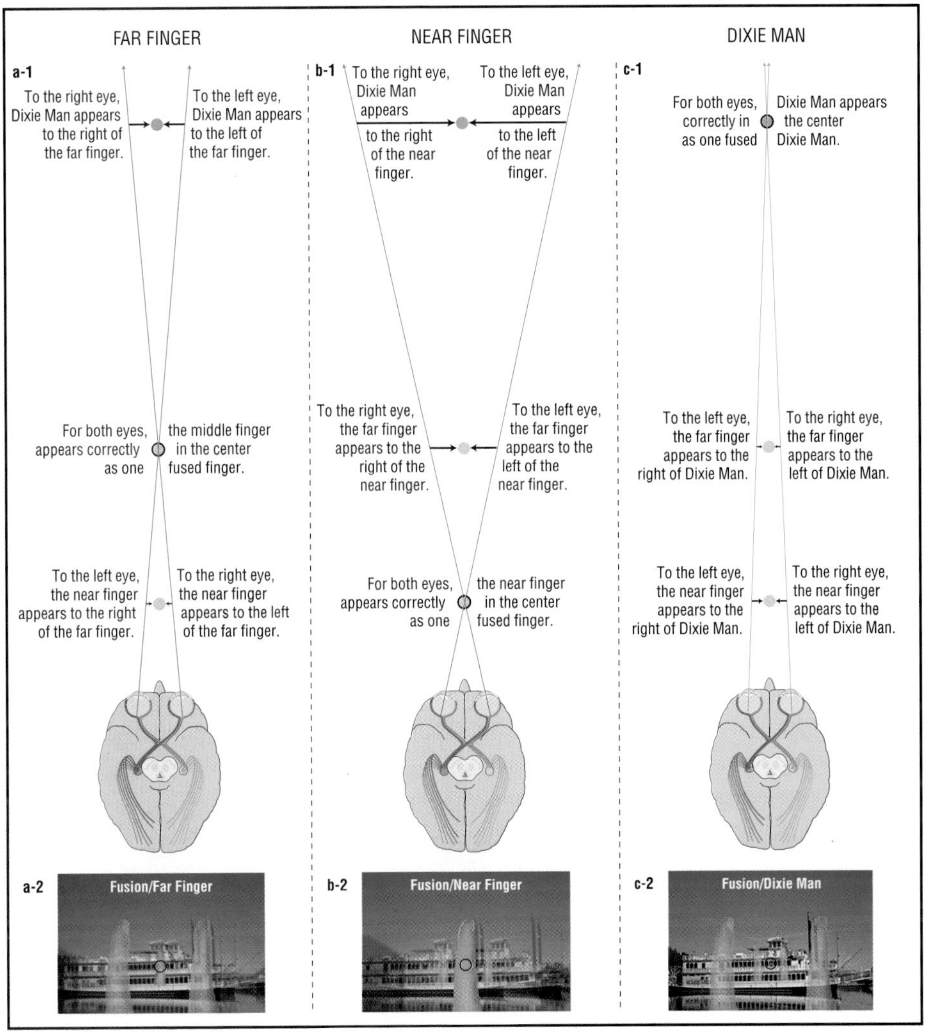

FAR FINGER

a-1

To the right eye, Dixie Man appears to the right of the far finger.

To the left eye, Dixie Man appears to the left of the far finger.

For both eyes, the middle finger appears correctly in the center as one fused finger.

To the left eye, the near finger appears to the right of the far finger.

To the right eye, the near finger appears to the left of the far finger.

a-2

Fusion/Far Finger

NEAR FINGER

b-1

To the right eye, Dixie Man appears to the right of the near finger.

To the left eye, Dixie Man appears to the left of the near finger.

To the right eye, the far finger appears to the right of the near finger.

To the left eye, the far finger appears to the left of the near finger.

For both eyes, the near finger appears correctly in the center as one fused finger.

b-2

Fusion/Near Finger

DIXIE MAN

c-1

For both eyes, Dixie Man appears correctly in the center as one fused Dixie Man.

To the left eye, the far finger appears to the right of Dixie Man.

To the right eye, the far finger appears to the left of Dixie Man.

To the left eye, the near finger appears to the right of Dixie Man.

To the right eye, the near finger appears to the left of Dixie Man.

c-2

Fusion/Dixie Man

Plate 53. Fusion 1.

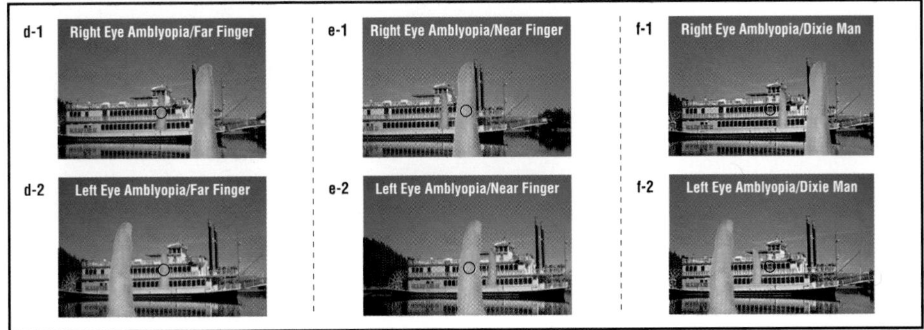

Plate 54. Amblyopia.

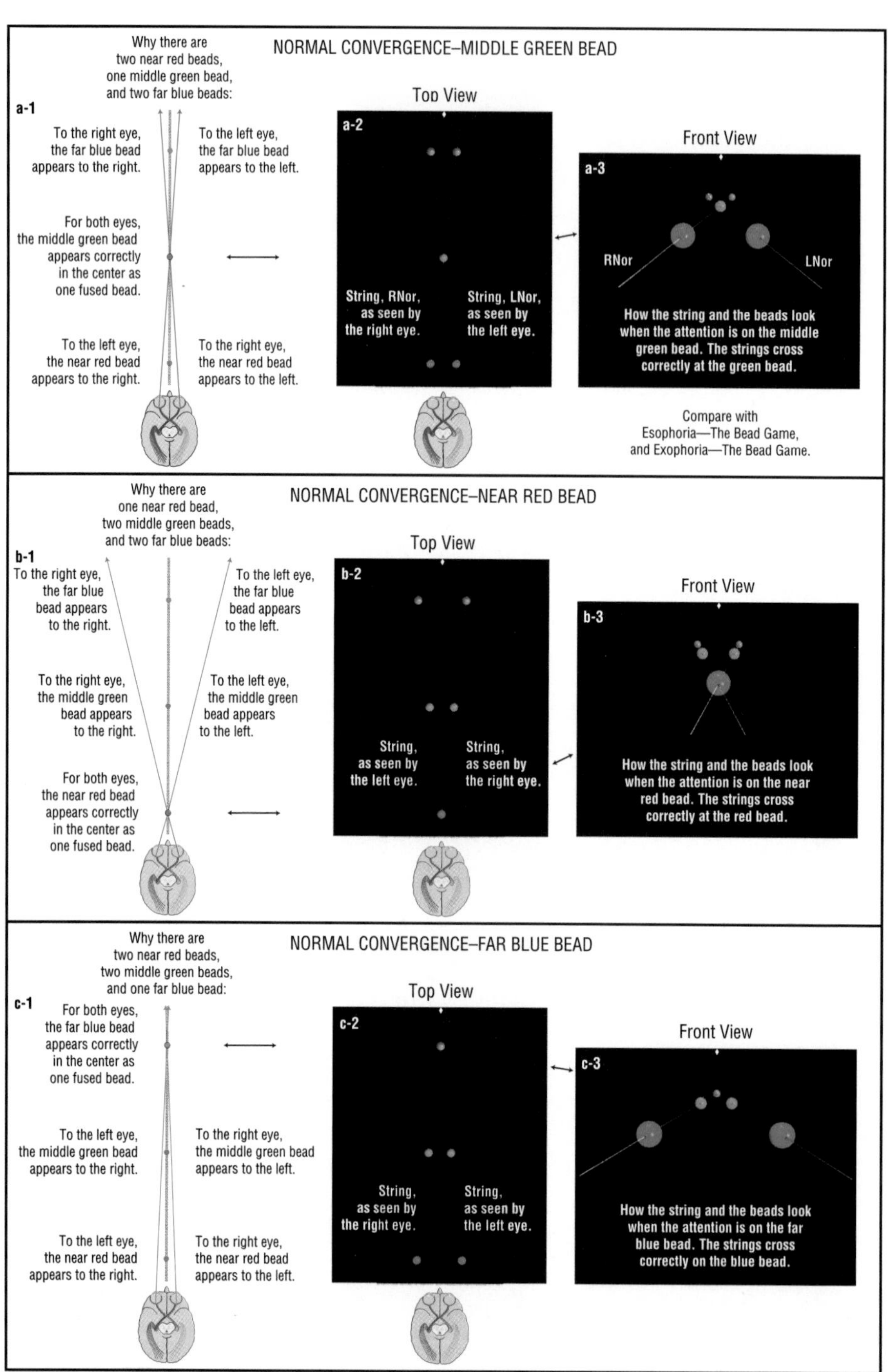

Plate 55. Fusion 2—The Bead Game.

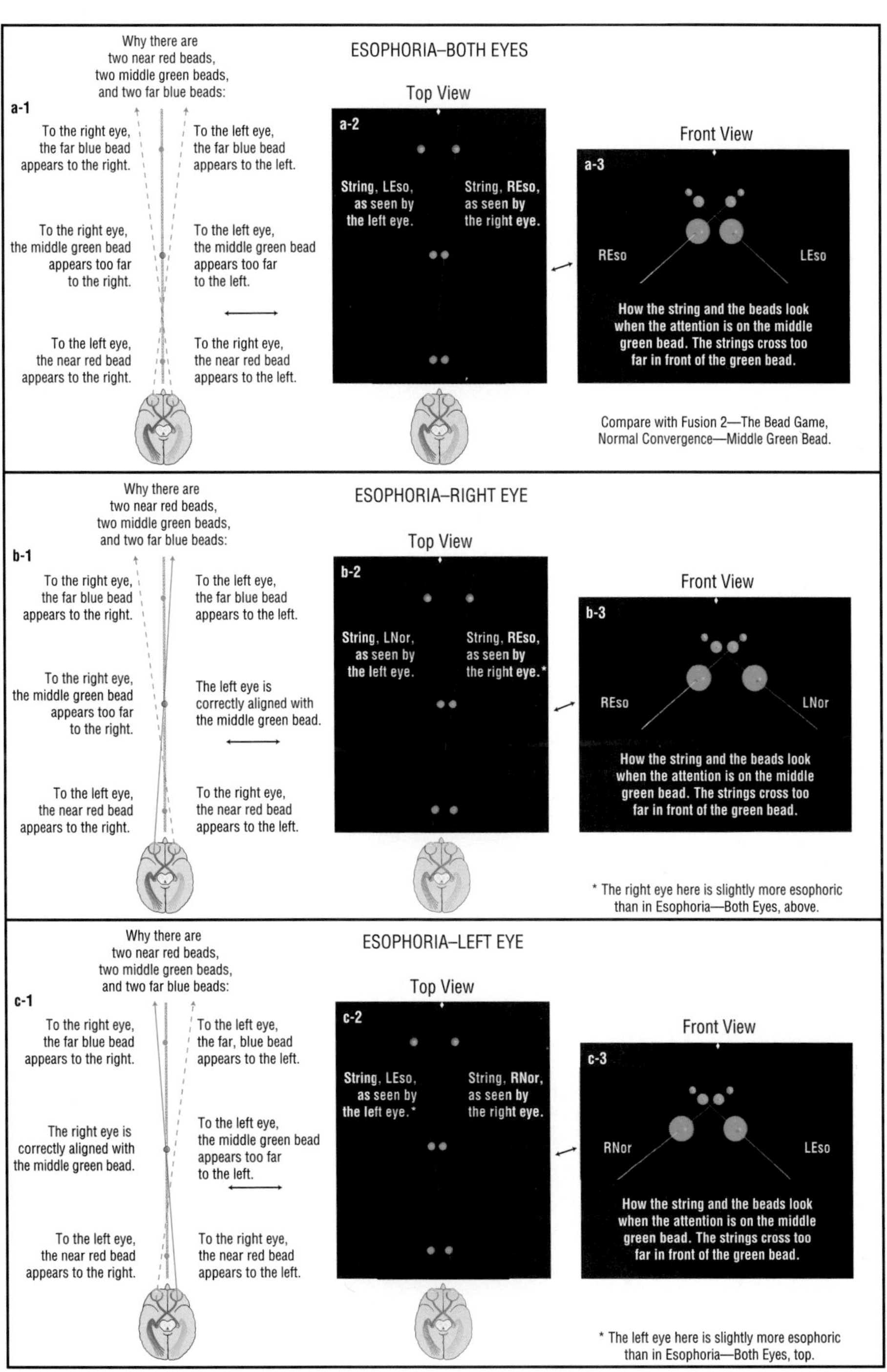

Plate 56. Esophoria—The Bead Game.

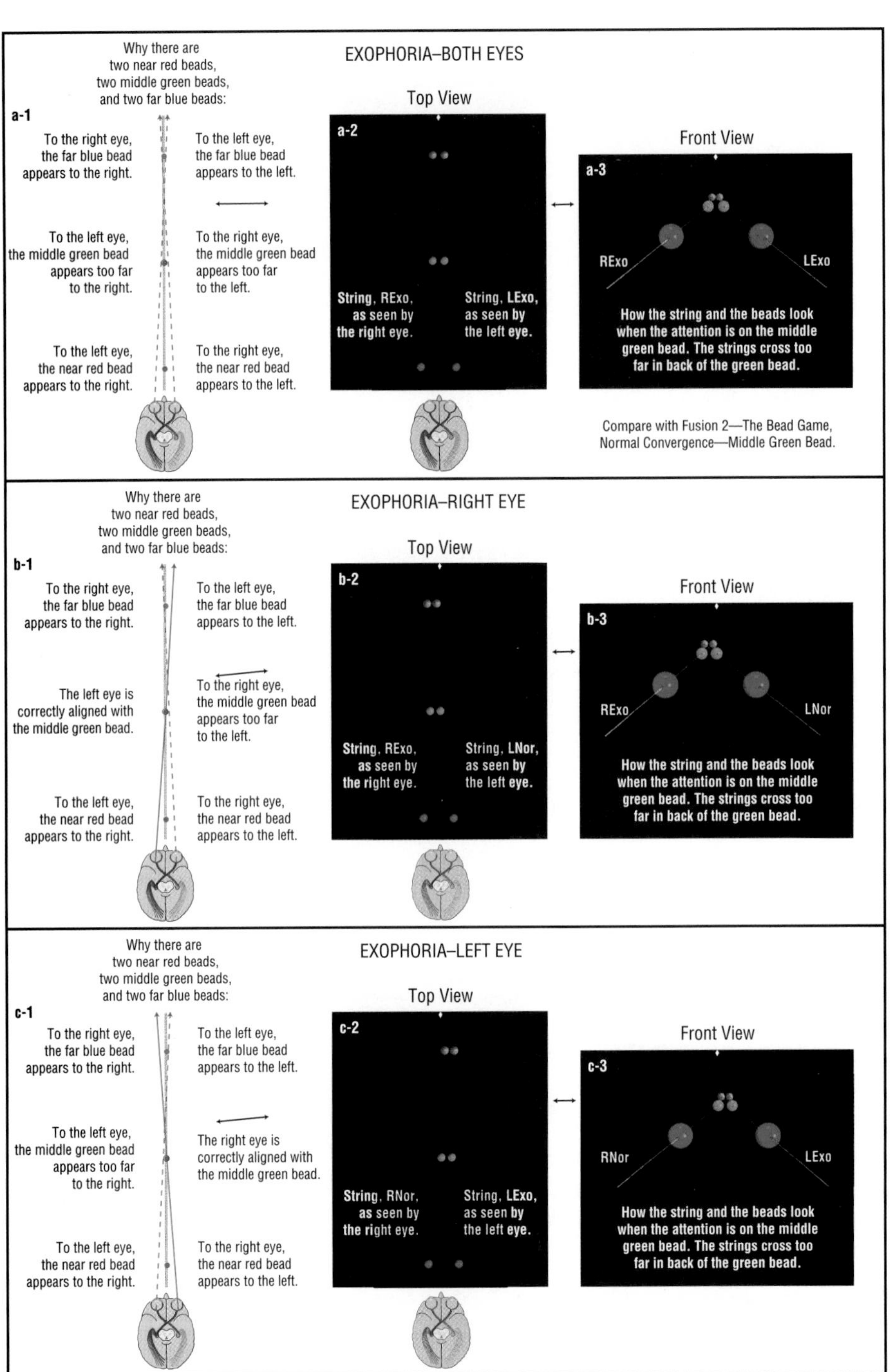

Plate 57. Exophoria—The Bead Game.

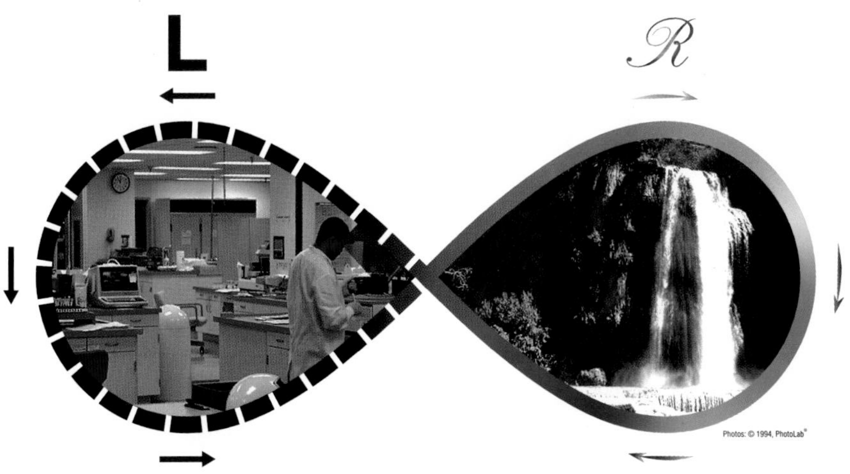

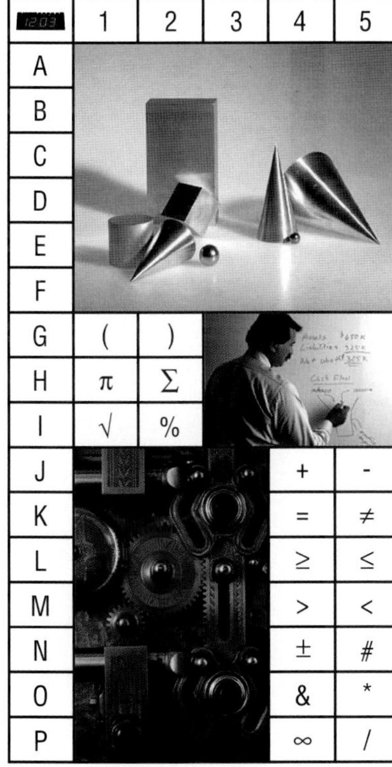

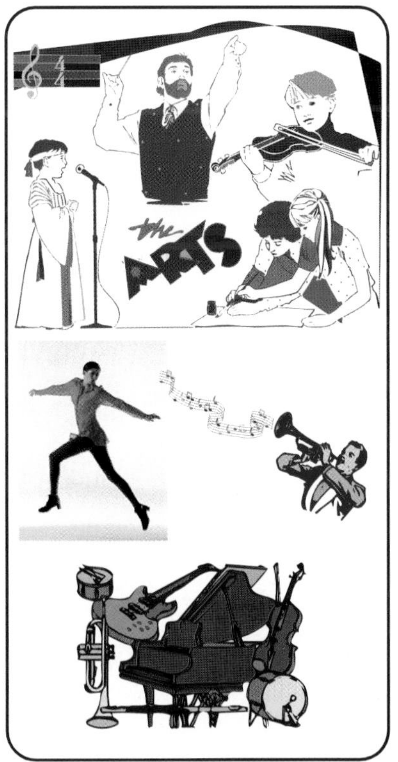

Plate 58. Infinitely Right and Left.

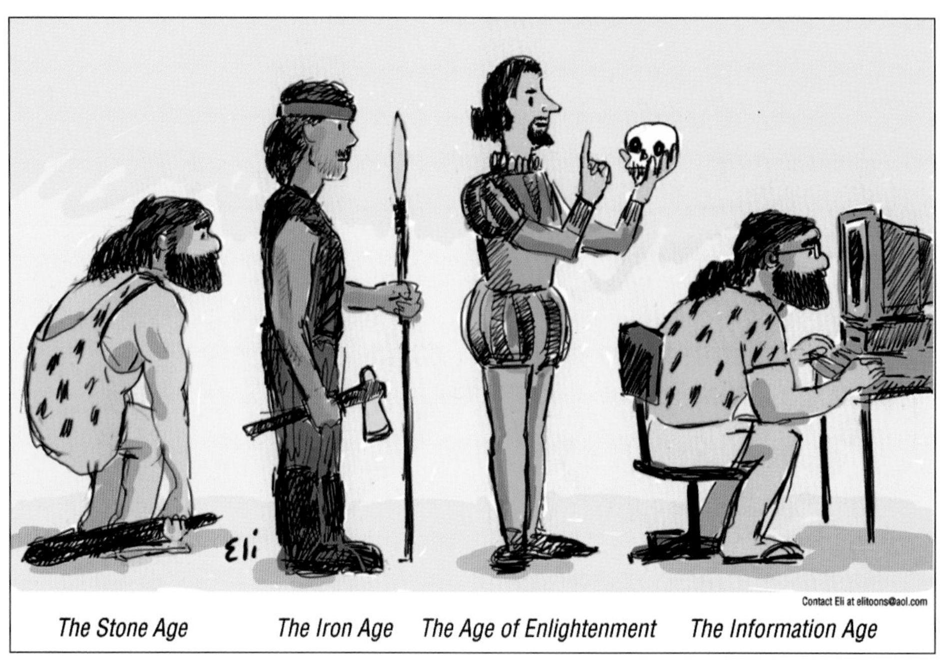

Plate 59. "Evolution."

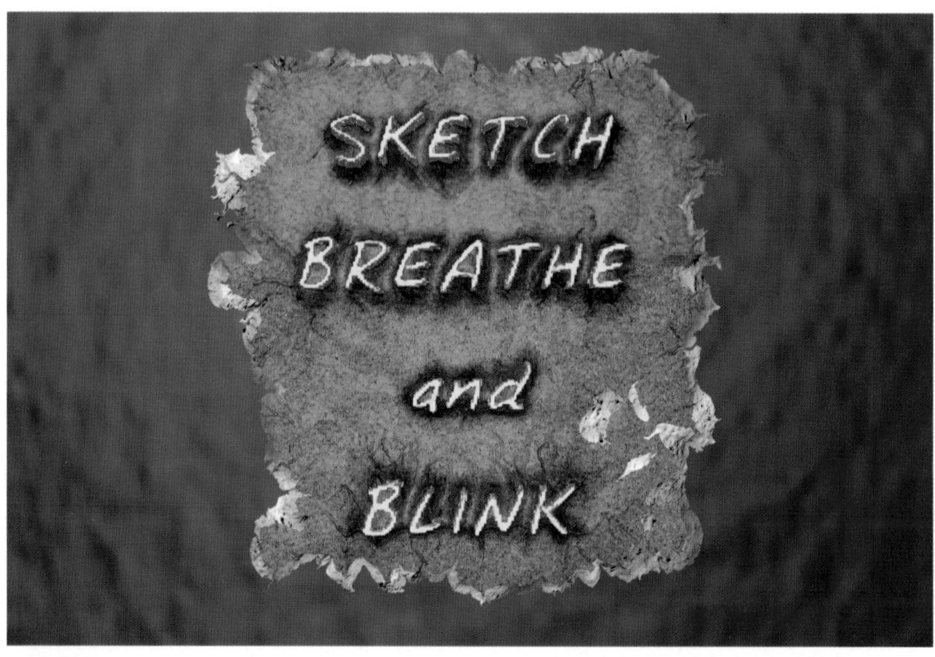

Plate 60. The Land of Sketch, Breathe, and Blink.

shown in *Plate 55: Normal Convergence—Middle Green Bead, a-1.* To help align the string, touch your nose with the thumb holding the string, and then move the thumb and string straight out one inch. Have someone check your alignment if needed.

Do not turn your head to the left or right. Do not align the string with one eye. Students, especially those with strabismus and amblyopia, often align the head and/or string incorrectly. If this is done, it will be difficult or even impossible to experience the Bead Game correctly. The alignment of the head and string is very important.

The red bead should be positioned about six inches out from the forefinger holding the string. The green bead should be positioned about ten inches beyond the red bead. The blue bead should be about ten inches beyond the green bead.

If a second person is holding the other end of the string, the blue bead should be about six inches from her nose.

Be sure there is adequate lighting, and that the lighting is fairly equal on both sides of the string.

Normal Convergence with the Bead Game

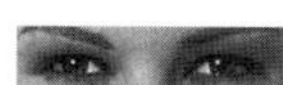

Refer to *Plate 55: Fusion 2—The Bead Game, Normal Convergence—Middle Green Bead, a-1, a-2,* and *a-3*.

Sketch the middle green bead. Remember to breathe abdominally and blink frequently during the Bead Game.

How many strings are there?

If there is only one string, study *a-1, a-2,* and *a-3*.

A person who has both eyes switched on experiences two strings as if they were aligned in *a-2*. What is actually seen is shown in *a-3*. The right eye sees string *RNor,* extending from the near left out to the far right. The left eye sees string *LNor,* extending from the near right out to the far left.

If two strings do not appear, return to the Amblyopia activities, above, to switch on the amblyopic eye. Also, read the following to gain a better idea of the experiences you want to have during the Bead Game.

If you have two strings, where do they cross? The two strings should cross through a single middle green bead—the bead you are sketching. The two strings, *RNor* and *LNor,* should form an "X" with the center of the X crossing through the middle green bead.

Where the X crosses is where the two eyes are intersecting their lines of sight (from the fovea out to the bead). Where the X crosses is the only place the string fuses into one string. Experiencing the X crossing at the middle green bead is equivalent to sketching the single fused far finger in *Fusion 1, Far Finger, a-1* and *a-2*.

By experiencing the X crossing through the middle green bead, we know both eyes are switched on (because there are two strings). Additionally, we know both eyes are properly converging on the middle green bead (because the X crosses through the single fused green bead).

Continue sketching the middle green bead. There should be two near red beads, and two far blue beads. This is equivalent to seeing two near fingers and two Dixie Men in *Fusion 1, Far Finger, a-1* and *a-2*.

Remember to take a break and rest if you become tired doing this Bead Game.

TOM'S PERSONAL LOG: In the beginning, I could only do the Bead Game for a very short time. I found it very uncomfortable and annoying. Two strings flashed off and on alternately. I had very high tension in my visual system. Now it is easy to do.

If you see two strings, but they do not cross through the middle green bead, note where the strings cross. They may cross in front of or in back of the green bead.

Refer to *Plate 55: Normal Convergence—Near Red Bead, b-1, b-2,* and *b-3*.

Sketch the near red bead.

The two strings should now cross through a single red bead. There should now be two middle green beads and two far blue beads. This experience is equivalent to *Fusion 1, Near Finger, b-1* and *b-2*.

Refer to *Plate 55: Normal Convergence—Far Blue Bead, c-1, c-2,* and *c-3*.

Sketch the far blue bead.

The two strings should now cross through a single far blue bead. There should be two near red beads, and two middle green beads. This experience is equivalent to *Fusion 1, Dixie Man, c-1* and *c-2*.

When sketching the far blue bead, the strings may look more like an inverted "V" than an "X." The two strings seem to join at the far blue bead.

If the X crosses through each bead, you do not need to do any more activities in this chapter.

If the X does not cross on one or more beads, continue with the next section.

STRABISMUS

Strabismus is the condition in which the eyes are not aligned to see the same point simultaneously. For example, the right eye correctly sees a book across the room, but the left eye turns out to the side, seeing a door on the left side of the room.

In cases of strabismus, the initial tendency is to experience double vision. The visual system wants to maintain binocular vision, but because prolonged double vision is very stressful, the brain usually turns off one of the pictures, creating amblyopia. This is why most people who have strabismus become amblyopic.

STRABISMUS AND THE BEAD GAME

If one or both eyes are not converging correctly on a bead in the Bead Game above, a student will not experience the X crossing at a bead being sketched.

There are many non-convergence experiences possible during the Bead Game. The more common types are discussed below.

Conventionally, the strabismic eye has been called the "deviating" eye, and the normal eye the "fixating" eye. Since the words used in vision training can affect the student's sight, it is better to refer to the strabismic eye as simply the "strabismic" eye, or the "turning" eye. The "fixating" eye is better called the "centralizing" eye for reasons discussed in Chapter 9, "The First Principle—Movement."

In esophoria the X crosses in front of the bead of interest. In exophoria, the X crosses in back of the bead of interest. Fusion occurs where the X crosses. But, since at least one eye is not converging properly to the bead of interest, fusion is not occurring at the correct location. The mind's interest is on a bead, but only one eye is seeing the bead with correct convergence and centralizing. A student is usually aware if he has strabismus.

Common Types of Strabismus

The four most common types of strabismus are esophoria, exophoria, hyperphoria, and hypophoria.

Esophoria

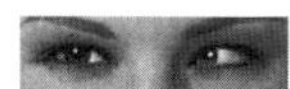

Esophoria (from the Greek *eso,* meaning "inward," and *phoria,* meaning "direction") is also called crossed eye, esotropia, and convergent. (The term convergent here means the eye is turning inward abnormally; it does not mean the eye has normal "convergence.") Typically, one eye turns inward, and the other eye is straight. If one or both eyes turn inward toward the nose, the X will cross in front of the bead you are sketching.

Compare *Plate 56: Esophoria—The Bead Game, Esophoria—Both Eyes,* with *Plate 55: Fusion 2, Normal Convergence—Middle Green Bead.*

In *Esophoria—Both Eyes,* both eyes turn inward too far. The right eye turns too far to the left, and the left eye turns too far to the right. As a result, the two strings appear to cross in front of two green beads.

In *Esophoria—Right Eye,* the right eye turns inward, too far to the left. The left eye converges and centralizes normally on the middle green bead. (In these diagrams, the right eye is slightly more esophoric than in *Esophoria—Both Eyes.*)

Compare the positions of the strings in *Esophoria—Right Eye, b-2* and *b-3,* with the strings in *Esophoria—Both Eyes, a-2* and *a-3,* and in *Normal Convergence—Middle Green Bead, a-2* and *a-3.*

In *Esophoria—Right Eye* and *Esophoria—Both Eyes,* the esophoric right eye turns inward too far to the left. As a consequence, the string seen by the right eye, *REso,* appears to angle too far to the right compared to the string seen by the right eye in *Normal Convergence—Middle Green Bead, RNor.* The string seen by the normal left eye, *LNor,* is the same in *Esophoria—Right Eye* and *Normal Convergence—Middle Green Bead.*

In *Esophoria—Left Eye,* the left eye turns inward, too far to the right. The right eye converges and centralizes normally on the middle green bead. (In these diagrams, the left eye is slightly more esophoric than in *Esophoria—Both Eyes.*)

Compare the positions of the strings in *Esophoria—Left Eye, c-2* and *c-3,* with the strings in *Esophoria—Both Eyes, a-2* and *a-3,* and in *Normal Convergence—Middle Green Bead, a-2* and *a-3.*

In *Esophoria—Left Eye,* the left eye turns inward too far to the right. As a consequence, the string seen by the left eye, *LEso,* appears to angle too far to the left compared to the string seen by the left eye in *Normal Convergence—Middle Green Bead, LNor.* The string seen by the normal right eye, *RNor,* is the same in both *Esophoria—Left Eye* and *Normal Convergence—Middle Green Bead.*

Exophoria

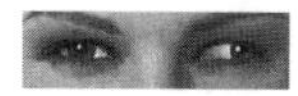

Exophoria (from the Greek *exo,* meaning "outward") is also called "wall eye," exotropia, or divergent. Typically, one eye turns out too far toward the temple, while the other is straight. If one or both eyes turn outward, the X will cross in back of the bead you are sketching. If one or both eyes turn too far outward, there may be two strings, but they may not cross anywhere. At least one eye must have some convergence in order to have the strings cross each other. If both eyes are parallel or divergent, the strings will not cross.

Compare *Plate 57: Exophoria—The Bead Game, Exophoria—Both Eyes* with *Plate 55: Fusion 2, Normal Convergence—Middle Green Bead.*

In *Exophoria—Both Eyes,* both eyes turn outward too far. The right eye turns too far to the right, and the left eye turns too far to the left. As a result, the two strings appear to cross in back of two green beads.

In *Exophoria—Right Eye,* the right eye turns outward too far. The left eye converges and centralizes normally on the middle green bead. (In these diagrams, the right eye is slightly more exophoric than in *Exophoria—Both Eyes.*)

Compare the positions of the strings in *Exophoria—Right Eye, b-2* and *b-3,* with the strings in *Exophoria—Both Eyes, a-2* and *a-3,* and in *Normal Convergence—Middle Green Bead, a-2* and *a-3.*

In *Exophoria—Right Eye* and *Exophoria—Both Eyes,* the exophoric right eye turns outward too far to the right. As a consequence, the string seen by the right eye, *RExo,* appears to angle too far to the left compared to the string seen by the right eye in *Normal Convergence—Middle Green Bead, RNor.* The string seen by the normal left eye, *LNor,* is the same in *Exophoria—Right Eye* and *Normal Convergence—Middle Green Bead.*

In *Exophoria—Left Eye,* the left eye turns outward, too far to the left. The right eye converges and centralizes normally on the middle green bead. (In these diagrams, the left eye is slightly more exophoric than in *Exophoria—Both Eyes.*)

Compare the positions of the strings in *Exophoria—Left Eye, c-2* and *c-3,* with the strings in *Exophoria—Both Eyes, a-2* and *a-3,* and in *Normal Convergence—Middle Green Bead, a-2* and *a-3.*

In *Exophoria—Left Eye,* the exophoric left eye turns outward too far to the left. As a consequence, the string seen by the left eye, *LExo,* appears to angle too far to the right compared to the string seen by the left eye in *Normal Convergence—Middle Green Bead, LNor.* The string seen by the normal right eye, *RNor,* is the same in both *Exophoria—Left Eye* and *Normal Convergence—Middle Green Bead.*

Hyperphoria

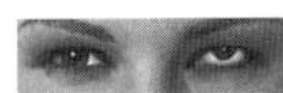

Hyperphoria (from the Greek *hyper,* meaning "above" or "over") is also called hypertropia. Convergence may not be possible during the Bead Game, as the string seen by the hyperphoric eye may appear lower than the string seen by the normal eye. As a consequence, the two strings seem to "miss" crossing each other because they appear to be at different heights.

Refer to *Figure 18–5: Head Balancing, b* and *c.* Noticing the heights of the two near fingers (or pencils) while sketching the far finger can give some clues as to hyperphoria.

If the right eye is hyperphoric—*without* tilting the head—the near left finger may appear too low. If the left eye is hyperphoric—*without* tilting the head—the near right finger may appear too low.

Hypophoria

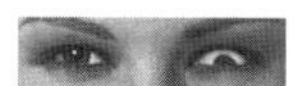

Hypophoria (from the Greek *hypo,* meaning "under" or "down") is also called hypotropia. Like hyperphoria, convergence may not be possible during the Bead Game, as the string seen by the hypophoric eye may appear higher than the string seen by the normal eye.

Refer to *Figure 18–5: Head Balancing, b* and *c.* Noticing the heights of the two near fingers (or pencils) while sketching the far finger can give some clues as to hypophoria.

If the right eye is hypophoric—*without* tilting the head—the near left finger may appear too high. If the left eye is hyperphoric—*without* tilting the head—the near right finger may appear too high.

Infinite Possibilities

There is an infinite number of possibilities involving strabismus and amblyopia. One eye can be esophoric while the other eye is both exophoric and hyperphoric. And, as pointed out by Bates, the degree and type of strabismus can be a function of time, particularly in relation to stress.

ACTIVITIES FOR STRABISMUS

Phoria (Directional) Swings

In strabismus, the muscle(s) is too tight in the direction the eye is turning. The idea behind phoria swings is to teach the strabismic eye to relax by coaxing it to move in the direction *opposite* to the direction it is turning.

For esophoria and exophoria, do the Bead Game, described above, to determine where the X is crossing when sketching the near red bead, the middle green bead, and the far blue bead. To review, the X usually crosses:

1. at each bead you are sketching, in which case the student already has the experiences he wants to have and there is no need to continue; or,
2. the X crosses in front of the bead (esophoria); or,
3. the X crosses in back of the bead (exophoria).

For hyperphoria and hypophoria, sketch a distant object while holding a finger or pencil in front of you as described above. Notice whether one finger or pencil is too high or too low.

Phoria Swing for Esophoria

Do the Bead Game. If the X crosses in front of the middle green bead, and if only the left eye is esophoric:

1. Cover or patch the right eye. Then move an object (e.g. your finger, a ball, a small light) in a circular pattern toward the left. The head remains facing straight ahead, while the left eye follows the moving object. The idea is to coax the left eye outward so that it will converge correctly on the middle green bead. Do this for three minutes.
2. Then cover only the left eye. Sketch objects normally with only the right eye. (If the right eye is also esophoric, keep the head facing straight ahead and move an object in a circular pattern over to the right, following the object's movement with the right eye.) *Important:* Never activate only one eye; both eyes must be activated, even if one eye has normal convergence. Do this for one minute. (Do this for three minutes if both eyes are esophoric.)

3. Remove the patch and sketch objects normally, using both eyes, for three minutes.

(If only the right eye is esophoric, simply reverse the above directions.)

4. Return to the Bead Game to see if the X is crossing closer, or even on, the middle green bead. When first doing the phoria swing, the X may appear either closer to, or exactly on, the middle green bead for a moment or two. Then the X may move back to the position it was in before doing the phoria swing. In time, the X can move closer to and on the middle green bead for longer periods of time.

Phoria Swing for Exophoria

Do the Bead Game. If the X crosses in back of the middle green bead, and if only the left eye is exophoric:

1. Cover or patch the right eye. Then move an object (e.g. your finger, a ball, a small light) in a circular pattern over toward the right. The head remains facing straight ahead, while the left eye follows the moving object. The idea is to coax the left eye inward so that it will converge correctly on the middle green bead. Do this for three minutes.
2. Then cover only the left eye. Sketch objects normally with only the right eye. (If the right eye is also exophoric, keep the head facing straight ahead and move an object in a circular pattern over to the left, following the object's movement with the right eye.) *Important:* Never activate only one eye; both eyes must be activated, even if one eye has normal convergence. Do this for one minute. (Do this for three minutes if both eyes are exophoric.)
3. Remove the patch and sketch objects normally, using both eyes, for three minutes.

(If only the right eye is exophoric, simply reverse the above directions.)

4. Return to the Bead Game to see if the X is crossing closer, or even on, the middle green bead. When first doing the phoria swing, the X may appear either closer to or exactly on the middle green bead for a moment or two. Then the X may move back to the position it was in before doing the phoria swing. In time, the X can move closer to and on the middle green bead for longer periods of time.

Phoria Swing for Hyperphoria

If the right finger (or pencil) is too low and the left eye is hyperphoric:

Follow the same directions as for the other phoria swings above, except in Step 1, move the object downward a few inches and follow it with the hyperphoric eye. Remember to keep the head facing forward. The idea here is to coax the eye downward, so that it is horizontal and level with the right eye. When it is horizontal, the two fingers will be at the same height.

If the left finger is too low, and the right eye is hyperphoric, coax the right eye downward, and continue with the same themes described above.

Phoria Swing for Hypophoria

If the right finger (or pencil) is too high and the left eye is hypophoric:

Follow the same directions as for the other phoria swings above, except in Step 1, move an object upward a few inches and follow it with the hypophoric eye. Remember to keep the head facing forward. The idea here is to coax the eye upward, so that it is horizontal and level with the right eye. When it is horizontal, the two fingers will be at the same height.

If the left finger is too high, and the right eye is hypophoric, coax the right eye upward, and continue with the same themes described above.

Phoria Swings for Other Types of Strabismus

If an eye is turning at any angle, cover the eye that does not have strabismus, and move an object opposite to the direction the strabismic eye is turning. Follow the same themes described above. The idea is to relax the eye back to the straight, normal position.

Straining is Not the Solution

Students with strabismus can be (and some have been) taught to "straighten" their eyes with a conscious effort. With this approach, the student then has a double strain—the initial tight muscle which pulled the eye out of alignment, and another tight muscle on the other side of the eye pulling the eye straight.

There was a girl who had strabismus (crossed eye) who was very proud of the "progress" she had made with her straining approach she was taught. While sitting in a chair, she gripped the side of the chair, and with the greatest of effort and straining, she forced her crossed eye to align straight with the other eye for a few seconds. When she ceased straining, her eye crossed again.

This is not the answer to strabismus.

Improvements with Strabismus

The *Better Eyesight* magazine for November 1920 is dedicated to the topic of strabismus. Several case histories of improvements are described.

Clara Hackett, in her book *Relax and See,* writes of her strabismus students:

> There were 179 crossed eye students. Seventy-one have achieved straight eyes and also have good fusion; 96 have straight eyes and good fusion except that there is a slight deviation from the norm when they are ill, emotionally upset or fatigued. Twelve had no enduring improvement.[8]

Final Chapter Notes

One of my students said she had "Stress-bismus."

Strabismus can be created by an unconscious strain—especially by staring. An indication that relaxation is the solution to strabismus problems is that many children are able to "cross" their eyes at will by straining hard enough. As soon as they stop straining, the eyes return to normal.

This chapter introduced some of the issues involved with binocular vision, stereopsis, and fusion. Only some of the causes of and solutions to strabismus and amblyopia have been presented here.

The activities presented in this chapter are a support for these specific vision problems. The relearning of correct vision principles and habits is the key to removing the underlying strain causing nearsightedness, farsightedness, astigmatism, and strabismus.

Those who have strabismus and/or amblyopia need to do these specific activities along with practicing correct vision habits better each day. The Long (Elephant) Swing is especially beneficial in strabismus cases. The oppositional movement releases tension from the visual system.

If you need help in understanding or doing the activities presented in this chapter, consult with a Natural Vision teacher. A student should consult with an eye doctor for any serious vision problems.

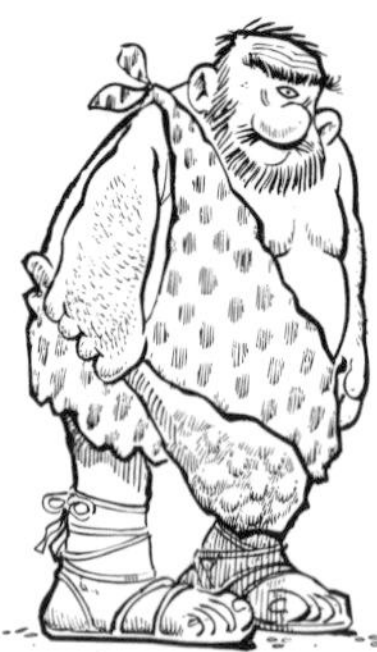

Figure 18-7: Cyclops.
"Well, Mr. Cyclops, before today's class, I could claim I had taught twice as many 'pupils' as students."

Notes

1 Lael Wertenbaker and the Editors of U.S. News Books, *The Eye: Window to the World* (Washington, D.C.: U.S. News Books, 1981), pp. 73–74.

2 Dr. Agarwal was an enthusiastic teacher of the Bates method in India. The title of his book, *Mind and Vision,* is the title of Chapter XXIX in *Perfect Sight Without Glasses.*

3 R. S. Agarwal, *Mind and Vision* (Pondicherry, India: Sri Aurobindo Ashram Press, 1983), p. 146.

4 Ibid., p. 208.

5 These graphics, caption, and text are from *Perfect Sight Without Glasses.*

6 John N. Ott, *Health and Light* (New York: Simon & Schuster, 1976), pp. 58, 68–69.

7 These graphics, caption, and text are from *Perfect Sight Without Glasses.*

8 Clara A. Hackett and Lawrence Galton, *Relax and See* (London: Faber and Faber, Limited, 1957), p. 25.

PART SIX

Brains, Health, and Healing

Chapter Nineteen

Brains and Vision

From *Better Eyesight* magazine, July 1920:

> Not only is keen sight a great convenience, but it reflects a condition of mind which reacts favorably upon all the other senses, upon the general health and upon the mental faculties.

Better Eyesight magazine, December 1925:

> Not only does the sight become imperfect [due to strain], but also the memory, imagination, judgment, and other mental faculties are temporarily lost....

Better Eyesight magazine, December 1925, from a testimonial submitted by ophthalmologist Dr. E. F. Darling:

> I feel more and more strongly that a person will not have full control of his mental faculties until he gets rid of his glasses.[1]

Aldous Huxley's *The Art of Seeing:*

> The eye and nervous system do the sensing, the mind does the perceiving ... It is a highly significant fact that, in Dr. Bates' method for re-educating sufferers from defective vision, these mental elements in the total process are not neglected. On the contrary, many of his most valuable techniques are directed specifically to the improvement of perception.... [2]

George Vithoulkas, in *The Science of Homeopathy,* discusses the mental, emotional, and physical levels of our being. He writes:

> These levels are not in reality separate and distinct, but rather there is a complete interaction between them.[3]
>
> ...The highest and most important level through which the human being functions is the mental and spiritual level.[4]

Bates proved that mental strain can create blur. Modern right-brain/left-brain concepts provide an interesting and valuable perspective on Bates' discoveries regarding normal sight, errors of refraction, and natural vision re-education.

The reader will find exceptions to some of the general discussion presented below because the model of brain characteristics presented here is simplified. Right-brain/left-brain concepts are very complex. For example, some people do not have right-brain characteristics located in their right brain—they are located in the left brain.

RIGHT TO THE BASICS

See *Figure 19–1: Left and Right Brains.* We have two brains—a right brain and a left brain. Each specializes in particular functions. See *Figure 19–2: Corpus Callosum.* The two brains are connected in the middle by a bundle of nerves called the *corpus callosum* (from Latin, meaning "callous body").

BRAIN CHARACTERISTICS

In the 1950s and 1960s, research was carried out by Roger W. Sperry and his associates at the California Institute of Technology. They determined that the right and left brains engage in different modes of processing information.

The modern right-brain/left-brain model is only our young society's re-discovery of the ancient principles of the duality of nature, called yin/yang. These principles have been used by Western holistic practitioners to help re-establish a balance in the health of their clients.

See *Plate 58: Infinitely Right and Left* and *Figure 19–3: Brain Characteristics.*

HOW THE BRAINS PROCESS THE PICTURES WE SEE

See *Figure 19–4: Left Sides to the Right Brain/Right Sides to the Left Brain.*

The entire picture from each eye (LVF' + RVF' + LVF" + RVF") travels along the optic nerves to the optic chiasm. At this junction, the messages from the left visual fields (light areas; LVF' + LVF") of each eye are sent to the right brain, while the messages from the right visual fields (dark areas; RVF' + RVF") of each eye are sent to the left brain.

See Figure 19–5: "Vision."

When the eyes look to the left, we tend to emphasize the characteristics of the right brain. When the eyes look to the right, we tend to emphasize the characteristics of the left brain.

One practical consequence of these facts

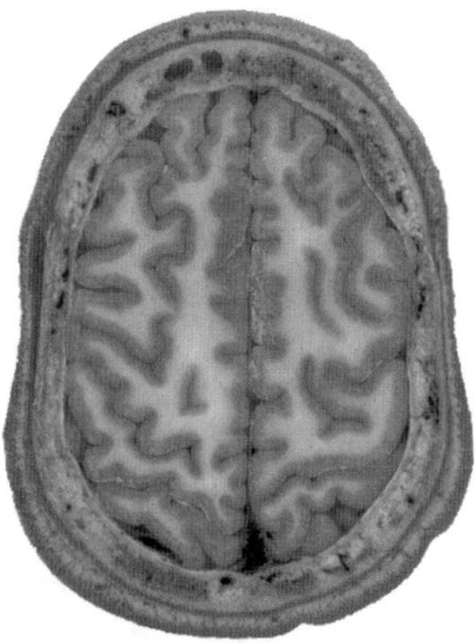

Figure 19–1: Left and Right Brains.

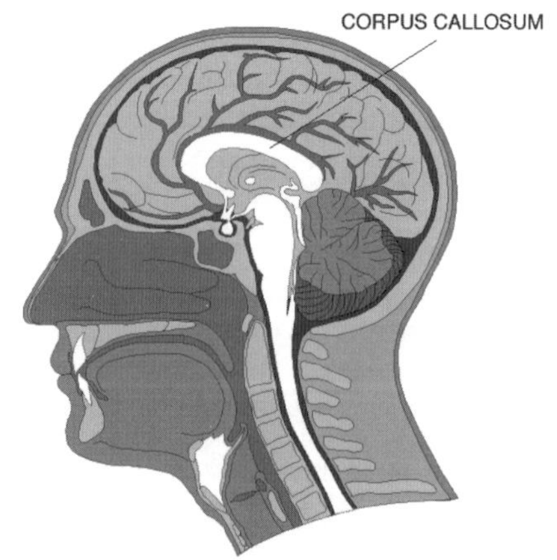

Figure 19–2: Corpus Callosum.

is the importance of "shifting" our attention to the right and to the left with a head movement. Crossing the midline of the body helps integrate the two brains, and is one reason the Long Swing and Infinity Swing (described in Chapter 9, "The First Principle—Movement") and the "Cross-Crawl" (described below) are so beneficial.

A VERY LEFT-BRAIN ORIENTED SOCIETY

The characteristics listed in *Figure 19–3: Brain Characteristics* indicate we live in a highly left-brain oriented society. Most people in our society are paid for, supported by, and praised for excelling in left-brain activities, especially reading, writing, and math. (Of course, the characteristics of the two brains overlap in many areas. Writing can be used to create poetry, while most music contains structure.)

Chérie Carter-Scott, in *Negaholics: How to Overcome Negativity and Turn Your Life Around,* writes:

> Transportation, communication, and technology have turned the modern world upside down. Rapid pace, pressure, and ambiguity have changed our lives from being steady, consistent, and stationary to being fraught with confusion, disillusionment, and disconnection. . . . We are living in a turbulent, chaotic, and perplexing era. Never before in the history of mankind have there been so many options, with so few tools with which to cope.[5]

Natural vision is primarily a right-brain function and is based on relaxation. The epidemic of blurred vision in this society is only one of the many serious consequences of switching off, or "dimming," our right-brain characteristics. Our vision problems reflect an imbalanced way of living. As stated in the Introduction, *blurred vision is a message from the mind and body that a person's visual system is out of balance with nature.* Bates discovered how to bring the visual system back into balance, with relaxation of the mind being the most important key.

Eighty Percent Right-Handed—A Clue to an Imbalanced Society

Research shows that 50% of animals are right-pawed (left-brain) dominant, and 50% are left-pawed (right-brain) dominant. These animals include chimpanzees and gorillas, whose anatomy is closely related to that of humans.

Paul Dennison and Gail Hargrove, in their book *Personalized Whole Brain Integration,* state their research proves that there are 50% right-brain-dominant individuals and 50% left-brain-dominant individuals in our society.[6]

It seems as if nature intends each species to have a perfect balance of right-brain (left-pawed) dominant individuals and left-brain (right-pawed) dominant individuals.

If 50% of our population is supposed to be right-handed and 50% left-handed, why are approximately 80% of the people in the US right-handed? Some experts say that many naturally left-handed/right-brain-dominant individuals have switched to using their right hand as their dominant hand—unnaturally. Why?

Many left-handed children in this society are forced to favor their right hand. Some have had their left hand tied behind their back until they learn to use their right hand. Some are punished for not using their right hand. Many tools are designed to be used with the right hand only. Left-handed individuals using tools designed for right-handers

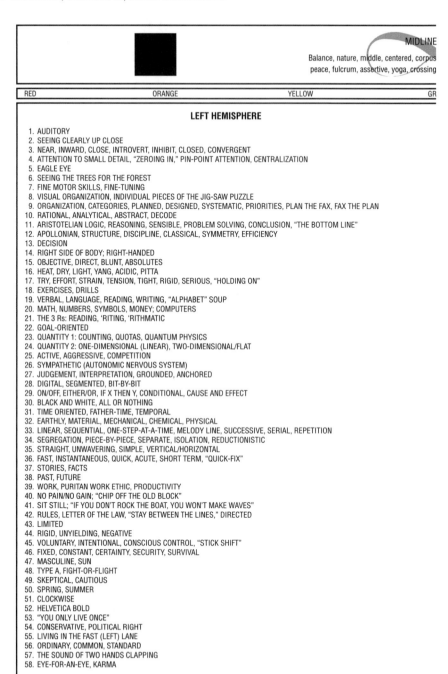

Figure 19–3: Brain Characteristics.

CHARACTERISTICS

callosum, self-actualization, equilibrium,
the midline, movement, the third-eye, love

EEN BLUE INDIGO VIOLET

RIGHT HEMISPHERE

1. Visual
2. Seeing clearly in the distance
3. Far, outward, distant, extrovert, exhibit, open, divergent
4. The whole picture, scan large areas, peripheral vision
5. Seeing the trees and the forest, the Gestalt: the whole is more than the sum of the parts
6. Night owl
7. Large movements
8. Scattered, diffused, the whole jig-saw puzzle
9. Random, aimless, disorder, entropy, Brownian motion, secondary
10. Intuitive, insight, instinct, "gut feeling"
11. Emotional, intuitive, psychic
12. Dionysian, wine, romantic, asymmetry
13. Choice
14. Left side of body; left-handed
15. Subjective, indirect, subtle, nuance, finesse, echo
16. Cold, wet, dark, yin, alkaline, kapha
17. Letting go, effortless, "going with the flow," "easy going," reflex, casual
18. Activities, games, habits
19. Poetry; non-verbal communications
20. Art, music, opera, piano, sculpture, painting, singing, humming
21. Artistic, images, pictures, color
22. Process-oriented
23. Quality 1: feelings, textures, tone, patterns
24. Quality 2: 3-D, spatial relationships
25. Passive, yielding, cooperation
26. Parasympathetic (autonomic nervous system)
27. Suspended judgement, irrational, dreams, floating
28. Analog, continuous
29. More/less, "more or less", if x/maybe y and/or z
30. Shades of gray, sliding-scale, fuzzy-logic, spectrum of the rainbow
31. Timeless, ageless, when time stands still
32. Spiritual, esoteric, mystical
33. Simultaneous, harmony, chords, multiple, parallel
34. Integration, holistic, "see the big picture," global, associations, synthesis, union, together
35. Curves, rhythmical, complex, diagonal
36. Slow, contemplative, chronic, long-term, "slow and steady wins the race"
37. Feelings, pretending, ideals, platonic
38. Present time, "in the here and now"
39. Play, fun, magic
40. No pain/no pain
41. Dance
42. Free, spirit of the law, creativity, imagination, inspiration
43. Infinite
44. Fluid, flexible, positive
45. Spontaneous, involuntary, unconscious, automatic, reflex
46. Variable, change, the Heisenberg Uncertainty Principle
47. Feminine, moon
48. Type B
49. Trust
50. Fall, Winter
51. Counter-clockwise
52. Calligraphy
53. Reincarnation
54. Radical, liberal, political Left
55. "Slow traffic keep right"
56. Innovation, strange, peculiar
57. The sound of one hand clapping
58. Forgiveness, detachment

Figure 19–3: Brain Characteristics.

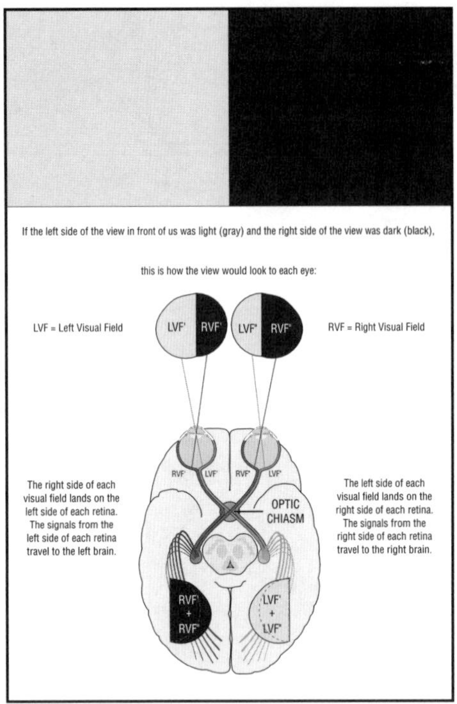

Figure 19–4: Left Sides to the Right Brain/ Right Sides to the Left Brain.

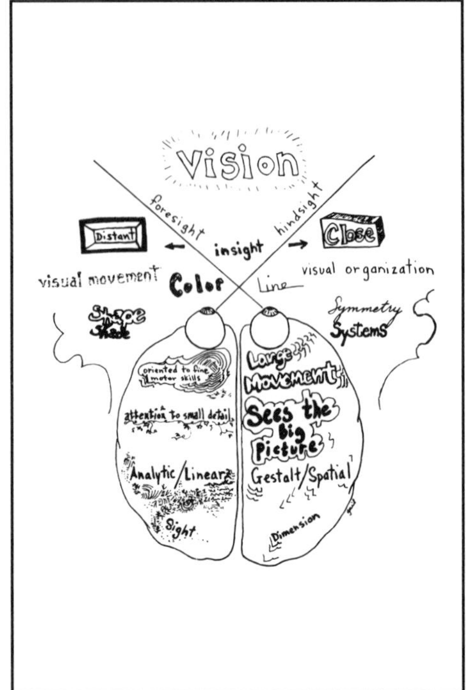

Figure 19–5: Vision." Reprinted from Personalized Whole Brain Integration, by Paul E. Dennison, Ph.D., and Gail E. Hargrove, 1985, Edu-Kinesthetics, Inc., Ventura, CA. Used with permission of the artist, Gail E. Hargrove.

may partially explain why almost twice as many left-handers as right-handers need medical attention for accidents.

If a right-brain-dominant individual is supposed to be left-hand-dominant, what adverse effects does the unnatural switching to favoring the right hand have on the mental functions of this individual?

Many conclusions about behavior drawn from research data are presented as *normal* because a specific behavior is found in the *majority* of a population. Case in point: some researchers have erroneously concluded that left-handedness is an aberration of nature because the majority of Americans are right-handed.

Are conclusions based on an *imbalanced* sample population valid? Erroneous conclusions drawn from studying unhealthy people seem to create, support, and even promote a *more* imbalanced population. This is especially the case in regards to eyesight in excessively left-brain oriented societies. One of the major reasons people believe they need to wear corrective lenses is because so many people wear them.

Bias Favoring Right-Handed (Left-Brain Dominant) Individuals

- Dictionaries define "right" as just, good, and proper (conduct), genuine, real; conforming to facts or standards.
- The Latin word for right is *rectus,* meaning straight.
- Dexterity comes from the Greek word *dexios,* meaning toward the right, or a good omen.
- You are right!
- I have my rights.
- You will see it right before your very eyes.
- You are an upright and righteous person.
- Be sure your socks are right side out.
- Would you like to meet right now, or right after lunch?
- We need to right the injustices done.
- Mr. Dexter is my right-hand man.
- The car on the right has the right-of-way.
- According to the Bible, Christ is seated at the right hand of God.

Bias Against (Right-Brain Dominant) "Lefties"

1. Dictionaries define "left-handed" as clumsy, awkward, insincere, backhanded, dubious, and ironical.
2. The word "left" in:
   - Old English means weak or worthless;
   - Latin is *sinister,* meaning covert;
   - French is *gauche,* meaning crude, awkward, clumsy, or lacking in social grace;
   - German is *linkisch,* meaning unhandy;
   - Italian is *mancion,* meaning dishonest;
   - Spanish is *zurdas,* meaning wrong way.
3. Tomorrow night we will have leftovers.
4. Hurry up, or you will be left out, southpaw.
5. Your views are way out in left field.
6. In the early 1980s, US Postal Service employees were forbidden to sort mail with their left hand.
7. Placing the wedding ring on the left hand comes from the morganic tradition in which European royalty gives the left hand in marriage to a person of inferior rank. Neither the lesser ranked spouse, nor their children, obtain estate or title rights after marriage.
8. In a left-brain society, it is said to be "efficient" for products to be made the same. Scissors, children's school desks, etc., are manufactured mainly for the right-handed people. Efficiency is a left-brain characteristic. Left-handed people are expected to "adapt" to a right-handed society.

Famous lefties include the *creative* geniuses Thomas Edison, Leonardo da Vinci, Michaelangelo, and the world figures Alexander the Great, Charlemagne, and Napoleon. Creativity is a right-brain characteristic.

Too Much Left-Brain Emphasis = Distress

Are the above biases against "lefties" and for "righties" just a coincidence, or do they reflect a society that is extremely left-brain oriented?

One might conclude that left-brain dominant people who live in a very left-brain dominant society would be happy and healthy. This is not necessarily the case. The pitfall for left-brainers is to become so saturated with left-brain activities that the right-brain characteristics are switched off or dimmed. Overworking to the point of ruining health is a common occurrence in fast-paced left-brain societies.

Healthy options for right-brain dominant individuals seem limited. Unless they are brilliant and successful artists (painters, musicians, etc.), right-brainers often must find a way to cope with primarily left-brain activities taught in primarily left-brain school, and end up working in primarily left-brain occupations. Many of my right-brain dominant students have told me they are in left-brain occupations only because they have not found occupations which support and reward right-brain activities as well.

"Slow Down, You Move Too Fast ... "

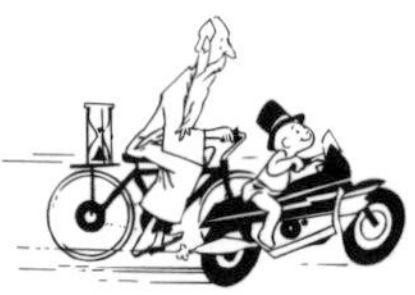

One indication of an excessively left-brain oriented society is the emphasis on speed. We live in a fast-paced, impatient culture. "Hurry to meet the deadline." "Time is money." Is profit the bottom line in our society—even at the cost of our health?

We have countless fast-food restaurants, speedy microwave ovens for TV dinners, fast music, speed reading of instant books, and fast cars. And your "machines of seeing" (corrective lenses) will be ready "in about an hour."

Computer companies keep designing faster and faster computers, which are then used to design even faster computers. Analysts now say a current "state of the art" computer is obsolete in only six months. And the period of time to obsolescence keeps getting shorter.

George Vithoulkas, M.D., writes in *A New Model for Health and Disease,* "The pressures of modern life place a premium on rapid [healing] and the speedy elimination of symptoms."[7] The pervasive use of unnecessary "quick fix" surgeries and drugs is discussed in the next chapter.

A man visiting my booth at a health fair once asked me how long it takes to improve vision naturally. I told him some people have taken several years to free themselves completely from glasses. In that case, he said, he was not interested in my classes, and he was going to have his corneas cut because the refractive surgical procedure only takes a few minutes.

Perhaps impatience, and moving too fast, is to be expected in a very young society like the US.

I used to be semi-apologetic regarding how long it takes students to improve vision. Now, I am proud to tell people it can take a long time. In regards to natural vision, "slow and steady wins the race." When the momentum of natural vision habits is re-established over a long period of time, it is not lost quickly. The long-term approach is a right-brain characteristic.

It is true some natural vision students have succeeded fairly quickly, especially those who have had low blur for only a short time. But I prefer to give conservative examples.

Bates reported some fast improvement of sight in the 1920s. I believe it takes students a longer time to improve sight today because we live in a much more stressful and imbalanced society. It takes more energy and time to re-establish the balance required for normal vision.

Re-Activating the Right Brain

Our young, technological society has led many people so far into left-brain activities that they have switched off many right-brain characteristics. As a result, many people are now discovering they need to switch back on the right brain.

Many holistic self-improvement programs emphasize right-brain characteristics, e.g., feelings, intuition, trust, "letting go," "seeing the large picture," etc., as vehicles for healing and achieving goals.

Regarding feelings, Chérie Carter-Scott, founder of Motivation-Management-Service, Inc., writes in her book *The New Species:*

> The basic point of view about feelings in our society is that they get in the way. They are a problem for those who feel them and for the people around them. They are unnecessary and bothersome. They are embarrassing and do not promote progress or profit.[8]
>
> ...The first step in discovering your being [true self] is to allow yourself to have and to experience the multitude of deep emotions that run through you. One reason so few people are in touch with their beings is that feelings and deep emotions are not encouraged in our society, and the inroad to the being is blocked.[9]
>
> ...Allowing yourself to have all of the feelings you experience requires tremendous trust in yourself.[10]

Many of the imbalances in our "Just give me the facts, Ma'am" society are due to our mechanical way of living, including the suppression and invalidation of feelings. The feelings of others do not need to be understood (assuming they could be), but they need to be validated as real and meaningful to the person experiencing them if that person is to grow.

T. Ribot, in *The Psychology of Attention,* wrote:

> ...just as everything that comes from the external senses constitutes the primal subject-matter of intelligence: and just as, physiologically, vegetative life precedes animal life, which rests upon it, so also, psychologically, emotional life precedes intellectual life, which rests upon it. The states designated as needs, appetites, inclinations, tendencies, and desires are the direct and immediate results of very animal organization. They constitute the true basis of emotional life.[11]

Kenneth R. Pelletier, in this book *Mind as Healer, Mind as Slayer,* writes:

> ...stress itself is difficult to identify and individuals are conditioned to ignore its sources and effects. Many people tend to suppress their feelings of stress because the current norm of social behavior is to tolerate extraordinarily high levels of stress. There is a martyrlike quality in this attitude which is not constructive.[12]

Dyslexia—Too Much Left-Brain Stress for the Right Brain

One choice the right-brain dominant person has in a left-brain oriented society is to "adapt" to living in a left-brain mode, in which case, things "just don't *feel* right."

The unnatural option of switching to primarily left-brain activities is so stressful for some right-brain dominant individuals, they switch off the left brain. This occurs with many children in our society.

One of the consequences of switching off the left brain can be the loss of verbal and math skills. Many people in our society lose the ability to speak, write, or do math correctly—and become dyslexic.

TOM'S PERSONAL LOG: Being a left-brain dominant, chess playing, analytical chemist, one might guess I would be the last person to become dyslexic.

When I started natural healing in 1980, I participated in many right-brain oriented programs. One program, which I participated in for about two years, was based a great deal on feelings, intuition, and trust.

After this program, I quit my chemistry job and attended school to become a Natural Vision teacher. The training I received was very right-brain oriented.

Upon graduation and moving to San Francisco to begin teaching vision classes, I found I had become dyslexic. When speaking, I left words out of sentences, and I switched the order of words within a sentence—somewhat embarrassing for someone who teaches clarity. Even simple math, like adding two numbers, had become difficult—very embarrassing and perplexing for a former chemist!

What happened? I emphasized right-brain characteristics to the point where I had switched off many of my left-brain verbal and math skills. During this dyslexic period, I was told by a right-brain/left-brain expert that I was *right-brain* dominant. This was interesting, because my true dominance is left brain.

By studying books on right-brain/left-brain characteristics, I recognized how I had then become imbalanced in an excessive right-brain manner. By giving more attention to left-brain characteristics, I began to re-establish a balance between the two brains—and eliminated the dyslexia.

Within the last few years I again experienced short periods of dyslexia when beginning work on the creative parts (graphics, etc.) of this book.

TOM'S PERSONAL LOG: In my first several years of holistic healing I had many reactions on the left side of my body.

The first stress reduction workshop I took resulted in a large red rash forming on my left leg. Left side reactions were related to healing (re-activating) my right brain. In the last ten years of healing, my remaining symptoms have become fairly even on both sides of my body.

It is interesting that in homeopathy, which side of the body a symptom appears on can be an important factor in determining the correct remedy.

THE BATES METHOD EXPLAINED BY THE RIGHT-BRAIN/LEFT-BRAIN MODEL

Decades before the characteristics of the two brains were formally presented by Sperry and others, Bates discovered that vision is primarily a right-brain function. This was the true brilliance of Bates' work. The majority of people in this society do not have normal sight because they use their vision in primarily a strained, left-brain manner.

If a person uses his visual system primarily in the way he is taught to live in this excessively left-brain oriented society, he will not keep normal, clear vision. The majority of people living in this society strain their vision and create their blur.

Bates' advanced model of vision—linking

the functions of the visual system to the mind—was too far ahead of his contemporaries' theories on eyesight.

The Machines of Seeing

Vithoulkas, in *A New Model for Health and Disease,* writes:

> Since the eighteenth century a mechanistic way of thinking has prevailed in the scientific method which has led to a mechanical approach to the whole problem of health and disease. The body, separated from the rest of the organism, was considered a machine.... [13]

And, unfortunately, still is.

As a result, we are given machines to wear when our machinery of sight malfunctions. *"Corrective" lenses are the left-brain mechanical solutions to excessive left-brain stress on the visual system.* And, as Bates pointed out, "corrective" lenses do not correct vision at all; they only "compensate" for the blurred vision.

And now we have sophisticated machines to cut and shape the corneas. Perhaps this development was only to be expected in this mechanically oriented society.

What's It All About, William?

Bates discovered how nature intends us to use our body (blinking, breathing, head movement, etc.), and more importantly, our mind (centralization, interest, the illusion of oppositional movement, a relaxed and receptive attitude toward vision, etc.) to see the world.

Bates' research and experiments explain the causes of errors of nearsightedness, farsightedness, astigmatism, strabismus, and many other problems of sight. However, it is not necessary to understand the physical mechanisms involved with eyesight to improve eyesight. The student only needs to understand the key habits of normal vision, and to re-integrate them more each day until they are subconscious habits—once again.

Still, it is interesting to delve deeper into the possible relationships between Bates' research and modern right-brain/left-brain concepts, discussed next.

Normal Vision

See *Figure 19–3: Brain Characteristics.*

Normal Distance Vision

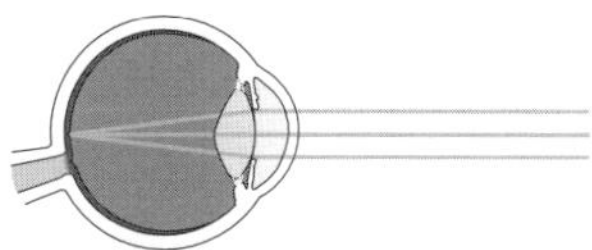

Bates stated that when the normal eye is "at rest," the oblique muscles are relaxed and expanded, the eyeball is in a spherical shape, and the eye is adjusted to see clearly in the distance. The relaxed, expansive right brain is responsible for seeing clearly in the distance.

Normal Near Vision

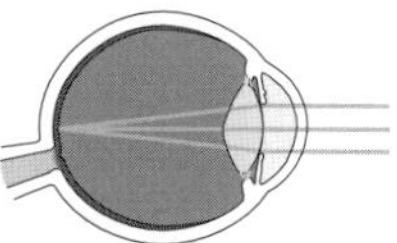

Bates stated that when the two oblique muscles contract, the eyeball elongates and accommodates to see clearly up close. The contractive, effort-oriented left brain is responsible for seeing clearly up close.

As stated before, the "effort" of the oblique muscles is minimal and automatic. There is no excessive strain involved during normal accommodation, just as there is no abnormal strain involved when the recti muscles move the eyes to see objects to the left, right, up, down, and to converge on near objects.

Abnormal Vision

Left-Brain Nearsights

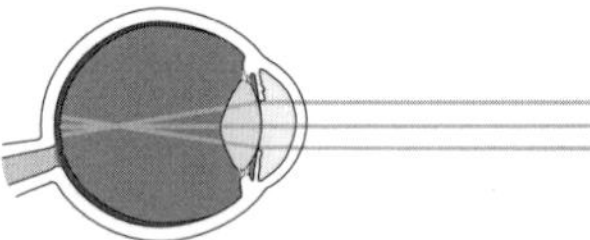

Bates demonstrated that when a person strains to see objects in the distance, the oblique muscles contract tight and elongate the eyeball, producing nearsightedness. An elongated eyeball see clearly up close. The problem in nearsightedness is that the obliques muscle *remain chronically* tight.

The right-brain/left-brain model allows us to explore more possibilities between the mind and Bates' discoveries.

Because a left-brain dominant individual is more "inner" oriented, she is more likely to strain while seeing distant objects than near objects. Nearsights have better vision habits when doing activities involving near objects. The nearsight tends to diffuse, strain, and become rigid when the attention is in the distance.

Our society places a great deal of attention on where the blur occurs for nearsights, while almost no attention is given to the fact that the near vision *remains* clear.

Myopes are *near*sighted. It appears that *when left-brain dominant people form incorrect, strained vision habits, they keep the clarity of their dominant personality—near orientation.* Stated the opposite way, when nearsights strain their vision, they lose the clarity associated with their subdominant personality—right-brain far vision.

Left-brain dominant individuals are relatively introverted and interested more in objects close to them. Myopes are usually content being alone, reading a book in their lap, working with machinery, and are more interested in details. Generally, myopes have less interest in what is going on "out there," especially when "out there" involves other people.

Nearsights are "seemingly" placid and tend to do activities slowly compared to farsights. Nearsights tend to be very sensitive and sit extremely still. They are good at hiding any nervousness or fear they feel. They do not become bored with near objects anywhere as quickly as farsights.

Bates teacher Janet Goodrich presents a very interesting discussion of the personalities of nearsights, farsights, and astigmatics in her book *Natural Vision Improvement.*

When vision is strained, blur must result. In myopia, the fact that the clarity remains up close is more interesting than the fact that the distance vision becomes blurred.

Earlier, the concern was raised about possible adverse effects of left-handed, right-brain dominant individuals unnaturally favoring their right hand. Now the question arises: What are the adverse effects on the personalities of many formerly nearsighted individuals who have become artificially farsighted as a result of corneal refractive surgeries, like RK and PRK? According to the model presented here, left-brain dominant individuals who strain their vision *should be myopic, not farsighted.* This may be the first time in history left-brain dominant individuals who have incorrect, strained vision habits have become farsighted instead of "correctly" nearsighted. (Of course, physically the eyeball is still elongated.)

Even seeing clearly through compensating lenses is an aberration. The blur is nature's way of telling (warning?) us to return to relaxed, normal vision habits. Could so-called "progressive myopia" be at least partially caused by the mind's rejection of the clarity provided by compensating lenses?

Right-Brain Farsights

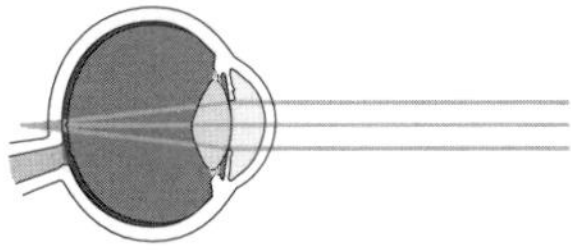

Bates demonstrated that when a person strains to see objects up close, the recti muscles contract tight and foreshorten the eyeball, producing farsightedness. The problem in farsightedness is the recti muscles *remain chronically* tight.

Because a right-brain dominant individual is more "outer" oriented, he is more likely to strain while seeing close objects than distant objects. Farsights have better vision habits while doing activities involving far objects than near objects. They tend to diffuse, strain, and become rigid when the attention is with near objects.

Hyperopes are *far*sighted. It appears that *when right-brain dominant people form incorrect, strained vision habits, they keep the clarity of their dominant personality—far orientation* (at least in beginning farsightedness). Stated the opposite way, when farsights strain their vision, they lose the clarity associated with their subdominant personality—left-brain near vision.

Right-brain dominant individuals are relatively extroverted and more interested in objects and especially people "out there" in the distance. Generally, farsights are less interested in what is going on "up close." Right-brain farsights are more interested in the "large picture" than in details. Farsights like large movements and tend to do most activities quickly.

Generally, farsights are highly emotional, want to talk, and ask for advice. Farsights become bored relatively quickly with close objects.

Again, when vision is strained, blur results. In beginning farsightedness, it is more interesting that clarity remains in the distance than the fact that vision becomes blurred up close. (As farsightedness increases, the close vision is *more* blurred than the distance vision.)

Hemispheric, Not Genetic, Predisposition

When a person is healthy and balanced, the left brain functions correctly to see clearly up close, and the right brain functions correctly to see clearly in the distance. Both brains are being used correctly, and the person has normal sight.

When a person becomes imbalanced and strains his visual system, neither brain is used correctly. Both brains are strained and the person acquires blur. (More on this below.)

Rather than nearsightedness and farsightedness being "genetically predisposed," as is often erroneously stated, it appears that functional vision problems are "hemisphere-predisposed."

When we encounter a problem, we tend to rely on our strengths. When an individual strains her visual system, she maintains clarity at the distance associated with her dominant brain, and acquires blur at the distance associated with her subdominant brain.

Bates discovered that *the key to normal sight is not to strain the visual system.* It appears that *hemisphere dominance is irrelevant as long as an individual does not interfere with the natural, normal, relaxed vision habits learned automatically and subconsciously early in life.*

Younger Left-Brain Nearsights, Older Right-Brain Farsights

Why, in literate societies, does nearsightedness often occur at a young age, and farsightedness often occur around "mid-life"? Some possible answers to this question are presented here.

Many Younger Nearsights

Of the left-brain dominant people and the right-brain dominant people, which of the two groups would be more likely to strain their sight *earlier* in life? Left-brain dominant people—especially in an excessively left-brain oriented society.

Why? The tendency of left-brain dominant individuals is to try too hard. If abnormal effort is applied to the vision system, e.g. straining to see the blackboard at school, vision will become blurred. Some left-brain dominant children *try so hard* to "succeed" in school, they become fatigued. It is very easy to fall into incorrect vision habits, especially the staring habit, under these conditions.

It should be noted here that blur first formed by a person around age forty is *not always farsightedness.* A small number of left-brain dominant individuals strain their vision for the first time *around age forty* and become "appropriately" *nearsighted,* not farsighted.

Many Older Farsights

Many people in this society become farsighted later in life. Of the left-brain dominant people and the right-brain dominant people, which of the two groups would be *more* likely to strain their sight *later* in life?

Before answering this question, let's ask it in a better way: Of the left-brain dominant people and the right-brain dominant people, which of the two groups would be *less* likely to strain their sight *earlier* in life? Right-brain dominant individuals. Why? It appears that they are more likely to remain *right-brain relaxed* earlier in life and not strain their visual system as children and young adults.

A relatively small number of right-brain dominant individuals *do* strain their vision *early* in life and become "appropriately" *farsighted* as children.

If vision is primarily a right-brain activity, why does a right-brain dominant person acquire any blur at all? Right-brain dominant people can, and often do, strain their visual system by forming incorrect vision habits—especially in a very left-brain oriented society.

Why do so many right-brain dominant people in our society form incorrect vision habits around age forty? There are many physical, emotional, and some say spiritual changes that occur around age forty. It appears that *if* a right-brain dominant person—in this society—is going to strain his vision, it will most likely occur around age forty.

Astigmatism—An Ambiguity of Brain Dominance?

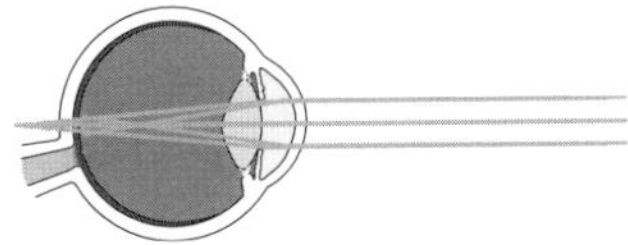

Astigmatism seems to occur when a left-brain dominant myope engages in primarily right-brain activities, and when a right-brain dominant farsight engages in primarily left-brain activities.

In astigmatism, usually an oblique *and* a rectus muscle are chronically tight. (In nearsightedness, both oblique muscles are chronically tight; in farsightedness the four recti muscles are chronically tight.) In astigmatism both near and far vision are blurred or distorted. The light rays entering the eye in one plane fall in front of the retina—as in nearsightedness—while the light rays entering the eye in another plane fall in back of the retina—as in farsightedness. From one point of view, astigmatism is a combination of nearsightedness and farsightedness.

If a left-brain dominant person who has incorrect vision habits engages in primarily right-brain activities, according to the ideas just presented, she should be farsighted! Astigmatism may be the visual system's attempt to transition from tight oblique muscles (left-brain dominant myopia) to tight recti muscles (right-brain dominant farsightedness). The opposite could be the case for right-brain dominant farsights who acquire astigmatism—tight recti muscles may be attempting to switch to tight oblique muscles.

Practicing circular motions with the nose-feather is important for those with astigmatism.

Tom's Personal Log: My astigmatism started (on top of my long-standing and increasing nearsightedness) at about the same time I began to play the bass instrument while attending college for my chemistry degree.

A Funny Thing Happened On My Way to My Other Personality

Some researchers have studied the vision of individuals with multiple personalities. Esophoria has been observed when an adult switches back to his five-year-old personality. When he returns to his adult personality, the esophoria disappears.

Some people with multiple personalities keep a drawer full of different prescription glasses—using the power of glasses associated with their current personality!

Note that the changes in sight are solely a consequence of a *shift in the mind.*

Could it be that nearsightedness, farsightedness, astigmatism, and strabismus are only physical manifestations or "reflections" of various forms of imbalance in the mind? *Are all functional vision problems determined by the individual's current personality, brain dominance, and incorrect vision habits?*

The *person*ality of the person with blurred vision needs to return to a certain degree of balance to return to normal sight. This is one of the main reasons improving eyesight naturally is not an overnight process.

The Principles of Natural Vision Explained by Right-Brain/Left-Brain Concepts

Though vision is primarily a right-brain function, when a person has normal sight, both brains are being used correctly to see.

The three principles of natural vision—relaxation, centralization, and movement—are the correct, natural ways of using the mind and body to see clearly.

Right-Brain Relaxation

Right-brain concepts teach us the principle of relaxation. Natural vision is a receptive, automatic, subconscious, and most importantly, *relaxed* activity. Bates proved relaxation is the key to normal sight. When effort or strain is applied to the visual system, sight lowers.

Straining to see is an interference with the right brain's natural, relaxed way of seeing.

In our "no pain, no gain, you didn't try hard enough" society, the majority of people have applied effort to the non-effort activity of natural vision. As a consequence, the majority of people in this society have blur.

The right brain teaches us to trust our vision, especially the unclear peripheral vision. People with blur do not trust their peripheral vision to pick up moving objects automatically and quickly. People with blur diffuse, "trying" to see everything clearly at once. As explained earlier, it is impossible to see the peripheral vision clearly. Diffusion is a strain. The eye muscles contract tight, and blurred vision or strabismus is created.

In terms of the field of vision, the right brain is responsible for seeing "the whole picture"—both the peripheral and the central vision. Of course it is correct to see the entire picture at one time—*but not clearly*.

Because vision is suggestible, the beliefs we carry can have a major impact on our sight. Many people in this society are told to expect the blur experienced by the *majority.* This simply reinforces, perpetuates, and increases the imbalances already present.

When a person with normal sight is told by an authority he will lose his clarity (for example, "due to the aging process"), this person may stop trusting his normal, clear vision. If worry about and distrust of his sight result in straining to see, blur will result. The prediction becomes true—a self-fulfilling prophecy. If strong corrective lenses are worn, the vision is strained even further. It is also predicted that vision will get worse, and it usually does.

The right-brain principle of relaxation is especially important for the left-brain nearsights, because their tendency is to *try* too hard.

Left-Brain Centralization

Left-brain concepts teach us the natural vision principle of centralization. The left brain "zeros in" to the center of the large picture to pick up sharp details and the best color. As we have learned, only the center of the visual field is clear and most colorful.

Parents often tell their children, "Do one thing at a time." This is excellent advice.

Diffusion is an interference with the left brain's natural, centralized way of seeing.

The left-brain principle of centralization is especially important for right-brain farsights, because their tendency is to avoid details.

Both Brains Connected by Movement

The natural vision principle of *movement* connects the right-brain principle of relaxation to the left-brain principle of centralization. See *Figure 19–5: "Vision."*

Rigidity interferes with the dynamic exchange of energy between the two brains. *Rigidity is an interference with both brains' continual movement through 3-D space:* near and far, left and right, and up and down.

Two Perspectives on Oppositional Movement

While we are moving, the left brain regards stationary objects as stationary. But the right brain regards stationary objects as moving in the opposite direction of our movement. Which brain is correct? Both.

The left brain is the absolute, stable, grounding brain. "Stationary objects do not move—by definition!" The right brain is the relative, flexible, floating brain. "Stationary objects seem to move in the opposite direction of my movement."

Both mental attitudes are correct *and necessary* for normal sight. A well-constructed bridge is both stable and flexible. We want both stability and flexibility. We are meant to have a balance.

Relaxation = Centralization = Movement

The universal principles of relaxation, centralization, and movement are intimately related to, and support, each other. Relaxation, movement, and centralization create and maintain clarity. Strain, rigidity, and diffusion create and maintain blur.

I find the right- and left-brain perspectives on the principles of natural vision to be one of the most exciting parts of teaching students how to improve their vision.

The Cross-Crawl

See *Figure 19–6: The Cross-Crawl.*

When a baby first learns to crawl, she moves the right arm forward with the right leg, and then the left arm forward with the left leg. This homolateral form of crawling requires the use of only one brain at a time. Later, the baby learns to move the right arm forward with the left leg, and then the left arm forward with the right leg. This advanced, balanced form of crawling requires the integrated use of both brains.

Generally, the right brain controls the left side of the body, and the left brain controls the right side of the body. The cross-crawl

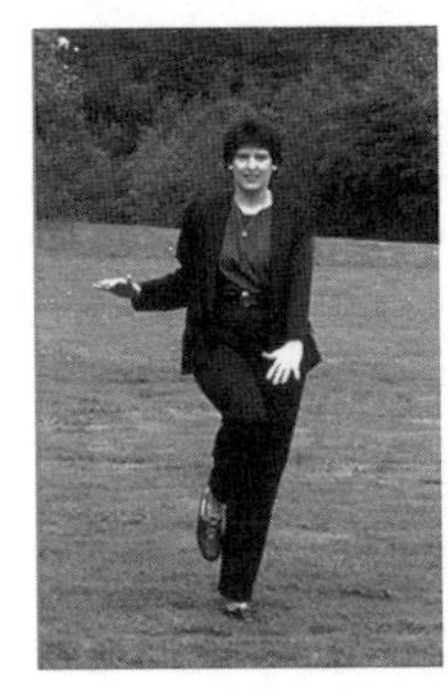
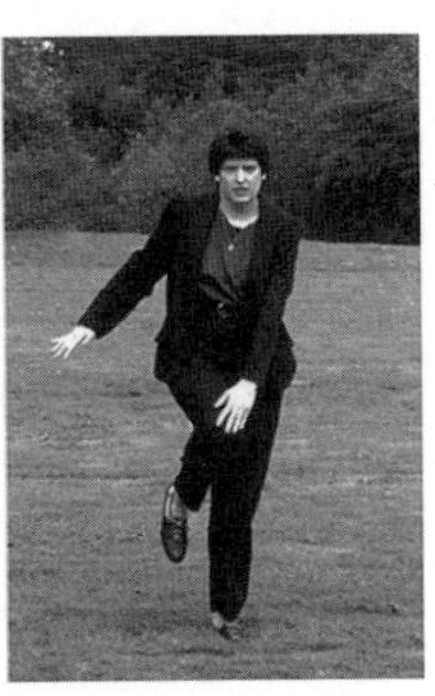
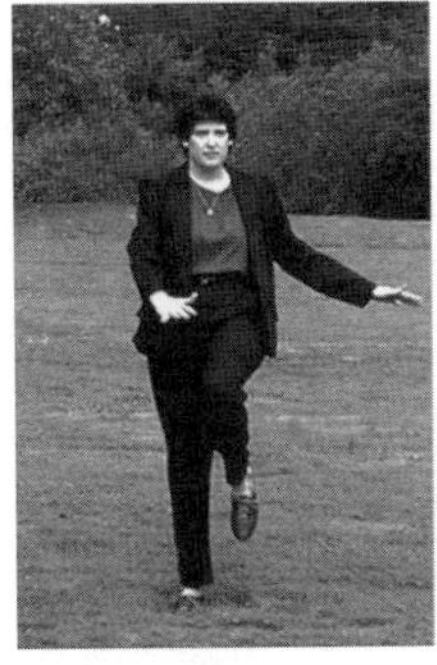
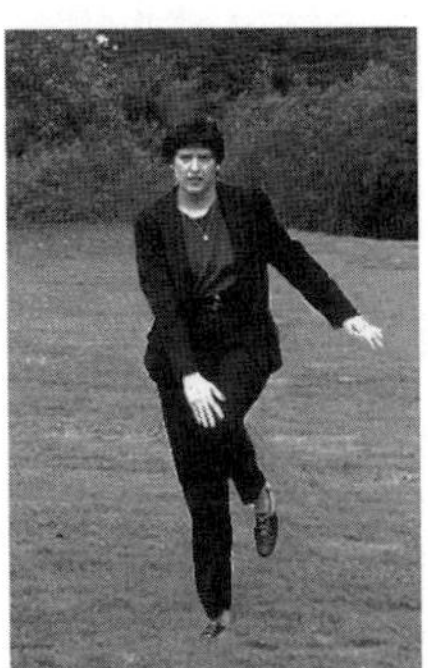

Figure 19–6: The Cross-Crawl.

emphasizes movement with the right side of the body *together* with movement of the left side of the body. Both brains are used in an integrative way. The cross-crawl is an excellent, simple activity for balancing (to a certain degree) the right and left brains.

HOW TO CROSS-CRAWL:
While lifting the left knee, simply reach over and touch it with the right hand. Then, while lifting the right knee, reach over and touch it with the left hand. While cross-crawling, remember to sketch, breathe, and blink.

The principles within the cross-crawl can be integrated into many daily activities. For example, when walking you can touch the right forefinger and thumb together as the left foot moves forward. Then touch the left forefinger and thumb together as the right foot moves forward. One jogger stated he could jog much farther, and with less discomfort, by including this variation of the cross-crawl.

The cross-crawl can also be performed during closed-eyelids sunning.

For a super balancing activity, move your nose-feather in the shape of the infinity sign (up through the middle, down on the outsides) while doing the cross-crawl. This powerful activity may require some practice before the student can do it comfortably.

Habits, Not Exercises

The emphasis of this book is on natural vision *habits*. Unfortunately, many people erroneously perceive the Bates method to be a series of "eye exercises."

There are three main reasons why the Bates method is not about eye exercises:

1. The underlying philosophy of eye exercises is to strengthen supposedly weak eye muscles. The eye muscles are not weak; they are chronically tense, squeezing the eyeball out of shape and/or out of alignment. Relaxation, not work, is needed to improve sight.
2. The eyes and eye muscles are not the main issue. Babies and animals do not even know they have eyes, yet they see clearly. It is how we use our entire mind and body that determines how well we see. At least 95% of the processes involved in seeing occur in the *mind*. The eyes and eye muscles respond to messages from the brain. Mental strain is the cause of blurred vision. Bates discovered relaxation of the mind is the single most important factor in natural sight.
3. The process of improving sight naturally is not limited to twenty minutes per day of exercises. Shortly before he died in 1931, Bates concisely stated that the natural, correct vision "habits" are to be used "all day long." If students do eye exercises for twenty minutes a day, and then revert to incorrect habits the remainder of the day, they will not succeed. Integration of the habits and principles of seeing as a "renewed visual lifestyle" is the key.

Many people, including many eye doctors, correctly state, "Eye exercises don't work" or "They only provide temporary benefit." I agree. The "eye exercise" presentation of the Bates method is an inappropriate left-brain presentation of Bates' work.

The Bates method is not about "eye exercises." It is about relearning normal vision habits permanently. It is important that natural vision students understand this distinction.

It should be acknowledged here that some eye exercise approaches to eyesight improvement do contain some correct principles and/or habits of natural vision. To the degree these correct habits and principles of natural vision are relearned while doing eye exercises, there can be some benefit. But the benefit is usually temporary because most students do not integrate all of the habits and principles permanently.

It is helpful to note that blurred vision is not caused by a person failing to do eye exercises. Therefore, eye exercises are not the solution to blurred vision. People and animals with normal sight do not do eye exercises. They have normal, relaxed vision habits.

Oftentimes I like to use the heart as an analogy to the eyes. The heart is a large muscle, but a person does not "try" to pump their blood with conscious effort. In fact, if you attempted to do so, you could interfere with the normal functioning of your heart. If a person has a healthy diet, exercises, reduces stress, and has a balanced lifestyle, the heart takes care of itself—automatically. The same is true with sight. The correct approach to improving sight is *indirect*—another right-brain characteristic.

Bates taught swings and shifting activities to demonstrate to students correct vision habits. They are *not* exercises.

Sketching, breathing, and blinking are the normal, natural vision habits we are meant to have our entire lifetime. Once the vision student understands this and begins to integrate correct vision habits, he is well on the way to success.

Bates also taught palming and sunning. These activities are not exercises. They are optional self-healing activities which can accelerate the release of strain put on the visual system by incorrect vision habits—habits which many people have had for many years.

TOM'S PERSONAL LOG: When I first became interested in improving my vision, I read many books on the Bates method. I thought this program was a series of eye exercises. (Some books even refer to them as drills!) I did not perceive any improvement of my sight by doing eye exercises.

I did not understand that relearning vision habits—all day long—was the key to improving my vision. I was fortunate enough to find an excellent vision teacher who taught me correct vision *habits.* Only then did my vision begin to improve.

One reason Bates' work is perceived as eye exercises is because Bates' most concise summaries of natural vision habits were not presented in his 1920 book *Perfect Sight Without Glasses.* They appeared later—in his monthly *Better Eyesight* magazines. The key vision habits were concisely summarized in the September 1927 issue of *Better Eyesight* magazine. (This summary was presented earlier, at the end of Chapter 15, "The Three Habits—Sketch, Breathe, and Blink.") My discovery of this summary in 1986 created an important shift in my understanding and teaching of natural vision.

Additionally, Bates' 1920 book was revised after his death in 1931. Most of the original illustrations, along with a significant amount of his writings, were removed.

Will the reader of *this* book succeed in improving his sight? This partly depends on how well he understands the habits and principles described herein, and how well he practices and re-integrates them.

A teacher of natural vision is especially valuable in helping the student relearn the *spirit* of natural seeing. When it comes to relearning the subtle mental aspects of natural vision, books can be limiting. If a person chooses to learn to play the piano, he may obtain many books on the topic. Most likely he will also seek instructions from an experienced piano teacher.

The best approach I have found is to receive instructions from an experienced and knowledgeable Natural Vision teacher and to read several books on this topic. (There is a large Bibliography of vision books in Appendix A.)

OTHER ASPECTS OF NATURAL VISION IMPROVEMENT

Forgetting About Your Eyes—Naturally

Not only are straining with effort and eye exercises not needed to improve sight, but students should forget their eyes exist. (Of course if there is a serious problem with the eyes, the student should consult with an eye doctor.) People with normal vision almost never think about their eyes.

What we see is conscious, but *how* we see is meant to be subconscious. This is why the imaginary nose-helper is attached to the *nose* and not the eyes—to encourage the student not to strain with their eyes.

As Bates pointed out, *there is nothing to do to see clearly.* Clarity is automatic, natural, subconscious, casual, and effortless.

The real issue in improving vision is *what not to do.* Blur is caused by interfering with normal, natural vision habits. The incorrect vision habits we have formed need to be unlearned. Remove the interferences, and improvement is automatic. This idea is difficult for many people in this society to grasp, because we often think that effort is required to obtain a goal.

If we eat harmful food, we become ill. Simply return to normal (not average!) food, and again we become healthy. There is nothing to do. There is only the harmful food to eliminate.

It can be valuable to reflect on the fact that the picture we are moving through is not "out there." Only atoms and light rays emanating from those atoms are "out there." The picture we see is created in the mind from the light rays striking the light receptors in the retina. It is primarily our relationship to this internal picture that determines how, and how well, we see. One of my students told me that some photographers who specialize in black and white or gray photographs begin to see the world in shades of gray instead of color. He has experienced this in his work with photography.

If we are living under mental strain, the mental picture will likely be blurred. If we live in a balanced, relaxed manner, the mental picture will likely be clear. Vision is primarily an *internal* process.

The Qualities of Natural Vision

As discussed earlier, there are many right-brain *qualities* of vision that are re-activated when a student relearns natural vision habits. Some of these qualities include full 3-D vision, color variations, texture awareness, and contrast. The popular solution to vision problems—compensating lenses—brings back artificial acuity. Natural vision involves much more than just acuity.

Vision Dreams

Many students have vision dreams. Vision dreams are dreams which are related to the process of improving sight. Dreaming is primarily a right-brain activity.

One of my students said she was in a dream without her glasses on. The dream was blurred. When she practiced correct vision habits in the dream, the dream cleared up! Some vision students begin remembering their dreams for the first time. Others begin dreaming in color for the first time, where before their dreams were seen in black and white or gray.

Vision dreams are an indication the right brain is being reactivated. This is a positive sign.

Right-Brain/Emotional Connection

Emotional connections to vision were discussed in previous chapters. Emotional issues surfacing while improving vision can be another positive sign. Emotions are primarily right-brain characteristics.

There is some form of stress present when vision becomes blurred. Most often, there is some emotion connected with that stress.

Some students have memories of tragic experiences resurface while improving their sight. Some vision students have sought professional counseling to help resolve issues related to the blurring of their sight.

Improving sight can be used as a tool for self-healing on many levels, including the emotional level. The alternative is to allow the strain associated with blurred vision to continue. Sometimes it takes courage and determination to improve our vision and health.

Vision and Memory

There is a high correlation between vision improvement and memory improvement. How many details do you remember of a room in which you were spaced-out and staring most of the time? Probably not many. How many details do you remember of a room where you were very interested in seeing the objects there? Probably many more.

Bates taught memory activities to his students. He understood the connections among movement, interest, memory, imagination, and normal vision. A simple way to improve memory skills is to sketch an object with your nose-pencil, and then continue to sketch the same object in your mind with the eyelids closed. Alternate back and forth a few times. This is very beneficial to sight.

By the way, most students with blurred vision are more relaxed when their eyelids are closed.

Tom's Personal Log: A college class I attended was taught by a man and a woman. The woman had a wonderful, lively energy, standing and moving most of the time while she was teaching. After all thirty students in the room said their names one after another, this teacher correctly named every person in the room! Her less lively partner (her former husband) sat behind the desk, staring with his head down much of the time. He did not repeat the woman's amazing feat of memory. She did not wear glasses; he wore thick, coke-bottle glasses.

Right-Brain Subjectivity and Beliefs

Vision, being primarily a right-brain function, is primarily a subjective and subconscious process. Therefore, the student's attitudes and beliefs about his vision improvement process are very important.

It is so ingrained in our society that vision cannot improve, when most people start to experience blurred vision, they do not even ask the question, "Is there a way I can improve my eyesight?" It is simply *assumed* that vision cannot get better—otherwise, why would so many people (in our society) be wearing corrective lenses? Many people conclude glasses must be worn for the rest of their lives.

Students need to be very strong and determined to follow their own choices about their vision. This is an essential ingredient for success, especially for people living in left-brain oriented societies. How well you see is highly dependent upon your *beliefs* about your vision.

Attitudes and Language

One of the problems of nearsightedness is that myopes often begin to think of themselves as *a nearsighted person.* Students with nearsightedness often say, "I *am* nearsighted." I reply, "The prescription given to you by your eye doctor indicates you have a correction for nearsightedness."

What a student *says* is, generally, what she *thinks*—and vision is primary a *mental* activity. When the student thinks and says, "I currently have nearsightedness," she opens up the possibility of *not* having nearsightedness.

Another problem with nearsightedness is the myope now seldom bothers to have interest in objects in the distance when not wearing corrective lenses. "Why should I bother noticing distant objects without my glasses on? They are not clear." This "mental set" needs to change to improve sight. The student is re-learning visual interest!

Similar issues apply to farsightedness, astigmatism, and crossed eye.

"It Makes Sense"

The key to normal sight is correct vision habits. The ideas and facts presented in this chapter simply help us to better understand why the correct vision habits and principles Bates discovered *are* correct.

Nature teaches us how to see clearly in the first few years of our life. Bates taught his students not to interfere with this natural process. The Bates method is only a *formal* educational program that provides the student with the opportunity to return to natural vision habits—and clear sight.

Those who take the time to explore what the Bates method of natural vision truly involves often remark how much sense it makes. Bates' own students stated this frequently, and my students have stated this for over thirteen years: "It makes sense."

Notes

1 Dr. Darling's entire testimonial can be found in Chapter 29, " 'This Method Has Been Proved.' " It is one of the finest testimonials of natural vision improvement I have encountered.

2 Aldous Huxley, *The Art of Seeing* (New York: Harper & Brothers Publishers, 1942), pp. 49, 51.

3 George Vithoulkas, *The Science of Homeopathy* (New York: Grove Press, 1980), p. 23.

4 Ibid., p. 25.

5 Chérie Carter-Scott, *Negaholics: How to Overcome Negativity and Turn Your Life Around* (New York: Ballantine Books, 1989), p. 67.

6 Paul E. Dennison and Gail E. Hargrove, *Personalized Whole Brain Integration* (Ventura, California: Edu-Kinesthetics, Inc., 1985), p. 13.

[7] George Vithoulkas, *A New Model for Health and Disease* (Berkeley, California: Health and Habitat, and North Atlantic Books, 1991), p. 27.

[8] Chérie Carter-Scott, *The New Species* (New York: Coleman Graphic, Inc., 1980), p. 62.

[9] Ibid., p. 9.

[10] Ibid., pp. 9–10.

[11] T. Ribot, *The Psychology of Attention* (Chicago: The Open Court Publishing Company, 1890), pp. 106–7.

[12] Pelletier, Kenneth R. *Mind as Healer, Mind as Slayer: A Holistic Approach to Preventing Stress Disorders* (New York: Dell Publishing Co., Inc., 1977), p. 35.

[13] Vithoulkas, *A New Model for Health and Disease,* p. 24.

CHAPTER TWENTY

The Two Sides of Health and Healing

Since natural vision is based largely on a healthy balance of the mind and body, it is worthwhile discussing some of the larger issues and problems of health and healing in our society.

As with the preceding chapter on right-brain/left-brain concepts, health issues are very complex. They are also closely related to each other. I view the serious health problems in our society as a subset of our extremely left-brain, imbalanced way of living. The student of natural health is encouraged to read the books referred to in this chapter for a more thorough explanation of these issues.

Scientific Assumptions of the Empirical and Rational Schools of Health and Healing

Empirical School		*Rational School*
Observation and experience are source of knowledge	**Premise**	Logical analysis is the source of knowledge
Studies growth or balance of "life force" or vital energy	**Object**	Studies disease entities
Workings of life force unknowable	**Hypothesis**	Established hypothesis of causation
Studies peculiar symptoms to determine uniqueness of individual	**Subject**	Classifies common symptoms into disease entities
Subjective sources of data	**Source**	Objective sources of data
Individual is energetic and has a spiritual dimension	**Nature**	Individual is material or mechanistic, chemical
Treatment by similars sometimes creating healing crisis	**Treatment** (or treatment approach)	Treatment by contraries sought removal of symptoms
Health is internal and environmental balance	**Context**	Health is absence of disease
Holistic methodology	**Methodology**	Atomistic or reductionistic methodology
Client	**Authority**	Doctor

***Figure 20–1:** "Scientific Assumptions of the Rational and Empirical Schools of Health and Healing." The above table is reprinted with permission from an article by Jerry Green entitled "The Health Care Contract: A Model For Sharing Responsibility."*

THE EMPIRICAL AND RATIONAL SCHOOLS OF HEALTH AND HEALING

Jerry Green's article summarizes the scientific assumptions of medicine and holistic practice.[1] The table in this article provides a succinct summary of the two complementary approaches to health and healing.

Breaking an arm, you may have an allopathic doctor take x-rays and set the broken bone. You may also have a homeopathic practitioner administer the energetic remedy *Symphytum* to accelerate the natural internal mechanisms already at work healing the fracture.

Few would argue the great advances Western civilization has made in some fields of medicine. Our ability to save the lives of accident victims and repair injured limbs and organs with great medical skills and drugs is marvelous.

But, these are acute care issues.

Robert S. Mendelsohn, M.D., states in *Confessions of a Medical Heretic:*

> I believe that Modern Medicine has gone too far, by using in everyday situations extreme treatments designed for critical conditions....[2]

The Shift to Rational Medicine

With the invention of the printing press, and the education of the masses in the skills of reading, writing, and math, industrialized societies evolved. Scientists began emphasizing the 3-Rs, logic, and cause and effect. Objective, rational data was decreed as the only valid source of knowledge.

Bates performed his research and presented his concepts on natural vision at a time when this society was spiraling (and continues to spiral) deeper into an overly left-brain, rationalist, myopic tunnel vision of health and healing.

Chiropractic has been attacked by the orthodox for decades,[3] as have osteopathy, naturopathy, the Bates method, and many other natural approaches to health and healing.

"Why Haven't I Heard of the Bates Method Before?"

The Bates method and Natural Vision teachers have been attacked, threatened, and ridiculed by the orthodox for over seventy-five years.

In the Preface to *Eye Education by Bates Method,* Natural Vision teacher Margaret Corbett, who studied with Bates, wrote:

> The development of civilization is a series of conflicts, some consisting of wars but most of them arising from a clash of ideas. Each step forward has been opposed by those who cling to the outworn thoughts and antiquated methods, and progress has been slowed. Fortunately, the retarding of the tempo of progress has not been wholly detrimental. For a new idea to be accepted, it must first be tested in the searing fires of criticism, ridicule and invective. To survive these ordeals the new idea must be correct, as the fallacious and unsound ones are destroyed by the attacks made upon them.
>
> So it has been with the Bates system of eye education. Though it was developed through long and sound research, it was nevertheless novel ... and when it was presented to the public, it immediately met with the opposition of those who believed that if glasses were good enough for their forefathers they are good enough for us. Some of this antagonism was sincere and came from those who were still unconvinced that Dr. Bates' discoveries would benefit mankind. Some of the attacks undoubtedly were inspired by less admirable reasons.

Regardless of the motives activating those opposing us, they were energetic in their assaults and soon we were being set upon from all sides. The hostilities grew in intensity and finally culminated in criminal prosecution. To the casual observer it appeared to be charged against me, but actually not only was I on trial, but also the entire system of eye education developed by Dr. Bates. Facing the criminal charge was a bitter ordeal, but since our cause was just and our system of eye education meritorious, we prevailed. The jury found me not guilty of practicing medicine or optometry.[4]

In 1943, George A. Posner wrote about Corbett's trial in *SIR!* magazine:

> ... They took her to court, all right, but try as they might, they could not obtain a conviction. And why? Because the charge was merely a sham. A cover-up of the good doctors' attempt to restrain Mrs. Corbett from ... teaching a certain method of eye education of proven success, because *they* had decreed it was verboten!!
>
> Why were the doctors up in arms about this so-called "pernicious activity"? Because of complaints of persons injured or defrauded by the defendant? Not at all!
>
> Three hundred witness clamored for the privilege of testifying. They thronged into the courtroom, told of the healing of practically every eye disorder known to ophthalmological practice ... *without the use of medicine or the wearing of glasses!* They ranged in age from four to 84; they sat for days in the anteroom of the court waiting for a chance to "have their say." ...
>
> [Aldous Huxley's testimony received special attention, as he demonstrated he could read without glasses though he had been totally blind in one eye and only had 20% sight in the other eye before taking lessons from Corbett. In two months he was reading without glasses.]
>
> Not one iota of adverse testimony was uncovered or proven. Although the doctors had used every endeavor, even to the sending of two female spies to take Mrs. Corbett's purported "treatments" for the sake of gathering evidence, they weren't able to procure a single instance whereby "medical practice" could be proven. Nor could anyone be found who considered himself injured or defrauded. In fact, the female spies were found in the side-room during the trial, practicing some of Mrs. Corbett's eye techniques!
>
> The court had no alternative but to dismiss the case against Mrs. Margaret Darst Corbett. And the publicity of it served her well. A number of the jurors and many of the spectators signed up for Mrs. Corbett's course.
>
> The Los Angeles trial revealed that there had been similar prosecutions of adherents of this new teaching throughout the country over a period of years. ...
>
> For over 30 years organized medicine has fought with every possible means to keep the news of this revolutionary discovery from the world![5]

Natural vision teacher Janet Goodrich, Ph.D., in discussing possible reasons why many people have not heard of the Bates method, writes in her book *Natural Vision Improvement:*

> ... the professional, technically trained eye practitioners ... were taught that the Bates method was ineffective, to be derided and distained. ...
>
> Margaret Corbett admonished the hundreds of teachers she trained in the 1940s and 1950s never to advertise, lecture or publish articles ... More understanding is generated by the knowledge that she was

> arrested (and acquitted) twice for practicing optometry without a license....
>
> In 1974, my colleague in San Francisco, Mrs. Anna Kaye, who'd been quietly transmitting Bates method principles for several decades, was visited by two undercover agents. She was told she was breaking the law on sixteen counts....
>
> You may now realize why substantiated object proof is scarce.[6]

Many people are not aware of the facts, or, if they are, they choose not to support them. Some orthodox are afraid of being ostracized (like Bates was ostracized) by their colleagues if they were to support Bates' work. I have talked with several such individuals, and many such references are made in the literature.[7]

From *Better Eyesight* magazine, July 1920:

> A small number of physicians, including a few eye specialists who have improved, or seen members of their families improve, eye troubles, without glasses, operations, or medication, have been convinced that the old theories about the eye ... are wrong; but very few have had courage to endorse the new education method publicly.

While completing the final parts of this book, I received a series of letters from an optometry student after he called me requesting my brochure. In his first letter, he invited me to "defend" my business practices and the Bates method of eyesight improvement or else he would assume his "allegations" that the Bates method is invalid, etc., are correct. In his second letter he suggested that my work and the Bates method were "medical schemes." In his attempts to support his position, he quoted from optometrist Gruman's book, *New Ways to Better Sight*—a book *supporting, teaching, and praising* the Bates method!

Margaret Y. Ferguson, D.C., wrote in the December 1945 *Journal of the California Chiropractic Association:*

> [Bates'] revolutionary principles have never been found to be in error, but for purely commercial reasons they are not generally accepted. In the last few years, all of Dr. Bates' experiments were twice repeated and confirmed.[8]

As Bates stated accurately in *Perfect Sight Without Glasses* (repeated):

> The fact is that, except in rare cases, man is not a reasoning being. He is dominated by authority, and when the facts are not in accord with the view imposed by authority, so much the worse for the facts. They may, and indeed must, win in the long run; but in the meantime the world gropes needlessly in darkness and endures much suffering that might have been avoided.

This is not just true of Bates' discoveries. It has been true of many, if not most, progressive discoveries since the beginning of civilization.

The recent emergence of more and more eye doctors supporting—and even teaching—the Bates method lends powerful validation to the truth of this educational method.

Due to suppression and ignorance[9] of the Bates method, it is likely its benefits, including "the prevention of an incalculable amount of human misery" (Bates), may not be known by the majority of people for many years to come.

What's Going On?

Mendelsohn, using a religion analog to orthodox medicine, warns in *Confessions of a Medical Heretic:*

> ... Modern Medicine has started to become *more than defensive.* It must rely on *force* to maintain itself and grow ... and has grown more oppressive and violent.... What was once the option of a free people is becoming an enforced obligation.[10]

Kenneth R. Pelletier, in his book *Holistic Medicine: From Stress to Optimum Health,* writes:

> Rather than emphasizing prevention and self-care, the United States has placed its faith in hospitals, biomedical technology, and medical expertise while ignoring destructive life-style habits until too late....
>
> Overall, the data illustrate quite clearly that most health hazards for most age groups are both predictable and related to life-style.[11]

SYMPTOMS—MESSAGES OF IMBALANCE

When a person becomes imbalanced, there are usually uncomfortable symptoms associated with that imbalance.

If a person overworks, fatigue may set in. The body requires rest to re-establish a balance. If a person digests harmful food, the stomach may ache. Physical symptoms can also be caused by emotional, mental, and/or spiritual stress.

The question is, "What do I do with my symptoms?"

OUR LEGALLY DRUGGED SOCIETY

In 1965, Henry G. Bieler, M.D., wrote in *Food is Your Best Medicine:*

> I came to the conclusion that I, personally, must give up the use of drugs and henceforth rely solely on food as my medicine. It wasn't long until (after repeated verified results) I discarded drugs in treating my patients....
>
> Today we are not only in the Atomic Age, but also the Antibiotic Age. Unhappily, too, this is the Dark Age of Medicine....
>
> Far too many of these new "miracle" drugs are introduced with fanfare and then revealed as lethal in character, to be silently discarded for newer and more powerful drugs.[12]

One of the consequences of the rationalist approach to health problems has been the mass production, marketing, and use of powerful and oftentimes dangerous drugs. Some of the so-called "side effects" of drugs are worse than the symptoms the drug is supposed to eliminate. Could it be that the "side effects" are actually the *primary* effects, lowering the overall health of the individual in the long term?

The norm in this society is to demand "quick fixes" when health symptoms appear. "Fix me quick, Doc, I am a busy person with a tight schedule." Americans often choose to eliminate uncomfortable symptoms as fast as possible—regardless, and often ignorant, of both short- and long-term consequences.

A recent survey showed that more than 70% of the parents in one large California city demand antibiotics from doctors to eliminate their child's illness symptoms quickly. If a doctor refuses to give the child an antibiotic, the parent simply finds another doctor who will. The parent wants to return the child to school quickly so the parent can return to work as soon as possible. As of 1994, over

25% of American children live in single-parent families. It appears there is little time for natural healing.

June Biermann and Barbara Toohey write in their book *The Woman's Holistic Headache Relief Book:*

> Drugs may work for acute, short-lived pain, but for the chronic pain we're involved with here, they have the dual problem of quickly losing their effectiveness and of causing addiction. On top of these negatives, they can have harmful to disastrous side effects, especially when they interact with other drugs. In short, your headaches can't kill you, but the drugs you take to relieve them can.
>
> Our main objection to using painkillers, tranquilizers, mood elevators, antidepressants, antihistamines, and all the rest of the chemical crutches many sufferers lean on is that drugs do not heal.[13]

SURGERIES 'R US

In 1992, more than 22,000,000 surgical procedures were performed on Americans—an average of 60,000 surgeries per day. Many of these surgeries are unnecessary.

Surgeries are a relatively easy, "quick fix" option for many Americans because many insurance companies pay most or all of the medical costs. How quickly would Westerners change their approach to health and healing if insurance companies stopped paying for drugs and surgeries?

Refractive corneal surgeries like radial keratotomy (RK) and photorefractive keratectomy (PRK) are now being mass-marketed and performed on hundreds of thousands of eyes. None of the commercials and ads I have seen give *all* the facts a person should know regarding the possible risks involved in these surgeries.

For example, none of the ads I have seen mention the following facts: In the 1950s, over 100 people in Japan underwent an early form of RK surgery. All of these people needed to have corneal transplants within ten years of the operation. The long-term development of degenerative corneal diseases was described by one ophthalmologist as "catastrophic complications." For the most part, even the corneal transplants were unsuccessful in restoring their sight. According to a local ophthalmologist, "essentially all" of these people became blind. As late as 1992, a California man was described as being "functionally blind" due to RK surgery. He won a $5.4 million lawsuit.

Military academies and some flight training programs have disqualified pilots who have had RK. The FBI refuses application to become an agent for anyone who has had RK. A person considering RK may want to investigate why these policies have been established if he, or someone he knows, is thinking of letting someone cut or laser beam his corneas.

Perhaps RK and PRK surgeries are appealing to some because they represent the epitome of the "quick fix," reductionistic, left-brain approach to eyesight—a super hi-tech, million-dollar machine approach to improving acuity artificially. The technology may be exceptional, but the healing of the scars is unpredictable from one patient to the next. There are many potentially serious risks involved with these surgeries. One fact has been established: any individual undergoing corneal surgery risks losing his eyesight—permanently.

A primary tenet of orthodox medicine has been never to perform surgery on healthy tissue. It appears this tenet has now changed.

Obviously, many people have better acuity soon after these surgeries—but what about the long-term consequences?

Most importantly from the holistic perspective: even if temporarily freed from "corrective" lenses, the underlying cause of blurred vision—mental strain—remains. And what happens to the acuity if the patient relaxes and the chronically tight eye muscles release their tension around the eyeballs? (This is discussed more later.)

I do not accept registrations from individuals who have had RK, PRK, or similar types of refractive corneal surgeries.

THE CONSEQUENCES—FROM THE PHYSICAL TO THE EMOTIONAL PLANE

Vithoulkas in *The Science of Homeopathy* and *A New Model for Health and Disease* presents a remarkable perspective on the mental-emotional-physical interrelationships of progressive illnesses, and healing.

Generally, physical symptoms (the outer plane) are relatively less important than emotional or mental symptoms. A person can live a happy, productive life without a leg. Emotional symptoms (the middle plane) are more important than physical symptoms. Anxiety can be handled. Mental symptoms (the inner plane) are the most important in regards to overall health. Destructive delirium is a very serious mental problem.

An individual's history of chronic health problems often shows a trend from the physical, through the emotional, toward the mental symptoms.

A person may have skin eruptions (physical) when young. Many teenagers use drugs and/or surgeries to "correct" acne. Later, a liver dysfunction may develop. With enough drugs, the liver symptoms may diminish or disappear, after which irrational mood swings (emotional level) may develop.

If powerful drugs are used to "fight" emotional disturbances, the "disease" can then shift into the mental realm. One drug used to control panic disorder causes some people to develop both short-term and long-term memory loss.

Some psychotics have had a prior history of physical and emotional disturbances before becoming psychotic. During psychosis, many of their physical and emotional symptoms can disappear.

The shifting from one state of illness to another makes it difficult to identify any one drug or surgery as the cause of the worsening state of health. The *energetic* state of the illness keeps shifting. A new, different "totality of symptoms" often emerges.

As a result, different disease states seem to be unrelated. A drug used to "control" high blood pressure is not connected to the later appearance of Crohn's disease. The drugs and surgeries used to combat Crohn's disease are not connected to the appearance of cancer.

In the attempt to "defeat" the cancer, chemotherapy, radiation treatments, and powerful drugs are used to "fight the enemy." Even when these solutions eradicate the cancerous cells, how do they affect the *person?* Is the underlying *cause* of the cancer eliminated?

Many patients are blindly shuffled from one specialist to another, until, finally, they are told, "There is nothing more Western medicine can do for you." This is true.

It appears that the overall disease state of our nation is shifting from the physical level into the emotional level.

Mortimer Zuckerman, editor-in-chief of *U.S. News & World Report,* writes:

> The youthful world has become dramatically more violent. Consider this piece of anecdotal evidence turned up by CBS News: The seven top problems in public schools in 1940 were identified by teachers as talking out of turn, chewing gum, making noise, running in the halls, cutting in line, dress-code infractions and littering. By 1980, the seven top problems had been identified as suicide, assault, robbery, rape, drug abuse, alcohol abuse and pregnancy.[14]

What is the explanation for the grave health problems confronting industrialized nations today? Could the increasingly serious health problems in our society be due to the relentless chemical and mechanical assaults on the human organism in the last forty years?

The wanton use of powerful drugs and surgeries constitutes the two major causes, if not *the two greatest* causes, of the health crisis we are now in.

AN ISSUE OF AWARENESS AND SELF-RESPONSIBILITY

> *I'm alive, I'm awake, I'm aware.*
>
> —Lyrics from the song "I'm Beginning to See the Light"

Natural vision student Dr. Shoichi Aoyagi, D.C., a San Francisco chiropractor and Ayurvedic practitioner of eleven years, writes:

> I have seen far too many people relinquish their responsibility for good health and hand it over to the health care practitioner. Optimum health begins and ends with responsibility. There are no magic drugs or cures that will totally resolve a health issue.
>
> If a person does not take the responsibility to eat right, breathe properly, exercise regularly, and actively reduce distress, the disease will return or manifest in a different form. The only lesson the person learns is: When another problem arises, it is time to return to the doctor for more drugs and surgeries. This is simply another version of the Pavlovian dog response.
>
> Unfortunately, many people have gone from human *beings* to human *doings.* We allow the medical profession to *do* all sorts of unnatural and harmful procedures to us—from vaccinations to chemotherapy.
>
> This is not to say that orthodox medicine does not have its place; it does. But with proper attention and care to one's own body, many health problems may be avoided. If good health is a concern, begin by becoming aware of what enters your body as well as your mind. From there, your mind and body will only want what is most beneficial and nurturing.
>
> Twentieth-century medicine has been—for the most part—about cutting out, irradiating, and suppressing unwanted diseases from the body—a violent form of health care. But twentieth-century health care will revert back to the wisdom of the past when people took responsibility for their own well-being and lived in peace and harmony with nature.[15]

SYMPTOMS—HOW TO ANSWER THE MESSAGES

Mendelsohn writes:

> I believe that more than ninety percent of Modern Medicine could disappear from the face of the Earth—doctors, hospitals, drugs, and equipment—and the effect on our health would be immediate and beneficial.[16]

One of the advantages of improving vision naturally is that the individual often becomes aware of other parts of his life that are out of balance. With awareness, changes can begin.

Symptoms are usually messages of imbalance.

How a person deals with current symptoms can have major consequences on his long-term health. If the person supports the body in healing naturally, the symptoms can pass, and the person can return to his former state of health. Oftentimes the individual becomes even stronger after healing naturally.

If the person suppresses the symptoms with drugs or removes a part of the body by surgery, his health will likely lower. The problem is: even though a specific symptom may no longer be present, its *cause* can remain. And if the cause remains, the person is still ill.

This is where the Western, reductionistic (left-brain) approach to health and healing has failed. Our health system is not balanced with the empirical (right-brain) approach to health and healing—especially in respect to long-term health problems.

Psychiatrist M. Scott Peck, M.D., writes in his bestseller *The Road Less Traveled:*

> The other development that is assisting us to escape from scientific tunnel vision is the relatively recent discovery by science of the reality of paradox. A hundred years ago paradox meant error to the [rational] scientific mind. But exploring such phenomena as the nature of light, electromagnetism, quantum mechanics and relativity theory, physical science has matured over the past century to the point where it is increasingly recognized that at a certain level reality is paradoxical.[17]

Peck then quotes the nuclear physicist J. Robert Oppenheimer:

> To what appears to be the simplest questions, we will tend to give either no answer or an answer which will at first sight be reminiscent more of a strange catechism than of the straightforward affirmations of physical science. If we ask, for instance, whether the position of the electron remains the same, we must say "no"; if we ask whether the electron's position changes with time, we must say "no"; if we ask whether the electron is at rest, we must say "no"; if we ask whether it is in motion, we must say "no." The Buddha has given such answers when interrogated as to the conditions of a man's self after his death; but they are not the familiar answers for the tradition of seventeenth- and eighteenth-century science.[18]

More and more Westerners are availing themselves of empirical approaches to health and healing—because, in the proper hands, they can be more effective. A few insurance companies now cover some "alternative" health care modalities. They are discovering these modalities can be cost-effective.

TWO PARTS TO NATURAL HEALING

> *The doctor of the future will give no medicine but will interest his patients in the care of the human frame, in diet and in the cause and prevention of disease.*
>
> —Thomas Edison

> *The art of medicine consists of amusing the patient while nature heals the disease.*
>
> —Voltaire

Two major parts of natural healing are: 1) removing the causes of the imbalances, and 2) accelerating healing.

Removing the Causes

In order to truly heal, the original cause or causes of the imbalance need to be removed.

It is often helpful if the cause can be identified. If poor diet, including overeating, is the cause of an illness, the diet must change. Many types of cancer have now been correlated to poor diet. If over-working is the cause of an illness, rest is needed. If excessive emotional, mental, or spiritual strain or trauma is the cause, it must be resolved. If harmful drugs are the cause, they must (eventually) be eliminated.

The *cumulative* effect of different stresses can create a critical health problem. This can explain why one modality of natural healing might be just as effective as another—when the total strain on the system is lowered, the illness may heal.

Of course, removing the real cause is usually easier said than done. True healing of chronic health problems often requires changes in the person's lifestyle.

Sometimes, the underlying cause is never identified but can still be removed by natural healing. In fact, one of the assumptions of the empirical school of health and healing is: "Workings of life force unknowable." See *Figure 20–1: "Scientific Assumptions of the Rational and Empirical Schools of Health and Healing."*

Accelerating Healing

The period of time required to heal severe imbalances may be unacceptably long if only the original causes are removed. A person may want to access holistic healing modalities to accelerate the rate of healing.

Some modalities of natural healing are described briefly here. For a larger presentation, refer to Richard Grossinger's *Planet Medicine: Modalities,* listed in the Bibliography.

Homeopathy

Dr. Samuel Hahnemann, 1755–1843, was the first physician to fully recognize the principles of homeopathy. G. Kent Smith, M.D., in *Homeopathy: Medicine for Today's Living,* writes:

> Hahnemann soon decided that he was doing his patients and family more harm than good by treating them according to the accepted medical practice of the day. For this reason he gave up the practice of medicine …
>
> Homeopathy has no medicine for the name of a disease. Each patient, regardless of the name of his complaint, must be treated according to his individual symptoms …
>
> Homeopathy treats the patient and not the disease.[19]

Vithoulkas, in *Homeopathy, Medicine of the New Man,* writes:

> Finally, after centuries of stumbling and experimenting, we have a system of medicine that not only recognizes the presence of the healing powers of the body and of Nature, the vital force, but actually bases its entire system upon the stimulation of that force.[20]

Basically, homeopathy works by stimulating the specific life-force energy currently at work within an individual which is attempting to heal that individual.

The set of physical-emotional-mental symptoms created in a healthy person by taking a large dosage of Substance A is the same set of symptoms an energized dilution of Substance A will heal in an ill person. This *law of similars* is based on philosophies of healing dating back more than 2000 years to Hippocrates.

Maesimund Panos, M.D., and Jane Heimlich, in *Homeopathic Medicine at Home,* write:

> Hahnemann did not claim to discover the concept. In the tenth century BC, Hindu sages described the law, as had Hippocrates, who wrote in 400 BC: "Through the like, disease is produced and through the application of the like, it is cured." Paracelsus, a sixteenth-century German physician, reiterated the law. Hahnemann, as an erudite thinker, was undoubtedly familiar with these writings, but he was the first to test the principle and establish it as the cornerstone of a system of medicine.[21]

Western critics have long ridiculed diluted homeopathy remedies as worthless. Yet, sophisticated scientific instruments have now shown that the energetic property of a solvent changes after diluting and succussing a solute *beyond the point that any solute atoms remain in the solute.*[22]

G.P. Barnard and James H. Stephenson state, "... in homeopathy one may be giving to a patient the informational content of a chemical without any actual chemical mass...."[23]

Critics also state the diluted homeopathic remedies are of value only because of the placebo effect. Yet remedies are effective when used with animals and babies. Additionally, rigorous double-blind tests have proven homeopathy is effective.

Acupuncture

Like homeopathy (I like to refer to homeopathy as "needleless acupuncture"), acupuncture is based on the flow of energy through the body. Many imbalances can be corrected with an experienced acupuncturist.

Chinese healing philosophy connects the visual system to the liver and kidneys. Chinese doctors say if a person has liver or kidney problems, that person can have vision problems. One Eastern healer I talked with said that many of her clients who wear corrective lenses have "classic liver-yin deficiency." Yin is a right-brain characteristic.

Couldn't the opposite also be true? If a person chronically strains his visual system, could he have liver or kidney problems?

I met one acupuncturist who, by reading natural vision books and receiving acupuncture, eliminated his need for corrective lenses.

Herbs

Herbs can help detoxify and restore balance to the body.

The acupuncturist just mentioned said the herb *Ming Mu Ti Huang Wan* has been used by many Eastern healers to nourish "yin-deficient" liver and kidneys and to improve eyesight. Benefits reported by others include increased lacrimation (tearing) for dry eyes and reduction of sensitivity to bright light.

Iridology

Classical iridology focuses much of its attention on imbalances caused by poor diet. These imbalances can be "read" in the iris. See *Figure 20–2: "Chart to Iridology"* by Bernard Jensen, D.C., Ph.D.

On the physical level, the colon is considered to be the "hub" of the nutritional system. The area of the iris that corresponds to the colon encircles the pupil like the hub of a wheel. The areas related to the organs of the body extend out from the central colon area, like the spokes of a wheel, to the outer edges of the iris.

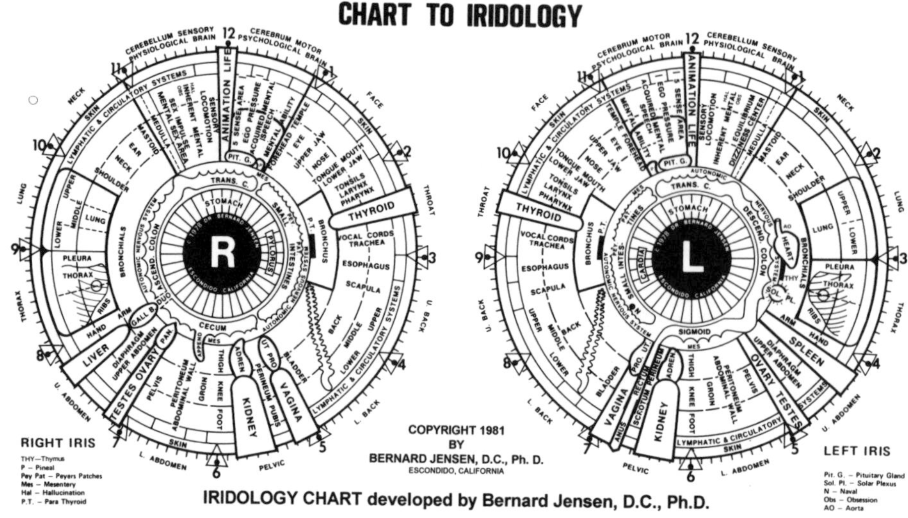

Figure 20–2: "Chart to Iridology."
Permission granted to reprint the "Chart to Iridology" by Bernard Jensen, D.C., Ph.D., that appears in his book The Science and Practice of Iridology.

Normal bowel movements and proper elimination are very important in iridology. The classical iridologist often recommends changes in diet, detoxification, herbs, supplements, fasts, enemas, and colonics, if needed.

Tom's Personal Log: Iridology has been one of my most important healing modalities. My iridologist/nutritionist, who was trained by Dr. Bernard Jensen, helped me discover I had an impacted colon, among several other serious problems.

Massage Therapy/Bodywork

Professional massage therapy and bodywork are often helpful in releasing chronic tension in the body. They can also educate the client about how she is living, providing her with the opportunity to make adjustments in her lifestyle. Since the neck and shoulders are tight for people who have blurred vision, have the masseuse give special attention to these areas.

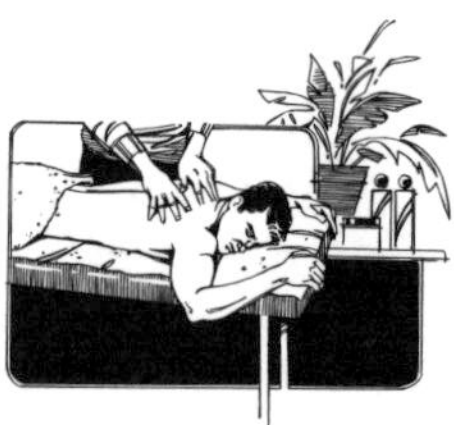

Tip: Schedule a one-and-a-half-hour massage, not just one hour. The extra half-hour makes a big difference.

Color Healing

See *Figure 19–3: Brain Characteristics.*

The colors red, orange, and yellow are associated with the left hemisphere. Blue, indigo, and violet are associated with the right hemisphere. Green is the "balancing" color.

Psychologists have known for many years the impact of colors on the mind. Have you ever seen a fast-food restaurant which does not use the colors red, orange, and yellow? These colors activate the hunger centers in the body.

In respect to healing, left-brain dominant individuals can use right-brain colors, for example, blue, to help re-establish a balance. Right-brain dominant individuals can use left-brain colors, for example, red and orange, to help re-establish a balance.

Stanley Burroughs, in his book *Healing for the Age of Enlightenment,* states:

> All hot (acute/left-brain) disorders are corrected or balanced by use of the cold colors. All cold (chronic/right-brain) disorders are corrected or balanced by the use of the warm colors.[24]

The color red is a hot, or warm, color; blue is a cold, or cool, color.

The color red is associated with near vision; the color blue is associated with far vision. Many nearsights have derived benefits from right-brain colors, and many farsights have derived benefits from left-brain colors. *Light: Medicine of the Future,* by Jacob Liberman, contains a list of color work (syntonic) practitioners.

Other Healing Modalities

In addition to the above holistic modalities, many people have received benefit from the following incomplete list:

- Stress reduction programs
- Osteopathy
- Naturopathy
- Cranial-mandibular orthopedics (TMJ)
- Craniosacral therapy
- Chiropractic
- Acupressure
- Ortho-bionomy
- Retreats
- Applied Kinesiology
- Breathing education
- Yoga
- Rolfing (Structural Integration)
- Exercise
- Meditation
- Natural vision training

All of the above have contributed significantly to the improvement of my health.

The Feldenkrais Method and Alexander Technique, and many other holistic modalities, can also be beneficial. All types of holistic health support each other. Holistic modalities are opportunities to return to, and maintain, a balance.

MESSAGES OF PROGRESS—AGGRAVATIONS AND REVERSALS

HEALING AGGRAVATIONS

It is sometimes difficult to distinguish between symptoms caused by doing something unhealthy, and symptoms caused by natural healing. If a person begins natural healing, and then feels uncomfortable, he might conclude he is doing something incorrect—when, in fact, he may finally be giving his body an opportunity to truly heal.

A *healing aggravation* is a period in which the mind, emotions, and/or body experience symptoms *because of* natural healing.

In his *Doctor-Patient Handbook: Dealing with The Reversal Process and The Healing Crisis through Elimination Diets and Detoxification,* Dr. Bernard Jensen emphasizes

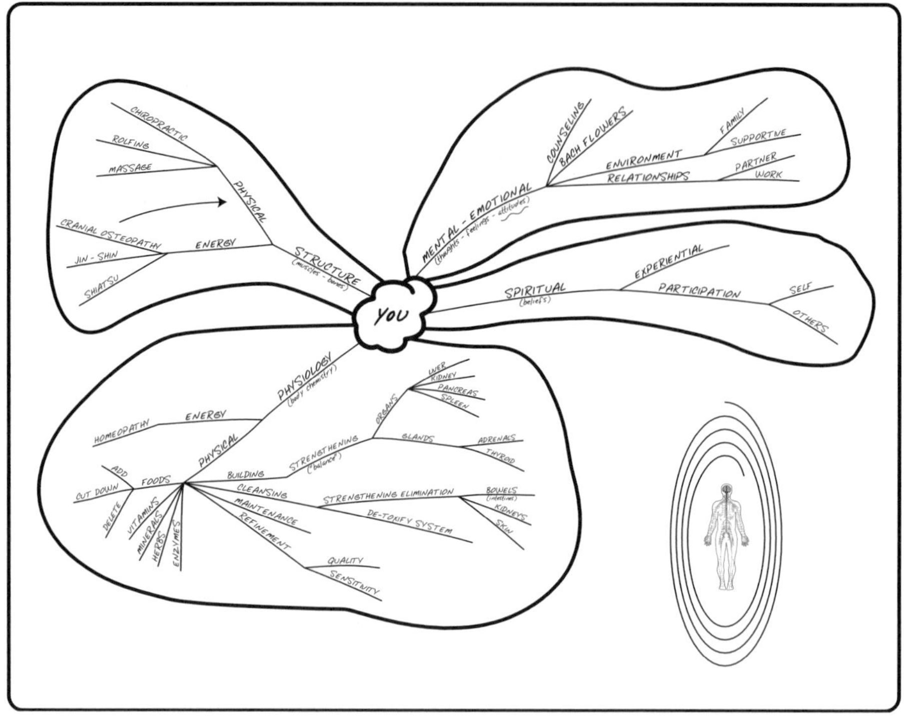

Figure 20–3: "Georgia's View of Holistic Health." Reprinted with permission from Georgia Dow.

proper nutrition and detoxification. In regards to nutritional healing, he states there are two ways a person can know if they are experiencing a "healing crisis":

1. Usually the person feels stronger just before a healing crisis; and
2. Elimination is perfect.

Figure 20–4: "Homeopathic Aggravation and Healing" is a graph from Vithoulkas' *The Science of Homeopathy.* ("Homeopathic Aggravation and Healing" is my [TQ] caption.) This ideal case shows the intensity of symptoms *increasing* slightly after the homeopathic remedy is administered, followed by a dramatic decrease in symptoms.

Many vision students have had a tight neck for many years. When correct vision habits are practiced, the chronic tension begins to release. One student experienced soreness in her neck after a few weeks of practicing correct vision habits. In the sixth week of the course, she said that she had previously gone to many different holistic healers for her health problems. She stopped visiting every holistic practitioner after the first visit because she felt uncomfortable symptoms after their work. She had concluded that their work was making her worse. She now believes her reactions were healing aggravations.

Tom's Personal Log: The first treatment I received from a holistic doctor (an M.D.) resulted in excruciating back pain. By the

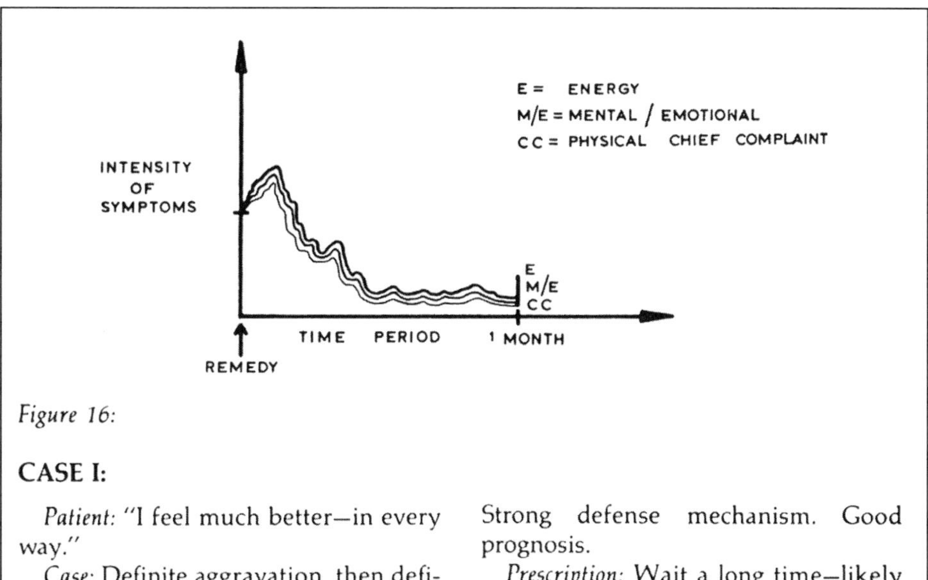

Figure 16:

CASE I:

Patient: "I feel much better—in every way."

Case: Definite aggravation, then definite improvement of all symptoms.

Interpretation: Remedy was precise. Strong defense mechanism. Good prognosis.

Prescription: Wait a long time—likely six months or more.

Figure 20–4: "Homeopathic Aggravation and Healing."
Graph reprinted with permission from Grove Press, Inc.

time I returned to work, I felt nauseated and dizzy. I called the doctor and he explained that such reactions can occur for some people. I felt so "ill" I had to go home.

The healing aggravations I experienced were proportional to my critical health problems. Not everyone experiences such painful aggravations. Over the next several months, I had significant improvement in my health.

The experience of uncomfortable healing aggravations may cause a person to approach holistic healing patiently. It takes time and energy to heal. A very ill person does not have a lot of energy.

Education and understanding may be the most important part of natural healing. When one identifies and uses true, natural modalities of healing, the healing aggravations from those modalities can be regarded as correct. If healing aggravations are suppressed, the illness can continue and become worse.

Of course, a person must not allow a serious symptom to go unattended when it is *not* part of a healing aggravation. This is where the study of holistic books can be helpful, along with consulting experienced natural health practitioners.

In regard to long-term health issues, I have come the conclusion that:

- With conventional approaches to health problems, a person often feels better right away (due to the suppression of symptoms), but becomes less healthy in the long term.

- With natural approaches to health problems, a person often feels worse right away (due to a healing aggravation), but becomes more healthy in the long term.

Not only *can* a person feel worse temporarily, some holistic practitioners *anticipate* healing aggravations. They can be a sign of true healing.

Another clue to natural healing is re-experiencing the same (or similar) symptoms we had in the past. These are known as reversals. Reversals often occur during a healing aggravation.

Reversals—A Clue to True Healing

Healing occurs from within out (the most important inner organs heal first), from above down (head down to the feet), and in the reverse order in which they were acquired.

—Hering's Law of Healing

When an imbalance from the past is addressed by natural methods, some of the mental, emotional, spiritual, and/or physical manifestations of that strain can return temporarily. This is known as a reversal. A *reversal* is a full or partial return of symptoms of a former imbalance that did not fully heal in the past. Reversals are very common when a person begins natural healing.

For example, a person may take correct action to heal his cancer by eliminating harmful foods from his diet. If this person eliminates his cancer, he does not necessarily become 100% healthy immediately. Rather, a previous—but less serious—illness from the past may take the cancer's place.

Jensen, in his *Doctor-Patient Handbook,* describes the progression of illnesses, and the reversal experiences his patients go through when they improve their diet and/or fast. This book is one of the most important I have read on health and healing.

Tom's Personal Log:

A. When I was born, casts and braces were immediately put on my deformed legs, so that I would be able to walk in the future.

After the first eight months of natural healing (about age 30), my legs started to bow back in again. I walked around awkwardly for about three days, after which my legs felt fine again. My holistic doctor told me he had found the cause of my leg problem in my spinal column, and he was correcting the imbalance with cranial-sacral manipulations.

B. Because of my illnesses as a child, I liked the rain because I did not have to go outdoors. Every winter, when others complained, I would say how much I liked the rain.

In the winter of 1993, after many years of holistic healing, I began to tell my osteopath/chiropractor/acupuncturist how much I liked the rain. But something strange occurred this time. I said, "I like the ra—. Wait a minute. No, I don't. I was going to say, 'I like the rain.' But I don't anymore. I am healthier now, and I want to be outside in the sunshine."

Reversals can occur on all levels.

I discovered that to move *forward* with my health problems, I needed to go *backward* temporarily. The old tension and strain were still in my body/mind, and needed to be released in order to truly heal. The alternative was to remain ill.

Reversals do not always appear in exactly

the reverse order in which they developed. Which symptoms return at a specific time depends to some degree on the timing and type of the natural healing the individual is receiving. For example, if a person had flues in early childhood, and neck problems later due to a car accident, the flu symptoms may return before the neck symptoms if the person begins changing her diet. The neck symptoms may resurface later during chiropractic adjustments.

Reactions may be exaggerated during a healing aggravation or reversal. Natural healing can be powerful, and the mind-body wants to eliminate any imbalances as quickly as possible.

In the case of chronic neck tension, a person's neck may have become tighter more each year for many years. While improving vision, a healing aggravation in the neck may be exaggerated because the healing process occurs in a relatively short period of time (a few months for some people). Compare this to the time it took for the neck to become chronically tight.

The student of natural health may appreciate the importance of healing health problems in the correct manner when they first occur. If problems are suppressed, the life-force energy of that individual can lower, and the symptoms may need to be experienced again in the future when true healing is used.

During a natural vision course, one of my students remembered how she diffused when a swarm of bees surrounded her. She tried to see all of the bees at the same time. This is an example of a vision reversal. Reversals related to vision are common experiences during natural vision improvement. They are a sign of true healing.

Tom's Personal Log: After about two years of improving my vision, a memory returned to me of being in the yard of my home as a child. I was watching a bee fly from one flower to another flower. I was moving my head naturally, and centralizing perfectly. I had normal vision and excellent vision habits at that time.

This return of the memory of normal vision and correct vision habits was an important part of my vision improvement process. I now practiced better vision habits more each day—not just because my vision was improving—but because these vision habits are *exactly* the same ones I used to have when I had normal, clear sight long ago. The vision habits I am relearning are natural and normal. I am now relearning to see.

"Health Returns in Cycles"

Figure 20–5: "Health Returns in Cycles" shows various factors involved as health becomes worse, and when it gets better.

As health becomes worse, as shown on the left side of the graph, there are times when a person feels better—the body wants to heal. Notice on the right side of the graph that there are temporary setbacks when improving health. Some of these setbacks can be caused by healing aggravations.

Some students take a rigid approach to their vision improvement process. They expect the vision to improve constantly every day—linearly, without any setbacks. This will not happen. Vision improvement is no different from other forms of relearning or learning processes. There will be fluctuations and temporary setbacks. Unpredictable fluctuation is primarily a right-brain characteristic and is part of the natural vision improvement process.

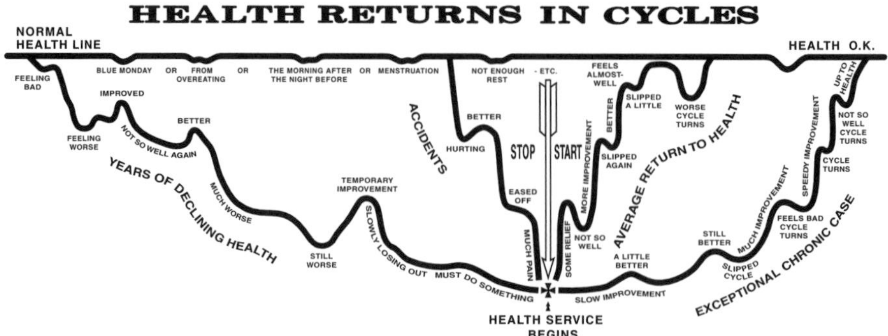

Figure 20–5: "Health Returns in Cycles."
Reprinted with permission from Share International, Inc.

When learning to play tennis, your skills improve over time. But on some days, it seems like you never played tennis at all, missing almost every shot. The same is true while learning to play a musical instrument. Yet, with continued practice, your skills improve. The key to success is to *continue* practicing. Do not quit because of temporary setbacks. Temporary setbacks are a natural part of any improvement process.

An important difference with the vision improvement process is that we were not born playing tennis or the piano. Virtually all of us had clear vision and proper vision habits at a very young age. In this process, we are literally *re*learning to see. *Anyone can relearn to do something they used to do perfectly.* Another difference is that one does not play tennis or the piano all day long. Correct vision habits are meant to be used our entire lifetime.

Changes in weather and the seasons can create fluctuations in vision and affect the rate of improvement. One vision teacher noted that in winter (in New York) it took three lessons for her students to have the same benefit they received with only one lesson in the spring or fall. High humidity and heat can also slow down vision improvement. In fact, *anything* that interferes with relaxed vision habits can slow progress.

HOLISTIC EDUCATION AND PRACTITIONERS

A person who wants to improve his health through natural methods may need to read many books, attend classes, and consult with holistic practitioners before the main cause or causes of his problems can be addressed. Studying a specific holistic modality can help you choose a practitioner that approaches that modality in the way you feel is correct.

I have seen and experienced several variations of holistic practices that I do not recommend. For example, some homeopathic remedies are now being combined, or mixed. In classical homeopathy, only single remedies have been "proven." I am not aware of any research in which mixtures have been proven. Homeopathic mixtures are a diffused, "shotgun" approach to homeopathy.

Maesimund Panos and Jane Heimlich write in *Homeopathic Medicine at Home:*

> This is a controversial issue ... But many of us believe that far better results are obtained in the long run by adhering strictly to fundamental laws of homeopathy, which include the single remedy.[25]

The classical, single-remedy approach is especially important in constitutional homeopathic healing. Using a single remedy at a time is a form of centralization.

Accessing an experienced health practitioner who understands his profession can sometimes be more important than the specific modality chosen. All forms of holistic health, when understood and applied correctly, move the individual toward a higher level of health. If possible, obtain a referral from someone you trust.

Even if the first holistic modality chosen is not the one most needed, oftentimes the benefits and awareness from that modality can lead the individual to the one most needed.

It is possible to "overdose" on holistic health. If a person engages in too many modalities at one time, the system can become confused. "Diffusion is confusion" even in holistic healing. Those individuals engaging in natural healing may choose to limit the number of modalities during a particular period of time.

CHAPTER COMMENTS

Many of the issues briefly touched on in this chapter are complex and serious. I realize they may be new to the reader.

I am not against Western medicine. The Western approach to accidents and injuries is often outstanding. But I am forced to agree with many of the world's leading natural health practitioners that people living in industrialized societies are—as a whole—extremely unhealthy. The Western, mechanical, left-brain, "quick-fix" approach to long-term health simply does not work. Worse, people become more ill. More and more people are realizing this fact and are seeking natural, holistic methods—methods that work. We need a balanced approach to our health.

As natural vision is a holistic process, many natural vision students have used holistic modalities to support their vision improvement process. Natural healing can require time, energy, trust, and patience. The reward is better health—especially in the long term.

Hippocrates, from *Regimen in Health, Book IX:*

> A wise man should consider that health is the greatest of human blessings, and learn how by his own thought to derive benefit from his illnesses.

Notes

1 Jerry Green is an attorney in Marin County, California, specializing in laws pertaining to holistic health and holistic practitioners, and is a natural vision improvement student. For a complimentary copy of the introduction to the consulting format "Holistic Practice Forum," send a self-addressed, stamped envelope to Jerry Green, P. O. Box 5094, Mill Valley, CA 94942.

2 Robert S. Mendelsohn, *Confessions of a Medical Heretic* (Chicago: Contemporary Books, Inc., 1979), p. xi.

3 At the 1966 clinical convention, the American Medical Association House of Delegates stated "chiropractic is an unscientific cult" and "chiropractic constitutes a hazard to rational health care...." One AMA official described chiropractors as "rabid dogs" and "killers." This same AMA official lectured to young physicians across the country, telling them chiropractic was stealing their money. Yet, in court, the defendants told the judge that chiropractic is efficient,

effective, therapeutic, and there is even scientific evidence for some portions of chiropractic. The judge stated, "the AMA knew of scientific studies implying that chiropractic care was twice as effective as medical care in relieving many painful conditions of the neck and back as well as related musculo-skeletal problems."

In 1987, Federal District Judge Susan Getzendanner found the defendants, the American Medical Association and two other medical groups, guilty of "overtly and covertly" trying to eliminate the profession of chiropractic in the United States. Judge Getzendanner ruled, "As early as September 1963, the AMA's objective was the complete elimination of the chiropractic profession ... In 1966 the AMA adopted an anti-chiropractic resolution ... In 1967, the AMA Judicial Council issued an opinion under Principle 3 specifically holding that it was unethical for a physician to associate professionally with chiropractors ... Keeping chiropractors out of hospitals was one of the goals of the boycott." Judge Getzendanner also stated that the AMA conducted "systematic, long-term wrongdoing and the long-term intent to destroy a licensed profession." The AMA engaged in numerous activities to maintain a medical physician monopoly over health care in this country. Judge Getzendanner issued a permanent injunction against the AMA, and two other medical groups, ruling they had violated Sherman Antitrust laws.

Source: The Summary of Opinion and Order and Permanent Injunction in *Wilk, et al., v. AMA, et al.,* and Complete Copy of Opinion and Order and Permanent Injunction Order in *Wilk, et al., v. AMA, et al.,* written by Federal District Judge Susan Getzendanner. An overview of this case can be found in "Wilk et al *vs.* AMA et al: DCs Win: Judge Finds AMA Guilty of Conspiracy, Issues Permanent Injunction," in *ICA International Review of Chiropractic* (October 1987).

Thanks to Dr. Michael D. Pedigo, D.C., one of the plaintiffs in this case, and his staff for providing me with this information. Dr. Pedigo is listed in the Resources/Holistic Health Appendix under San Leandro Chiropractic Center.

4 Margaret D. Corbett, *Eye Education by Bates Method* (Los Angeles: DeVorss & Co., 1943), p. 7.

5 George A. Posner, "Are Eye Glasses a Racket ... ?" in *SIR!* (August 1943).

6 Janet Goodrich, *Natural Vision Improvement* (Berkeley, California: Celestial Arts, 1985), pp. 184–85.

7 For example, see Bates' introduction to ophthalmologist E. F. Darling's testimonial in Chapter 29, " 'This Method Has Been Proved.' "

8 Margaret Y. Ferguson, "The Dr. Bates Method of Eye Training," in *Journal of the California Chiropractic Association* (December 1945), p. 13.

9 See "Ophthalmologist Darling's Testimonial" in Chapter 29, " 'This Method Has Been Proved,' " for one example.

10 Mendelsohn, *Confessions of a Medical Heretic,* p. 149.

11 Pelletier, Kenneth R., *Holistic Medicine: From Stress to Optimum Health* (New York: Dell Publishing Co., Inc., 1979), pp. 57–58.

12 Henry G. Bieler, *Food is Your Best Medicine* (New York: Random House, 1965), p. xiii.

13 June Biermann and Barbara Toohey, *The Woman's Holistic Headache Relief Book* (Los Angeles: J. P. Tarcher, Inc., 1979), p. 113.

14 Mortimer Zuckerman, editor-in-chief, "Editorial: The Victims of TV Violence," *U.S. News & World Report* (August 2, 1993), p. 64.

15 Personal communication to the author on July 26, 1996. Sho Aoyagi is planning to write a book on the topic of self-responsibility for health and healing.

16 Mendelsohn, *Confessions of a Medical Heretic,* p. xi.

17 M. Scott Peck, *The Road Less Traveled* (New York: Simon and Schuster, 1978), p. 227.

18 J. Robert Oppenheimer, *Science and the Common Understanding* (New York: Simon and Schuster, 1953), p. 40.

19 G. Kent Smith, *Homeopathy: Medicine for Today's Living* (Glendale, California: private printing, 1978), pp. 5–7.

[20] George Vithoulkas, *Homeopathy, Medicine of the New Man* (New York: Arco Publishing, Inc., 1979), p. 27.

[21] Maesimund B. Panos and Jane Heimlich, *Homeopathic Medicine at Home* (New York: G. P. Putnam's Sons, 1980), p. 11.

[22] James Stephenson, "On the Possible Field Effects of the Solvent Phase of Succussed High Dilutions," *Journal of the American Institute of Homeopathy* (September/October, 1966), pp. 9–10.

[23] G. P. Barnard and James H. Stephenson, "Fresh Evidence for a Biophysical Field," *Journal of the American Institute of Homeopathy* (April/May/June, 1969): Vol. 62.

[24] Stanley Burroughs, *Healing for the Age of Enlightenment* (Kailua, Hawaii: self-published, 1976), p. 114.

[25] Panos and Heimlich, *Homeopathic Medicine at Home,* p. 47.

Chapter Twenty-One

Palming and Acupressure

PALMING

A reminder from the beginning of this book: The reader assumes responsibility for choosing to do any of the activities mentioned in this book, and the responsibility for any responses from doing them. Any person with a disease, pathologies, or accidents with the eyes should consult with an eye doctor before doing any activity in this book.

Have you ever watched a mother put her hand on a child's bruised knee? Have you ever seen a person under emotional distress put his palms over his eyes? Have you ever seen a person put his hand on an upset stomach? This is called *palming*.

There are subtle energy fields that flow through the body. These energy fields are the basis of many holistic practices including acupuncture, foot reflexology, homeopathy, and Reiki healing. Some of these energy fields flow out from the palms and can be used for healing yourself or others.

The purpose of palming is to bring relaxation to the visual system, especially the mind. Although Bates was probably not aware of these energy fields, he *was* aware of the benefits of "palming." Bates taught palming as a self-healing technique to bring relaxation to the eyes and mind.

Palming, performed in the correct manner, can bring a great amount of rest, relaxation, and circulation to the visual system—often in a surprisingly short time. Palming can aid in removing the excessive, chronic tension put on the visual system by the many years of incorrect vision habits. Although palming is not essential, it is valuable for the great majority (~95%) of vision students.

How to Palm

See *Figure 21–1: Palming*.

To palm correctly, sit in a comfortable chair, with proper posture, giving special attention to correct alignment of the head, neck, and shoulders. Rest your elbows on a cushion, pillow, or some other support. If a cushion or pillow are not available, you can use a table or desk, but do not lean over forward. Rest your feet flat on the floor. Do not cross your feet or legs.

Self-healing energy emanates from the center of the palms. You can increase this energy

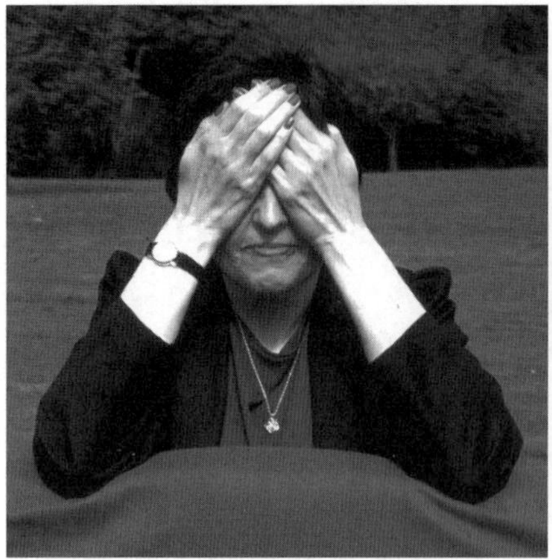

CORRECT PALMING

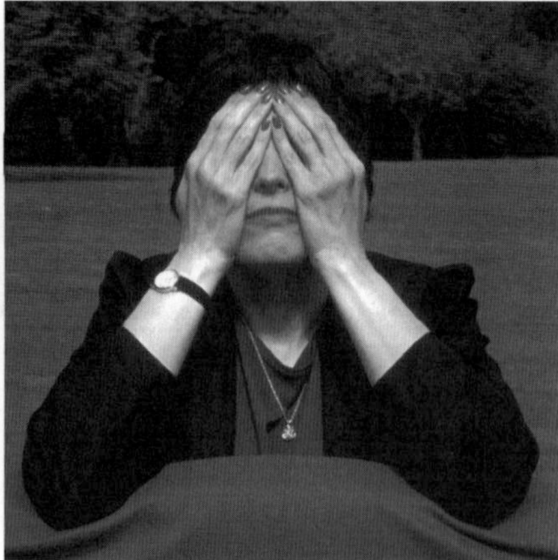

INCORRECT PALMING

Figure 21–1: Palming.

flow before palming by "rubbing your hands an inch apart"; in other words, without actually touching your hands together. While doing this, some students feel a tingling on their hands, or a warming of the hands. When the hands are moved slowly away from and toward each other, some students feel a magnet effect. Not all students feel these effects in the beginning.

Do not touch your eyes.

"Cup" your hands slightly. The fingers are relaxed, not stiff. The left hand is placed first, with the center of the "cupped" palm over the left eye. The base of the hand rests softly on the cheek, without putting pressure on the nose. The hand is angled slightly, so that the fingers extend toward the center of the forehead. Next, the right hand is placed with the fingers extending over the fingers of the left hand.

Breathe abdominally. It is important that the neck is loose. The neck has a small movement during palming. The eyelids are closed during palming.

Continue to centralize while palming; do not diffuse.

Figure 21–1 also shows the incorrect way of palming. The palms are not over the eyes, and they do not cross over the forehead. Also, the chin is jutting forward, with the top of the head pulled back too far. The fingers and hands should not be parallel to each other, i.e., they should not be vertical.

Also, do not place the heel of the hand too high.

From *Better Eyesight* magazine, April 1928:

> *Question:* Is it all right to palm while lying down? Is it better to sit or stand while doing so? If the arms get tired is it all right to rest the elbows on a desk or something like that while palming? Or is it best to hold the elbows up free from all support?
>
> *Answer:* It is all right to palm while lying down. Palming should not be done while one is standing. The elbows should rest on a desk or table or on a cushion placed in the lap. One should be in as comfortable a position as possible while palming, in order to obtain the most benefit....

What To Do While Palming

While palming, pretend you are sketching any object that is relaxing to you. Do not "space out" or stare while palming. Nose-pencil or -feather objects that are interesting, colorful, and textured. Add details and movement. Have fun being creative!

Palming is an excellent time for nearsights to pretend they are sketching clear objects in the distance. Farsights can sketch clear objects up close. People with astigmatism can sketch clear objects both near and far.

When one Bates teacher told a student to think of something relaxing while palming, the student said, "Nothing is relaxing for me!" The teacher asked, "Nothing?" Then the student replied, "Well, there is this butter-dish my grandfather gave to me, and I like it. So, I will think about my butter-dish." Think of pleasant things while palming—otherwise it is of little value.

Positive Affirmations

Palming provides an excellent opportunity to practice positive vision affirmations. One of the most important parts of natural vision improvement is to begin thinking like a person who has clear vision. Vision is primarily mental. Affirmations are usually more powerful when spoken out loud.

Here are some sample positive affirmations:

- I have the potential to see clearly with my own eyes.
- I can see the feathers of an eagle on a hilltop.
- I can read Shakespeare written on a sunflower seed.
- I can watch a beautiful horse trotting along a forest path.
- I can see a mosquito floating on a pond.
- I can watch ducks migrating to the south.
- I can read the small print in a phone book.
- I can read the words on the school blackboard easily and clearly.
- I can read microprint ten inches away.
- I can see anything clearly in the distance.
- I can see anything clearly up close.
- And everything in-between is a piece of cake.
- All without glasses, drugs, or surgery.
- I *want* to see clearly with my own eyes.
- I used to.
- I can relearn to do something I used to do perfectly—called sketching, breathing, and blinking.
- My vision is improving more each day.

Create your own positive affirmations, too! They will be the best ones!

A Palming Story

Pretend you are sitting in a beautiful, sunny meadow in a comfortable chair. You can hear the rustling of the leaves of the tall cottonwood trees at the edge of the meadow. You can also hear the bluejays singing and woodpeckers tapping on trees.

In your hand you hold a large, yellow lemon, with lots of little dimples sparkling in the sunshine. While feeling the lemon with your fingers, brush the smooth skin of the lemon with your nose-feather. Smell the lemon. Taste the lemon!

Now, in slow motion, toss the lemon out in front of you into the air. Continue to brush the lemon with your nose-feather as it floats out—five feet, ten feet, fifteen feet. At about twenty feet, the lemon lands softly on top of a tall, white, picket fence.

Continuing to brush the lemon with your nose-feather, you now notice it has fluorescent purple letters on it, which say "Grown Organically." Brush the shapes of the letters on the lemon.

Now, sweep your nose-feather along the picket fence. Sweep casually to the left, then back to the middle, and then to the right, back to the middle, over to the left again, and so on. Tap all of the pickets with your nose-feather as you sweep left and right.

Now, take a deep breath in. While exhaling, remove your hands from your head and open your eyelids. With frequent, soft butterfly blinks, brush the objects in your room or environment in a very relaxed, casual manner. Yawn.

With any palming story, you can add the sense perceptions of smell, taste, hearing, and touch. Add a variety of details and colors; near, middle, and far objects; objects high and low, left and right; textures, dimension, and motion. Natural vision thrives on interest, curiosity, and variety.

It is best to keep the palming stories simple in the beginning. You can add variations to the same palming story each time you palm, or you can create new stories.

Bates on Palming

From Chapter XII of *Perfect Sight Without Glasses:*

> All the methods used ... are simply different ways of obtaining relaxation, and most students, though by no means all, find it easiest to relax with their eyes shut. This usually lessens the strain to see, and in such cases is followed by a temporary or more lasting improvement in vision.
>
> Most students are benefited merely by closing the eyes; and by alternately resting them for a few minutes or longer in this way and then opening them ... But since some light comes through the closed eyelids, a still greater degree of relaxation can be obtained, in all but a few exceptional cases, by excluding it. This is done by covering the closed eyes with the palms of the hands (the fingers being crossed upon the forehead) in such a way as to avoid pressure on the eyeballs. So efficacious is this practice, which I have called "palming," as a means of relieving strain, that we all instinctively resort to it at times, and from it most students are able to get a considerable degree of relaxation ...
>
> Palming is one of the most effective methods of obtaining relaxation of all the sensory nerves.

Do Not Try to See Black

This section is added to help clarify the confusion regarding seeing "black" while palming. I add this information primarily for the sake of completeness, as many students have asked me about Bates' references to seeing black.

In *Perfect Sight Without Glasses,* Bates discussed the advantages of remembering pure black during palming. Later, in his *Better Eyesight* magazines, he basically told his students not to try to remember or see black.

Better Eyesight magazine, July 1923:

> *Question:* I still cannot visualize "black"—what else can I use as a substitute?
>
> *Answer:* ... If it is an effort to visualize

black, think of something that is pleasant, for instance, a field of daisies, a sun-set, etc. The result will be just as beneficial.

Better Eyesight magazine, February 1924:

Question: To palm successfully is it necessary to remember black or try to see black?

Answer: No. When one palms successfully the eyes and mind are relaxed and black is usually seen, but any effort to see black is a strain which will always fail.

Better Eyesight magazine, December 1927:

REST

The student is then directed to either close his eyes or palm for half an hour, whichever is more comfortable for him. In palming, the student closes both eyes and covers them with the palms of both hands, in such a way as to exclude all light. To palm successfully, he should make no effort to remember, imagine or see black. If black cannot be seen perfectly, the student is told to let the mind drift from one pleasant thought to another.

A "half an hour" is not essential. Generally the more time given to palming, the more benefit is received.

Do not be concerned if some light enters through your hands.

It is clear that remembering black is not essential for improving sight. Most students will do better by ignoring the entire issue of seeing black, white, or any other color. The principles of movement, centralization, and relaxation, and the habits of natural seeing are far more important than any issue of blackness.

More on Palming by Bates

From *Perfect Sight Without Glasses:*

When palming is successful it is one of the best methods I know of for securing relaxation of all the sensory nerves, including those of sight ... the greater the degree of the relaxation produced by palming, the more of it is retained when the eyes are opened and the longer it lasts. If you palm perfectly, you retain, when you open your eyes, all of the relaxation that you gain, and you do not lose it again. If you palm imperfectly, you retain only part of what you gain and retain it only temporarily—it may be only for a few moments. Even the smallest degree of relaxation is useful, however, for by means of it a still greater degree may be obtained ...

A very remarkable case ... was that of a man nearly seventy years of age with compound hypermetropic astigmatism and presbyopia, complicated by incipient cataract. For more than forty years he had worn glasses to improve his distant vision, and for twenty years he had worn them for reading and desk work. Because of the cloudiness of the lens, he had now become unable to see well enough to do his work, even with glasses; and the other physicians whom he had consulted had given him no hope of relief except by operation when the cataract was ripe. When he found palming helped him, he asked:

"Can I do that too much?"

"No," he was told. "Palming is simply a means of resting your eyes, and you cannot rest them too much."

A few days later he returned and said:

"Doctor, it was tedious, very tedious; but I did it."

"What was tedious?" I asked.

"Palming," he replied. "I did it continuously for twenty hours."

"But you couldn't have kept it up for twenty hours continuously," I said incredulously. "You must have stopped to eat."

And then he related that from four o'clock in the morning until twelve at night he had eaten nothing, only drinking large quantities of water, and had devoted practically all of the time to palming. It must have been tedious, as he said, but it was also worthwhile. When he looked at the reading card, without glasses, he read the bottom line at twenty feet. He also read fine print at six inches and at twenty. The cloudiness of the lens had become much less, and in the center had entirely disappeared. Two years later there had been no relapse ...

After resting the eyes by closing [the eyelids] or palming, shifting and swinging are often more successful.

Note: Some students will find frequent, short periods of palming to be more beneficial than one long period.

Better Eyesight magazine, November 1921:

It is a good thing to go to sleep swinging or palming....

Question: How long should one palm at a time ... ?

Answer: The length of time you should palm depends entirely on the results you obtain from the practice. Some students can palm for hours with benefit; others cannot keep it up for more than a few minutes.

Better Eyesight magazine, November 1923:

The student is directed to rest his eyes and to forget them as much as possible by thinking of other things ... The length of time necessary to palm to obtain maximum results varies with individuals. Most persons can obtain improvement in fifteen minutes while others require a longer time, a half hour ... With improvement of the vision it usually follows that a shorter period of palming may obtain maximum results.

Better Eyesight magazine, January 1925:

Question: While palming is it necessary to close the eyes?

Answer: Yes.

Although it is possible, of course, to palm with the eyelids opened and blinking, this is not as beneficial as closed-eyelids palming. Open-eyelid palming is not recommended.

Optometrist Harris Gruman wrote in his book *New Ways to Better Sight:* " ... palming. Dr. Bates was the first to suggest it, and for this he deserves the fullest credit."[1]

The Palming/Sunning Sandwich

Alternating palming with sunning is very relaxing and beneficial to the visual system and aids in the student's ability to adjust from bright to dark, and dark to bright light situations. The student can sun for two minutes, palm for two minutes, sun for two minutes, and so forth. Of course, the eyelids are always closed during sunning.

You can also alternate palming and sunning with the acupressure points described below. These are three excellent optional activities for removing strain from the visual system.

Variations on Palming

You can palm the back of your neck. In fact, palming can be used with any part of the body.

GENERAL DIRECTIONS

In acupressure activities 1-3, gently and slowly massage each area indicated for a few minutes. In acupressure activity 4, gently slides your curled fingers over the acupressure points as shown.

The purpose of these self-healing activities is to increase the flow of energy associated with the visual system.

Rest your elbows on a table for support. Do not touch your eyes.

Remember to keep your neck released and to breathe abdominally. Though the eyelids can remain open or closed, closed eyelids is best. If they are open, remember to blink.

1

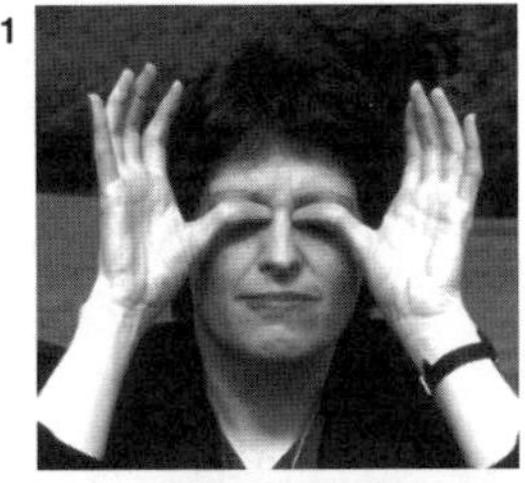

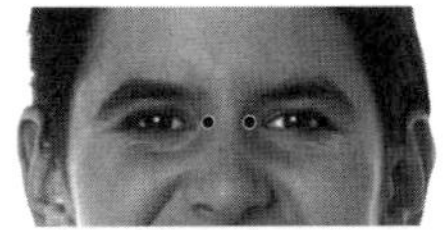

1. Jing-ming points. These two acupressure points are located on both sides of the bridge of the nose. You can use your forefingers as an alternative to the thumbs if desired.

2

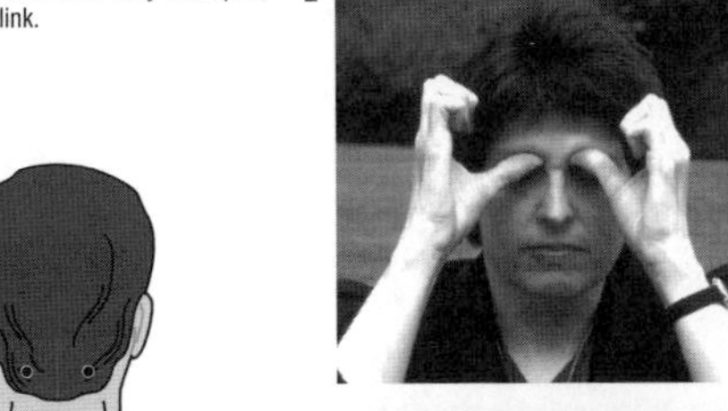

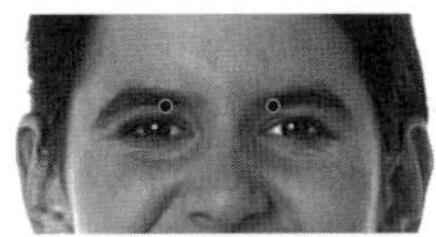

2. Zheng-guang points. These two acupressure points are located in the indentations underneath the eyebrow bones approximately one-half inch away from the bridge of the nose. These points are associated with superior oblique muscles.

5

5. Feng-chi points. These two points are located in the two hollow areas just below the occipital bone. Place your fingers on the back of the head and use your thumbs to massage theses points.

3

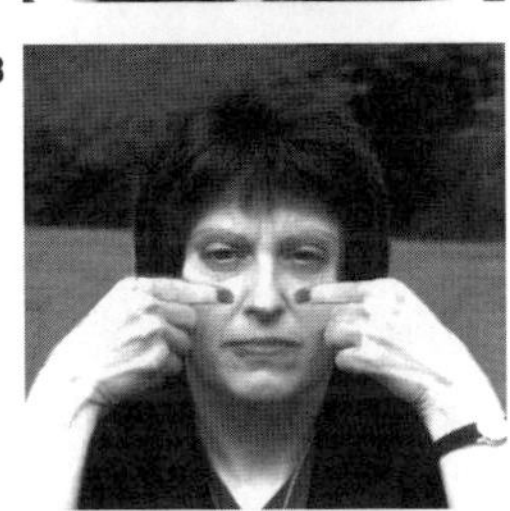

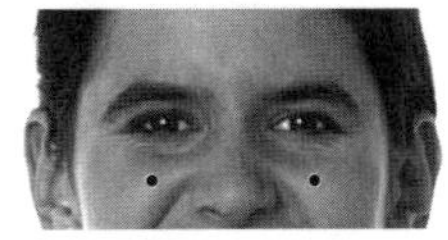

3. Si-bai points. These two acupressure points are located on the cheekbones as shown.

4

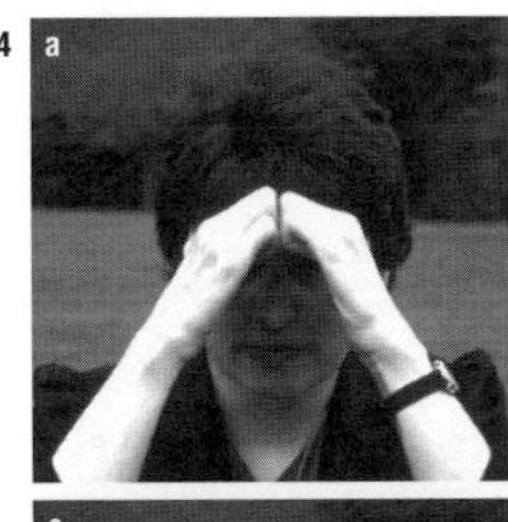

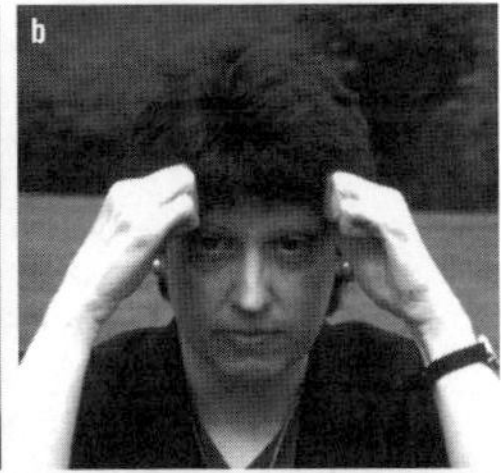

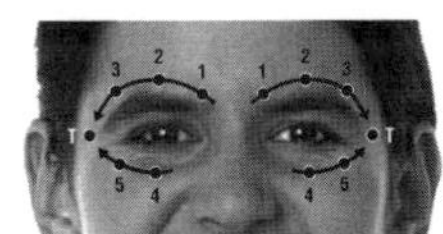

4. These twelve acupressure points are located as shown—six above the two eyebrows, four below the eyes and two on the temples. The two points on the temples (T) are associated with recti muscles. Place your thumbs on the two temple points. (The thumb remain on the two temple points at all times.) Then slide your curled forefingers from the middle of your forehead out to the temples—paths 1-2-3-T. Next, slide your curled forefingers from your nose out to the temples—paths 4-5-T. Then repeat several times.

c

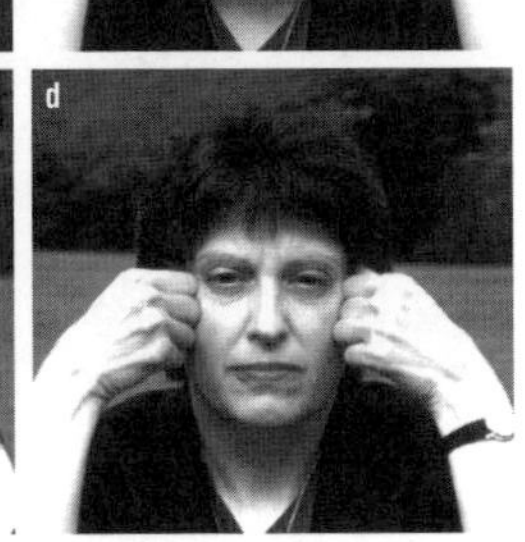

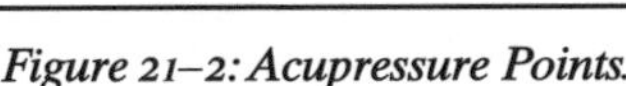

Figure 21–2: Acupressure Points.

Margaret Corbett, in her book *Help Yourself to Better Sight,* writes:

> Ear training consists of . . . stimulation of the aural nerves by relaxation, that is by the total exclusion of *all* sound, ear-palming.[2]

ACUPRESSURE

Applying a gentle, slow, massaging pressure to the acupressure points associated with the visual system increases the circulation of meridians related to eyesight, and releases tension from the visual system.

See *Figure 21–2: Acupressure Points.*

Notes

[1] Harris Gruman, *New Ways to Better Sight* (New York: Hermitage House, 1950), p. 183.

[2] Margaret D. Corbett, *Help Yourself to Better Sight* (North Hollywood, California: Wilshire Book Co., 1949), p. 205.

PART SEVEN

Reading, Children, Schools, and More

Chapter Twenty-Two

Reading—For All Ages

Better Eyesight magazine, October 1920:

> *Question:* How young a person can you teach with this method, and up to what age can you expect results?
>
> *Answer:* The age is immaterial. It is a matter of intelligence. People as old as eighty-two have improved. Children can be taught as soon as they are able to talk.

Better Eyesight magazine, November 1920:

> *Question:* Is it possible to regain the ability to read without glasses when it fails after the age of forty, the sight at the distance being perfect?
>
> *Answer:* The failure of the sight at the near point after forty is due to the same cause as its failure at any other point and at any other age, namely strain. The sight can be restored by practicing at the near point the same methods used to improve the vision at the distance—palming, shifting, swinging, etc. The sight is never perfect at the distance when imperfect at the near point, but will become so when the sight at the near point has become normal.

INTERFERENCES TO CLEAR READING

Many people read frequently and for long periods of time. If a person becomes fatigued or bored during these times, he may interfere with normal vision habits. When fatigued, many people do not rest, but continue reading. It is easy to fall into a "spaced out" staring habit in this situation.

Have you ever had the experience of still moving the eyes along the sentences, while your attention is on something else? Then, when the staring has stopped, did you need to go back and find out where your comprehension left off?

As mentioned earlier, research studies have linked myopia to *literate* cultures. It is not the activity of reading itself that strains vision—it is the formation of incorrect vision habits during reading that strains vision.

A Locked Neck

Many people lock their head and neck when they read—only the eyes are moving. Locking the neck will create fatigue. This can create a vicious cycle: fatigue creates staring, which creates more fatigue, and so on.

After the head stops moving, the eyes can also stop moving, as the person drifts into the staring habit. This is the worst form of staring because the person is both rigid and diffused.

Diffused Speed Reading

There are several "speed reading" programs that teach their students to look at large areas at a time. This is diffusion training.

If you diffuse your vision, you will strain it. In previous chapters, we proved that a person can only see clearly in a small area in the center of the visual field. A person attempting to see a large area of print clearly simultaneously will strain their vision. Diffusion is confusion and a strain—and it lowers vision.

One instructor of a speed reading program told me that many of her students get headaches when they are taught speed reading techniques.

It is possible to read very rapidly once correct vision habits are re-established.

Posture and Reading

Use correct posture while reading.

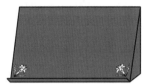

Figure 22–1: Book Support.

Tip: A book support for your desk can support better posture while reading.

READING NATURALLY

To read clearly, a person needs to have correct vision habits. The principles of movement, centralization, and relaxation allow a person to read comfortably and clearly for long periods of time.

How to Read Naturally

When reading, simply move your nose-pencil—with a head movement—from left to right though the middle of each sentence. At the end of a sentence, move your nose-pencil (and head) down and to the left, between the two sentences, to the next sentence. This releases the neck. Blink frequently, softly, and quickly. Breathe abdominally.

The eyes move also, but it is best to forget about your eyes. Your *interest* is what really moves through each line you are reading. So, you do not need to think about your eyes. If you practice the correct habits and principles of natural vision, the eyes will take care of themselves—automatically.

One way to practice reading with head movement and centralization is by using a straightened paper clip. Simply move the tip of the paper clip exactly through the center of the words as shown in *Figure 22–2*.

A "high-tech" alternative to the paper clip is a laser beam, like the ones used for lectures and presentations. Simply move the (usually) red beam through the middle of each line. Vision students like the laser beam a lot!

Since there are some cones that pick up the letters close to the letter your nose-pencil is touching at any particular moment, the visual system is able to determine what an entire word is—without diffusing.

For example, if the nose-pencil is on the letter "o" in the word "dog," the letters "d" and "g" are so close to the letter "o" the visual system can tell this word is "dog." But do not try or expect to see all of the letters of a word, or

RELEARNING TO READ—NATURALLY

When reading, move your nose-pencil through each line as if you are actually drawing a pencil line from left to right directly through the words. At the end of each line, the nose-pencil moves quickly down and to the left to the beginning of the next line. This is called shifting or sketching.

Remember to blink frequently and to breathe abdominally. Never stare. Never strain or squint. Move both the eyes and the head from left to right as you read. The head movement releases the neck.

Have correct posture when reading. Do not bend your head over looking downward at a page. Tilt the book up at an angle so that the head and neck can turn easily.

Centralize. Do not try to see an entire paragraph simultaneously clear. This is impossible to do and strains vision.

Remember to sketch objects in the distance occasionally. If you become tired, take a break.

Apply these same habits and principles to computer work also!

Figure 22–2: Reading Naturally.

all the words of a paragraph equally clearly at one moment. This would be a form of diffusion.

Never strain to see the letters on a page.

You do not need to "sketch" every letter as you read.

Oppositional Words

From *Better Eyesight* magazine, July 1920: "In reading, the page appears to move in a direction opposite to that of the eye [and head]."

Imagine the words and the entire page are moving in the opposite direction of your head and eye movements. This illusion is essential for normal sight.

Children Read Naturally—Until ...

Learning to read is a complex activity. Have you ever watched a child when she first learns to read? The child moves her finger along the line she is reading. She uses her finger—naturally—to help keep her attention on one word at a time. "It helps me keep my place." The main principles involved here are centralization and movement.

Unfortunately, many children are scolded for pointing, especially at other people. "Don't point; it is rude!" A child who is told not to point might assume that diffusion is correct.

A child also naturally moves her head when reading. Movement is natural.

Yet many children are told to "sit still" or "be still." Some are even told not to move their head when reading. This is incorrect and very harmful.

If the messages from adults that movement and centralizing are not correct translate into incorrect vision habits, the child's sight will lower. Many children are unwittingly *taught* how to lose their sight.

Additionally, many children are put under a lot of pressure to perform well at school. If this pressure translates into straining to see, vision will lower.

When a person has normal vision, there is no difference between the vision habits used during reading and during other activities. *The habits and principles of normal vision are the same at all times and during all activities.*

BATES ON READING

Bates: "The Menace of Large Print"

Bates believed that the large print put in children's schoolbooks could—and did—strain vision. Why? Large print can teach children to diffuse. If a child attempts to see a very large word clearly simultaneously, the vision will be strained.

Bates emphasized the importance of centralizing when regarding any type of print, and, for that matter, *all objects!*

Better Eyesight magazine, December 1919:

> THE MENACE OF LARGE PRINT
>
> If you look at the big "C" on the Snellen card (or any other large letter of the same size) at ten, fifteen, or twenty feet, and try to see it all alike, you may note a feeling of strain, and the letter may not appear perfectly black and distinct. If you now look at only one part of the letter, and see the rest of it worse, you will note that the part seen best appears blacker than the whole letter when seen all alike, and you may also note a relief of strain. If you look at the small "c" on the bottom line of the card, you may be able to note that it seems blacker than the big "C." If not, imagine it as forming part of the area of the big "C." If you are able to see this part blacker than the rest of the letter, the imagined letter

will, of course, appear blacker also. If your sight is normal, you may now go a step further and note that when you look at one part of the small "c," this part looks blacker than the whole letter, and that it is easier to see the letter in this way than to see it all alike.

If you look at a line of the smaller letters that you can read readily, and try to see them all alike—all equally black and equally distinct in outline—you will probably find it to be impossible, and the effort will produce discomfort and, perhaps, pain. You may, however, succeed in seeing two or more of them alike. This, too, may cause much discomfort, and if continued long enough, will produce pain. If you now look at only the first letter of the line, seeing the adjoining ones worse, the strain will at once be relieved, and the letter will appear blacker and more distinct than when it was seen equally well with the others. If your sight is normal at the near point, you can repeat these experiments with a letter seen at this point, with the same results. A number of letters seen equally well at one time will appear less black and less distinct than a single letter seen best, and a large letter will seem less black and distinct than a small one; while in the case of both the large letter and the several letters seen all alike, a feeling of strain may be produced in the eye. You may also be able to note that the reading of very fine print, when it can be done perfectly, is markedly restful to the eye.

The smaller the point of maximum vision, in short, the better the sight, and the less the strain upon the eye. This fact can usually be demonstrated in a few minutes by anyone whose sight is not markedly imperfect; and in view of some of our educational methods, is very interesting and instructive.

From the earlier explanations of the distribution of cones in the fovea centralis, we know that a person sees more distinctly the smaller the area of centralizing. The corollary to this is: the farther away another object, or part of an object, is from the central vision, the less distinct it is.

The same holds true for contrast. Above, Bates highlights the difference between blacker, sharper images in the central vision and less black, less clear images in the peripheral vision. People with blurred vision try to see everything sharp and with the same high contrast simultaneously. This is impossible to do and strains the visual system, whether attempted while reading or any other time. Again, the principles of natural vision are the same for all activities.

Bates gave a lot of attention to reading because we live in a literate society—and many people form incorrect habits when reading.

Better Eyesight magazine, December 1919, continued:

> Probably every man who has written a book upon the eye for the last hundred years has issued a warning against fine print in school books, and recommended particularly large print for small children. This advice has been followed so assiduously that one could probably not find a lesson book for small children anywhere printed in ordinary reading type, while alphabets are often printed in characters one and two inches high.
>
> The British Association for the Advancement of Science does not wish to see children read books [with small type] at all before they are seven years old, and would conduct their education previous to that age by means of large printed wall-sheets,

blackboards, pictures, and oral teaching. If they must read, however, it wants them to have 24- and 30-point type, with capitals about a quarter of an inch in height. This is carefully graded down, a size smaller each year, until at the age of twelve the children are permitted to have the same kind of type as their elders. Bijou editions of Bible, prayer-book and hymnals are forbidden, however, to children of all ages.[a]

In the London myope classes, which have become the model for many others of the same kind, books are eliminated entirely, and only the older children are allowed to print their lessons in one- and two-inch types.[b] ...

... [Yet] the reading of fine print, when it can be done with comfort, has been found to be a benefit to the eyes.

---

[a] Report on the Influence of School-Books upon Eyesight, second revised edition, 1913.

[b] Pollock: The Education of the Semi-Blind, Glasgow Med. Jour., Dec., 1915.

From Chapter XV in *Perfect Sight Without Glasses:*

SHIFTING AND SWINGING

When the eye with normal vision regards a letter either at the near point or at the distance, the letter may appear to pulsate, or move in various directions, from side to side, up and down, or obliquely. When it looks from one letter to another on the Snellen card, or from one side of a letter to another, not only the letters, but the whole line of letters and the whole card may appear to move from side to side. This apparent movement is due to the shifting of the eye [and the head], and is always in a direction contrary to its movement. If one looks at the top of a letter, the letter is below the line of vision, and therefore appears to move downward. If one looks at the bottom, the letter is above the line of vision and appears to move upward. If one looks to the left of the letter, it is to the right of the line of vision and appears to move to the right. If one looks to the right, it is to the left of the line of vision and appears to move to the left.

Persons with normal vision are rarely conscious of this illusion, and may have difficulty in demonstrating it; but in every case that has come under my observation they have always become able, in a longer or shorter time, to do so. When the sight is imperfect the letters may remain stationary, or even move in the same direction as the eye.

It is impossible for the eye to fix [on] a point longer than a fraction of a second. If it tries to do so, it begins to strain and the vision is lowered. This can readily be demonstrated by trying to hold one part of a letter for an appreciable length of time. No matter how good the sight, it will begin to blur, or even disappear, very quickly, and sometimes the effort to hold it will produce pain. In the case of a few exceptional people a point may appear to be held for a considerable length of time; the subjects themselves may think that they are holding it; but this is only because the eye shifts unconsciously, the movements being so rapid that objects seem to be seen all alike simultaneously.

[Even some people with normal vision think that what Bates is teaching is incorrect. Many people with normal sight *think* that stationary objects *appear* to be stationary. But we know stationary objects *appear to move* in the opposite direction of our movement.]

The shifting of the eye with normal vision is usually not conspicuous, but by direct examination with the ophthalmoscope[a] it can always be demonstrated. If one eye is examined with this instrument while the other is regarding a small area straight ahead, the eye being examined, which follows the movements of the other, is seen to move in various directions, from side to side, up and down, in an orbit which is usually variable. If the vision is normal, these movements are extremely rapid and unaccompanied by any appearance of effort. The shifting of the eye with imperfect sight, on the contrary, is slower, its excursions are wider, and the movements are jerky and made with apparent effort.

It can also be demonstrated that the eye is capable of shifting with a rapidity which the ophthalmoscope cannot measure. The normal eye can read fourteen letters on the bottom line of a Snellen card at a distance of ten or fifteen feet, in a dim light, so rapidly that they seem to be seen all at once. Yet it can be demonstrated that in order to recognize the letters under these conditions it is necessary to make about four shifts to each letter. At the near point, even though one part of the letter is seen best, the rest may be seen well enough to be recognized; but at the distance it is impossible to recognize the letters unless one shifts from the top to the bottom and from side to side. One must also shift from one letter to another, making about seventy shifts in a fraction of a second....

OPTIMUMS AND PESSIMUMS

In nearly all cases of imperfect sight due to errors of refraction there is some object, or objects, which can be regarded with normal vision. Such objects I have called *optimums.* On the other hand, there are some objects which persons with normal eyes and ordinarily normal sight always see imperfectly; an error of refraction being produced when they are regarded, as demonstrated by the retinoscope. Such objects I have called *pessimums.* An object becomes an optimum, or a pessimum, according to the effect it produces upon the mind, and in some cases this effect is easily accounted for.

For many children their mother's face is an optimum, and the face of a stranger a pessimum. A dressmaker was always able to thread a No. 10 needle with a fine thread of silk without glasses, although she had to put on glasses to sew on buttons, because she could not see the holes. She was a teacher of dressmaking, and thought the children stupid because they could not tell the difference between two different shades of black. She could match colors without comparing the samples. Yet she could not see a black line in a photographic copy of the Bible which was no finer than a thread of silk.... An employee in a cooperage factory, who had been engaged for years in picking out defective barrels as they went rapidly past him on an inclined plane, was able to continue his work after his sight for most other objects had become very defective, while persons with much better sight for the Snellen card were unable to detect the defective barrels. The familiarity of these various objects made it possible for the subjects to look at them without strain—that is, without trying to see them. Therefore the barrels were to the cooper optimums; while the needle's eye and the colors of silk and fabrics were optimums to the dressmaker. Unfamiliar objects, on the contrary, are always pessimums.

In other cases there is no accounting for

[a] An instrument for viewing the interior of the eye. When the optic nerve is observed with the ophthalmoscope, movements can be noted that are not apparent when only the exterior of the eye is regarded.

the idiosyncrasy of the mind which makes one object a pessimum and another an optimum. It is also impossible [for me] to account for the fact that an object may be an optimum for one eye and not for the other, or an optimum at one time and at one distance and not at others. Among these unaccountable optimums one often finds a particular letter on the Snellen card. One person, for instance, was able to see the letter K on the forty, fifteen and ten lines, but could see none of the other letters on these lines, although most people would see some of them, on account of the simplicity of their outlines, better than they would such a letter as K.

Pessimums may be as curious and unaccountable as optimums. The letter V is so simple in its outlines that many people can see it when they cannot see others on the same line. Yet some people are unable to distinguish it at any distance, although able to read other letters in the same word, or on the same line of the Snellen card. Some people again will not only be unable to recognize the letter V in a word, but also to read any word that contains it, the pessimum lowering their sight not only for itself but for other objects. Some letters, or objects, become pessimums only in particular situations. A letter, for instance, may be a pessimum when located at the end, or at the beginning of a line, or sentence, and not in other places. When the attention of the person is called to the fact that a letter seen in one location ought logically to be seen equally well in others, the letter often ceases to be a pessimum in any situation.

A pessimum, like an optimum, may be lost and later become manifest. It may vary according to the light and distance. An object which is a pessimum in a moderate light may not be so when the light is increased or diminished. A pessimum at twenty feet may not be one at two feet, or thirty feet, and an object which is a pessimum when directly regarded may be seen with normal vision in the eccentric field—that is, when not directly regarded.

For most people the Snellen card is a pessimum. If you can see the Snellen card with normal vision, you can see almost anything else in the world. *People who cannot see the letters on the Snellen card can often see other objects of the same size and at the same distance with normal sight.* [TQ emphasis.] When letters which are seen imperfectly, or even letters which cannot be seen at all, or which the person is not conscious of seeing, are regarded, the error of refraction is increased. The person may regard a blank white card without any error of refraction; but if he regards the lower part of a Snellen card, which appears to him to be just as blank as the blank card, an error of refraction can always be demonstrated, and if the visible letters of the card are covered the result is the same. The pessimum may, in short, be letters or objects which the person is not conscious of seeing. This phenomenon is very common. When the card is seen in the eccentric field it may have the effect of lowering the vision for the point directly regarded. For instance, a person may regard an area of green wallpaper at the distance, and see the color as well as at the near point; but if a Snellen card on which the letters are either seen imperfectly, or not seen at all, is placed in the neighborhood of the area being regarded, the retinoscope may indicate an error of refraction. When the vision improves, the number of letters on the card which are pessimums diminishes and the number of optimums increases, until the whole card becomes an optimum.

A pessimum, like an optimum, is a manifestation of the mind. It is something asso-

> ciated with a strain to see, just as an optimum is something which has no such association. It is not caused by the error of refraction, but always produces an error of refraction; and when the strain has been relieved it ceases to be a pessimum and becomes an optimum.

Right-brain/left-brain experts may now be able to explain some of the "unaccountable" observations mentioned by Bates. Looking to the left activates right-brain characteristics, and looking to the right activates left-brain characteristics. See *Figure 19–5: "Vision."*

An optimum is anything that promotes correct vision habits. A pessimum is anything that promotes incorrect vision habits. The process of improving vision involves the transformation of objects or thoughts we now regard to be pessimums into optimums. Optimums are relaxing.

Again quoting from *Perfect Sight Without Glasses:*

> THE FUNDAMENTAL PRINCIPLE
>
> Do you read imperfectly? Can you observe then that when you look at the first word, or the first letter, of a sentence you do not see best where you are looking; that you see other words, or other letters, just as well as or better than the one you are looking at? Do you observe also that the harder you try to see the worse you see?
>
> Now close your eyes and rest them, remembering some color, like black or white [or anything else that is relaxing] that you can remember perfectly. Keep them closed until they feel rested, or until the feeling of strain has been completely relieved. Now open them and look at the first word or letter of a sentence for a fraction of a second. If you have been able to relax, partially or completely, you will have a flash of improved or clear vision, and the area seen best will be smaller....
>
> If your trouble is with distant instead of near vision, use the same method with distant letters.

From Chapter XVII of *Perfect Sight Without Glasses,* Bates writes the following:

> According to accepted ideas of ocular hygiene, it is important to protect the eyes from a great variety of influences which are often very difficult to avoid, and to which most people resign themselves with the uneasy sense that they are thereby "ruining their eyesight." Bright lights, artificial lights, dim lights, sudden fluctuations of light, fine print, reading in moving vehicles, reading lying down, etc., have long been considered "bad for the eyes," and libraries of literature have been produced about their supposedly direful effects. These ideas are diametrically opposed to the truth. When the eyes are properly used, vision under adverse conditions not only does not injure them, but is an actual benefit, because a greater degree of relaxation is required to see under such conditions than under more favorable ones ...
>
> ... [If] persons with imperfect sight practice centralization, they become accustomed to them [i.e., the adverse conditions] and derive great benefit from them....
>
> The universal fear of reading or doing fine work in a dim light is, however, unfounded. So long as the light is sufficient so that one can see without discomfort, this practice is not only harmless, but may be beneficial.
>
> ... fine print cannot be read in a dim light and close to the eyes unless the eyes are relaxed, whereas large print can be read in a good light and at ordinary reading distance although the eyes may be under a

strain. When fine print can be read under adverse conditions, the reading of ordinary print under ordinary conditions is vastly improved....

FACTS VERSUS THEORIES

Reading fine print is commonly supposed to be an extremely dangerous practice, and reading print of any kind upon a moving vehicle is thought to be even worse. Looking away to the distance, however, and not seeing anything in particular is believed to be very beneficial to the eyes. In the light of these superstitions the facts contained in the following letter are particularly interesting:

"On reaching home Monday morning I was surprised and pleased at the comments of my family regarding the appearance of my eyes. They all thought they looked so much brighter and rested, and that after two days of railroading. I didn't spare my eyes in the least on the way home. I read magazines and newspapers, looked at the scenery; in fact, I used my eyes all the time. My sight for the near point is splendid. I can read for hours without tiring my eyes. I went downtown today and my eyes were very tired when I got home. The fine print on the card [diamond type] helps me so much I would like to have your little Bible. [Bates gave many students a card with diamond type print, and a photographic reduction of the Bible printed in type smaller than diamond.] I'm sure the very fine print has a soothing effect on one's eyes, regardless of what my previous ideas on the subject were."

It will be observed that the eyes of this student were not tired by her two-day railroad journey, during which she read constantly; they were not tired by hours of reading after her return; they were rested by reading extremely fine print; but they were very much tired by a trip downtown during which they were not called upon to centralize upon small objects.

Better Eyesight magazine, May 1923:

Question: Why are books for small children printed in large type?

Answer: Because Boards of Education have not yet learned that it is a strain for anyone to look at big print and a relaxation to read fine print.

Better Eyesight magazine, June 1923:

Question: ... Does age make any difference?

Answer: ... No, age does not make any difference.

Better Eyesight magazine, September 1923:

Question: If fine type is beneficial, why do they print children's school books in large type?

Answer: For the same reason that people wear glasses—Ignorance of the proper way.

Better Eyesight magazine, April 1928:

Question: I have attained normal vision, but after reading for a while, my eyes feel strained. Would you still consider I had normal sight?

Answer: If your eyes feel strained you are not reading with normal vision.

The Fine Print

Type Size	Vision Acuity (at 14")
7 point	20/40 (14/28)
6 point	20/35 (14/24)
5 point	20/30 (14/21)
4 point	20/25 (14/18)
3 point	20/20 (14/14)
1.5 point	20/10 (14/7)

The reduced-size paragraphs on the next two pages are provided so you can practice reading small print.

"But I Feel Like I Am Straining When I Read Small Print"

When the sight is imperfect, there is always a strain involved—by definition. The practice of reading small print may feel like a strain when relearning centralization. This is because the person with imperfect sight has learned to diffuse.

A person who argues that reading small letters is harmful logically needs to agree that the eyes are being harmed every time a person has their sight tested by an eye doctor, because the person is often asked to read the *smallest* line. Similarly, people who have their vision tested at the California Department of Motor Vehicles are asked to read small letters in the distance. Certainly these activities would not be allowed if reading small size letters was believed to be harmful.

It takes time to unlearn incorrect, strained ways of seeing. Ultimately, only centralization and movement are relaxing.

A Temporary Lowering of Comprehension

Some students comment that they experience a lowering in comprehension while practicing the correct vision habits during reading. This is common. Usually, a person does not think about *how* they are supposed to read. While improving sight, *how* to read with correct vision habits requires some conscious attention. This can temporarily diminish, to some degree, comprehension while reading.

As the habits of natural vision become more automatic, the comprehension increases again. Also, you can read for longer periods of time when you have relaxed vision habits.

Tip: To practice natural vision habits without comprehension, turn your book upside down, and move your nose-pencil through the lines for half a minute or so. Remember abdominal breathing and frequent, soft blinking.

Palm and rest if you become tired while reading.

Lighting and Reading

Many people believe reading small print and reading in dim light is a strain to their eyes. Parents often tell their children they will ruin their eyes if they read in bed at night using a flashlight.

If a person strains to see in dim light, his sight will lower. Similarly, if a person strains to read small print, sight will lower. Bates discovered that the only way a person can read small print in dim light is by relaxing and using correct vision habits.

When first improving vision, a student can use bright light while reading. Bright light usually gives the student better acuity because of the pinhole effect. The better sight will allow the student to be more relaxed as she improves her sight. This relaxation supports faster improvement.

As vision improves, the intensity of light can be lowered. The vision will be less clear

7 Point

THE MENACE OF LARGE PRINT

If you look at the big "C" on the Snellen test card (or any other large letter of the same size) at ten, fifteen, or twenty feet, and try to see it all alike, you may note a feeling of strain, and the letter may not appear perfectly black and distinct. If you now look at only one part of the letter, and see the rest of it worse, you will note that the part seen best appears blacker than the whole letter when seen all alike, and you may also note a relief of strain. If you look at the small "c" on the bottom line of the test card, you may be able to note that it seems blacker than the big "C." If not, imagine it as forming part of the area of the big "C." If you are able to see this part blacker than the rest of the letter, the imagined letter will, of course, appear blacker also. If your sight is normal, you may now go a step further and note that when you look at one part of the small "c" this part looks blacker than the whole letter, and that it is easier to see the letter in this way than to see it all alike.

If you look at a line of the smaller letters that you can read readily, and try to see them all alike—all equally black and equally distinct in outline—you will probably find it to be impossible, and the effort will produce discomfort and, perhaps, pain. You may, however, succeed in seeing two or more of them alike. This, too, may cause much discomfort, and if continued long enough, will produce pain. If you now look at only the first letter of the line, seeing the adjoining ones worse, the strain will at once be relieved, and the letter will appear blacker and more distinct than when it was seen equally well with the others. If your sight is normal at the near-point, you can repeat these experiments with a letter seen at this point, with the same results. A number of letters seen equally well at one time will appear less black and less distinct than a single letter seen best, and a large letter will seem less black and distinct than a small one; while in the case of both the large letter and the several letters seen all alike, a feeling of strain may be produced in the eye. You may also be able to note that the reading of very fine print, when it can be done perfectly, is markedly restful to the eye.

The smaller the point of maximum vision, in short, the better the sight, and the less the strain upon the eye. This fact can usually be demonstrated in a few minutes by any one whose sight is not markedly imperfect; and in view of some of our educational methods, is very interesting and instructive.

6 Point

THE MENACE OF LARGE PRINT

If you look at the big "C" on the Snellen test card (or any other large letter of the same size) at ten, fifteen, or twenty feet, and try to see it all alike, you may note a feeling of strain, and the letter may not appear perfectly black and distinct. If you now look at only one part of the letter, and see the rest of it worse, you will note that the part seen best appears blacker than the whole letter when seen all alike, and you may also note a relief of strain. If you look at the small "c" on the bottom line of the test card, you may be able to note that it seems blacker than the big "C." If not, imagine it as forming part of the area of the big "C." If you are able to see this part blacker than the rest of the letter, the imagined letter will, of course, appear blacker also. If your sight is normal, you may now go a step further and note that when you look at one part of the small "c" this part looks blacker than the whole letter, and that it is easier to see the letter in this way than to see it all alike.

If you look at a line of the smaller letters that you can read readily, and try to see them all alike—all equally black and equally distinct in outline—you will probably find it to be impossible, and the effort will produce discomfort and, perhaps, pain. You may, however, succeed in seeing two or more of them alike. This, too, may cause much discomfort, and if continued long enough, will produce pain. If you now look at only the first letter of the line, seeing the adjoining ones worse, the strain will at once be relieved, and the letter will appear blacker and more distinct than when it was seen equally well with the others. If your sight is normal at the near-point, you can repeat these experiments with a letter seen at this point, with the same results. A number of letters seen equally well at one time will appear less black and less distinct than a single letter seen best, and a large letter will seem less black and distinct than a small one; while in the case of both the large letter and the several letters seen all alike, a feeling of strain may be produced in the eye. You may also be able to note that the reading of very fine print, when it can be done perfectly, is markedly restful to the eye.

The smaller the point of maximum vision, in short, the better the sight, and the less the strain upon the eye. This fact can usually be demonstrated in a few minutes by any one whose sight is not markedly imperfect; and in view of some of our educational methods, is very interesting and instructive.

Figure 22–3: The Menace of Large Print: 7 and 6 point.

5 Point

THE MENACE OF LARGE PRINT

If you look at the big "C" on the Snellen test card (or any other large letter of the same size) at ten, fifteen, or twenty feet, and try to see it all alike, you may note a feeling of strain, and the letter may not appear perfectly black and distinct. If you now look at only one part of the letter, and see the rest of it worse, you will note that the part seen best appears blacker than the whole letter when seen all alike, and you may also note a relief of strain. If you look at the small "c" on the bottom line of the test card, you may be able to note that it seems blacker than the big "C." If not, imagine it as forming part of the area of the big "C." If you are able to see this part blacker than the rest of the letter, the imagined letter will, of course, appear blacker also. If your sight is normal, you may now go a step further and note that when you look at one part of the small "c" this part looks blacker than the whole letter, and that it is easier to see the letter in this way than to see it all alike.

If you look at a line of the smaller letters that you can read readily, and try to see them all alike—all equally black and equally distinct in outline—you will probably find it to be impossible, and the effort will produce discomfort and, perhaps, pain. You may, however, succeed in seeing two or more of them alike. This, too, may cause much discomfort, and if continued long enough, will produce pain. If you now look at only the first letter of the line, seeing the adjoining ones worse, the strain will at once be relieved, and the letter will appear blacker and more distinct than when it was seen equally well with the others. If your sight is normal at the near-point, you can repeat these experiments with a letter seen at this point, with the same results. A number of letters seen equally well at one time will appear less black and less distinct than a single letter seen best, and a large letter will seem less black and distinct than a small one; while in the case of both the large letter and the several letters seen all alike, a feeling of strain may be produced in the eye. You may also be able to note that the reading of very fine print, when it can be done perfectly, is markedly restful to the eye.

The smaller the point of maximum vision, in short, the better the sight, and the less the strain upon the eye. This fact can usually be demonstrated in a few minutes by any one whose sight is not markedly imperfect; and in view of some of our educational methods, is very interesting and instructive.

4 Point, Diamond Type

THE MENACE OF LARGE PRINT

If you look at the big "C" on the Snellen test card (or any other large letter of the same size) at ten, fifteen, or twenty feet, and try to see it all alike, you may note a feeling of strain, and the letter may not appear perfectly black and distinct. If you now look at only one part of the letter, and see the rest of it worse, you will note that the part seen best appears blacker than the whole letter when seen all alike, and you may also note a relief of strain. If you look at the small "c" on the bottom line of the test card, you may be able to note that it seems blacker than the big "C." If not, imagine it as forming part of the area of the big "C." If you are able to see this part blacker than the rest of the letter, the imagined letter will, of course, appear blacker also. If your sight is normal, you may now go a step further and note that when you look at one part of the small "c" this part looks blacker than the whole letter, and that it is easier to see the letter in this way than to see it all alike.

If you look at a line of the smaller letters that you can read readily, and try to see them all alike—all equally black and equally distinct in outline—you will probably find it to be impossible, and the effort will produce discomfort and, perhaps, pain. You may, however, succeed in seeing two or more of them alike. This, too, may cause much discomfort, and if continued long enough, will produce pain. If you now look at only the first letter of the line, seeing the adjoining ones worse, the strain will at once be relieved, and the letter will appear blacker and more distinct than when it was seen equally well with the others. If your sight is normal at the near-point, you can repeat these experiments with a letter seen at this point, with the same results. A number of letters seen equally well at one time will appear less black and less distinct than a single letter seen best, and a large letter will seem less black and distinct than a small one; while in the case of both the large letter and the several letters seen all alike, a feeling of strain may be produced in the eye. You may also be able to note that the reading of very fine print, when it can be done perfectly, is markedly restful to the eye.

The smaller the point of maximum vision, in short, the better the sight, and the less the strain upon the eye. This fact can usually be demonstrated in a few minutes by any one whose sight is not markedly imperfect; and in view of some of our educational methods, is very interesting and instructive.

3 Point

THE MENACE OF LARGE PRINT

If you look at the big "C" on the Snellen test card (or any other large letter of the same size) at ten, fifteen, or twenty feet, and try to see it all alike, you may note a feeling of strain, and the letter may not appear perfectly black and distinct. If you now look at only one part of the letter, and see the rest of it worse, you will note that the part seen best appears blacker than the whole letter when seen all alike, and you may also note a relief of strain. If you look at the small "c" on the bottom line of the test card, you may be able to note that it seems blacker than the big "C." If not, imagine it as forming part of the area of the big "C." If you are able to see this part blacker than the rest of the letter, the imagined letter will, of course, appear blacker also. If your sight is normal, you may now go a step further and note that when you look at one part of the small "c" this part looks blacker than the whole letter, and that it is easier to see the letter in this way than to see it all alike.

If you look at a line of the smaller letters that you can read readily, and try to see them all alike—all equally black and equally distinct in outline—you will probably find it to be impossible, and the effort will produce discomfort and, perhaps, pain. You may, however, succeed in seeing two or more of them alike. This, too, may cause much discomfort, and if continued long enough, will produce pain. If you now look at only the first letter of the line, seeing the adjoining ones worse, the strain will at once be relieved, and the letter will appear blacker and more distinct than when it was seen equally well with the others. If your sight is normal at the near-point, you can repeat these experiments with a letter seen at this point, with the same results. A number of letters seen equally well at one time will appear less black and less distinct than a single letter seen best, and a large letter will seem less black and distinct than a small one; while in the case of both the large letter and the several letters seen all alike, a feeling of strain may be produced in the eye. You may also be able to note that the reading of very fine print, when it can be done perfectly, is markedly restful to the eye.

The smaller the point of maximum vision, in short, the better the sight, and the less the strain upon the eye. This fact can usually be demonstrated in a few minutes by any one whose sight is not markedly imperfect; and in view of some of our educational methods, is very interesting and instructive.

2 Point

THE MENACE OF LARGE PRINT

If you look at the big "C" on the Snellen test card (or any other large letter of the same size) at ten, fifteen, or twenty feet, and try to see it all alike, you may note a feeling of strain, and the letter may not appear perfectly black and distinct. If you now look at only one part of the letter, and see the rest of it worse, you will note that the part seen best appears blacker than the whole letter when seen all alike, and you may also note a relief of strain. If you look at the small "c" on the bottom line of the test card, you may be able to note that it seems blacker than the big "C." If not, imagine it as forming part of the area of the big "C." If you are able to see this part blacker than the rest of the letter, the imagined letter will, of course, appear blacker also. If your sight is normal, you may now go a step further and note that when you look at one part of the small "c" this part looks blacker than the whole letter, and that it is easier to see the letter in this way than to see it all alike.

If you look at a line of the smaller letters that you can read readily, and try to see them all alike—all equally black and equally distinct in outline—you will probably find it to be impossible, and the effort will produce discomfort and, perhaps, pain. You may, however, succeed in seeing two or more of them alike. This, too, may cause much discomfort, and if continued long enough, will produce pain. If you now look at only the first letter of the line, seeing the adjoining ones worse, the strain will at once be relieved, and the letter will appear blacker and more distinct than when it was seen equally well with the others. If your sight is normal at the near-point, you can repeat these experiments with a letter seen at this point, with the same results. A number of letters seen equally well at one time will appear less black and less distinct than a single letter seen best, and a large letter will seem less black and distinct than a small one; while in the case of both the large letter and the several letters seen all alike, a feeling of strain may be produced in the eye. You may also be able to note that the reading of very fine print, when it can be done perfectly, is markedly restful to the eye.

The smaller the point of maximum vision, in short, the better the sight, and the less the strain upon the eye. This fact can usually be demonstrated in a few minutes by any one whose sight is not markedly imperfect; and in view of some of our educational methods, is very interesting and instructive.

1.5 Point

THE MENACE OF LARGE PRINT

If you look at the big "C" on the Snellen test card (or any other large letter of the same size) at ten, fifteen, or twenty feet, and try to see it all alike, you may note a feeling of strain, and the letter may not appear perfectly black and distinct. If you now look at only one part of the letter, and see the rest of it worse, you will note that the part seen best appears blacker than the whole letter when seen all alike, and you may also note a relief of strain. If you look at the small "c" on the bottom line of the test card, you may be able to note that it seems blacker than the big "C." If not, imagine it as forming part of the area of the big "C." If you are able to see this part blacker than the rest of the letter, the imagined letter will, of course, appear blacker also. If your sight is normal, you may now go a step further and note that when you look at one part of the small "c" this part looks blacker than the whole letter, and that it is easier to see the letter in this way than to see it all alike.

If you look at a line of the smaller letters that you can read readily, and try to see them all alike—all equally black and equally distinct in outline—you will probably find it to be impossible, and the effort will produce discomfort and, perhaps, pain. You may, however, succeed in seeing two or more of them alike. This, too, may cause much discomfort, and if continued long enough, will produce pain. If you now look at only the first letter of the line, seeing the adjoining ones worse, the strain will at once be relieved, and the letter will appear blacker and more distinct than when it was seen equally well with the others. If your sight is normal at the near-point, you can repeat these experiments with a letter seen at this point, with the same results. A number of letters seen equally well at one time will appear less black and less distinct than a single letter seen best, and a large letter will seem less black and distinct than a small one; while in the case of both the large letter and the several letters seen all alike, a feeling of strain may be produced in the eye. You may also be able to note that the reading of very fine print, when it can be done perfectly, is markedly restful to the eye.

The smaller the point of maximum vision, in short, the better the sight, and the less the strain upon the eye. This fact can usually be demonstrated in a few minutes by any one whose sight is not markedly imperfect; and in view of some of our educational methods, is very interesting and instructive.

Figure 22–4: The Menace of Large Print: 5 to 1.5 point.

for a period of time because of the larger pupil size. As the vision continues to improve, the light can be lowered further.

When vision is normal, the pupil size has much less of an effect on acuity (assuming, of course, lights at night are sufficiently bright to activate the cones in the fovea).

NEAR PRINT FOR FARSIGHTS; FAR PRINT FOR NEARSIGHTS

In general, farsights strain their vision more when seeing close objects, like reading a book. Bates said that straining to see close objects produces farsightedness. So, farsights are learning to relax their vision when regarding close objects.

Nearsights strain their vision more when seeing distant objects, like reading a street sign. Bates said that straining to see far objects produces nearsightedness. So, nearsights are learning to relax their vision when regarding far objects.

Reminder: Wear reduced glasses only if they are essential. Remember to practice correct vision habits when wearing reduced glasses.

THE WHITE GLOW!

See *Figure 22–5: The White Glow!*

From *Perfect Sight Without Glasses:*

> The normal eye usually sees the background of a letter whiter than it really is. In looking at the letters on the Snellen card it sees white streaks at the margins of the letters, and in reading fine print it sees between the lines and the letters, and in the openings of the letters, a white more intense than the reality. People who cannot read fine print may see this illusion, but less clearly. The more clearly it is seen, the better the vision; and if it can be imagined consciously—it is imagined unconsciously when the sight is normal—the vision improves. If the lines of fine type are covered, the streaks between them disappear. When the letters are regarded through a magnifying glass by the eye with normal sight, the illusion is not destroyed, but the intensity of the white and black is lessened. With imperfect sight it may be increased to some extent by this means, but will remain less intense than the white and black seen by the normal eye.

With normal sight, there is a white glow that appears around black letters on white paper. There is also a thin white stripe along the inside borders of a white page. The insides of the letter "O" appear to be whiter than the rest of the paper because of the glow in the inside edges of the letter "O" directed inward toward the center of the letter.

This white glow creates a higher contrast

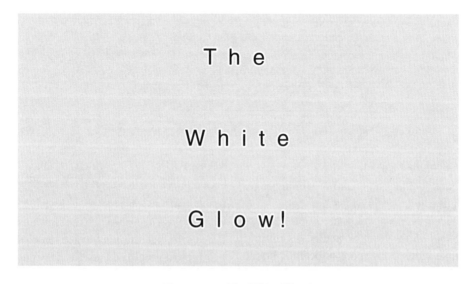

Figure 22–5: The White Glow!

between the black letter and the white paper. Much of the visual system functions by contrast and edges. (Imagine everything in the world was the same shade of gray. This would be very boring!)

Like the three-dimensional quality of normal vision, and the sense of the oppositional movement, the perception of this "glow" along edges diminishes with incorrect vision habits and wearing corrective lenses. The white glow returns when the student relearns natural vision habits. Almost all of my students have seen this white glow during vision classes.

Upon seeing the white glow around letters during a vision class, one of my students told the class how he had lost his normal eyesight: During the first two years of high school, he had normal vision. One day, he stopped reading a book and began to think about the letters on the page. He noticed the letters had white glows around them! Assuming that letters should not have white glows around them, he began to strain his eyes to get rid of this effect. Soon after, his vision became blurred and he was given prescription glasses for the first time.

The memory of how a person interfered with normal vision habits often returns when improving eyesight naturally.

Note: Do not move your attention below a sentence you are reading. Some teachers and books advocate moving along the white stripe that appears just below the baseline of a sentence. (This "white stripe" is created by the merging of the bottoms of the white glows of all of the letters along the baseline of the sentence.) Do not move your nose-paintbrush along this white stripe while reading. To do so would be a form of diffusion. Painting this white stripe with your nose-paintbrush when you are *not* reading is OK.

MORE BY BATES ON READING

From *Perfect Sight Without Glasses:*

> The fact is that when the mind is at rest nothing can tire the eyes, and when the mind is under a strain nothing can rest them. Anything that rests the mind will benefit the eyes. Almost everyone has observed that the eyes tire less quickly when reading an interesting book than when perusing something tiresome or difficult to comprehend. A schoolboy can sit up all night reading a novel without even thinking of his eyes, but if he tried to sit up all night studying his lessons he would soon find them getting very tired.

There is no strain present when correct vision habits are used.

Better Eyesight magazine, March 1925: "Blink consciously, whenever possible, especially when reading."

And, remember to take frequent breaks.

Chapter Twenty-Three

Children and Schools

As for putting glasses upon a child, it is enough to make the angels weep.

—William H. Bates

A CHILD'S NATURAL EYESIGHT— A PRECIOUS GIFT

Bates was especially interested in teaching children to improve their sight. A child can be shown how to improve her sight before the incorrect habits become deeply ingrained—as they have become for many adults. The progression of blurred vision can be reversed relatively quickly with most children.

From *Better Eyesight* magazine, July 1920:

> All parents should be told that they have it in their power to prevent and reverse defects of vision in their children and at the same time to improve their health and increase their mental efficiency. The same message should be carried to teachers and school boards.

Better Eyesight magazine, August 1920:

> The atmosphere of the average classroom is extremely irritating. It makes the children nearsighted, farsighted and astigmatic.

From *Perfect Sight Without Glasses:*

> Persons of all ages have been benefited by this educational process of relaxation; but children usually, though not invariably, respond much more quickly than adults. If they are under twelve years of age, or even under sixteen, and have never worn glasses, they ... [usually return to normal vision] ... in a few days, weeks, or months, and always within a year, simply by reading the Snellen card every day.

Children are often more receptive to the habits and principles of natural seeing because they have not been incorrectly influenced by the prejudices of our society regarding eyesight. To escape the torment and long-term harm caused by wearing corrective lenses is a precious gift for a child.

Natural vision education can also serve as a preventative measure.

A 65-year-old San Francisco woman related the following story to one of my colleagues:

> A man was taking lessons from Bates to improve his sight. During one of the

> lessons, he complained to Bates, "This is childish what you are teaching me." Bates replied, "Precisely!" In spite of his objections, this man continued to apply the correct vision habits, and improved his sight.
>
> This man's daughter had normal sight. When she was a child, he taught her the correct and incorrect habits of vision so that she would never strain her eyes.

This man was the father of the 65-year-old woman. She still has normal sight.

W.B. MacCracken, M.D., writes in his book *Use Your Own Eyes:*

> If this book succeeds only in arousing the attention of those who are interested in the welfare of children, I will feel that it has fulfilled a purpose sufficient for the effort. They are being wronged when their eyes are made the slaves of glass lenses for life.[1]

THE PREVENTION OF MYOPIA IN SCHOOL CHILDREN

As mentioned earlier, myopia has been correlated to literate societies. The prevention of myopia in school children was the subject of a paper Bates published in the *New York Medical Journal,* July 29, 1911:

> In 1903 I examined the eyes of 1,500 school children at Grand Forks, N. D., a city of 12,000 inhabitants, and found six percent myopic. The superintendent, Mr. J. Nelson Kelly, was interested in the facts and desired prevention. At my suggestion Snellen cards were placed in all the class rooms with directions for their use. The results were so encouraging that the method was employed continuously for eight years and is still in use. In 1910, among 2,000 children, less than one percent were myopic.
>
> The children were examined during a study period while sitting in their seats.
>
> After testing the sight of all the children in one classroom, the teacher asked me the character of the vision of one of the boys. I said his sight was normal—that he was slow in reading the letters of the test card; but, after some encouragement he read the smallest letters the normal eye should see at his distance from the card. The teacher was incredulous and told me very emphatically that she was positive the boy was "near sighted." She declared his vision for all distant objects was poor: he was unable to read the writing or figures on the blackboard, he did not recognize people at a distance, or see the maps, charts, or diagrams on the walls. The teacher told me that my conclusion was erroneous. She suggested that the boy might have learned the letters or had been prompted by another student. She asked me to test him again. The second examination was made carefully under her supervision, the sources of error she suggested were met, and I found the boy's sight was normal. Immediately afterward the teacher tested his sight with the writing on the blackboard and the boy read what she had written. Then she wrote additional words and figures which the boy read equally well. She asked him to tell the hour by a clock twenty-five feet distant which he did correctly. It was a dramatic situation. The children were intensely interested. I was impressed by her surprise when she was convinced that the boy's vision was normal.
>
> Three other cases in this class were similar and on examination yielded identical results. The teacher asked for an explanation. I told her that when the children looked at the blackboard or other distant objects and strained or made an effort to see better, they focused their eyes for a near

point and consequently could not see distant objects clearly; and, while testing the vision with Snellen's card, I educated them to use their eyes properly for distant vision. It was interesting also to me to find that the few moments devoted to testing them were sufficient to relieve these children so that their vision for distant objects became normal. This teacher at once realized that the Snellen card was valuable in relieving and preventing defective vision. At her request a Snellen card was given her which was placed permanently on the wall of the class room where all the children could see it from their seats.

NORMAL EYES WITH DEFECTIVE VISION FOR DISTANCE

...Why was the Snellen card better than other distant objects to improve the sight? It enabled the student to know when an improper strain or effort to see was made. It was only when the eyes were properly adjusted for distant vision that the small letters were read. With other distant objects, children had greater difficulty in knowing when the focus was adjusted accurately. Many persons with normal eyes believed erroneously that they saw better at the distance by partly closing the eyelids or by otherwise straining the eyes; but, when they looked at the Snellen card, they at once discovered that the effort made the letters indistinct.

Why did children strain their eyes when looking at distant objects? *They strained because their experience had taught them that to accomplish most things an effort was required.* [TQ emphasis.] They had learned that they saw near objects more distinctly [artificially] by making a voluntary effort [of squinting]. Naturally, most of them strained, when looking at distant objects, to improve their sight artificially....

THE PRINCIPAL FACTOR IN THE CAUSE OF MYOPIA IN SCHOOL CHILDREN

The normal eye could focus for near and distant objects.

The myopic eye could focus only for near objects.

Obviously, the principal difference between the two was in the ability of the normal eye to see at a distance.

When the normal eye acquired myopia it lost the ability to adjust its accommodation for distant vision, therefore: *All individuals with normal eyes who do not adjust their accommodation accurately* for distant vision become myopic.

Nothing else was possible. It was self-evident. The demonstration of temporary functional myopia is simple: Look at the letters of a distant sign and note their clearness. If one has normal eyes any effort or strain made by staring, partly closing the eyelids, or focussing a nearer point, is followed by a blurring of the distant letters. In 1910, I demonstrated this fact with the aid of the Snellen card to 2,000 school children whose ages ranged from six to twenty years....

PERFECT SIGHT WITHOUT GLASSES—SCHOOL CHILDREN

Bates addressed the same topic in *Perfect Sight Without Glasses:*

> Of twenty thousand school children examined in one year, more than half had normal eyes, with sight which was perfect at times; but not one of them had perfect sight in each eye at all times of the day. Their sight might be good in the morning and imperfect in the afternoon, or imperfect in the morning and perfect in the afternoon. Many children could read one Snellen card with perfect sight, while unable to see a different one perfectly. Many could also read

some letters of the alphabet perfectly, while unable to distinguish other letters of the same size under similar conditions. The degree of this imperfect sight varied within wide limits, from one-third to one-tenth, or less. Its duration was also variable. Under some conditions it might continue for only a few minutes, or less; under others it might prevent the subject from seeing the blackboard for days, weeks, or even longer. Frequently all the students in a classroom were affected to this extent.

... When the eye regards an unfamiliar object, an error of refraction is always produced. Hence the proverbial fatigue caused by viewing pictures, or other objects, in a museum. Children with normal eyes who can read perfectly small letters a quarter of an inch high at ten feet always have trouble in reading strange writing on the blackboard, although the letters may be two inches high. A strange map, or any map, has the same effect. I have never seen a child, or a teacher, who could look at a map at the distance without becoming nearsighted.

German type has been accused of being responsible for much of the poor sight once supposed to be peculiarly a German malady; but if a German child attempts to read Roman print, he will at once become temporarily hypermetropic. German print, or Greek or Chinese characters, will have the same effect on a child, or other person, accustomed to Roman letters. Cohn repudiated the idea that German lettering was trying to the eyes.[a] On the contrary, he always found it "pleasant, after a long reading of the monotonous Roman print, to return 'to our beloved German.'" ... Because the German characters were more familiar to him than any others he found them restful to his eyes. "Use," as he truly observed, "has much to do with the matter." Children learning to read, write, draw, or sew always suffer from defective vision, because of the unfamiliarity of the lines or objects with which they are working....

...A schoolboy was able to read the bottom line of the Snellen card at ten feet, but when the teacher told him to mind what he was about, he could not see the big C. Many children can see perfectly so long as their mothers are around; but if the mother goes out of the room, they may at once become myopic, because of the strain produced by fear.

... Parents who wish to preserve and improve the eyesight of their children should encourage them to read the Snellen card every day. There should, in fact, be a Snellen card in every family; for when properly used it always prevents myopia and other errors of refraction, always improves the vision, even when this is already normal, and always benefits functional nervous troubles.

Parents should improve their own eyesight to normal, so that their children may not imitate wrong methods of using the eyes and will not be subject to the influence of an atmosphere of strain. They should also learn the principle of centralization sufficiently well to relieve and prevent pain, in order that they may teach their children to do the same. This practice not only makes it possible to avoid suffering, but is a great benefit to the general health ...

...Attempts were made to minimize the supposed evil effects of the reading, writing and other near work which it demanded. Careful and detailed rules were laid down by various authorities as to the sizes of type to be used in schoolbooks, the length of the lines, their distance apart, the

[a] Eyes and School-Books, Pop. Sci. Monthly, May, 1881, translated from Deutsche Rundschau.

distance at which the book should be held, the amount and arrangement of the light, the construction of the desks, the length of time the eyes might be used without a change of focus, etc. Face-rests were even devised to hold the eyes at the prescribed distance from the desk and to prevent stooping, which was supposed to cause congestion of the eyeball and thus to encourage elongation. The Germans, with characteristic thoroughness, actually used these instruments of torture, Cohn never allowing his own children to write without one, "even when sitting at the best possible desk." ...

... Further study of the subject has only added to its difficulty, while at the same time it has tended to relieve the schools of much of the responsibility formerly attributed to them for the production of myopia. As the American Encyclopedia of Ophthalmology points out, "the theory that myopia is due to close work aggravated by town life and badly lighted rooms is gradually giving ground before statistics."[b]

In an investigation in London, for instance, in which the schools were carefully selected to reveal any differences that might arise from the various influences, hygienic, social and racial, to which the children were subjected, the proportion of myopia in the best lighted building of the group was actually found to be higher than in the one where the lighting conditions were worst, although the higher degrees of myopia were more numerous in the latter than in the former. It has also been found that there is just as much myopia in schools where little near work is done as in those in which the demand upon the accommodative power of the eye is greater.[c] It is only a minority of children, moreover, that become myopic; yet all are subject to practically the same influences, and even in the same child one eye may become myopic while the other remains normal. On the theory that shortsight results from any external influence to which the eye is exposed it is impossible to account for the fact that under the same conditions of life the eyes of different individuals and the two eyes of the same individual behave differently.

Owing to the difficulty of reconciling these facts on the basis of the earlier theories, there is now a growing disposition to attribute myopia to hereditary tendencies;[d] but no satisfactory evidence on this point has been brought forward, and the fact that primitive peoples who have always had good eyesight become myopic just as quickly as any others when subjected to the conditions of civilized life, like the Indian students at Carlisle,[e] seems to be conclusive evidence against it.

In spite of the repeated failure of preventive measures based upon the limitation of near work and the regulation of lighting, desks, types, etc., the use of the eyes at the near point under unfavorable conditions is still admitted by most exponents of the heredity theory as probably, if not certainly, a secondary cause of myopia. Sidler-Huguenin, however, whose startling

[b] American Encyclopedia and Dictionary of Ophthalmology, edited by Wood, 1913–1919, vol. xi, p. 8271.

[c] Lawson: Brit. Med. Jour., June 18, 1898.

[d] It seems to have been amply demonstrated, by the studies of Motais Steiger, Miss Barrington, and Karl Pearson, that errors of refraction are inherited. And while the use of the eyes for near work is probably a secondary cause, determining largely the development of the defects, it is not the primary cause.—Cyclopedia of Education, edited by Monroe, 1911–1913, vol. iv, p. 361.

[e] Fox (quoted by Risley): System of Diseases of the Eye, vol. ii, p. 357.

conclusions as to the hopelessness of controlling shortsight were quoted earlier, has observed so little benefit from such precautions that he believes a myope may become an engineer just as well as a farmer, or a forester; and as a result of his experiences with anisometropes, persons with an inequality of refraction between the two organs of vision, he even suggests that the use of myopic eyes may possibly be more favorable to their well-being than their non-use. In 150 cases in which, owing to this inequality and other conditions, the subjects practically used but one eye, the weaker organ, he reports, became gradually more and more myopic, sometimes excessively so, in open defiance of all the accepted theories relating to the matter.

The prevalence of myopia, the unsatisfactoriness of all explanations of its origin, and the futility of all methods of prevention, have led some writers of repute to the conclusion that the elongated eyeball is a natural physiological adaptation to the needs of civilization. Against this view two unanswerable arguments can be brought. One is that the myopic eye does not see so well even at the near point as the normal eye, and the other that the defect tends to progression with very serious results, often ending in blindness. If Nature has attempted to adapt the eye to civilized conditions by an elongation of the globe, she has done it in a very clumsy manner. It is true that many authorities assume the existence of two kinds of myopia, one physiological, or at least harmless, and the other pathological; but since it is impossible to say with certainty whether a given case is going to progress or not, this distinction, even if it were correct, would be more important theoretically than practically.

Into such a slough of despond and contradiction have the misdirected labors of a hundred years led us! But in the light of truth the problem turns out to be a very simple one. In view of the facts given in Chapters V and IX [of *Perfect Sight Without Glasses*], it is easy to understand why all previous attempts to prevent myopia have failed. All these attempts have aimed at lessening the strain of near work upon the eye, leaving the strain to see distant objects unaffected, *and totally ignoring the mental strain which underlies the optical one.* [TQ emphasis.]

There are many differences between the conditions to which the children of primitive man were subjected, and those under which the offspring of civilized races spend their developing years, besides the mere fact that the latter learn things out of books and write things on paper, and the former did not. In the process of education civilized children are shut up for hours every day within four walls, in the charge of teachers who are too often nervous and irritable. They are even compelled to remain for long periods in the same position. The things they are required to learn may be presented in such a way as to be excessively uninteresting; and they are under a continual compulsion to think of the gaining of marks and prizes rather than the acquisition of knowledge for its own sake. Some children endure these unnatural conditions better than others. Many cannot stand the strain, and thus the schools become the hotbed, not only of myopia, but of all other errors of refraction.

Better Eyesight magazine, October 1920:

That imperfect sight is a fruitful cause of retardation in school is well known. According to the New York City Board of

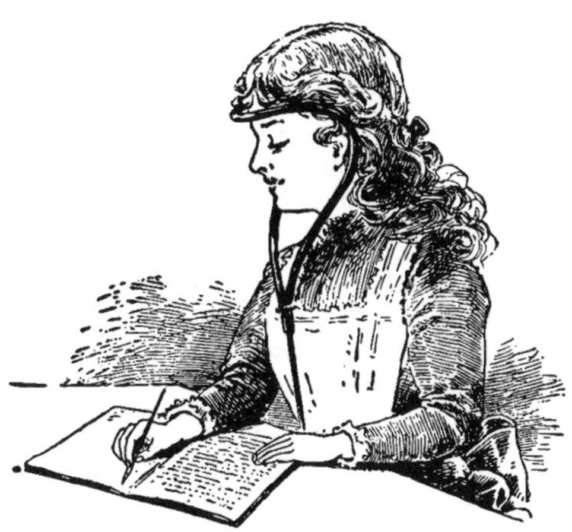

Figure 23–1: Face-Rest Designed by Kallman, a German Optician[2].

Health, it is responsible for a quarter of the habitually left backs.[a] But that this condition cannot be solved by glasses has not been generally observed. By making the person more comfortable glasses do often improve his mental condition, but since they cannot relieve the mental strain that underlies the visual one, they cannot improve it to normal and by confirming it in a bad habit they may make it worse.

[a] Archiv. f. Augenh. vol. IXXIX, 1915, translated in Arch. Ophth., vol. XLV, Nov. 1916.

Paul E. Dennison states, "the juvenile delinquent population is 80% farsighted.... "[3]

Clara Hackett, in *Relax and See,* writes:

Vision difficulties can affect a child in many ways. Poor posture, inferior manual skills and personality disturbances are often linked with it. Specialists of the Dyslexia Institute at Northwestern University estimate that fully 70 percent of school failures are the result of reading difficulties, which, very often, trace back to poor sight.

The problem of inadequate vision in our children is enormous.[4]

Continuing with Bates' discussion in *Perfect Sight Without Glasses:*

A Snellen card was hung in the classroom where all the children could see it, and the teacher carried out my instructions literally. At the end of six months all but two had normalized, and these had improved very much, while the worst incorrigible and the worst truant had become good students. The incorrigible, who had previously refused to study, because he said it gave him a headache to look at a book or at the blackboard, found out that the test card, in some way, did him a lot of good; and although the teacher had asked him to read it but once a day, he read it whenever he felt uncomfortable. The result was that in a few weeks his vision had become normal and his objection to study had disappeared. The truant had been in the habit of remaining away from school two or three days every week, and neither his parents nor the truant officer had been able to do anything about it. To the great surprise of his teacher he never missed a day after having begun to read the Snellen card. When she asked for an explanation, he told her that what had driven him away from school was the pain that came in his eyes whenever he tried to study, or to read the writing on the blackboard. After reading the Snellen card, he said, his eyes and head were rested and he was able to read without any discomfort.

To remove any doubts that might arise as to the cause of the improvement noted in the eyesight of the children, comparative tests were made with and without cards. In one case six students with defective sight were examined daily for one week without the use of the test card. No improvement took place. The card was then restored to its place, and the group was instructed to read it every day. At the end of a week all had improved and five normalized. In the case of another group of defectives the results were similar. During the week that the card was not used no improvement was noted; but after a week of practice in distant vision with the card all showed marked improvement, and at the end of a month all were normal. In order that there might be no question as to the reliability of the records of the teachers, some of the principals asked the Board of Health to send an inspector to test the vision of the students, and whenever this was done the records were found to be correct.

One day I visited the city of Rochester, and while there I called on the Superintendent of Public Schools and told him about my method of preventing myopia. He was very much interested and invited me to introduce it in one of his schools. I did so, and at the end of three months a report was sent to me showing that the vision of all the children had improved, while quite a number of them had obtained normal vision in both eyes.

The method has been used in a number of other cities and always with the same result. The vision of all the children improved, and many of them obtained normal vision in the course of a few minutes, days, weeks, or months.

It is difficult to prove a negative proposition, but since this system improved the vision of all the children who used it, it follows that none could have grown worse. It is therefore obvious that it must have prevented myopia. This cannot be said of any method of preventing myopia in schools which had previously been tried. All other methods are based on the idea that it is the excessive use of the eyes for near work that causes myopia, and all of them have admittedly failed.

It is also obvious that the method must have prevented other errors of refraction, a problem which previously had not even been seriously considered, because hypermetropia is supposed to be congenital, and astigmatism was until recently supposed also to be congenital in the great majority of cases. Anyone who knows how to use a retinoscope may, however, demonstrate in a few minutes that both of these conditions are acquired; for no matter how astigmatic or hypermetropic an eye may be, its vision always becomes normal when it looks at a blank surface without trying to see. It may also be demonstrated that when children are learning to read, write, draw, sew, or to do anything else that necessitates their looking at unfamiliar objects at the near point, hypermetropia, or hypermetropic astigmatism, is always produced. The same is true of adults. These facts have not been reported before, so far as I am aware, and they strongly suggest that children need, first of all, eye education. They must be able to look at strange letters or objects at the near point without strain before they can make much progress in their studies, and in every case in which the method has been tried it has been proven that this end is attained by daily practice in distant vision with the Snellen card. When their distant vision has been improved by this means, children invariably become able to use their eyes without strain at the near point.

The method succeeded best when the teacher did not wear glasses. In fact, the effect upon the children of a teacher who wears glasses is so detrimental that no such person should be allowed to be a teacher, and since errors of refraction can be eliminated, such a ruling would work no hardship on anyone. Not only do children imitate the visual habits of a teacher who wears glasses, but the nervous strain of which the defective sight is an expression produces in them a similar condition. In classes of the same grade, with the same lighting, the sight of children whose teachers did not wear glasses has always been found to be better than the sight of children whose teachers did wear them.

In one case I tested the sight of children whose teacher wore glasses, and found it very imperfect. The teacher went out of the room on an errand, and after she had gone I tested them again. The results were very much better. When the teacher returned she asked about the sight of a particular boy, a very nervous child, and as I was proceeding to test him she stood before him and said, "Now, when the doctor tells you to read the card, do it." The boy couldn't see anything. Then she went behind him, and the effect was the same as if she had left the room. The boy read the whole card.

Still better results would be obtained if we could reorganize the educational system on a rational basis. Then we might expect a general return of that primitive acuity of vision which we marvel at so greatly when we read about it in the memoirs of travellers. But even under existing conditions it has been proven beyond the shadow of a doubt that errors of refraction are no necessary part of the price we must pay for education.

There are at least ten million children in the schools of the United States who have defective sight. This condition prevents them from taking full advantage of the educational opportunities which the State provides. It undermines their health and wastes the taxpayers' money. If allowed to continue, it will be an expense and a handicap to them throughout their lives. In many cases it will be a source of continual misery and suffering. And yet practically all of these cases could be reversed and the development of new ones prevented by the daily reading of the Snellen card.

Why should our children be compelled to suffer and wear glasses for want of this simple measure of relief? It costs practically nothing. In fact, it would not be necessary, in some cases, as in the schools of New York City, even to purchase the Snellen cards, as they are already being used to test the eyes of the children. Not only does it place practically no additional burden upon the teachers, but, by improving the eyesight, health, disposition and mentality of their students, it greatly lightens their labors. No one would venture to suggest, further, that it could possibly do any harm. Why, then, should there be any delay about introducing it into the schools? If there is still thought to be a need for further investigation and discussion, we can investigate and discuss just as well after the children get the cards as before, and by adopting that course we shall not run the risk of needlessly condemning another generation to that curse which heretofore has always dogged the footsteps of civilization, namely, defective eyesight....

CHAPTER XXIX
MIND AND VISION

Poor sight is admitted to be one of the most fruitful causes of retardation in the schools. It is estimated[a] that it may reasonably be held responsible for a quarter

[a] School Health News, published by the Department of Health of New York City, February 1919.

of the habitually "left-backs," and it is commonly assumed that all this might be prevented by suitable glasses.

There is much more involved in defective vision, however, than mere inability to see the blackboard, or to use the eyes without pain or discomfort. Defective vision is the result of an abnormal condition of the mind; and when the mind is in an abnormal condition it is obvious that none of the processes of education can be conducted with advantage. By putting glasses upon a child we may, in some cases, neutralize the effect of this condition upon the eyes, and by making the student more comfortable may improve his mental faculties to some extent; *but we do not alter fundamentally the condition of the mind, and by confirming it in a bad habit we may make it worse.* [TQ emphasis.]

It can easily be demonstrated that among the faculties of the mind which are impaired when the vision is impaired is the memory; and as a large part of the educational process consists of storing the mind with facts, and all the other mental processes depend upon one's knowledge of facts, it is easy to see how little is accomplished by merely putting glasses on a child that has "trouble with its eyes." The extraordinary memory of primitive people has been attributed to the fact that owing to the absence of any convenient means of making written records they had to depend upon their memories, which were strengthened accordingly; but in view of the known facts about the relation of memory to eyesight it is more reasonable to suppose that the retentive memory of primitive man was due to the same cause as his keen vision, namely, a mind at rest.

The primitive memory, as well as primitive keenness of vision, has been found among civilized people; and if the necessary tests had been made it would doubtless have been found that they always occur together, as they did in a case which recently came under my observation. The subject was a child of ten with such marvelous eyesight that she could see the moons of Jupiter with the naked eye, a fact which was demonstrated by her drawing a diagram of these satellites which exactly corresponded to the diagrams made by persons who had used a telescope. Her memory was equally remarkable. She could recite the whole content of a book after reading it, as Lord Macaulay is said to have done, and she learned more Latin in a few days without a teacher than her sister, who had six diopters of myopia, had been able to do in several years. She remembered five years afterward what she ate at a restaurant, she recalled the name of the waiter, the number of the building and the street in which it stood. She also remembered what she wore on this occasion and what every one else in the party wore. The same was true of every other event which had awakened her interest in any way, and it was a favorite amusement in her family to ask her what the menu had been and what people had worn on particular occasions.

When the sight of two persons is different it has been found that their memories differ in exactly the same degree. Two sisters, one of whom had only ordinary good vision, indicated by the formula 20/20, while the other had 20/10, found that the time it took them to learn eight verses of a poem varied in almost exactly the same ratio as their sight. The one whose vision was 20/10 learned eight verses of the poem in fifteen minutes, while the one whose vision was only 20/20 required thirty-one minutes to do the same thing. After palming, the one with ordinary vision learned eight more verses in twenty-one minutes, while the one with 20/10 was able to reduce her time by only two minutes, a variation clearly within the limits of error. In other words, the mind of the latter being already in a normal or nearly normal condition, she could not improve it appreciably by palming, while the former, whose mind was under a strain, was able to gain relaxation, and hence improve her memory, by this means.

Even when the difference in sight is between the two eyes of the same person it can be demonstrated, as was pointed out in the chapter on "Memory as an Aid to Vision," that there is a corresponding difference in the memory, according to whether both eyes are open, or the better eye closed.

Under the present educational system there is a constant effort to compel the children to remember. These efforts always fail. They spoil both the memory and the sight. The memory cannot be forced any more than the vision can be forced. We remember without effort, just as we see without effort, and the harder we try to remember or see the less we are able to do so.

The sort of things we remember are the things that interest us, and the reason children have difficulty in learning their lessons is because they are bored by them. For the same reason, among others, their eyesight becomes impaired, boredom being a condition of mental strain in which it is impossible for the eye to function normally.

Some of the various kinds of compulsion now employed in the educational process may have the effect of awakening interest. Betty Smith's interest in winning a prize, for instance, or in merely getting ahead of Johnny Jones, may have the effect of rousing her interest in lessons that have hitherto bored her, and this interest may develop into a genuine interest in the acquisition of knowledge; but this cannot be said of the various fear incentives still so largely employed by teachers. These, on the contrary, have the effect, usually, of completely paralyzing minds already benumbed by lack of interest, and the effect upon the vision is equally disastrous.

The fundamental reason, both for poor memory and poor eyesight in school children, in short, is our irrational and unnatural educational system. Montessori has taught us that it is only when children are interested that they can learn. It is equally true that it is only when they are interested that they can see. This fact was strikingly illustrated in the case of one of the two pairs of sisters mentioned above. Phebe, of the keen eyes, who could recite whole books if she happened to be interested in them, disliked mathematics and anatomy extremely, and not only could not learn them but became myopic when they were presented to her mind. She could read letters a quarter of an inch high at twenty feet in a poor light, but when asked to read figures one to two inches high in a good light at ten feet she miscalled half of them. When asked to tell how much 2 and 3 made, she said "4" before finally deciding on "5"; and all the time she was occupied with this disagreeable subject, the retinoscope showed that she was myopic. When I asked her to look into my eye with the ophthalmoscope, she could see nothing, although a much lower degree of visual acuity is required to note the details of the interior of the eye than to see the moons of Jupiter.

Shortsighted Isabel, on the contrary, had a passion for mathematics and anatomy, and excelled in those subjects. She learned to use the ophthalmoscope as easily as Phebe had learned Latin. Almost immediately she saw the optic nerve, and noted that the center was whiter than the periphery. She saw the light-colored lines, the arteries; and the darker ones, the veins; and she saw the light streaks on the blood-vessels. Some specialists never become able to do this, and no one could do it without normal vision. Isabel's vision, therefore, must have been temporarily normal when she did it. Her vision for figures, although not normal, was better than for letters.

In both these cases the ability to learn and the ability to see went hand in hand with interest. Phebe could read a photographic reduction of the Bible and recite what she had read verbatim, she could see the moons of Jupiter and draw a diagram of them afterwards, because she was interested in these things; but she could not see the interior of the eye, nor see figures even half as well as she saw letters, because these things bored her. When, however, it was suggested to her that it would be a good joke to surprise her teachers, who were always reproaching her for her backwardness in mathematics, by taking a high mark in a coming examination, her interest in the subject awakened and she contrived to learn enough to get seventy-eight percent. In Isabel's case letters were antagonistic. She was not interested in most of the subjects with which they dealt, and, therefore, she was backward in those subjects, and had become habitually myopic. But when asked to look at objects which aroused an intense interest her vision became normal.

When one is not interested, in short, one's mind is not under control, and without mental control one can neither learn nor see. Not only the memory but all other mental faculties are improved when the eyesight becomes normal. It is a common experience with [students who normalize] defective sight to find that their ability to do their work has improved.

The teacher whose letter is quoted in a later chapter testified that after gaining perfect eyesight she "knew better how to get at the minds of the students," was "more direct, more definite, less diffused, less vague," possessed, in fact, "centralization of the mind." In another letter she said: "The better my eyesight becomes the greater is my ambition. On the days when my sight is best I have the greatest anxiety to do things."

Another teacher reported that one of her students used to sit doing nothing all day long, and apparently was not interested in anything. After the test card was introduced into the classroom and his sight improved, he became anxious to learn, and speedily developed into one of the best students in the class. In other words his eyes and his mind became normal together....

From all these facts it will be seen that the problems of vision are far more intimately associated with the problems of education than we had supposed, and that they can by no means be solved by putting concave, or convex, or astigmatic lenses before the eyes of the children.

SPONTANEOUS VS. VOLUNTARY ATTENTION

T. Ribot wrote in *The Psychology of Attention:*

> There are two well-defined forms of attention: the one spontaneous, natural; the other voluntary, artificial. The former—neglected by most psychologists—is the true, primitive, and fundamental form of attention. The second—the only one studied by most psychologists—is but an imitation, a result of education, of training, and of impulsion.[5]

SPONTANEOUS ATTENTION

Spontaneous attention is the only existing form of attention until education and artificial means have been employed. There exists no other kind in most animals and in young children. It is a gift of nature....

... whether strong or weak, everywhere and always, *it is caused by emotional states.* This rule is absolute, without exceptions....[6]

... spontaneous attention is natural and devoid of effort....[7]

Every intellectual state is accompanied by definite physical manifestations....[8]

The movements of the body, which are said to express attention, are ... of paramount importance....[9]

Are the movements of the face, the body, and the limbs, and the respiratory modifications that accompany attention, simply effects, outward marks, as is usually supposed? Or, are they, on the contrary, *the necessary conditions, the constituent elements, the indispensable factors of attention?* Without hesitation we accept the second thesis. Totally suppress movements, and you totally suppress attention.... The fundamental role of movements in attention is to *maintain* the appropriate state of consciousness and to *reinforce* it....[10]

The motor manifestations are neither effects nor causes, but elements; together with the state of consciousness, which constitutes their subjective side, *they are* attention....[11]

... a close observer of children, Sikorski has shown that their activity and attention are mainly developed through play.[a]

VOLUNTARY ATTENTION

Voluntary or artificial attention is a product of art, of education, of direction, and of training. It is grafted, as it were, upon spontaneous or natural attention ... voluntary attention is always accompanied by a certain feeling of effort. The maximum of spontaneous attention and the maximum of voluntary attention are totally antithetic ...

The process through which voluntary attention is formed may be reduced to the following single formula: To render attractive, by artifice, what is not so by nature; to give an artificial interest to things that have not a natural interest.... During the earliest periods of its life the child is only capable of spontaneous attention....

The birth of voluntary attention, the power of fastening the mind upon non-attractive objects, can only be accomplished by force, under the influence of education, whether derived from men or things external....[12]

Acquired attention has thus become a second nature, and the artificial process is complete.[13]

... Voluntary attention, in its durable form, is really a difficult state to sustain....

But if, as we have attempted to show, the higher form of attention is the work of the education that we have received from our parents, teachers, and surroundings, as well as the education which later we have ourselves acquired in imitating that which we earlier experienced, this explanation, nevertheless, only forces the difficulty further back; for our teachers have only acted upon us, as others had previously acted upon them, and so on back through the generations. This, accordingly, does not explain the primordial genesis of voluntary attention.

How then does voluntary attention originate? It originates of necessity, under the pressure of need, and with the progress of intelligence. *It is an instrument that has been perfected—a product of civilization.*

... Onward movement, in the intellectual world, has also effected the transition from spontaneous attention to the dominance of voluntary attention. The latter is both

[a] *Revue Philosophique,* April 1885.

the cause and effect of civilization.

In the preceding chapter it was pointed out that in the state of nature the power of spontaneous attention, both for animals and men, is a factor of the foremost order in the struggle for life. In the course of man's development from the savage state, so soon as (through whatever actual causes, such as lack of game, density of population, sterility of soil, or more warlike neighboring tribes) there was only left the alternatives of perishing or of accommodating oneself to more complex conditions of life—in other words, to go to work—voluntary attention also became a foremost factor in this new form of the struggle for existence. So soon as man had become capable of devoting himself to any task that possessed no immediate attraction, but was accepted as the only means of livelihood, voluntary attention put in an appearance in the world. It originated, accordingly, under the pressure of necessity, and of the education imparted by things external.

It is easily shown that before civilization voluntary attention did not exist, or appeared only by flashes and then of short duration. The laziness of savages is well known; travelers and ethnologists are all agreed on this point, and the proofs and instances are so numerous that it would be idle to quote authorities. The savage has a passion for hunting, war, and gambling; for the unforeseen, the unknown, and the hazardous in all its forms; but sustained effort he ignores or contemns. Love of work is a sentiment of purely secondary formation, that goes hand in hand with civilization. And we may note, now, that work is the concrete, the most manifest form of [voluntary] attention.

Continuous work is repugnant even to half-civilized tribes ... [14]

Everyone knows by experience that voluntary attention is always accompanied by a feeling of effort, which bears a direct proportion to the duration of the state and the difficulty of maintaining it.[15]

This means that [voluntary] attention is an abnormal, a transient state, producing a rapid exhaustion of the organism; for after effort there is fatigue, and after fatigue there is functional inactivity.... [16]

CONCLUSION

We have endeavored to establish, in the present work, the thesis that the immediate and necessary condition of attention in all its forms is interest—that is, natural or artificial emotional states—and that, further, its mechanism is motor. Attention is not a faculty, a special power, but a predominantly *intellectual state,* resulting from complex causes that induce a shorter or longer adaptation.... [17]

"DEFINITE, IRREFUTABLE PROOF"

From *Better Eyesight* magazine, September 1922:

AN EDUCATOR OFFERS PROOF

Received too late for publication in the special August School number of Better Eyesight *is the following report by Professor Husted, Superintendent of Schools of North Bergen, N. J., of the astounding results in the improvement of children's vision achieved through the use of Dr. Bates' methods. This report, made independently by Professor Husted to the school commissioners of his locality, is definite, irrefutable proof, from an unquestionably neutral observer of the efficacy of those methods.*

In the schools of North Bergen, New Jersey, are some six thousand children. They are, besides being children of a typical near metropolitan community and a part of the coming generation of our citizens, men and women, a representative living laboratory of childhood. And in that laboratory has been performed a practical test by Professor Husted, Superintendent of Schools, the results of which are stated by him in the subjoined extract from a regular report to his school commissioners.

They are of vital significance.

Professor Husted's report says:

High Spot Normal Eye Health
Crusade a Successful
Three Years' Experiment

Early in October, 1919, under the direction of our school nurse, Miss Marion McNamara, a Snellen test of the eyes of all our students was made. A novel health experiment was begun, a campaign for "*Better Eyesight*." In June a second test was made in order to verify the value and progress in this phase of health work. The June test shows marvelous, practical, successful results....

The following summary shows the remarkable results of the North Bergen experiment in the use of the Bates System. The first grades are omitted because of the difficulty in making accurate tests.

Grades II to VIII

Schools	**No. Tested**			**No. Absent 2nd Test**		
	1920	**1921**	**1922**	**1920**	**1921**	**1922**
Grant	72	100	133	0	4	19
Robert Fulton	359	498	672	11	4	122
Franklin	341	339	418	17	3	54
Lincoln	388	585	873	21	21	135
Hamilton	211	225	204	12	1	8
Jefferson	526	542	609	33	16	41
Washington	353	543	538	11	15	67
Horace Mann	335	319	446	5	19	45
McKinley	144	157	312	17	5	36
Totals	**2729**	**3308**	**4205**	**127**	**88**	**527**

Schools	**No. Below 20/20**			**No. Absent 2nd Test**			**% Improved**		
	1920	**1921**	**1922**	**1920**	**1921**	**1922**	**1920**	**1921**	**1922**
Grant	36	31	31	30	16	19	83.3	51.6	61.3
Robert Fulton	112	127	11	76	84	56	75.2	66.1	36.8
Franklin	103	102	152	53	53	53	61.6	51.8	53.0
Lincoln	169	131	100	103	90	71	69.4	68.6	43.8
Hamilton	78	60	162	48	40	22	72.7	66.6	52.4
Jefferson	216	181	42	109	117	86	59.5	64.6	58.5
Washington	184	134	147	107	84	80	63.4	62.6	58.8
Horace Mann	96	70	136	66	42	61	72.5	60.0	61.0
McKinley	75	38	100	55	21	52	94.8	55.2	57.1
Totals	**1049**	**874**	**961**	**647**	**547**	**500**	**70.1**	**62.5**	**52.0**

This is a remarkable demonstration of the priceless values of this method of education. That 647 or 70.1% of the 922 students below normal (20/20) should have been improved in eyesight in 1920, that 547 or 62.5% should have been improved in 1921, and that 500 or 52% should have been improved in 1922, is surely a marvelous showing. The record of improvement is suggestive of what a very faithful and systematic application of these health principles may accomplish. In 1920 there were 1,049 or 38% students out of 2,729 tested that were below 20/20 or normal standard, while in 1921 but 874 students or 26% out of 3,308 were found below normal, and in 1922 only 961 students or 23% were below standard.

This cumulative improvement is credited to our health work of 1920 and 1921. This reduction from 38% to 26% and then 23% must be due to those students who are benefited and remain in the North Bergen system. We have enrolled 389 new students from other systems this year. As the percentage of students below standard becomes less (38%, 26%, 23%), the percentages of improvement has become less (70.1, 62.5, 52). This suggests that many cases remaining in our schools are less amenable to improvement and should, therefore, receive persistent and systematic attention.

Not only does this work place no additional burden upon the teachers, but, by improving the eyesight, health, disposition and mentality of their students, it surely lightens their labors.

BETTER EYESIGHT MAGAZINES—SCHOOL CHILDREN

From *Better Eyesight* magazine, August 1921:

SIGHT SAVING IN THE SCHOOLROOM

By Edith F. Gavin

It seemed so wonderful to me to be able to lay aside my glasses and have eye comfort after wearing them for twenty-two years with discomfort the greater part of the time! I could scarcely wait to get back home to talk to the other teachers about it and try to help a few of the children.

I began with Gertrude, who was so nearsighted that from a front seat she was unable to see very black figures one and one-half inches high printed on a white chart and hanging on the front board. Her vision January 11, 1921, was 20/70 in both eyes, but by March 10th she had improved to 20/70 with the right eye and 20/30 with the left and could read the chart from the last seat in the row.

Matilda had complained of headaches since last September. Glasses were obtained last December, and after a two months' struggle to get used to them, she refused to wear them, saying that they made her head and eyes feel worse. I then told her how to palm and practice with the chart. She had no more headaches in school, and her mother said she didn't complain at home. Her vision also improved from 20/30 to 20/15.

I next took Walter in hand. His mother would not get glasses for him, although advised to do so by the school nurse and doctor. His vision February 18th was 20/200. Three weeks later his mother decided to get glasses for him, but his vision had improved to 20/20 in the right eye and 20/30 in the left.

A teacher brought Helen to me, saying she was so nervous and read in such a halting manner that she felt sure that her glasses did not fit her. Her mother said that she might lay aside her glasses and Helen could hardly wait to begin. Shortly after she was taken ill with scarlet fever and did not return, but her vision improved from 20/40 to 20/15, and her teacher said that her reading had improved noticeably.

Mollie, age six, was sent in to me February 18th. She tested 20/70 in the right eye and 20/50 in the left. Her vision in May was 20/30, right, and 20/20, left.

When Rae came to my room, May 15th, her vision was 20/70. Her father was very much opposed to her wearing glasses and readily gave permission for me to help her. She remained in the district only two weeks, but she had improved to 20/20 in the right eye and 20/30 in the left.

Bennie, mentally defective, required a great deal of patience, but he improved from 20/50 February 9th to 20/15 March 4th.

Leo, a fifth grade student, was sent to me February 20th by his teacher. She said he wouldn't wear his glasses and was a poor student. He tested 20/50 in the right eye and 20/30 in the left. By March 15th his vision was 20/30, right eye, and 20/15, left, and his teacher said that he showed a marked improvement in his scholarship.

The children needing help came to me fifteen minutes before the afternoon session began. If I was busy with one, the others would work quietly by themselves, seeming to take great pride in their improvement. The chart hangs on the front wall at all times. I taught the class how to palm and often different ones would come up early to practice. Several children with apparently normal vision told me that they were able to read two or three lines more at the end of the term. To my mind there is no limit to the good that might be accomplished if this method were in general use in the schools.

THE SCHOOL CHILDREN AGAIN

By Emily C. Lierman

We have so many interesting cases among the children sent to us from the schools to be fitted with glasses that one hardly knows where to begin when trying to tell about them. Little Agnes, eight years old, comes to my mind, not because she was more remarkable than a good many others, but because she came recently. Her mother came with her, and told me that Agnes suffered from frequent headaches and that for the past year her teachers had been saying that she needed glasses, as she had great difficulty in seeing the blackboard. The mother had hesitated to take her to an oculist, however, as two of her children were already wearing glasses and she did not want to see them on a third.

I could easily see that Agnes was suffering, and when I tested her eyes with the Snellen card I found that her vision was very poor. At fifteen feet she could not read more than the seventy line. This was so surprising in so young a child that I thought at first she did not know her letters; but when I tested her with pothooks she did no better. I now showed her how to palm, and in a few moments she read the bottom line. The mother was thrilled and said:

"My goodness! When I first entered this room my hope was gone. I could think of nothing but glasses for my child. When she first read the card and I saw how bad her eyes were, I was convinced that there was no escape for her. But now that I see her vision improved so quickly I have hope indeed."

I told the mother that I was thrilled myself, and added that she could help me to improve the sight of the child if she would.

"What I do for her here you can do for her at home," I said. "Encourage her to rest her eyes. Nature requires rest for the eyes, but your little girl, instead of closing her eyes when they are tired, strains to keep them open."

The mother promised to do all she could, and as she was leaving she said:

" . . . I will send my two boys to be rid of their glasses also."

The next clinic day Agnes brought with her brother Peter, who was wearing glasses for astigmatism and headaches. He was very attentive while I taught Agnes, who told me that she had not been having her usual headaches. Peter's vision I found to be 15/40, right eye, and 15/15, left eye. After palming only a few minutes, his right eye improved to 15/15 and his left to 15/10. He was very happy when told that he did not need glasses any more, and that I could teach him during vacation. As children are reversed very quickly when one helps the other at home, I expect that Agnes and Peter will soon be reading 20/10, which is twice what the normal eye is expected to do....

A very remarkable case still under education is that of a girl with nystagmus, a condition in which the eyes vibrate from side to side. The child is now so much improved that ordinarily her eyes are normal, but when anything disturbs her the vibration returns. This always happens, she tells me, when the teacher asks her a question, and at the same time she loses her memory. But the teacher allows her to cover her eyes to rest them, and in a few minutes the vibration ceases and her memory improves. Before she came to the clinic she often became hysterical and was obliged to leave the classroom. Now she is never troubled in this way.

One of the most puzzling cases I ever had was sent by the school nurse for glasses. A student who came from the same school told me that she was stupid, and she certainly appeared to be so. I asked her if she knew her letters, and in trying to reply she stuttered painfully. I tried to reassure her by speaking as gently as I could, but without avail. I could not get her to answer intelligently. I tried having her palm, but it did not help. I held the test card close to her eyes, and asked her to point out certain letters as I named them, but only in a few cases did she do this correctly. Completely baffled I appealed to Dr. Bates. He asked the child to come to him and touch a button on his coat, and she did so. He asked her to touch another button, but she answered:

"I don't see them."

"Look down at your shoes," he said. "Do you see them?"

"No," she answered.

"Go over and put your finger on the door-knob," he said, and she immediately did so.

"It is a case of hysterical blindness," the doctor said.

The child came for some time very regularly, and now reads 15/10 with both eyes. She has stopped stuttering, and has lost her reputation for stupidity. She has become a sort of Good Samaritan in her neighborhood, for every once in a while she brings with her some little companion to reverse imperfect sight. She never has any doubts as to our capacity to do this, and so far we have never disappointed her. I hope she never brings anyone who is beyond our power to help, for I would be sorry to see that sublime faith which we have inspired in her shattered.

Two of our students graduated in June, and after the final examinations they told me that they had been greatly helped in these tests by the memory of a swinging black period. One of them was told by the principal that if she failed to pass it would not be because of her stupidity, but because she refused to wear glasses. She gave him Dr. Bates' book, and after that, though he watched her closely, he did not say anything more about her eyes.

"I made up my mind to pass without the aid of glasses," she said, "and put one over on the principal, and you bet I never lost sight of my precious swinging period. The book has become a family treasure," she continued. "When one of us has a pain in the head or eyes, out it comes. It is a natural thing to see mother palming after her work is done. She enjoys her evenings with us now, because palming rests her and she does not get so sleepy."

The other graduate said: "I did not have to think of a black period when the subject was easy, but when I had to answer questions in the more difficult branches I certainly did find the period a lifesaver. I know I would have failed without it."

Bates taught students to imagine a black period. While shifting to the right side of the period, the student imagines the period moves to the left, and vice versa. The principles involved, once again, are centralization and movement.

From *Better Eyesight* magazine, November 1921:

THE SENSE OF TOUCH AN AID TO VISION

Just as Montessori has found that impressions gained through the sense of touch are very useful in teaching children to read and write, persons with defective sight have found them useful in educating their memory and imagination.

... [One student] found that when he lost the swing [the illusion of oppositional movement], he could get it again by sliding his forefinger back and forth over the ball of his thumb. When he moved his fingers it seemed as if his whole body was moving.

Better Eyesight magazine, April 1923:

DR. BATES' LECTURE

By L. L. Biddle, 2nd

... [Bates] told us of a specific case: A woman wearing very strong glasses brought her daughter to him, because the little girl's eyes were getting so bad that she could not continue at school. When the woman, in her usual cross manner, told her daughter to take off her glasses and read the test card, she was only able to read the top letter. Doctor Bates then very kindly asked the child to close her eyes and rest them. After a little while he asked her to open her eyes, and tell what she could see. Much to their surprise the little girl read the whole card. Her mother was very happy and said that she would see that her daughter would practice every day with the test card as Doctor Bates instructed. In a few days, however, they returned very discouraged and the mother said that her child was only able to read the top letter on the test card. Doctor Bates said that he asked her who had tested the girl's sight, and the woman admitted that it was she. He remonstrated with her, and reminded her that he especially asked her to stay out of the room when her daughter was practicing, and to have someone with normal sight test her. He then took his little student as before and speaking to her kindly, had her rest her eyes, and she again read the whole card.

Doctor Bates stated that he cited this example to show how the strain which this woman was under from wearing very strong glasses was contagious, and harmed her daughter's sight. Moreover, he said that it showed how the child's state of mind directly affected her ability to see. For when she was spoken to kindly and her mind was relaxed, her eyes were rested and she read the whole card. He explained that when one's mind was under a strain one unconsciously tightened the muscles which encir-

> cle the eyeball, and consequently squeeze it out of shape and out of focus. But when the mind is at rest these muscles are relaxed and the eyeball is allowed to assume its proper shape and focus.... He said that all children under 12 years of age not wearing glasses can obtain perfect sight by reading the Snellen Card once a day, first with one eye and then with the other.

"Great Imitators"

Many parents have contacted Bates teachers for classes for their children. Oftentimes, the parent(s) has been wearing glasses for many years. Many parents choose to improve their vision to set a correct example for their children. If the parents are staring rigidly, "spaced out," blinking infrequently, squinting, breathing shallowly, this can obviously impact the child's sight in a negative manner. Children are "great imitators" of other people's habits, especially their parents.

Better Eyesight magazine, July 1923:

> The father of the son disturbed the mind of the son, and I have found during all these years that one of the greatest difficulties with teaching children is to counteract the harmful influence of the parents wearing glasses. *Nearsightedness is contagious.* Children are great imitators, and they consciously or unconsciously imitate the habits of their parents, even to the smallest detail. I have talked until I was all talked out trying to explain this fact to the parents of children who were wearing glasses. I have tested the sight of many thousands of children in public schools, and was very much impressed to find that in those classes presided over by teachers wearing glasses the percentage of imperfect sight in the students was very much increased, while in those classes where teachers did not wear glasses imperfect sight was less frequent.

Better Eyesight magazine, July 1923:

> I feel the principal duty of every man, of every woman, is the business of looking after the children. Of what use is it to accumulate many dollars when your child goes around half blind wearing glasses?

Better Eyesight magazine, March 1924:

> Since perfect sight is contagious, and imperfect sight is contagious, consider it your duty as a teacher to acquire normal eyesight without the use of glasses.

So many parents and teachers wear glasses today, it is not a trivial task for children to escape the influence of their poor vision habits. The importance of adults—who are with children many hours per day—improving their own vision becomes clear.

Better Eyesight magazine, August 1927:

> SCHOOL CHILDREN
>
> by Emily C. Lierman
>
> Davey, eight years old, was very nearsighted, and the glasses he was wearing made him nervous and irritable. His father had been told about the Bates method and what could be done to restore perfect sight without wearing glasses. Davey's father brought the boy to me, although he was skeptical and his mother was even more so. I could tell by the little boy's attitude toward me that the Bates method had been much discussed in the home circle, and that I was considered a sort of mystic worker.
>
> The first question Davey asked me was, "What are you going to do to me?"
>
> I answered, "I am not going to do any-

thing to you, but I will try to do a whole lot for you. I will help you to get rid of your thick glasses that I am sure you don't like."

His answer was, "Oh, yes, I would like my glasses if I could see out of them. Father said that if you don't help me, he will try to find other glasses that will help."

I let the little fellow talk for a while, because I thought it would help me to understand him better. I told him I was especially interested in children and that it was always my delight to give school children better sight. I said I would not interfere with him, if glasses were what he wanted most. He said that he was afraid to play baseball or other games which might not only break his glasses, but perhaps hurt his eyes.

... With his glasses on ... at ten feet from the test card, he could see only black smudges on the white, but no letters. ... All he could see at [six feet] was the letter on the top of the card, seen normally at two hundred feet. ... Without his glasses ... he could not see anything at all on the card. I asked him to follow me to the window and to look in the distance and tell me what he could see. To the right of me, about one hundred feet away, there was a sign. The letters of this sign appeared to be about three feet square. One word of the sign had four letters. The first letter was straight and the last was curved, and had an opening to the right. I explained this to Davey, as I told him to look in the direction in which I was pointing, and then to a small card with fine print that I had given him to hold. I told him to read what he could of the fine print. He read it at two inches from his eyes. Under my direction, he alternately followed my finger as I pointed to the fine print and then to the building sign. He told me he could not see anything in the distance.

Davey felt very uncomfortable because of his poor sight and became rather restless. [I gave him some more instructions and told him] to blink often. He shifted from the ... fine print to the sign in the distance, watching my finger as I pointed, first to the near point and then to the distance. Suddenly, he got a flash of the first letter of the first word on the sign. This practice was continued for twenty minutes, and then we had a rest period. Davey sat comfortably in a chair and palmed his eyes. Children are very apt to become bored with anything that takes time and patience, and I know that Davey had little patience with anything regarding his eyes.

I asked him questions about his school work, and what subjects he liked best. He said he just loved arithmetic. I asked his father to give him an example to do while he palmed. The little fellow thought this was great fun, and without hesitation he gave his father the correct answer for each example. This gave Davey a rest period of fifteen minutes. His mother remarked that this was the first time she had ever noticed him sit quietly for so long a time.

Davey was then shown how to swing, by moving his body slowly from left to right, and getting only a glimpse of the letters on the card, at six feet. When he looked longer than an instant at the card, he leaned forward and strained to see better, but failed each time. When he learned not to stare, but to shift and blink while he swayed, his vision improved to 6/50. We returned to the window. I told him to shift from ... the fine print, which I held close to his eyes, then to the distant sign, and he became able to read all of the sign without any difficulty.

Much had been accomplished in one lesson and both parents were grateful. Davey was given a card with instructions for home practice. He returned three days each week for further lessons. Every time he visited me, I placed the ... card one foot farther away. Eight weeks after his first lesson, he read all of the ... card letters at ten feet. This was accomplished by reading fine print close to his eyes, then swinging and shifting, as he read one letter of the card at a time.

This boy has sent other school children to me as well as a school teacher with progressive myopia, who practiced faithfully until she was seeing clearly. Every week, she sent me a report about her eye lessons and the progress she made. Her students noticed that she had discarded her glasses, and after school hours she invited some of them, who had trouble with their eyes, to practice the Bates method with her. In eight weeks' time, her vision became normal, and all her students, with the exception of three, are improving their vision without the use of glasses....

Natural Speech Improvement

Better Eyesight magazine, August 1927:

A SCHOOL TEACHER'S REPORT

June 12, 1927

As a teacher of Speech Improvement I have found that some of the teachings that are used by Dr. Bates in the improvement of poor vision are very helpful in the improvement of stammering. Those who stammer are invariably nervous, and the palming and swaying activities calm the nerves and help the children to speak more quietly and slowly and therefore without stammering. In all cases where I have introduced the swaying in my stammering classes, the result has been a greater calmness both in reading and speaking and I believe that in this age of nerve tension, relaxation activities are a boon even for children of school age.

Poor speech and poor sight often go together, and it is a happy circumstance that Dr. Bates has devised activities that will help both defects at the same time. An outstanding case of a child suffering both from defective speech and very poor eyesight was a little Italian boy who was in one of my stammering classes. I asked him to read a sentence from the blackboard and he immediately bent his body away over to one side and stretched his neck as far forward as he could, straining to see the letters. I directed him to cover his eyes for a few minutes and then to sway for a while. He soon found that he could see much better and that he could read without stammering. He was very backward in reading and spelling. Although in the second year of school, he did not even know the names of all the letters of the alphabet. I believe that this was largely due to his poor vision and that the stammering came as he became aware of his inability to keep up with the rest of his class. During the short time that he was with me, his speech and sight greatly improved.

Posture is another thing that may be improved by the swaying activity. Ordinarily, when you ask a child to stand in good posture he will place his feet close together like an Egyptian statue. In the sway, he is shown that by putting his feet apart he has a broader base for standing and more ease and comfort for moving. I hope that some day we may be able to bring all these beneficial activities to all the children in the schools who need them.

CHILDREN'S VISION STORIES

From *Better Eyesight* magazine, June 1924:

SINBAD THE SAILOR

By George Guild

Why Sinbad? Of what benefit to the readers of this magazine or to people who

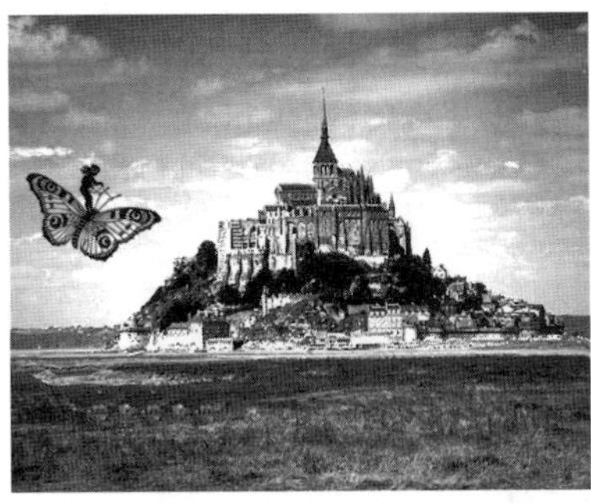

desire to see clearly without glasses can a reference to Sinbad be? In Arabian Nights tales, he occupies a prominent place. In his many voyages he described many extraordinary things which happened and which were very wonderful, although not always probable or true. Being a sailor, he used his eyes principally for distant vision. He had good eyesight, but after one of his numerous voyages he returned to his home in Baghdad and complained to his friends that his sight for distance had become poor, so poor that he was unable to recognize people ten feet away. An Egyptian astrologer sold him a pair of glasses for a price which made a big hole in his savings. For a time he was happy because his vision was decidedly improved by the glasses, but it was not long before his imperfect sight required stronger glasses, and the strength of his glasses was frequently increased. In a shipwreck he had difficulty in reaching the shore because the water clouded his glasses so that they became useless. Whenever it rained the glasses became too clouded to help him to see. In many emergencies, when he most needed his glasses, they failed him. When swimming he could not see any better than without his glasses. It embarrassed him very much when trying to reach land, because he was unable to locate it. Other sailors would throw water in his face, fog his glasses, and tease the blind man without risk to themselves. With his glasses he suffered great pain and fatigue.

While visiting a city in a foreign land and walking the streets without seeing much, a stranger handed him a parchment on which was written:

"Go where all things are moving,
Watch and think the livelong day;
The truth is always proving
Your sight will return, I say."

The words gave him some hope and he believed that in one of his voyages he would find some land or country where all things would be moving and nothing immovable or stationary. In a voyage to India he felt that in this country he would find a land where all things were moving. After a long day of traveling he entered a temple where many worshippers on their knees were alternately raising their arms and faces on high and then bowing to the ground, saying:

"Allah is Allah,
God is Allah."

To avoid attracting attention he imitated the others while remembering that the paper of instructions told him to watch and think. He noted that when he raised his head up that things in front of him and to one side seemed to move down or in the opposite direction, and that when he bowed his head down to the ground, things appeared to move up.

At last he believed that he had found a place were all things were moving. By going through the motions without prayer he found that it worked just the same. After he left the temple he was able to notice that when he walked straight ahead things to each side of him, and the ground in front of him appeared to move in the opposite direction. He was able to demonstrate then, without any effort, that the place where all things are moving was wherever he happened to be, and since he was always moving his eyes during the day it was possible for him to see things moving opposite all day long.

"Watch and think" was ever in his mind. He became able to demonstrate that when he imagined the movement easily that all pain, discomfort or fatigue in his eyes and in other parts of his body were prevented or relieved. It was not long before he found that the light became brighter; and, with this increased illumination, his vision improved.

When the swing was practiced with an effort, very little or no benefit followed. He discovered that the swing was of great help to his vision when practiced at night, and brought him more comfort than the same time devoted to sleep. All this time he believed that he had discovered a *truth;* that the cause of his imperfect sight was a strain or an effort to see, and that he improved by *rest* and not by *effort.*

He returned to Baghdad overflowing with the wonderful news. He called on the Egyptian astrologer who had sold him his glasses, and with a happy smile on his face reported the facts.

The astrologer was furious and screamed in a loud voice:

"Out upon you, you lying knave. I believed your story of the mammoth bird, the rock, your experiences with mermaids and many other of your strange tales, but this is too much. To eliminate poor sight by rest is too absurd. You must be crazy." Then he drove Sinbad from his house, announcing to the mob of people outside to shun him for a liar, a cheat, and a fool.

For many years later Sinbad held his peace but did not neglect to help those with poor sight until their number became sufficiently great to overwhelm the ignorant astrologer and others like him.

More stories from the *Better Eyesight* magazines are located in Appendix G, "Additional Vision Stories."

CHAPTER COMMENTS

Clara Hackett, in *Relax and See,* writes:

> Overcoming the handicap of defective vision, important at any age, is especially rewarding for a child. For better vision can play an important role throughout his lifetime—in personality and social development, in school work and, later in his whole career.
>
> ... Helping him to firmly establish sound habits of using his sight which will stand him in good stead all his life, are worthwhile goals.... [18]
>
> One of the most important assets you can endow your child with is an understanding of how to develop and maintain the good visual habits that will help to keep his sight perfect throughout his life.[19]

I am especially interested in training Natural Vision teachers who can teach children. (See Appendix E—Becoming a Natural Vision teacher.)

Ellen Raskin wrote a wonderful little children's book, called *Nothing Ever Happens on My Block,* which is all about interest. (See Bibliography.)

Notes

1 W. B. MacCracken, *Use Your Own Eyes* (Berkeley, California: Published by the author, 1937), p. 232.

2 Graphic and caption reprinted from *Perfect Sight Without Glasses.*

3 Paul E. Dennison, "Reading and Vision," *Brain Gym Magazine,* Vol. II, No. 3 (Fall 1988), p. 1.

4 Clara A. Hackett and Lawrence Galton, *Relax and See* (London: Faber and Faber, Limited, 1957), p. 262.

5 T. Ribot, *The Psychology of Attention* (Chicago: The Open Court Publishing Company, 1890), p. 2.

6 Ibid., p. 6.

7 Ibid., p. 8.

8 Ibid., p. 12.

9 Ibid., p. 15.

10 Ibid., p. 19.

11 Ibid., p. 23.

12 Ibid., pp. 29–32.

13 Ibid., p. 34.

14 Ibid., pp. 36–37.

15 Ibid., pp. 59–60.

16 Ibid., p. 66.

17 Ibid., p. 105.

18 Clara A. Hackett and Lawrence Galton, *Relax and See,* p. 254.

19 Ibid., p. 261.

CHAPTER TWENTY-FOUR

Computers, TVs, and Movie Theaters

COMPUTERS

See *Plate 59: "Evolution."*

COMPUTERS AND NATURAL VISION HABITS

The same principles—movement, centralization, and relaxation—and the same habits—sketch, breathe, and blink—are necessary during computer work and play.

Shift from one point to another with a head movement. Even a small head movement makes a big difference in releasing the neck. Do not lock your neck. This is probably the greatest problem. Move your body as you work. The human body is not designed to be stationary. Again, even a small movement is valuable. Do not lock your body.

Centralize. Do not try to see the whole screen at once, i.e., do not diffuse.

Do not stare and "space out" when you are thinking of something else. Either continue to sketch and blink, or close your eyelids.

Blink frequently and softly. Many people have dry eyes when using a computer because of infrequent blinking.

Breathe abdominally. Yawn!

Computer screens, like books and TV screens, are relatively "flat" or two-dimensional. Vision needs to move from near to far and back. Shift your attention into the distance (at least twenty feet) periodically. If you are in a small room, close your eyelids and pretend you are shifting your attention to a far-away object. Never "stare into the distance" as one computer magazine incorrectly suggests.

Take breaks. This is important. It is better to take a break *before* you feel uncomfortable. Stretch and yawn!

Note that computers and TVs did not exist when Bates taught his students in the 1920s. It is easy to acquire incorrect vision habits while using a computer—especially if used for long periods of time, and if you are not aware of correct vision habits. Keep the neck and shoulders loose and flexible. Computers do not lower vision—incorrect vision habits do.

If your computer work is somewhat boring, the correct vision habits will create more interest automatically. Boredom often leads to the harmful staring habit.

Tip: If you have a programmable screen saver, type in "Sketch, Breathe, and Blink!"

Computer Posture

See *Figure 24–1: Computer Posture.* The woman on the right has excellent posture. The wrist/forearm angle is straight, and the computer monitor is positioned at an excellent height.

All of the monitors on the left are too low—a very common mistake. A low monitor encourages poor posture. The body tends to bend over forward or even sideways. This puts a high strain on the neck and spinal column.

One of the simplest adjustments that can be made with a computer is to raise the monitor to a comfortable level. A good rule of thumb is to position the top of the active part of the screen (not the top of the monitor) slightly above eye level.

Correct posture supports a released, mobile neck and abdominal breathing. Incorrect posture creates tension, shallow breathing, fatigue, and strain.

It is easy to understand how computer work can be a strain on the visual system. With a few ergonomic adjustments and the practice of correct vision habits, one can support normal sight.

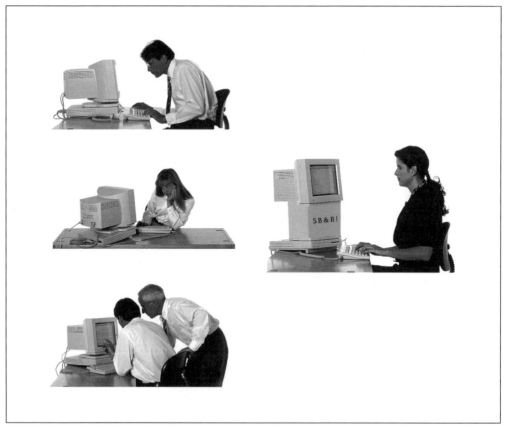

Figure 24–1: Computer Posture.

Annoying Monitor Flicker

Almost all monitors have a vertical scan frequency of 60–75 Hz. Vertical scan frequency is also known as vertical refresh rate (VRR).

It is mainly the VRR which determines whether a monitor has annoying flicker. This flicker is similar to the annoying 60-Hz flicker in fluorescent light fixtures with magnetic ballasts. Since the horizontal scan frequency, or horizontal refresh rate (HRR), is usually many thousands of Hz, there is no noticeable flicker created by the HRR.

Monitors with VRRs of 65 Hz or less can have noticeable flicker. The lower the rate, the more noticeable the flicker.

This "flicker" is perceived mainly by the rods from the peripheral parts of the monitor (relative to where you are centralizing). The cones in the fovea do not pick up movement as well as the rods. So, the point at which you are centralizing often appears to be stable, while the periphery may flicker annoyingly.

VRRs of 70 Hz or higher produce an essentially "flicker-free" monitor. Many modern monitors have a VRR of 70 Hz or higher. Some VRRs go as high as 79 Hz. On multi-resolution monitors, the VRR is often dependent upon the resolution selected. The manual or manufacturer should be able to provide this information.

Tom's Personal Log: My monitor has a VRR of 75 Hz with a HRR of 60,000 Hz at 1024 x 768 resolution. This provides flicker-free viewing on a large screen.

CRT Computer Monitor Radiation Concerns

One of the biggest concerns regarding computers is the potentially harmful effects of the radiation emitted from monitors. Many articles have been written in computer magazines and newspapers about the possible harmful biological effects of electromagnetic frequency (EMF) radiation from computer monitors, power lines, and other electrical devices. A computer monitor operates similar to a television. However, most people do not sit as close to a television[1] as a CRT.

Since this "invisible" energy could be a potential source of strain, it could be prudent to minimize possible risks.

Radiation 101

There are two main types of electric and magnetic radiation emitted by CRTs: Very Low Frequency (VLF), 10,000–300 Hz; and Extremely Low Frequency (ELF), 300 Hz and lower. See *Plate 22: Electromagnetic and Visible Spectrums.* Since VLF is not considered to be as potentially harmful as ELF, most research has been directed toward the ELF radiation.

Children who have prolonged exposure to low-level (2–3 milligauss), 60-Hz magnetic fields may have an increased risk of cancer. A gauss is a unit of measure of magnetic energy; a milligauss is 1/1000th of a gauss.

Brain chemistry of living cats has been changed by exposure to low-level EMF. Low-level EMF radiation, similar to the type found in CRTs, has produced malformations in developing chick embryos and mice. The development of cancer has been associated with workers, like some utility employees, in occupations in which they are frequently exposed to power lines. ELF has been identified as a possible cause of miscarriages, birth defects, and cancer.

The Environmental Protection Agency

issued a draft report in 1990 entitled "An Evaluation of the Potential Carcinogenicity of Electromagnetic Fields." In the summary of this report, the EPA states:

> The human evidence, as described in the next section, suggests that magnetic fields rather than electric fields are associated with cancer incidence, and mechanisms have been sought to explain how weak currents induced by ELF magnetic fields could interact with cells and body tissue in such a way as to induce a carcinogenic response ... With our current understanding we can identify 60 Hz magnetic fields from power lines and perhaps other sources in the home as a possible, but not proven, cause of cancer in people.

Robert O. Becker, M.D., in his book *Cross Currents: The Perils of Electromagnetic Pollution, The Promise of Electromedicine,* recommends "a maximum field strength of 1 milligauss for continuous exposure to 60-Hz fields."[2]

Most monitors appear to have maximum emissions at the top and sides. Some monitors have as high as 73 milligauss at a distance of four inches from the top. The front and back usually have less emissions.

Swedish MPR-II and TCO Low-Emission Standards

Not surprisingly, many government agencies and computer companies claim there is no proof radiation from monitors has had any detrimental effects on our health. Yet many computer companies have gone to great lengths to comply with MPR-II and TCO radiation standards—*even though there is no legal requirement for them to do so.* Hmmm.

A standard for low electromagnetic radiation from monitors, known as MPR-II, was set in 1990 by the Swedish Board for Measurements and Testing (MPR). The MPR-II guideline, which has gained international acceptance, limits ELF electromagnetic fields to 2.5 milligauss at 50 centimeters (approximately 20 inches) in all directions from the monitor. Many modern monitors meet the MPR-II standard, and they usually advertise this fact.

The Swedish Confederation of Profession Employees (TCO) determined that there was inadequate protection using the older MPR-II standard. So, in 1992, a stricter standard was set by the Swedes, called TCO. TCO limits ELF radiation to 2.5 milligauss at 30 centimeters from the front of the monitor, and (the same) 50 centimeters from other sides. Some monitors now meet the stricter TCO guidelines.

MPR-II and TCO guidelines set limits on VLF and electrical fields as well.

Radiation Solutions

Most ELF radiation does not come directly from the front of the monitor to the user, as one might guess. ELF radiation travels from the sides, top and bottom, *around* the front of the screen to the user sitting in front of the monitor. So, although radiation screens can dramatically reduce *electric* field emissions, they usually do little, or nothing, to block the magnetic VLF/ELF emissions in front of the monitor.

One way to lower ELF radiation is to add a special metal shield inside the monitor.

A large coil inside the monitor produces EMF radiation. Some computer companies and monitor manufacturers have taken steps to reduce this radiation by adding a second "reversed" coil. The second coil creates another electromagnetic field which, theoretically, cancels out the electromagnetic field created by the CRT's primary coil. This is the method used in many monitors to meet the Swedish MPR-II and TCO standards for low emissions.

Tip: Sit back at least an arm's length from your CRT. As discussed in Chapter 16, "Light," radiation (from an ideal point source) diminishes exponentially with distance. A monitor that has 30 milligauss at 4 inches may have only 7 milligauss at 12 inches, 1 milligauss at 28 inches, and 0.5 milligauss at 36 inches. As you can see, a small increase in distance from the CRT reduces radiation exposure by a large amount. One computer magazine reports that all ten monitors they tested had less than 1 milligauss from the front at a distance of 28 inches.

Note: Contrary to common belief, dimming the monitor's screen or using "screen saver" software does *not* reduce radiation from a monitor.

On the Horizon

Perhaps the best solution to avoiding radiation from monitors will be the new "flat" LCD (Liquid Crystal Display) monitors which have negligible radiation. These monitors do not use a magnetic coil to create the images on the screen.

Unlike their predecessors, the very latest LCD monitors have excellent performance and quality. Unfortunately, they are too expensive for most computer users. But prices should drop as they are produced in larger quantities. (TV screens will be flat LCD monitors in the future also.)

Radiation, Poor Vision Habits, or Both?

Many problems attributed to radiation from monitors have also been attributed by Bates to incorrect vision habits. These problems include headaches, eyestrain, blurred vision, red eyes, irritated eyes, dry eyes, nausea, sleeplessness, fatigue, neck and shoulder pain, etc.

While CRT radiation may be, and probably is, harmful, incorrect vision habits *are* harmful. Minimize the former and eliminate the latter.

Glare

The easiest way to reduce glare on a computer monitor is to orient it so that bright lights are not in front of the screen. Placing a monitor perpendicular to a window reduces glare, and lets you enjoy the light and scenery outside!

Another way to reduce glare is to place an opaque visor on top and/or on the sides of the monitor.

Glare screens can be used as an option, but they tend to distort the image and usually reduce the amount of light from the screen. Glare screens that use optical glass tend to have less distortion than other types. If you use a glare screen, avoid the mesh type.

Many monitors have an "etched" glass surface, or sprayed-on coating, which helps reduce glare. Etched screens can produce some loss of detail, but they are usually better, overall, than glare screens.

Never strain to see the images on the screen. Vision is always best when relaxed.

Smaller, Not Larger, Print is the Solution

Many computer users and software designers have read or assumed that larger letters on the computer screen result in less eyestrain. This is incorrect.

Magnifiers that fit over the front of the monitor have been used to enlarge the entire screen. "Computer glasses" enlarge the print and even claim to "protect" you from UV light. (Oh, no. Here we go again.) No UV light emanates from CRTs.

Some computer users have enlarged the size of print on the screen with software.

These solutions could encourage diffusion. As mentioned in Chapter 22, "Reading—For All Ages," Bates objected to large type. Centralizing in a *smaller* area is what is needed—not greater diffusion. A person who wears corrective lenses already diffuses. Increasing the size of print, by any method, only encourages more diffusion and increases the strain.

Tom's Personal Log: I set the type size to a small size (9 point is nice) on my monitor. This encourages centralization. (Now, if I can just convince my editor and designer to use smaller type. . . .)

Of course, one should never squint or strain to see. Remember to practice relaxed vision habits—especially when using a computer.

Other Computer Tips

If you use a computer for long periods of time, obtain a comfortable chair—preferably one that allows sufficient mobility.

Adjust your monitor controls to provide maximum contrast. Vision functions by contrast and edges.

Place paper holders on both sides of the monitor. Then, alternate your papers from left to right periodically. This helps keep the neck balanced.

Bifocals can create higher neck tension while using a computer. Often the head is forced unnaturally upward in order to look through the bottom part of the bifocal. Single-lense glasses (reduced) are the solution.

Palm occasionally to rest your eyes. Again, take breaks!

TELEVISION

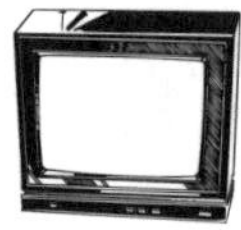

As with computers, televisions were not available to the masses in Bates' day. We live in a very different era than the 1920s.

Many of the issues discussed above regarding computer monitors apply to watching TV. One major difference is posture. Most people do not sit upright in a chair when watching TV. Correct posture is important when watching TV.

Do not lock your neck while watching TV. Do not stare.

Dr. Thomas H. David, D.C., in his 1951 booklet, *Improve Your Vision with Television!,* wrote:

> To STARE steadily at the television screen . . . can cause congestion which may result in eye-strain, headaches, a feeling of tiredness, or pressure behind the eyeballs, nerve tension . . . and other discomforts resulting from looking at the television incorrectly. If these conditions are allowed to go on, they could lead to more serious complications.[3]

> ... Do not squint; do not open the eyes widely ... Glance around the room from time to time for a few seconds....
>
> Shift ... from one part of the picture to another, and blink frequently....
>
> ... prevent stiffness and strain of neck muscles [by] turning the head....[4]

Sketch *with a head movement;* this keeps the neck released and mobile. Breathe abdominally. Yawn also.

Remember to blink frequently. Do not copy the incorrect habit of non-blinking taught to many actors and actresses! (See "TV and Movies—No Blinking Allowed," in Chapter 14, "The Third Habit—Blinking.")

Centralize. Do not diffuse over the whole TV screen. Shift from one point of the screen to another.

Notice that as the TV camera moves in one direction, all stationary objects move in the opposite direction—oppositional movement. The same is true at movie theaters.

There are some excellent programs on TV. Unfortunately, many programs and movies today do not support relaxation. Do not watch "negative, pessimum" programs. Perhaps the poor programs will encourage us to find other activities which include more movement. We live in a very sedentary (read: staring) society.

MOVIE THEATERS

Better Eyesight magazine, October 1920:

> GO TO THE MOVIES
>
> Cinematograph pictures are commonly supposed to be very injurious to the eyes, and it is a fact that they often cause much discomfort and lowering of vision. They can, however, be made a means of improving the sight. When they hurt the eyes it is because the subject strains to see them. If this tendency to strain can be overcome, the vision is always improved, and, if the practice of viewing the pictures is continued long enough, nearsight, astigmatism and other troubles are reversed.
>
> If your sight is imperfect, therefore, you will find it an advantage to go to the movies frequently and learn to look at the pictures without strain. If they hurt your eyes, look away to the dark for a while, then look at a corner of the picture; look away again, and then look a little nearer to the center; and so on. In this way you may soon become able to look directly at the picture without discomfort. If this does not help, try palming for five minutes or longer. Dodge the pain, in short, and prevent the eyestrain by constant shifting, or by palming.

Movie theaters provide an excellent opportunity to practice correct vision habits. Notice how many people do *not* move their head while watching the movie!

CHAPTER COMMENTS

There are people who read, use a computer, and watch TV and movies who have normal sight. It is not the activities of reading, doing computer work, and watching TV and movies which lower sight—it is the acquiring of incorrect vision habits.

Natural vision students can learn how to use their sight correctly—in all situations. Practice the correct habits and principles of eyesight more each day during *all* activities.

Notes

[1] See John N. Ott's *Light, Radiation and You: How to Stay Healthy* for more information regarding radiation from television sets.

[2] Robert O. Becker, *Cross Currents: The Perils of Electromagnetic Pollution, The Promise of Electromedicine* (Los Angeles: Jeremy P. Tarcher, Inc., 1990), p. 271.

[3] Thomas H. David, *Improve Your Vision with Television!* (Los Angeles: DeVorss & Co., 1951), p. 6.

[4] Ibid., pp. 11–12.

Chapter Twenty-Five

Commuting and Recreation

DRIVING

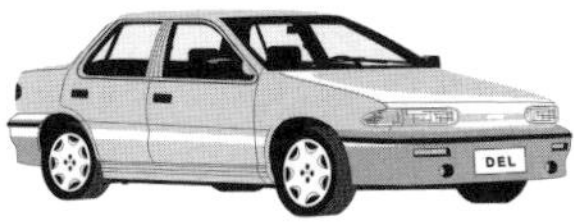

Natural Vision Habits = Safer Driving

Ninety percent of the information we receive while driving comes to us through sight. Natural vision habits help a person remain more alert—and therefore safer—while driving a car or other motor vehicles.

When someone has a car accident, oftentimes we hear the driver say, "I just never saw it"—"it" referring to another car or object the driver hit. Many accidents can be attributed to "spaced out" staring. The driver was simply "not paying attention." How many of us have had "close calls" due to "not paying attention"? The danger of unnatural staring while driving should be obvious. The fact that most Americans have blurred vision means most Americans practice "spaced out" staring—a good reason to be especially attentive while driving.

Enjoyable and Relaxing Commuting

Many of my students say how much more relaxed and comfortable they now are driving a car, especially when traveling long distances. Many vision students have experienced less eyestrain, fatigue, neckaches, and headaches by using correct vision habits while driving.

Head movement is important while driving. Head movement loosens and relaxes the neck. Abdominal breathing and butterfly blinking are also relaxing and energizing. Normal vision is a form of relaxed alertness.

Relearning Centralization and Movement While Driving

All people with blurred vision have mastered diffusion. Some of my students have told me they are willing to relearn centralization during all of their activities—except for driving. They think—erroneously—that in order to be safe, it is essential to diffuse. They say, "I have to see everything on the road equally at one time." Some students have also told me they think they must keep their head locked straight ahead in order to drive safely.

Some students tell me that—while driving

with their glasses on—they can see everything clearly simultaneously. This is, of course, impossible. As discussed in Chapter 10, "The Second Principle—Centralization," it is impossible to see everything clearly at one time. Only one central point is clear at any instant. *If a person diffuses while driving, he is unnaturally and dangerously taking his primary attention away from the only place he sees clearly—the center.*

Attempts to support the erroneous belief that diffusion is essential for safe driving are only made by those people who have mastered diffusion, i.e., those who have blurred vision.

The fact is people who have normal sight centralize when they drive—just as they do when they are *not* driving. They shift their attention from one point to another. This is *safe* driving.

Once again, the rods are designed to pick up movements in our peripheral vision. When a person locks their head and diffuses, peripheral movement perception is *lowered* not increased. Paradoxical as it may seem, the better and more a person centralizes (and moves the head), the better objects in the peripheral vision are picked up by the rods.

It takes practice, trust, and time to relearn natural vision habits while driving. By practicing correct vision habits more each day when you are *not* driving, the correct habits and principles will eventually become automatic while driving.

During the first few weeks of vision classes, one of my students said she was unwilling to centralize while driving her car. One day, while stopped at a stoplight, she was sketching a car on the other side of the intersection. To her surprise, she picked up the changing of the light signal in her peripheral vision. Prior to this experience, she *thought* she had to centralize on the light signal to see whether or not it had changed from red to green. Surprise! Now she was willing to centralize while driving. She learned to *trust* the rods' ability to pick up movement and changes in the peripheral vision—automatically.

Notice how, throughout this book, the *beliefs* a person holds about how eyesight should be used and how it functions are very often the opposite of the *facts*—even after the facts are clearly stated and repeated many times. One of the benefits of attending vision classes is the support the student receives in changing their incorrect beliefs into true beliefs.

As discussed in Chapter 10, "The Second Principle—Centralization," centralization does not mean the peripheral field is not seen, or is of no interest. To the contrary, peripheral vision is *essential* vision—*but it is never clear.* It is designed primarily for movement perception. It is our "protection" vision. If an object moves in the peripheral vision, the rods pick up its movement; then we shift our nose-pencil to that object to see its detail—to determine exactly what the moving object is.

Another student told me she perfected diffusion while living in New York City. She said she was so afraid of being attacked, she felt she needed to protect herself by *trying consciously* to see everything around her clearly—simultaneously. Her mastery of diffusion resulted in her not being able to drive a car. She was so diffused, she was not able to keep her attention in the center—"on the road." "Diffusion is confusion," and dangerous. About halfway through the vision course, she was able to drive a car again—for the first time in many years.

I have heard hundreds of "diffusion" stories like this one from students. The return from diffusion to centralization is one of the most important aspects of returning to clear vision. Sight, as Bates correctly stated, is primarily a mental process.

Patience is needed while relearning to see. The strain of incorrect vision habits from the past needs time to unwind itself.

Diffusion and rigidity are fatiguing. A person with incorrect habits will become fatigued sooner than someone who has correct vision habits.

Some of my students who only needed glasses for driving temporarily postponed driving while improving their sight. They wanted to stop wearing glasses completely and as soon as possible.

Unlike some of the students mentioned above, some students find driving the *easiest* time to practice correct habits. Each student associates correct or incorrect vision habits with different activities. For some, driving is an optimum; for others it is a pessimum. Change all visual pessimums into visual optimums!

Reading While Commuting

A person riding on a bus or train can read clearly and comfortably if objects, e.g., the books, are allowed to move. If an effort is made to hold objects rigid, sight will be strained.

Of course, a person would never read when she is the driver of a vehicle.

From *Perfect Sight Without Glasses:*

> Persons who wish to preserve their eyesight are frequently warned not to read in moving vehicles; but since under modern conditions of life many persons have to spend a large part of their time in moving vehicles, and many of them have no other time to read, it is useless to expect that they will ever discontinue the practice. Fortunately the theory of its injuriousness is not borne out by the facts. When the object regarded is moved more or less rapidly ... ultimately the vision is improved by the practice.

Driver's Education = Bates Method!

In the section entitled "Safe Driving Practices, Visual Search: Seeing Well," the State of California Department of Motor Vehicles' 1995 California Driver Handbook states:

> Keep your eyes moving. Look near and far. Turn your head before changing lanes ... Don't develop a "fixed stare." Look around. Keep your eyes moving. Check the rear view mirrors frequently (every 2 to 5 seconds) ... Keep shifting your eyes from one part of the road to another. Look at objects near and far, left and right.

Be sure to move your *head.* Moving *only* the eyes is incorrect. Head movement is especially important to check for cars or objects in the "blind spots" on either side of the car.

Similar to the DMV manual just quoted, many driver education schools teach their students natural vision habits. They frequently remind their students to shift their attention from one point to another. "Watch the traffic far ahead of you. Check traffic behind you in the rear view mirror. Watch carefully for a child who might dash out into the street, especially near schools, parks, and playgrounds."

Be attentive while driving—and while *not* driving!

While driving, notice how stationary objects in front of you move toward you, while in the rear view mirror they move away from you. Stationary objects on the sides of car move in the opposite direction of the car's movement. (See also *Figure 9–6: Oppositional Movement and Depth Perception* in Chapter 9, "The First Principle—Movement.") Natural clear eyesight is dependent upon movement and the illusion of oppositional movement.

Tip 1: Be sure to keep the windshields of your car clean. Dirt or smudges on the windshield can distract your sight away from the road and traffic.

Tip 2: For additional safety, drive with your car headlights on during the day. Studies have shown that it is easier for other drivers and pedestrians to see you if your lights are on during the day. In fact, some newer cars automatically turn on headlights when the car is started.

If you do not turn your headlights on during the day, at least turn them on at twilight. Most accidents occur at this time. Many people are driving home, tired from a long day at work, when their attention might not be their best. Additionally, the visual system is beginning to transition from daytime vision into nighttime vision.

"Motion Sickness" While Driving

Some people become sick when riding in a car. This can be caused by straining, usually subconsciously, to keep stationary objects from moving. Interfering with the illusion of stationary objects moving in the opposite direction of the car's movement is a strain.

Tips for Passing the Driver's Vision Test

If you currently have a restriction on your driver's license requiring you to wear corrective lenses, you can have it removed by passing the vision test without corrective lenses.

Here are some tips regarding the DMV (Department of Motor Vehicles) vision test:

- Since some testing environments are not very relaxing (to say the least), visit the DMV and walk around to get accustomed to the workers, desks, tables, and so on. Stand or sit for a while to become familiar with the total environment. Generally, we see familiar objects more clearly than unfamiliar objects. Practice correct vision habits. Watch the procedures of clerks and clients taking the vision test. Note the lighting level. Vision is highly dependent on the level of light. You can visit the DMV several times before actually taking the vision test. You can also take the test even if you do not think you might pass it yet.
- If possible, visit more than one DMV office. I have found a large difference in the levels of relaxation (read: stress) among DMV offices.
- Check with your eye doctor or DMV to find out what the vision requirements are in your state for safe, legal driving.

At home, place your Distance Eye Chart (located in Appendix F) twenty feet away. Adjust your lights to be approximately the same level as at the DMV. Practice the correct habits with the appropriate line of letters, imagining you are at the DMV. Imagine being very relaxed while seeing the letters at the DMV. Practice in your mind sketching or shifting from one letter to another.

Shift to the top of a letter, then to the bottom, then to the right, then to the left, then through the middle. Imagine the letter is moving in the opposite direction of your nose-pencil movement. Imagine you are seeing one part of a letter more clearly than the other parts of the letter—centralization. Do not "lock on," or strain to see a particular letter; this is staring. Continue to shift—even a tiny amount is correct. Do not diffuse.

Cover one eye at a time while reading the letters. Then use both eyes. Imagine taking the vision test and passing! Many natural vision students have done this, and you can too!

Student Case Histories

The following case histories are about some of my natural vision students who eliminated the restriction from their driver's license which required them to wear corrective lenses.

M. P.

M. P., 60, received glasses for nearsightedness at age 14. She had 20/70 in the right eye and 20/200 in the left eye when she started natural vision classes in January 1991. She passed her driver's vision test without corrective lenses by July 1992.

Her mother, 83, and sister, 66, who attended the vision classes with her, have also had excellent improvement of their sight.

S. C.

S. C., 31, had nearsightedness since age 17. His prescription had increased to –2.75 DS for nearsightedness, and +1.25 DC for astigmatism by the time he enrolled in the natural vision classes in September 1989. At the end of the vision course he saw 20/10 with the glasses that were 20/20 at the beginning of the course. By February 1991, he passed his driver's vision test, without corrective lenses.

T. L.

T. L., 33, had a prescription of –3.50 DS for nearsightedness and –1.00 DC for astigmatism. She attended natural vision classes in August 1984, and passed her driver's vision test, without corrective lenses, by December 1987.

T. L. also says she now looks ten years younger! The difference between her photos in the old and new driver's licenses is dramatic.

W. C.

W. C., 62, experienced nearsightedness beginning at age 32. He received bifocals in 1975. In January 1992, he attended natural vision classes. By August of 1992, he passed his driver's vision test without corrective lenses.

W. C. is also a graduate of the Natural Vision Center's 1992 Certified Teacher Training Program.

B. D.

> I am 42 years old and I have had radiation retinopathy in both of my eyes, and I had been wearing glasses with a correction of –1.75 in both eyes for the last seven years. The retinopathy in my eyes was caused by high-dose radiation treatments for a malignant tumor four years ago. Since that time I have had constant difficulties with my eyes, and reading for more than 15–20 minutes has become virtually impossible....

> I attended [natural vision] classes from September through November of 1995 and integrated the habits of natural vision into my life and daily activities. On January 22, 1996, I passed the California driver's license test without my glasses. In February of 1996, during an eye examination at an ophthalmologist, my vision was 20/30 without glasses. I still have many eye problems, but . . . I can see more clearly than when he and I first spoke in 1995.
>
> [Signed] B. D.
>
> *Permission to reprint*

None of these students have had artificial refractive corneal surgeries or ortho-keratology. Their vision improvement was by 100% natural means.

More testimonials are given in Chapter 29, " 'This Method Has Been Proved.' "

FLYING

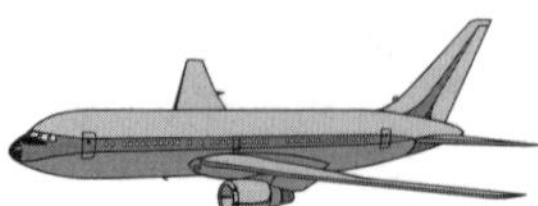

From *Perfect Sight Without Glasses:*

> To aviators, whether engaged in military or civilian operations, or whether they are flying merely for pleasure, eye education is of particular importance. Accidents to aviators, otherwise unaccountable, are easily explained when one understands how dependent the aviator is upon his eyesight, and how easily perfect vision may be lost amid the unaccustomed surroundings, the dangers and hardships of the upper air.
>
> It was formerly supposed that aviators maintained their equilibrium in the air by the aid of the internal ear; but it is now becoming evident from the testimony of aviators who have found themselves emerging from a cloud with one wing down, or even with their machines turned completely upside down, that equilibrium is maintained almost entirely, if not altogether, by the sense of sight. If the aviator loses his sight, therefore, he is lost, and we have one of those "unaccountable" accidents which, during the war, were so unhappily common in the air service.
>
> All aviators, therefore, should make a daily practice of reading small, familiar letters, or observing other small, familiar objects, at a distance of ten feet or more. In addition, they should have a few small letters, or a single letter, on their machines, at a distance of five, ten, or more feet from their eyes, arrangements being made to illuminate them for night flying and fogs, and should read them frequently while in the air. This would greatly lessen the danger of visual lapses, with their accompanying loss of equilibrium and judgment.

When the US entered WW2, hundreds of natural vision students were able to pass the air corps vision test by taking vision lessons. Margaret Corbett alone helped more than 200 men pass their tests.

Many military and commercial airline pilots are trained to use their sight in many of the same ways Bates taught his students to relearn to see correctly. Pilots are taught to have continual "situational awareness." They are trained to constantly scan and shift from one point to another—left, right, up, down, near and far. Their survival depends on it.

The US Air Force Academy requires pilots to have 20/20 sight, both near and far.

It is not a coincidence that Air Force pilots are required to have normal sight. In addition to excellent acuity, people with clear sight have the important *qualities* of seeing—3-D vision, excellent contrast perception, texture awareness, and superior color perception.

The best military pilots have 20/10 sight—eyes like hawks. They can see a 4x4-foot object nearly two miles away, and can spot another airplane fifteen miles away.

Fighter pilots say they see enemy planes long before the enemy sees them. The famous German Ace pilot "Red Baron" Manfred von Richthofen claimed that 80% of the enemy pilots he shot down never saw him.

General Charles "Chuck" Yeager was a WW2 Ace fighter pilot and the top US Air Force Test Pilot for nearly ten years. Electronic Arts' *General Chuck Yeager Air Combat* manual contains the following quotes from General Yeager:

> Concentration is total. You remain focused, ignoring fatigue or fear, not allowing static into your mind.... [1]
>
> In World War I, detecting the enemy was simply a matter of having good eyesight, knowing what to look for, staying alert....
>
> In a sky filled with airplanes, I needed to keep my head on a swivel to avoid getting hit, being shot down, or running into somebody. The best survival tactic always was to check your tail constantly and stay alert....
>
> My biggest tactical advantage was my eyes. I spotted him from great distances, knowing he couldn't see me because he was only a dim speck. Sometimes he never did see me—or when he did it was too late.... [2]
>
> THE MAKING OF AN ACE
>
> Electronic Arts: ... What characteristics make an ace?
>
> Chuck Yeager: Experience. You start from a baseline of very good eyesight ... I was always gifted with good eyesight, from a kid on up. Even to this day I have 20/10 eyesight ... In World War II, we learned to pick a piece of the sky and focus out to infinity and back, and then move over and do it again. You don't let your eyes focus on a set place. Normally, if your eyes relax they focus at about 18 feet—you've got to be able to focus them out and in.
>
> Radar caused the pilots to get lazy. They were using radar to look out 20 to 30 miles ahead. Before we had radar, you had to depend on your eyes to pick up things coming. But now with the ability to jam radars, and also stealth technology coming into the picture, we've got to teach the guys to start looking again....
>
> Electronic Arts: Would you describe most pilots as cool-headed?
>
> Yeager: "Cool-headed?" What you don't do is worry about the outcome of anything because you don't have any control over it. You concentrate on what you're doing. If you want to call that "cool-headed," fine.
>
> Electronic Arts: It's a matter of focusing, then?
>
> Yeager: There you are. You focus on what you're doing....
>
> One thing we saw in World War II was that only 11% of the fighter pilots involved in combat with the Germans shot down about 90% of the airplanes destroyed. That's a small number. If you look at the commonality of these guys, they were all rural kids—they understood deflection shooting—they had good eyesight, and were aggressive and self-sufficient.[3]

One magazine on flying states "make a *conscious effort* to focus." Following this advice will strain your vision. The correct method of seeing is to "shift constantly from one point to another," in a relaxed, attentive manner.

Many pilots maintain their normal sight during their flying careers. Their training and practice of correct vision habits keeps their vision clear. I have met and heard of pilots who lost their clear vision after they stopped flying.

So, have "Ace" pilot vision all day long!

SWIMMING AND BOATING

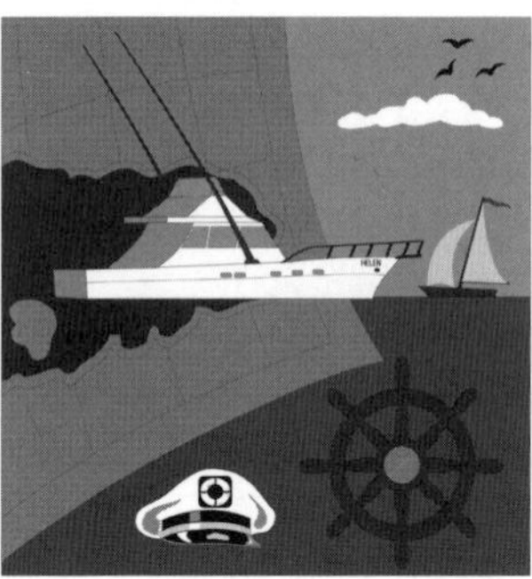

While swimming in a pool, stationary objects seem to move in the opposite direction of your movement.

Some people become "seasick" when boating. This can be caused by subconsciously trying to stop the illusion of the horizon "tilting." Strain is the result. Allow in your mind the illusion that stationary objects move.

SPORTS

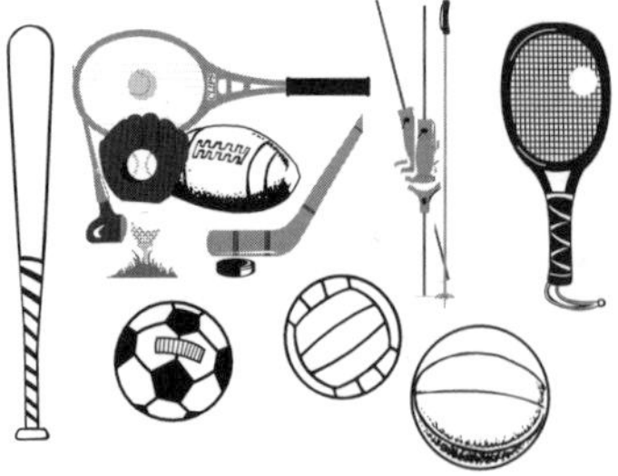

All sports involve movement.

When playing in the outfield in softball, some children "freeze" and diffuse when the ball is hit to them. In this state, catching the ball is nearly impossible.

One of my students, a fifty-year-old woman, told me she never could catch a ball. When she tossed a ball up into the air, she held her head very straight and stiff. When the ball went up, it went out of her visual field, so she never caught it.

Holding a ball in her hand, she practiced slowly moving and following a ball up and down with her nose-feather, with a head movement. Apparently it had never occurred to her she should, or could, move her head up when the ball went up. Finally, she tossed the ball upward and, by following it with her nose-feather for the first time, she caught it! She was extremely pleased!

It is said that one famous baseball player could see the threads on the spinning baseball as it was being pitched to him. He must have had excellent centralizing and movement vision skills. "Keep your nose-feather on the ball!"

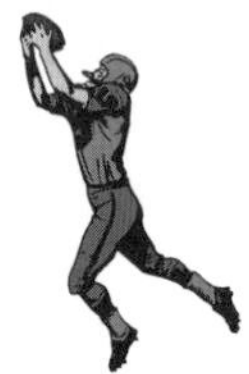

One of the greatest football receivers described how he not only kept his total attention on the football as it was soaring through the air toward him, he kept his attention on the *center* of the spiraling football.

As noted in Chapter 9, "The First Principle—Movement," the best tennis players are in constant motion. A tournament champion often states how relaxed and concentrated (centralized) she was during the tournament. Relaxation = Movement = Centralization =

Win; Strain = Rigidity = Diffusion = Lose.

Notice that most of the greatest tennis players do not wear sunglasses—even while playing in the brightest sunlight. They often wear a hat.

GAMES

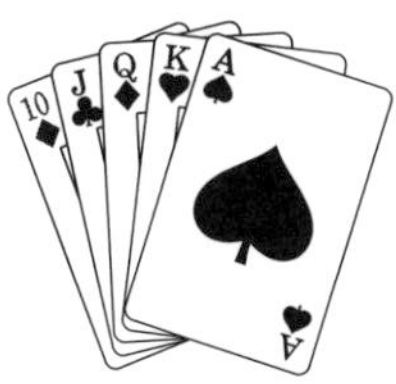

Do not keep a "poker face" while playing games. Keep the neck mobile. Sketch, breathe, and blink! Move your body.

Card games can be an excellent activity for practicing correct vision habits. Move your nose-feather with the card movements. The near and far movements from the cards in your hands to the table are especially beneficial.

TOM'S PERSONAL LOG: Reflecting on many years of playing chess in school and in tournaments, it seems that, for long periods of time, only the eyes moved.

CHAPTER COMMENTS

Practice the correct vision habits—sketching, breathing, and blinking—while commuting and "re-creating." Correct vision habits are meant for all day long, and all activities benefit from them.

NOTES

[1] Brent Iverson, *General Chuck Yeager Air Combat* manual (San Mateo, California: Electronic Arts, 1993), p. 46.

[2] Ibid., pp. 122–24.

[3] Ibid., pp. 171–73.

Chapter Twenty-Six

Nutrition

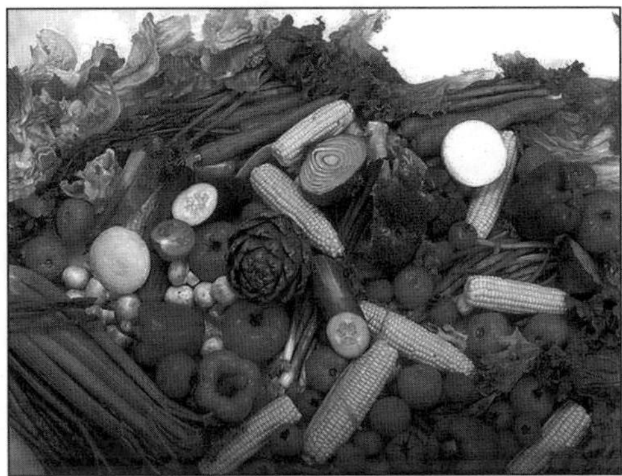

Figure 26–1: "See" Food.

THE NUTRITION CONNECTION

Many students have asked me which foods they should eat to benefit their eyesight. I do *not* recommend which foods a person should eat for improving sight or any condition.

Students are referred to a nutritionist or doctor for any concerns regarding diet.

There are many factors that influence vision habits—and, therefore, how well we see. One of these factors is nutrition.

Some individuals have improved their sight simply by improving their diet. This fact puzzled me when I first started teaching vision classes. I knew that it was not possible to improve sight naturally unless better vision habits were practiced.

Yet, these people did not know about correct vision habits. Their improvement was not related to an increased *ability* of the cones to see sharp detail, because these people could already see sharp detail by using compensating lenses. I also knew other people had improved their sight by initiating various types of lifestyle changes. How can these facts be explained?

I finally understood that all of these people *were* relearning correct, natural vision habits—but they were doing so *automatically and subconsciously.* As well as interfering with correct vision habits automatically and subconsciously during excessive stress, a person could also *cease* interfering with correct vision habits automatically and subconsciously when excessive stress is removed.

Most people have no idea of the incorrect vision habits they started when their vision first became blurred. What matters is which vision habits the person is using.

When a person takes steps to improve their health, they will be more relaxed, mobile, and centered. As a consequence, the tendency is to form better vision habits. These ideas fit observed facts—and coincide perfectly with Bates' discoveries on natural seeing. They also help form a large, complete holistic picture of natural vision.

So, to the degree that proper nutrition supports correct vision habits and principles, sight improves.

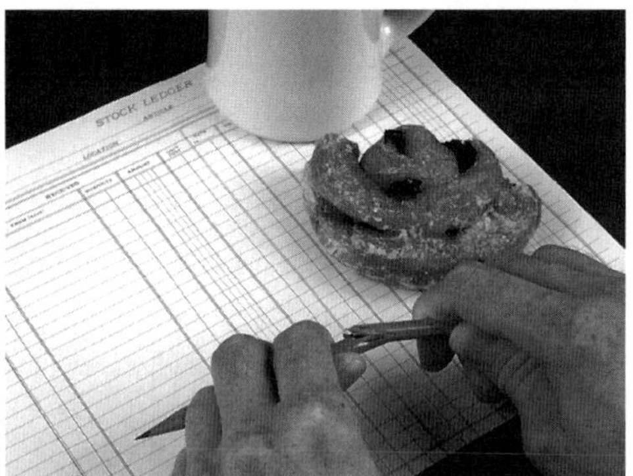

Figure 26–2: Typical American Diet.

Conversely, to the degree improper nutrition supports incorrect vision habits and principles, sight lowers.

It is simple. Most truths are.

For many students the relationship between nutrition and vision becomes obvious while improving their sight.

One student had a large milkshake during the third week of the vision course. He said his sight became blurred after drinking the milkshake. Many students discover how "wired," i.e., hyper, tense, and diffused, they become after drinking coffee or soft drinks. Many soft drinks contain caffeine.

THE VITAMIN A CONNECTION

As discussed in Chapter 17, "The Retina," Vitamin A is essential for normal functioning of the cones and rods. However, it is not essential to eat food that *contains* Vitamin A. We only need food that the body can *convert* to Vitamin A. Among other functions, the liver can convert carotene to Vitamin A.

Ann Wigmore, in *The Wheatgrass Book,* writes, "Vitamin A is not found in wheatgrass juice, or any other plant food, but its precursor, carotene, is."[1]

Carotene, also known as Provitamin A, can be converted to Vitamin A by the body.

GENERAL NUTRITION PRINCIPLES

Henry G. Bieler, M.D., writes in his book *Food is Your Best Medicine:*

> When I was a medical school student in the early days of the century, the study of nutrition was very sketchy; even today most doctors are painfully ignorant of the real advances in nutritional science....[2]
>
> The average American predilection for doughnuts and coffee, hot dogs with mustard, ice cream, fried meat, French-fried potatoes, pie à la mode, together with between-meal sweetened cola drinks, candy bars and coffee breaks, synthetic vitamins and aspirin cannot make for health.[3]

Here are some general tips on nutrition for better health:

- Eat the best *quality* food you can buy or grow. Organically grown food is the best. Minimize or eliminate left-brain, technologically processed "dead" food. The life-force energy, not just the chemicals, in food is important.
- Eat a variety of foods. The body needs many different nutrients.
- Learn "food combining." The digestive system is designed to take in similar groups of foods at one time. For example, eat starchy food together, eat pro-

tein foods together, and eat fruits together. The stomach creates different chemical environments to digest different groups of food. Incorrect food combinations result in food not being digested properly and fully. It is inefficient. Diffusion is confusion. Centralize your food!

- Tobacco is out. Period.
- If you consume alcohol, do so minimally.
- If you like vegetable juice, buy a juicer and juice your own. Many juices lose their nutritive powers within a day of being juiced. Freshly juiced carrot/beet/celery juice is outstanding.
- Wheatgrass juice must be consumed within 30 minutes of juicing. (See *The Wheatgrass Book,* by Ann Wigmore.)
- Eliminate refined white sugar, caffeine, and white flour. (Brown sugar is white sugar colored with molasses.)
- Minimize salt and spices.
- Minimize or eliminate milk, milk products, dairy products, meat, and wheat. Only fresh goat milk is compatible with the human body. Wheat would normally be fine, but Americans have consumed so many wheat products for so many years, our bodies have become allergic to it. Cow's milk and wheat create mucus and congestion.
- Have cool drinks in the summer and warm drinks in the winter.
- Do not miss breakfast, unless, of course, you are *fast*ing.
- Do not eat when you are not hungry. The body knows when it needs nutrients and when it doesn't.
- Never eat during highly emotional or stressful periods.
- Eliminate unnecessary artificial preservatives and other chemicals from your diet. "If you can't pronounce it, don't eat it." Read *The Chemical Feast* by James Turner.
- Think twice before putting *anything* into or on your body that is artificial.
- Do not eat late at night. The body detoxifies during the night. If a person eats late at night, the body will need to use its energy to digest rather than detoxify.
- Seek out a good iridologist/nutritionist. Many nutritional imbalances can be "read" in the eyes. Read the *Doctor-Patient Handbook* by Bernard Jensen.
- Be patient if you choose to change your diet. Dietary habits, like vision habits, take time to change. If you have a typical American diet, there is a lot to learn about correct nutrition.
- Continue improving your diet until you have normal bowel movements and stools.
- Avoid tap water.
- Eat 80% alkaline, non-acidic food. (Coffee is acidic.)
- Masticate your food.
- Study natural nutrition!
- Since individuals have different nutritional requirements, get individual counseling from a nutritionist.

Unfortunately, many Americans do not know what, how, or when to eat, and are unhealthy as a result.

TOM'S PERSONAL LOG: When I was a child, I assumed my body could easily handle anything I put in it. I ate literally tons of candy, colas, donuts, cakes, pastries, pizza, "fast foods," etc. I literally drank that "pink liquid" for my stomach aches. I had little appreciation of how important diet was to my health. During the period of my most serious health problems, I was 35 pounds overweight.

During the last fifteen years of healing, I have become much more "tuned in" to what I eat and its relationship to my health. I no longer eat anything that fights me back. I am happy to be free of my stomach aches *and* pink liquid. I am no longer overweight. Changes in my diet have been an essential part of my health recovery process. And they have accelerated my re-integration of correct vision habits.

As mentioned in Chapter 16, "Light," research has shown that there may be harm from sunlight *if* a person has poor nutrition.

For example, much attention has been given to beta-carotenes, a natural anti-oxidant found in many foods like carrots, tomatoes, wheatgrass, lettuce, spinach, and asparagus. Beta-carotene appears to protect the skin from harmful "free radicals." Since beta-carotene can be "used up" while we are in sunlight, it is important to have a diet that supplies adequate reserves.

For more information see Dr. Zane R. Kime's book *Sunlight Could Save Your Life.*

"OH, I DON'T EAT MUCH"

In *Better Eyesight* magazine, July 1920, Emily C. Lierman writes about one of her vision students:

> As she weighed over two hundred pounds and was sick in both mind and body, I asked her how much she ate every day.
>
> "Oh, I don't eat much—nothing to speak of at all," she said. "In the morning I eat eggs, or something like that, and rolls and butter and coffee. Then about ten I have a few slices of bread with more butter and more coffee. At noon I have soup, bread and butter and more coffee. For supper I have bread, butter, meat, vegetables and more coffee. That's all."
>
> ... Dieting ... helped her eyesight and nerves very much....

THE FINAL KEY TO NUTRITION

TOM'S PERSONAL LOG: After spending countless hours studying and changing my diet, someone mentioned that no matter how healthy my food was, the nutrients may not be *assimilated* by my body—due to excessive stress. So, *relaxation* became another key to my nutritional changes.

In silence, O dear one,
eat without haste.
With peace, delight,
and onepointedness,
thoroughly chew your food.
Don't eat merely for
the pleasure of taste.
—Swami Muktananda

CHAPTER COMMENTS

The body, mind, and spirit rejoice when nurtured with natural foods—and many serious health problems are avoided. A diet that supports the principles of relaxation, movement (circulation), and centralization will automatically support natural clear vision. The principles of natural health and natural vision fit together.

Notes

[1] Ann Wigmore, *The Wheatgrass Book* (Wayne, New Jersey: Avery Publishing Group, Inc., 1985), p. 34.

[2] Henry G. Bieler, *Food is Your Best Medicine* (New York: Random House, 1965), p. xiii.

[3] Ibid., p. xv.

Chapter Twenty-Seven

Serious Vision Problems

Students with serious vision problems such as diseases, pathologies, growths, injuries, accidents, etc., should seek the aid of an ophthalmologist.

The Bates method is educational in nature only. It is non-medical and non-optometric.

THE RISKS OF BLURRED VISION

Several references have been made previously to the relationship between blurred sight, compensating lenses, and the potential for more serious vision problems. Many serious eye problems are preceded by blurred vision.

From *Perfect Sight Without Glasses* (with some repetition from earlier chapters):

> For the prevailing method ... of compensating lenses, very little was ever claimed except that these contrivances neutralized the effects of the various conditions for which they were given, as a crutch enables a lame man to walk. It has also been believed that they sometimes checked the progress of these conditions; but every ophthalmologist now knows that their usefulness for this purpose, if any, is very limited. In the case of myopia (shortsight), Dr. Sidler-Huguenin of Zurich, in a striking paper recently published,[a] expresses the opinion that glasses and all methods now at our command are "of but little avail" in preventing either the progress of the error of refraction, or the development of the very serious complications with which it is often associated.
>
> ... It is fortunate that many people for whom glasses have been prescribed refuse to wear them, thus escaping not only much discomfort but much injury to their eyes....
>
> The idea that presbyopia is "a normal result of growing old," is responsible for much defective eyesight.... But once the glasses are adopted, in the great majority of cases, they produce the condition they were designed to relieve, or, if it already existed, they make it worse, sometimes very rapidly, as every ophthalmologist knows. In a couple of weeks sometimes, the person finds, as noted in the chapter on *What Glasses Do to Us*, that the large print which he could read without difficulty before he got his glasses can no longer be read with-

[a] Archiv f. Augenh, vol. lxxix, 1915, translated in Arch. Ophth., vol. xlv, No. 6, Nov., 1916.

> out their aid. In from five to ten years the accommodative power of the eye is usually gone; and if from this point the person does not go on to cataract, glaucoma, or inflammation of the retina, he may consider himself fortunate....
>
> The prevalence of myopia, the unsatisfactoriness of all explanations of its origin, and the futility of all methods of prevention have led some writers of repute to the conclusion that the elongated eyeball is a natural physiological adaptation to the needs of civilization. Against this view two unanswerable arguments can be brought. One is that the myopic eye does not see so well even at the near point as the normal eye, and the other is that the defect tends to progression with very serious results, often ending in blindness.

From *Better Eyesight* magazine, October 1920:

> THE PROBLEM OF IMPERFECT SIGHT
>
> Errors of refraction are so common that we have learned to take them lightly. They are usually reckoned among minor physical defects, and the average lay person has no idea of their real character. It is well known, of course, that they sometimes produce very serious nervous conditions, but the fact that they also lead to all sorts of eye diseases is known only to eye specialists, and not fully appreciated even by them. The complications of myopia (nearsight) constitute a large and melancholy chapter in the science of the eye, but most eye specialists say that no organic changes occur in hypermetropia (farsight). That this is very far from being the case was proven by Risley in the investigation alluded to above, and it is strange that this report on the subject has attracted so little attention. His studies also showed that these organic changes occurring in all states of refraction are very common among children and have often progressed to an extent that would be expected only after long years of eyestrain....
>
> My own experience is that errors of refraction are always accompanied by some organic change. It may be only a slight congestion, but this may be sufficient to lower the vision....
>
> From the foregoing facts it will be seen that in the condition of the eyesight of our people we have a health problem, an educational problem, and a military problem of the first magnitude, and one would think that if any method of either prevention or reversal that was even tolerably successful had been found, it would immediately be put into general use.

From *Better Eyesight* magazine, November 1927:

> It is an interesting fact that all diseases of the eyes and all diseases of the body are generally associated with eye tension.

Bates dedicated over thirty years of research to finding a way to improve sight naturally. It is clear his motivations were not limited to simply removing the "inconvenience" of compensating lenses. Was the "development of the very serious complications" what Bates was mainly referring to in his preface to *Perfect Sight Without Glasses*?

> The explanations of the phenomena of sight put forward by Young, von Graefe, Helmholtz and Donders have caused us to ignore or explain away a multitude of facts which otherwise would have led to ... the consequent prevention of an incalculable amount of human misery.

Bates is not alone in his concern about the potential long-term risks of blurred sight.

Joseph Kennebeck, O.D., a practicing optometrist for over fifty years, warns in *Why Glasses are Harmful for Children and Young People:*

> Wearing myopic glasses through life could lead to blindness from detachment of the retina, conical corneas, myopic cataracts or glaucoma, at middle age or past. Myopic cases are more subject to these conditions than other cases.[1]

Mary Dudderidge reports in *Scientific American:*

> For 100 years the medical profession has wrestled in vain with the problem [of defective sight], finding no means compatible with the conditions of modern life for preventing errors of refraction, and no means of relieving them except eyeglasses. These, at their best, are poor substitutes for natural sight and often fail to relieve discomfort or to stay the progress of the malady, which is a much more serious one than most people imagine. The oculist knows that present conditions are ominous of evil for the future, that the nearsighted, farsighted, or astigmatic eye is disposed to all sorts of ocular diseases.[2]

Most myopes have worn glasses much longer than most farsights.

Ophthalmologist R. S. Agarwal writes in his natural vision improvement book *Mind and Vision:*

> Not only do all errors of refraction and all functional disturbances of the eye disappear when it sees by [centralization], but many organic conditions are relieved or reversed.[3]

Natural vision teacher Clara Hackett, in *Relax and See,* writes, "No less important than improving vision defects is their prevention in the first place."[4]

Ophthalmologist Dr. Deborah E. Banker, M.D., stated at the 1995 Whole Life Expo in San Francisco:

> . . . your reading [farsighted] glasses are causing you to lose your ability to see for near [*sic*], accelerating cataracts, glaucoma, floaters, vitreous detachment, potentially retinal detachment, and perhaps macular degeneration. . . .[5]

RISKS *NOT* AVOIDED BY REFRACTIVE CORNEAL SURGERIES AND ORTHO-KERATOLOGY

As mentioned earlier, nearsights who have RK and PRK performed *are still myopic regardless of the results of the surgeries.* Refractive corneal surgeries and ortho-keratology do not decrease the risks mentioned above.

Optometrist Bruce May writes in his pamphlet *Rx for Nearsightedness—Stress-Relieving Lenses:*

> When processes like keratotomy or orthokeratology produce improved distance acuity without the use of glasses, they do not change the basic problem of myopia, only the refractive status.
>
> The change involves only the cornea, while the depth of the vitreous chamber remains increased, and so does the eyeball length. Thus, the person still has myopia and remains subject to all the risks of myopia.[6]

After a myope has had refractive corneal surgery in which sharp acuity is obtained, what would happen if extrinsic eye muscles then relax their chronic tension, and the eye returns to its normal shape? Presumably, "all the risks of myopia" would be eliminated—but wouldn't the vision then become blurred (in particular, farsighted)?

In short, after refractive corneal surgery, if the eye remains strained, serious risks remain; if the eye muscles relax, blur would theoretically result.

As mentioned earlier, I do not accept students who have had refractive corneal surgeries.

SERIOUS VISION PROBLEMS

Cataracts

Better Eyesight magazine, September 1927:

> In cataract, the pupil instead of being black becomes light gray or some other color, due to the opacity of the focusing lens of the eye, which is just behind the colored part of the eye, the iris. Rays of light which enter the eye pass through this lens and are focused on the back part of the eye, the retina. When the lens becomes opaque, the rays of light from different objects do not pass through the lens and the vision is consequently lowered and the person becomes more or less blind.
>
> If one places six sheets of glass, one on top of the other, so that all are parallel, it is possible to see through them. If, however, one or more of the glasses form an angle or is not parallel with the rest, the layers of glass become cloudy, just like the layers which form the crystalline lens in cataract.
>
> *Cause:* Cataract has been observed for many thousands of years by the people of India, Egypt, and in various countries of Europe. The theories of the cause of cataract are very numerous. The lens is composed of transparent layers. When these layers are squeezed or when the eyeball is squeezed, the layers which form the lens become cloudy or opaque. It is a very simple experiment to take the eye of some [dead] animal ... and to hold it with the tips of the fingers of one hand. By pressing the eyeball, the lens at once becomes cloudy, and a white mass, which can be seen twenty feet or farther, usually appears in the pupil. With the cloudiness of the lens, there may occur at the same time a cloudiness in the front part of the eye, the cornea. Just as soon as the pressure is removed from the eyeball, the area of the pupil becomes perfectly clear and the lens becomes perfectly transparent. It is such an easy thing to try and is so convincing that I wish that more ophthalmologists would study it.
>
> Pressure on the eyeball may come from the contraction of the muscles on the outside of the eye, which are quite capable of keeping up a continuous pressure for many years, without the person being conscious of it.
>
> Cataract has been produced in normal eyes by the memory or the imagination of imperfect sight. The memory of imperfect sight produces a strain of the outside muscles of the eyeball, which is accompanied by a contraction of these muscles, and cataract is produced.
>
> Almost any kind of opacity of the lens has been produced by pressure. The area of the pupil may become varicolored, due to the difference in pressure.

Better Eyesight magazine, April 1928:

> Some years ago a professor of anatomy was exhibiting the effect of pressure on the enucleated eyeballs of a dead cow and some other animals. At a distance of about twenty feet from the eye, the audience observed that the pupil was perfectly clear. Immediately after the eyeball was squeezed by the fingers of the professor, the area of

> the pupil became at once completely opaque, from the production of a cataract. Then when the pressure on the eyeball was lessened, the cataract at once disappeared and the eyeball became normal. Again squeezing the eyeball, a cataract was produced as before. And again, the cataract disappeared when the pressure was lessened. The experiment was repeated a number of times with the result that the pressure on the eyeball always produced a cataract, which was relieved by reducing the pressure....
>
> In animals the eyeball has been shortened experimentally by operations on each of the four straight [recti] muscles, which increased the pressure temporarily. These operations were performed after death. Similar operations on the two oblique muscles at the same time produced pressure and increased hardness of the eyeball, with cataract following.
>
> Persons suffering from cataract have increased the hardness of the eyeball, at the same time increasing the density of the cataract. While the cataract is being observed with the aid of the ophthalmoscope, it can be seen to change in size or density when the person consciously or voluntarily increases or diminishes the hardness of the eyeball with the aid of the memory or the imagination.

More than 30% of Americans over age 65 have cataracts. More than $3 billion is paid for over one million cataract surgeries each year.

One case history of cataract improvement by a student of Bates was given in Chapter 21, "Palming and Acupressure." More cataract references and/or case histories can be found in the following *Better Eyesight* magazines: March 1920, July 1920, January 1921, September 1923, January 1924, September 1927, April 1928. The entire January 1921 issue is dedicated to the topic of cataract, and includes several case histories.

Ophthalmologist R. S. Agarwal writes in *Mind and Vision,* "The opacity of the lens or cataract is caused by a strain in most of the cases.... " He gives case histories of improvement of senile, secondary, and black cataracts.[7]

W. B. MacCracken, M.D., gives case histories of cataract improvements in his natural vision book *Use Your Own Eyes.*

Clara Hackett, a Natural Vision teacher who had many students referred to her from medical doctors, writes in *Relax and See:*

> I have had the privilege of working closely with many physicians more recently, not only in cases of refractive loss, but also of serious eye disorders.
>
> It must be emphasized that the vision reeducation techniques presented in this book do not constitute a panacea. They are not intended to replace medical care. It is essential that people with actual diseases or growths in the eye seek medical aid.... Only an oculist [eye doctor] is qualified to detect and identify disease.
>
> In recent years, doctors who have encouraged individuals with such serious disorders as glaucoma and cataracts to undertake vision education have found that astonishing improvement often occurs.
>
> Thus far, I have worked with 312 people with cataracts. Of these, 278 had improvements ranging from 10 percent better sight to complete normality, while only 34 had no noticeable lasting improvement.[8]

Glaucoma

From *Better Eyesight* magazine, September 1927:

> Glaucoma is a serious disease of the eyes. In most cases, the eyeball becomes hard.... For the relief of this hardness, various operations have been performed to promote the escape of the fluids of the eyes. These operations have not always been satisfactory. Many cases of glaucoma have been relieved for a limited period of time, but sooner or later, become totally blind. When blindness occurs, operations have usually failed to restore the sight.
>
> *Cause:* The theory that the disease is caused by a hardening of the eyeball is incorrect, because we find cases of glaucoma in which the eyeball is not increased in hardness, and there are cases of hardening of the eyeball in which there is no glaucoma. The normal eye may be hardened temporarily by conscious eyestrain.

There are case histories of "spontaneous remissions" of people who had glaucoma. One such "spontaneous remission" occurred with the sister of one of my students.

References and/or case histories of glaucoma improvement can be found in the following *Better Eyesight* magazines: July 1920, December 1920, January 1924, July 1927, September 1927, January 1928. The entire December 1920 issue is dedicated to the topic of glaucoma, and includes several case histories.

Ophthalmologist R. S. Agarwal in *Mind and Vision* gives several case histories of improvement of glaucoma.[9]

Clara Hackett writes in *Relax and See:*

> Forty of my recent students have had glaucoma. Of these, 11 gained greater field of vision and increased sight; 18 had a lowering of tension according to their doctors; 11 had no great lasting improvement, although 5 do report less pain and discomfort.[10]

An 83-year-old student told me one year after the vision course that she no longer had glaucoma and her ophthalmologist had taken her off of the glaucoma medication she previously needed.

Another student had his glaucoma pressure checked by his ophthalmologist at the end of the eight-week natural vision course. His eye doctor told him glaucoma pressure had lowered.

Detached Retina

In humans, the ends of the cones and rods are not attached to the pigment epithelium very securely. With continuous strain placed on the retina by an "out of shape" eyeball and/or an accident or blow to the head, the upper nine layers of the retina can tear, or even detach. "Detached retina" can cause serious vision loss.

Oftentimes boxers experience detached retinas due to the many traumatic blows received to the head and eyes.

When the front third of a cow's eye, along with the vitreous humor, is removed, the retina easily "detaches" from the choroid. The retina then remains attached to the back of the eye only at the optic nerve.

Optometrist Bruce May states in his pamphlet *Rx for Nearsightedness—Stress-Relieving Lenses:*

> A Worthwhile Concern ... Most of the major causes of blindness (except a disease called diabetic retinopathy) seem to relate directly to increased inner eye or vitreous pressure, which is a common factor in myopia. Two-thirds of those persons who suffer detached retinas are myopic. The average age for retinal detachment for those myopes experiencing this problem is 29, while the comparable age for farsighted

> [individuals] is 62. There is real reason for concern and need for review of the general attitude toward myopia.... [11]

Ophthalmologist Charles H. May, M.D., writes in *Diseases of the Eye:*

> When [detached retina is] due to disease, it is most often found in myopia of high degree ... Unless the retina can be reattached by operation, the detachment generally *extends,* becomes *complete* and *blindness* results, though rare cases of spontaneous reattachment as well as stationary cases do occur.[12]

A guest at one of my Introductory Lectures had a very high degree of nearsightedness. His ophthalmologist told him he had no signs of detached retina—*but that he would have it someday because of his very high myopia.*

I have met many people who have detached retina. Most of them had very high degrees of myopia.

A reference to and/or case history of detached retina can be found in the March 1921 *Better Eyesight* magazine.

Conical Cornea (Keratoconus)

Better Eyesight magazine, September 1927:

> In conical cornea, the front part of the eye bulges forward and forms a cone-shaped body. The apex of the cone usually becomes the seat of an ulcer and sooner or later, the vision becomes very much impaired. In advanced cases, the person suffers very much from pain. Various operations have been performed, but the results have always been unsatisfactory.
>
> *Cause:* The cause of conical cornea is eyestrain.

The conical cornea protrusion is due to a "thinning" of the cornea. Conical cornea is also known as keratoconus.

May, in *Diseases of the Eye,* states in regard to conical cornea, "It may be important to improve the general health."[13]

A reference to and/or cases histories of conical cornea can be found in the July 1920, May 1924, and September 1927 *Better Eyesight* magazines.

Opacity of the Cornea

Better Eyesight magazine, September 1927:

> The cornea when healthy is perfectly transparent and does not interfere with the vision of the colored part of the eye, or pupil, but when the cornea becomes opaque, the opacity may be so dense that the color of the iris cannot be distinguished, and there is no perception of light.
>
> *Cause:* Opacities of the cornea are said to be caused by infections, ulcers or some general disease, but there are many cases which are caused by eyestrain....

A reference to and/or case history of corneal opacity can be found in the July 1920 and September 1927 *Better Eyesight* magazines.

Other Natural Improvements

References to and/or case histories of serious vision problems can be found in the following *Better Eyesight* magazines:

Iritis: January 1928
Retinitis pigmentosa: April 1920, July 1920, May 1921, June 1924, January 1928
Atrophy of the optic nerve: July 1920, October 1920, June 1924
Blindness: March 1921, June 1924, July 1924, September 1927

Clara Hackett writes in *Relax and See:*

> Fifty-seven persons with retinitis pigmentosa have had lessons. Of these, only 2 achieved 20/20 or normal sight; however, 38 had their field of vision and acuity helped appreciably even to the extent of driving a car again; 17 had no lasting benefit.
>
> Of 31 persons with progressive sight losses from such diseases as retinitis, conical cornea, chorioretinitis, 10 have stopped the progression ... One conical cornea case obtained 20/20 sight.
>
> There have been worthwhile results in vision losses due to other serious problems.... [14]

THREE CASE HISTORIES

Told to Learn Braille

Anna Kaye, a Natural Vision teacher trained by Clara Hackett, was told by four ophthalmologists to learn Braille. She had no useable vision due to atrophy of the optic nerves. She could not see a door, and no glasses gave her correction. When she moved from Europe to the US, she took vision lessons from Clara Hackett. In two and one-half years, she was seeing 20/30 without corrective lenses. At age seventy-five she still needed no corrective lenses. She had no restriction on her driver's license and could read small print without corrective lenses.

Aldous Huxley's Improvement

Author Aldous Huxley, due to a disease of his eyes, had critical eye problems as a teenager. For eighteen months he needed Braille to read and a guide to walk. "There is no doubt about it," he writes in his book, *The Art of Seeing,* "My capacity to see was steadily and quite rapidly failing."[15]

His wife Laura writes in the Foreword of his book:

> ... *The Art of Seeing* was Aldous' response to the fact that his sight was rapidly failing and that, in a matter of a short time, he would be blind. With an open mind he studied the Bates method which, still now especially in 1939, was unaccepted by the orthodox ophthalmologist. His eyesight and that of thousands of others was improved, even saved.[16]

Betsy's Testimonial

May 13, 1992

Dear Tom,

A note to thank you for continuing to do the work you're doing, and for making the monthly review classes available to us. It's great to hear others' stories.

I wanted to record for you what for me is a milestone this year. In 1983, a retinal hole with lattice degeneration was discovered in my right eye, and also some peripheral retinal degeneration (without hole formation) in my left eye. Although at first the ophthalmologist was going to seal the hole with laser surgery, he decided to wait and monitor the condition instead. The condition remained the same (but didn't worsen) for eight years.

In summer 1990, I began studying natural vision improvement. In February 1992, I started seeing a new eye doctor, one who is open to discussing N.V.I. (whereas the other was not, so I stopped seeing him). The new guy also specializes in retinal photography.

His examination of my retinas, and our observations of the developed photos, revealed *no retinal holes or lattice degeneration!* They had self-healed. I know that the healing took place as a result of relearning to relax my eyes. I also firmly believe in self-healing, and that *belief* had to be a big contribution.

The joys of using my own eyesight, and building on that, are endless. I emphasize what I *can* see, not what I cannot. The most comfortable pair [of glasses] is the weakest: R –4.50, L –3.75, and the astigmatism correction is gone.

It's a lifetime commitment. And it's fun! My whole outlook has changed: I have become a positive person—just knowing you have a choice about influencing your own vision makes a big difference in attitude. *Measurable* improvements are merely icing on the cake.

Thanks,
Betsy

Betsy attended the eight-week natural vision course from January to March 1991, and attended many Review classes after the course.

CHAPTER COMMENTS

TOM'S PERSONAL LOG: I have become highly motivated to improve my eyesight to avoid the possibility of serious eye problems in the future.

Bates associated mental strain with many serious vision problems. Many people who have serious vision problems are under very high stress, and have a tremendous staring habit. Also, many such people have worn compensating lenses for many years.

From the larger, holistic perspective, could "simple" errors of refraction be a warning to relax the mind and body? Do some of the more serious vision problems result from ignoring the initial message of blurred vision?

Improvement of many serious eye problems has been experienced by many people who have attended natural vision classes.

There are many causes of serious eye problems. A person should seek the care of an ophthalmologist for any serious eye problems.

NOTES

1 Joseph J. Kennebeck, *Why Eyeglasses are Harmful for Children and Young People* (New York: Vantage Press, 1969), pp. 91–92.

2 Mary Dudderidge, "New Light Upon Our Eyes: An Investigation Which May Result in Normal Vision for All, Without Glasses," in *Scientific American* (January 12, 1918), p. 53.

3 R. S. Agarwal, *Mind and Vision* (Pondicherry, India: Sri Aurobindo Ashram Press, 1983), pp. 56–57.

4 Clara A. Hackett and Lawrence Galton, *Relax and See* (London: Faber and Faber, Limited, 1957), pp. 25–27.

5 This quote is from a lecture given by Dr. Deborah Banker, M.D., on October 22, 1995, at the San Francisco Whole Life Expo.

6 Bruce May, *Rx for Nearsightedness: Stress-Relieving Lenses* (Optometric Extension Program Foundation pamphlet, 1981).

7 R. S. Agarwal, *Mind and Vision,* pp. 237–43.

8 Clara A. Hackett and Lawrence Galton, *Relax and See,* pp. 25–27.

9 R. S. Agarwal, *Mind and Vision,* p. 246.

10 Clara A. Hackett and Lawrence Galton, *Relax and See,* pp. 25–27.

11 Bruce May, *Rx for Nearsightedness: Stress-Relieving Lenses.*

12 Charles H. May, *Diseases of the Eye* (Baltimore, Maryland: William Wood and Company, 1943), pp. 314–15.

[13] Ibid., p. 165.

[14] Clara A. Hackett and Lawrence Galton, *Relax and See,* p. 26.

[15] Aldous Huxley, *The Art of Seeing* (Berkeley, California: Creative Arts Book Co., republished in 1982), p. 9.

[16] Ibid., p. 7.

CHAPTER TWENTY-EIGHT

Just For Fun!

Answers to questions are on the last page of this chapter.

1. Refer to the butterfly border around *Plates 14-21*. Which two butterflies are identical in detail, shape and color? (There are only two!)
2. In *Plate 45: A Difference Between Night and Day,* find all eight animals. Hint: There are two of each kind. Also, find the Big Dipper.
3. In *Plate 33: Daytime Cones Sensitivity Chart,* notice the color of the green border along the top of the "Green" Cones curve. Which part of the green border is darker—the part around 515 nm or the part around 550 nm?
4. Similar to *Plate 12: The Edge,* notice how the following solid bars appear to have a different shade of gray at the right and left edges of each bar.

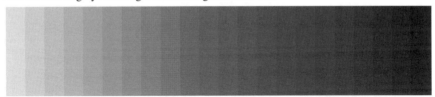

5.Which gray square box does not have the same shade of gray as the others?

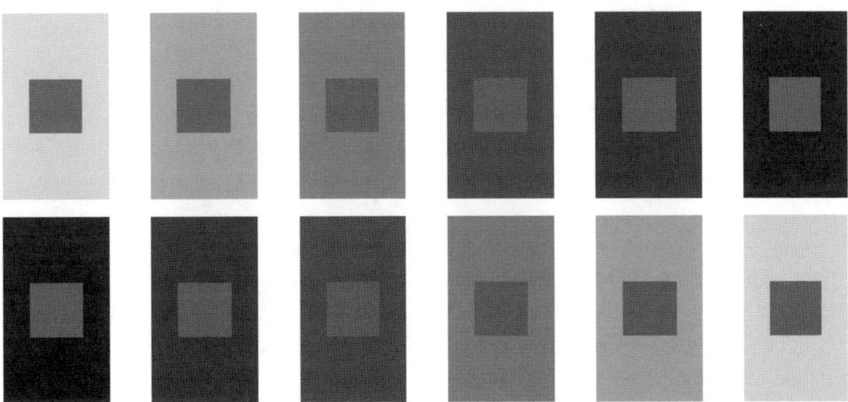

6. Which square is larger?

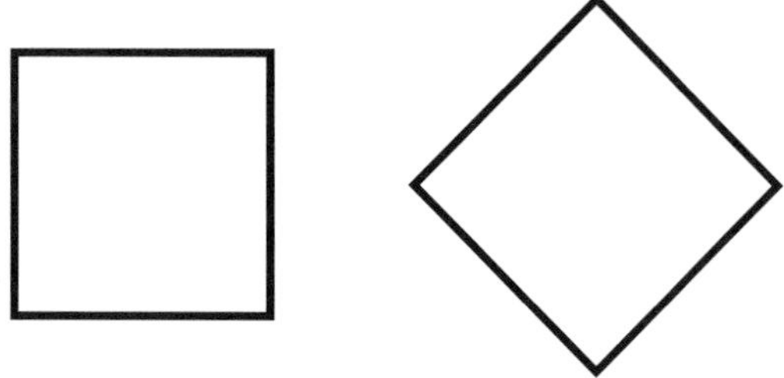

7. Which is longer, the horizontal or vertical line ?

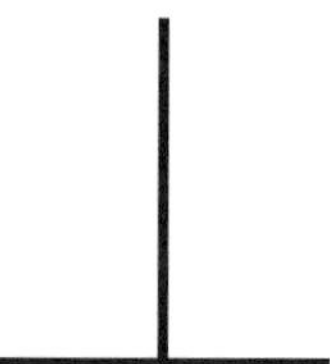

8. Which is longer, the line on the left or the right?

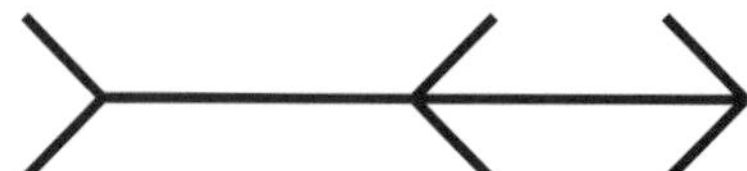

9. Which horizontal line is longer?

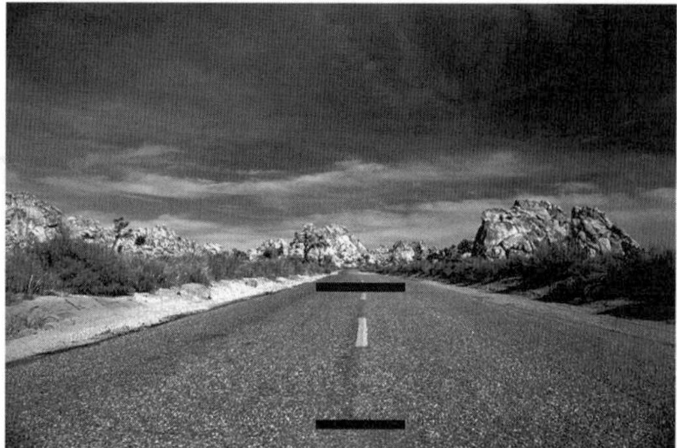

10. Which object is wider? Which is taller?

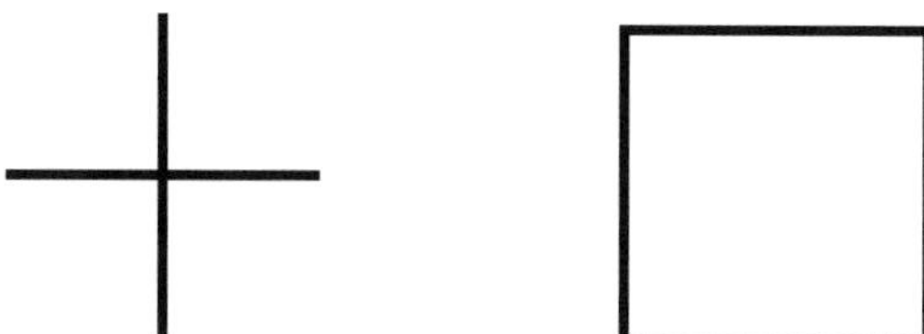

11. Are these vertical lines curved or straight?

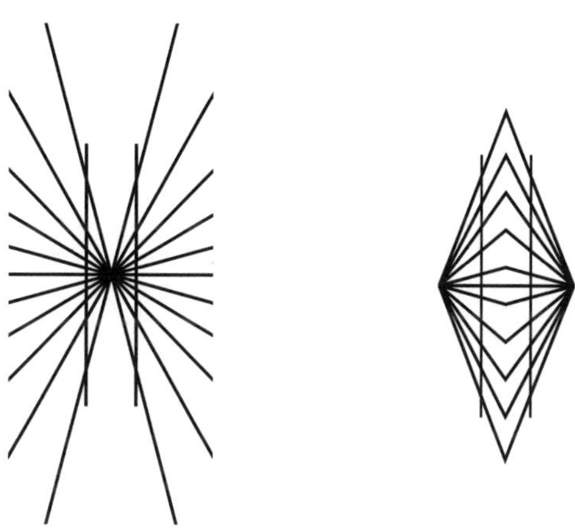

12a. Are the diagonal lines in the left box curved or straight?
12b. Are the black vertical lines in the right box curved or straight?

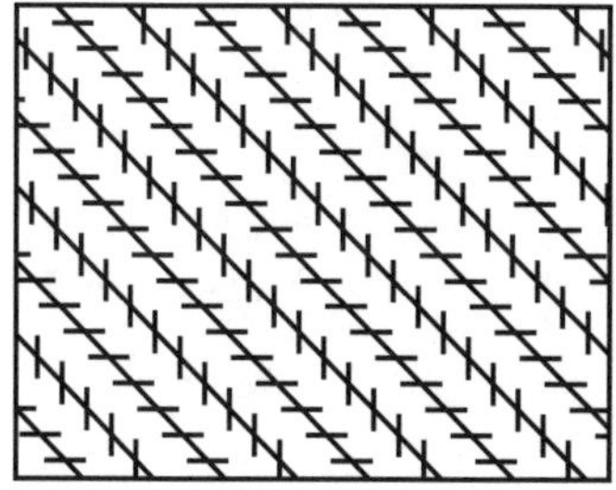

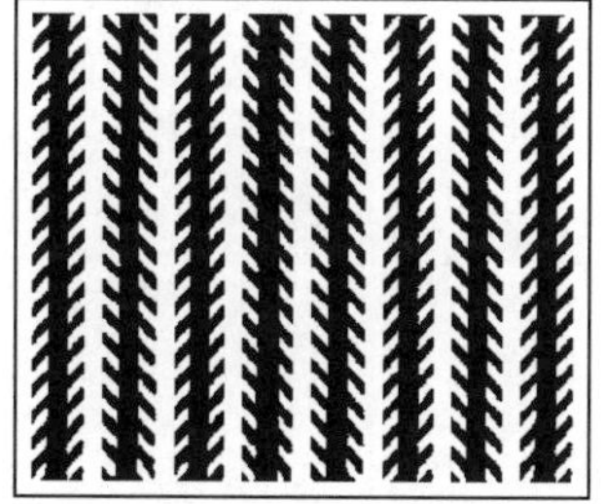

13. Is the diagonal line aligned?

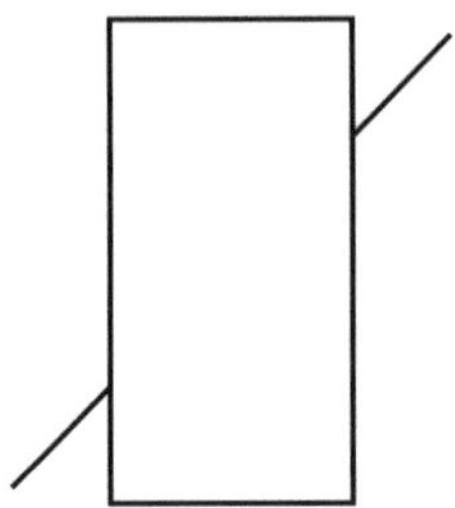

14. Shift between the boxes to notice flashing gray corners! Notice that when you centralize at one of the corners, the gray corner is not seen at that corner.

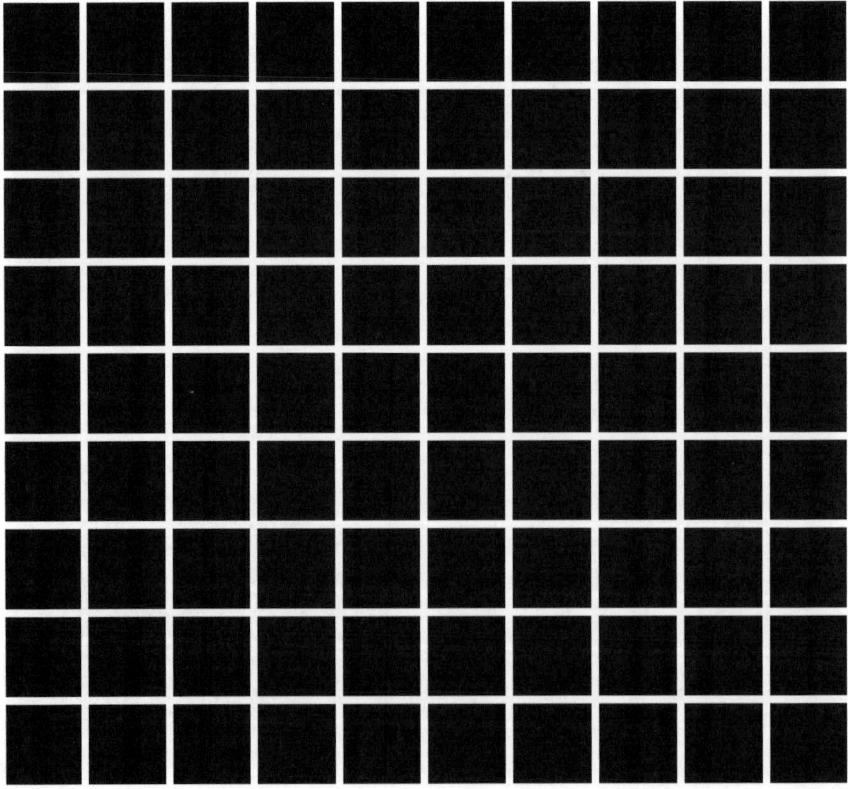

15. Do you see circles or spirals?

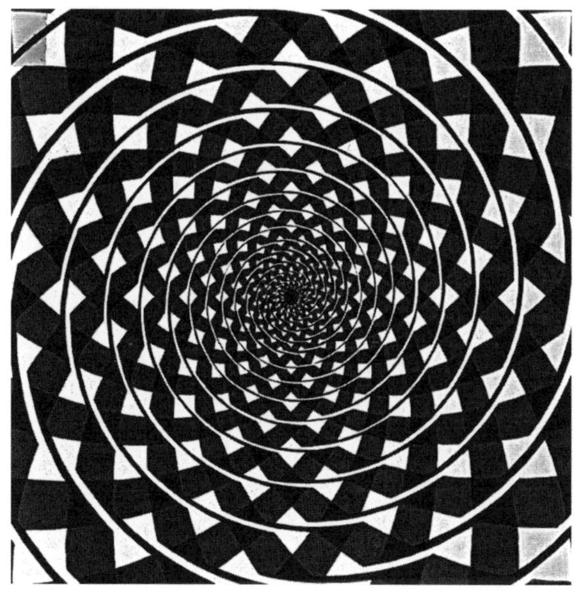

16. More 3-D fun:

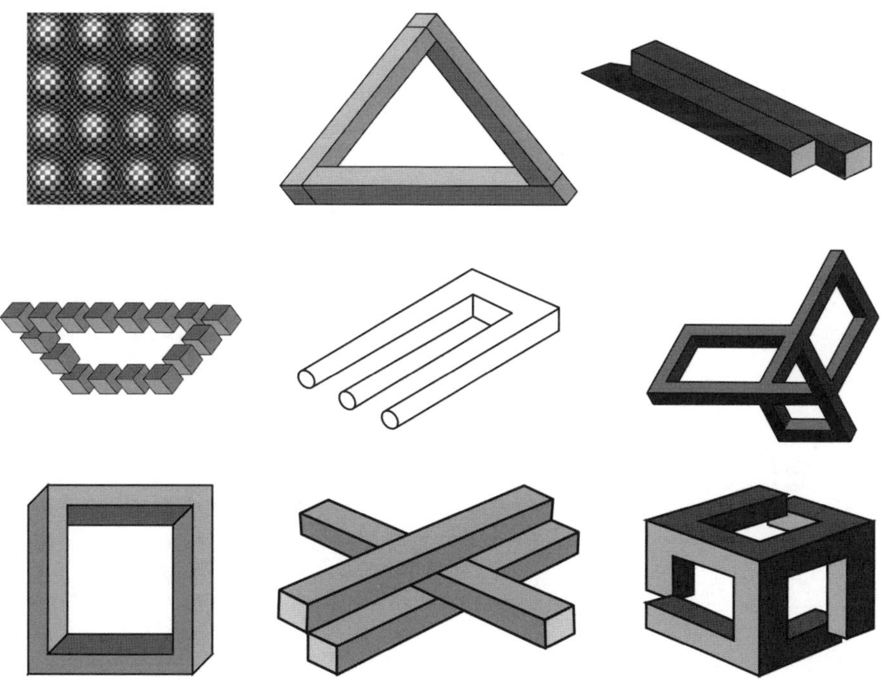

Answers:

1. The fourth small butterfly to the left from top right corner and the third small butterfly up from the bottom left corner are the only two butterflies that are identical.
2. There is a flying eagle, hen, sleeping bat and owl from top to bottom on the left side of the picture. On the right side there is flying bat, flying owl, eagle and sleeping hen. The Big Dipper? (I can't give you all the answers!)
3. You might have guessed that the green border near 515 nm appears lighter than the border near 550 nm. Actually, the entire (upper) green border is the same color. Different parts of the border appear to have different shades of green because the brain is comparing the green border to the colors in area underneath the border. Vision functions largely by comparisons of one object to another, and less by absolutes.
4. Each rectangle is one solid shade of gray. The brain compares the edges of two neighboring rectangles and interprets the left edge of the right rectangle to be darker than it actually is. Similarly, the brain interprets the right edge of each rectangle to be lighter than it actually is.
5. All gray square boxes are identical.
6. The squares are the same size.
7. Both are the same length.
8. Both are the same length.
9. Both are the same length.
10. Both objects have the same height and width.
11. All vertical lines are straight and parallel.
12a. All diagonal lines in the left box are straight and parallel .
12b. All vertical black lines in the right box are straight and parallel.
13. Yes!
14. N/A.
15. The thin lines are concentric circles. Follow them around to see how each is a circle.

Chapter Twenty-Nine

"This Method Has Been Proved"

There are truths which are not for all men, nor for all times.

—Voltaire, 1761

"IT IS SCIENTIFIC AND SUCCESSFUL"

W. B. MacCracken, M.D., trained with Bates and taught natural vision improvement in Berkeley, California. In his excellent 1937 book, *Use Your Own Eyes,* MacCracken writes:

> This method has been proved. It is scientific and successful. It requires, however, that the student be receptive, earnest, and confident.
>
> The story in this book is founded on these truths. Vision is the most precious of the senses, which feed the life and the happiness of the human....
>
> How long will it be before the minds of the children, who are beginning their lives, will be taught to use their own eyes, with the freedom and the power which belongs to them, and which will give them a new fullness of life? ...[1]
>
> The needless subjection of the eyes of the coming generation to the domination of glass lenses must have an absolute and malevolent influence on the mentality of any weak-eyed nation....
>
> In the United States the habit of wearing artificial lenses is increasing at such an astonishing rate, that it is fast becoming a remarkable national trait. A young woman from Australia, who came to me because she had heard of the Bates method there, told me that for the last three or four days on the ship, she was impatient, above every other thought, to get on the streets in San Francisco, to see if it was really true that almost everyone wore spectacles. She said she had tried to imagine how the people would look, and that in spite of her preparation, she never-the-less was astonished when she saw the procession of glasses. The shock made her more than ever determined to have the beginning trouble with her own eyes [reversed], so she would not be compelled to wear spectacles for the remainder of her life....[2]
>
> The subject of this book is not an abstract exposition. It is not an academic discussion of public policies or class interests. It is not offering theory. The issue is simple and clear, and of the most vital interest. It has been established, during a period of over twenty-five years, that most of those who

are wearing spectacles can use their natural eyesight, without any artificial assistance, and with perfect satisfaction....

Simply to deny that an eye which is finding some difficulty in seeing cannot be given any [restorative] assistance—to reply merely that "Bates has been discredited"—is not an answer worthy the medical profession....

[Bates] has met with the same old incredulity, skepticism, controversies, and opposition....

... the inevitable phases of reaction and consternation always provoked by new discoveries have not yet been passed....

The findings of Dr. Bates are as important as any other discovery, but they have never been investigated, nor weighed, nor tested. They are simply ignored. And will this always be so? ... I am not afraid to hazard a challenge that in due time the discovery of Dr. Bates will, likewise, come into its own.... The decision as to the value of the method of Dr. Bates will come from the men whose life work is the same as that of Dr. Bates....

Bates gave his life for a cause, battling against fate, during many years of magnificent struggle, when the unending disappointment finally broke in hopeless despair. His torch is still burning. There will come some other battler, who is fit, and who will hold it high until the people who are sitting in darkness have seen its great light.[3]

Optometrist Harris Gruman writes in his book *New Ways to Better Sight:*

The conservative methods of sight improvement outlined above are safe, time tested, and clinically proven. Everywhere people have benefited from them.[4]

... Certainly it is not to be denied that there are many who discard their glasses.[5]

THREE M.D. TESTIMONIALS

Dr. Woodward's Testimonial

From *Better Eyesight* magazine, November 1923:

A DOCTOR'S STORY

By H. W. Woodward, M.D.

About two years ago I visited New York for the purpose of investigating the claims made by Dr. Bates relative to the reversal of refractive errors ...

I visited his clinic at Harlem Hospital. Here I found most unusual methods taught by the doctor and Mrs. Lierman in the reversal of disorders of the eye. I was surprised at the cheerfulness of the students, particularly the children.

The doctor invited me to call at his office. I did so, and again I found his methods so different from the usual oculist that I was interested at once in finding out how he did his work. The first thing that impressed me was seeing so many students working in his waiting room. They seemed to be engaged in steadfastly regarding the letters of test cards placed upon the wall.

After I had seen the doctor teach several students, he turned to me and inquired about the condition of my own eyes. I replied that I had reached the age where most people require glasses for reading, but was just beginning to be annoyed by a blurring of vision when I consulted a telephone directory in a dimly lighted room. I knew that this symptom means in the almost universal experience of mankind, glasses, and more glasses, until one becomes dependent upon them. While I was contemplating this prospect, Dr. Bates explained to me that he had been through this experience, having had to wear quite strong lenses for reading and that he had healed himself.

He handed me one of his professional cards. On the back of this card was printed in small diamond type seven paragraphs stating seven fundamentals of perfect sight. He requested me to hold this card about six inches from my eyes, then close my eyes and form in my imagination or memory a small letter "o" and to see it in my mind, very black with a white center. After doing this for a few seconds, I was to open my eyes and look at the letters on the card. I did this, and to my surprise upon opening my eyes, the letters were jet black and remarkably distinct; but, for only a moment did this clear vision last. The letters soon faded away into a blur.

This experience of getting a flash of clear vision, though evanescent in character, was encouraging to me, because it suggested the possibility of conquering this tendency to blurring. In other words, if I could learn to sustain this primary normal position that my eyes relaxed into just before opening them, I would certainly achieve perfect vision. Dr. Bates instructed me to practice what I had just done twice a day. I did as he advised. At first I could not hold this flash of clear vision more than a second or two. It was too subtle. I could not get a hold on it. I continued, however, practicing night and morning for several weeks with but slight improvement. At last, however, I became able to sustain the clear vision for about thirty seconds; but if I would wink my eyes while seeing clearly, my vision would fade into a blur. In time my patience was rewarded by more improvement, for now I am often able to read the whole card without a blur.

Dr. Bates deserves much credit for the pioneer work which he is doing and for the way he keeps on doing it in spite of the hostile criticism continually directed toward him. To know him is a privilege and I am thankful to have had this experience.

Ophthalmologist Darling's Testimonial

From *Better Eyesight* magazine, December 1925:

[*Editor's Note:* This contribution from an oculist of twenty years' experience in one of the largest eye hospitals in the United States is of unusual interest. He is to be congratulated on his perseverance in going without glasses so long before his sight for reading had sufficiently improved to do his work properly. He has not told of the opposition and loss of many of his old friends, because he did not prescribe glasses for his clients. This is the article by Dr. Darling.]

AN OCULIST'S EXPERIENCE

by E. F. Darling, M.D.

I have been practicing medicine as an ophthalmologist for the last twenty years. During the period of eighteen years prior to 1923, I spent a large part of my time putting glasses on my helpless clients. However, for the last two years I have been trying to make amends by removing their glasses as rapidly as possible.

The first time I heard of Dr. Bates' work was from an article in one of the medical journals about fifteen years ago. The article made some impression on me because it was entirely at variance with our accepted views as to the cause and reversibility of defective vision. In the clinic I attend at one of the largest eye hospitals, most of the men seemed to know nothing about Dr. Bates. Some thought he was a quack, while others said he was insane.

About three years ago, I received notice of the publication of his book *Perfect Sight Without Glasses,* and at that time I decided to purchase the book and see what it was all about. The thing slipped my mind for another year or so, when one of my old clients came into my office without her glasses on, and said she had been working with Dr. Bates. Her vision was much improved, and she wanted to know if I could continue the same kind of education with her. I was obliged to confess that I knew nothing about his methods....

The next day I went over to the Central Fixation Publishing Company and bought the book. When I reached home, I started reading it and didn't stop until I had finished the whole thing. Here was a plain statement of facts accomplished, and I at once decided to test the matter with my own eyes.

I was wearing convex +2.25 DS for distance and convex +4.25 DS for reading. My distance vision had deteriorated in the eighteen years I had worn glasses from better than normal to about one-third of normal. My near vision had gone back so much that I was wearing the glasses that theoretically should suit a person sixty or seventy years old.

With the glasses off I could see only the largest headlines on the newspapers. While wearing the glasses, I had occasional headaches and eyeaches, and my near vision was at times very defective, so that I had difficulty in doing fine work of any kind.

The first day I went around without glasses, everything seemed blurred. But I felt somehow I had gotten rid of some particularly galling chains. It was pleasant to feel the air blowing against my eyes, and I walked around the whole afternoon trying to get used to the new condition.

In carrying out the suggestions in Dr. Bates' book, I had a great deal of trouble with the first week or so, especially with the mental images. This was simply due to my extreme eye strain. In spite of this, my vision steadily improved by palming, so that at the end of three weeks, I could read the 10/15 line instead of the 20/70 line. I had only an occasional eyeache when I had forgotten to use my eyes properly.

In improving my near vision, I had to make several visits to Dr. Bates, and he overcame most of my difficulties at once. I used many of the methods he advocates in this near work, but it was about three months before I could read fine print. It seemed an extremely long, long time to give up reading. But knowing now the advantages after an experience of two years without glasses, I would be willing to go without reading for a much longer period.

Many people the same age get results in a much shorter time than I did. I feel more and more strongly that a person will not have full control of his mental faculties until he gets rid of his glasses. Whether it takes two weeks or two years, the results will pay for the deprivation.

At present, I usually read an hour or so in the daytime, and three or four hours at night with no eyestrain whatever. Previously I used to walk along with my eyes fixed on the pavement because of the discomfort in taking note of passing people or objects. Now, it is a great pleasure to examine things minutely.

In my work I can go nine hours with about the same fatigue as I felt before in three or four hours. In other words, Dr. Bates' work has changed me from an old man of forty-eight to a young man of fifty. I now enjoy the practice of medicine for the first time since finishing my hospital internship. As I am absolutely certain that if students will carry out my directions, their whole condition will be improved.

In no case can the time required to obtain normal vision be definitely stated. People of the same age and wearing the same strength of glasses vary in time required as much as they differ in color

> of their hair or size of their appetites. Some get quick results; others drag along indefinitely before they get where they should be. These slow cases require lots of encouragement, and it sometimes takes all of their own and the teacher's perseverance to keep them going.

Note: It is not necessary to completely eliminate glasses immediately to succeed. However, the less glasses are worn, the faster the progress.

Ophthalmologist M. H. Stuart, M.D.—Improvement and Teaching

Better Eyesight magazine, September 1920:

> ... Slight as my error of refraction was, I was not able to leave off my glasses for more than an hour or two without suffering from nervousness and the feeling of tenseness in the spinal cord alluded to above.
>
> ... Recently I read, in the May (1920) number of *Better Eyesight,* Dr. Arnau's story of how his headaches were relieved, and I was so impressed by it that I determined to try the relaxation method upon myself. I palmed for five minutes and then read the card three times with each eye as far as I could without effort. I did this six times a day for five days, and at the end of this time I had gained a very decided degree of relaxation. I had, of course, discarded glasses, and, although this caused me a little discomfort at first, I was able, about a week later, to perform, without them, three tonsillectomies and one operation for cataract, and to remove two blind eyes. At the same time I went through my daily routine of treating ten to thirty patients, examining eyes, ears, noses and throats, much of which work requires extra good vision....
>
> I was so pleased with the results of the new method in my own case that I have since taught centralization to about forty of my patients, and in only about two did I fail to improve the vision at the first sitting....
>
> [After describing several case histories of improvements with students he taught, Dr. Stuart concludes with:]
>
> I was particularly pleased to be able to relieve these little girls of a disfigurement which means so much more to them than it would mean to a boy, and I was much interested to note how much prettier their eyes were, apart from the disappearance of strabismus, after a few sessions. They were wide open, softer-looking, in short, relaxed.

MORE PROOF

Janet Goodrich offers proof of vision improvement of her students in three different cases in her book *Natural Vision Improvement:*

1. A group of nine students monitored by optometrist H. H. Friend in Australia;
2. A group of eighteen students monitored by ophthalmologist Dr. J. Soorani in Los Angeles; and
3. A group of twelve students monitored by Coralie La Salle, who was awarded a master's degree from UCLA on her thesis, titled, "Some Psychophysiological Influences in Myopia."[6]

I have personally talked with one ophthalmologist and two optometrists who *teach* natural vision improvement.

Mary Dudderidge reports in *Scientific American:*

> The problem of [reversing] errors of refraction, therefore, is to induce the eyes

> to take it easy, and look at things without effort....
>
> More than one thousand children with defective sight have regained normal vision by [Bates' educational] means. In one class in which there had been 27 eye defectives, 25 were reported [reversed], while one truant and one incorrigible had become good students, because they were now able to study without pain.[7]

See also Chapter 23, "Children and Schools," section "Definite, Irrefutable Proof."

(ALMOST) 100 MESSAGES FROM NATURAL VISION STUDENTS

Following are parts of some messages left at or delivered to the Natural Vision Center of San Francisco by my natural vision students (a couple of exceptions are noted) between September 1984 and August 1996. They have been edited for clarity of understanding. Irrelevant and redundant parts have been removed.

Note that many of the improvements of sight have been validated by the student's eye doctor.

1. N. T.: I have very good news after having gone to my eye doctor to have my eyes checked yesterday. He says that out of the glasses that were reduced the middle of last April to 20/40, I am now seeing 20/25, so—I am so excited about this—I am now getting new glasses that are dropped one diopter in one eye and one and a quarter diopters in the other eye. So, I couldn't wait to tell you about that.
2. E. R.: On the way home I had some really nice clear vision flashes for a little while. (*Comment:* This student has had serious vision problems since birth.)
3. Z. R.: I just wanted to let you know I went back to my eye doctor and my vision has improved a whole lot. I now have four and a half diopters, and I started with seven diopters.
4. K. R. (Z. R.'s sister): I just wanted to tell you that I can see—and I am very happy! Thank you. Bye.
5. O. E.: I just called to tell you I am really excited. I went to my eye doctor today. I see 20/40 [without glasses] and he did not see the need for me to get any more glasses because he said there is no need to reduce them—which makes me think I have just thrown away my glasses that I have worn for twelve years ... I am really ecstatic and also really grateful. (O. E. is a Natural Vision teacher.)
6. O. C.: I saw my eye doctor this afternoon and my 20/80 glasses had turned into 20/30. So, I got reductions and he took out all of the astigmatism correction, and I am very, very happy!
7. D. T.: I went to see my eye doctor today, and he was quite impressed, and I got another reduced prescription. So, I am real excited about that. I was seeing better today just knowing that.
8. R. F.: I have improved one diopter in each eye, which was great news to me. I was so excited, I thought someone gave me a brand new gift of some kind. I am one step away from perfect vision, by the way. I catch myself staring more than I ever have before, so that must be a good sign. (*Comment:* Students become more aware of when they are staring as they improve.)
9. P. W.: I wanted to tell you that my 20/40s are 20/20⁻, and my 20/80s are now 20/50. So, I am so happy!

10. T. L.: I am calling to tell you that I took my driving test today, and I passed!
11. C. N.: I saw my eye doctor today and I am getting new glasses. I'm real excited. The new reduced glasses are both below –10 diopters. One is –8.5 and the other is –9.5. My optometrist is pretty excited. So, I'm pretty excited. (*Comment:* Before the classes, C. N. wore OD: –13, and OS: –12.)
12. K. I.: Wanted to let you know my eye doctor is again reducing my prescription. I started out at –3.50 and –1.50 for astigmatism. The first reduction was –2.75 and –0.75 for astigmatism. He is now moving me down to –2.00 and leaving the astigmatism correction the same. I am very pleased.
13. T. W.: My eyesight has really taken off. I just cannot get over it. Everything has become very three-dimensional and so much better as far as clarity goes. Thanks.
14. D. B.: I wanted to tell you the good news. I just went to see my eye doctor, and my 20/40 lenses are now 20/25. So we are reducing down the next step. The 20/80s only went to 20/60, so we are going to keep those for a while. I'm thrilled! I will be attending the next Review class.
15. R. G.: I am calling the "staring hotline," basically just to say that I am very excited with my vision this morning and all the bright colors that I have been seeing since I first opened my eyes.
16. O. N.: Thank you very much. I haven't reduced my glasses [for a second time] yet. My optometrist says my eyes have not improved that greatly to do another reduction. There was only a slight reduction during my trip. But I did not wear my glasses at all during my trip, which lasted about three weeks. And, I did a lot of fantastic things—without my glasses!
17. N. Z.: I am doing so well. I really don't need glasses that much in the house. And only when I go to strange places do I wear glasses, or when I am driving. Otherwise, I do not need glasses. I am doing so well. I am so thrilled. I just wanted to let you know. Thanks.
18. W. T.: I just saw two poles hanging from the Vision Halo. (*Comment:* W. T. only saw one pole when she first used the Vision Halo, which is discussed in Chapter 18, "Stereoscopic Vision.")
19. M. L.: I called to tell you I just got a reduction, and I'm just so excited, I don't know what to do. And I just thought you would like to know about it.
20. L. W.: Good news—I went to see my eye doctor, and my vision has improved from 20/300 to 20/200. Not bad, eh? Sketch, breathe, and blink!
21. R. D.: My vision tests at 20/20 now. See you tonight at the Review class. Thank you.
22. K. N.: I am definitely having the centralizing realization, and understanding that diffusion is confusion. As far as my close-up vision, I am seeing that if I really slooowww doooownnn, I can see close-up. So, I can actually read your phone number off of your flyer when I was calling you. If I don't strain, and if I just slooowww doooownnn, and take the time, then I can see. Thank you.
23. K. N., again: I can see in areas that I could not see before, not all the time,

but I do not have to put my glasses on always for close up. It is not as clear as I would like it to be.

24. K. N., again: I am brushing and breathing and blinking as I drive back to Lake Tahoe. I had a really good meditation last night, and part of what I see is the significance of reversals—beyond eyesight—just the significance of going back and healing, and then coming forward again.
25. K. N., again: I am really going through some stuff now. I'm seeing some of my patterns. Fear of authority. Fear of humiliation. And overwhelm. I have my little reminders around my house. And I am really seeing a lot better; not all of the time, but sometimes. It is very exciting. When I slooowww doooownnn enough to take the time to do them (the habits), if I really take the time I can read even the fine print on the page.
26. N. T.: Yesterday I went and had a massage. And when I was done with the massage and I came out into the light, I thought, "Wow! Everything just looks so bright!" But I thought it was because I had my eyes closed for an hour. And I just noticed everything was bright on the way home. And then I went on with my daily business, and then I noticed that objects just seemed to be jumping out at me. My depth perception is incredible! And, anyway, I went to bed last night, and I woke up this morning, and it is the same! I see colors so brightly that I can't get over it. Wow! I can't even tell you how exciting this is. Things have texture! (*Comment:* Many *qualities* of the visual system reactivate with natural vision improvement.)
27. K. N., again: I am doing very well—some total major breakthroughs, as far as self-love and self-confidence, and just feeling good about myself. I am, I must admit, forgetting sometimes to sketch, breathe, and blink, but like you said, previously I did not even know such things (habits) were available.
28. O. G.: I just wanted to call, and tell you for the first time I can see crystal clear out of my glasses that used to be 20/40. Now I think I can see 20/20 out of these glasses. I was so amazed. (*Comment:* O. G. is a Natural Vision teacher.)
29. K. G.: Although I stuck my glasses in my pocket to go to vision class last night, I don't think I got home with my glasses. I don't remember taking them out of my pocket at all during class. This will now be my seventh pair of *mysteriously disappearing glasses.* Hmmm, it is so strange. I am not quite ready to do without them yet. *But it's my old childhood story of losing my glasses.* And so, this is it, my seventh pair lost this year. Hmmm. I am just hoping I left them in your classroom, but I think you don't have them. I will just keep looking, but weird, weird things happen to me with this. (*Comment:* Losing the glasses again was a reversal process.)
30. D. F.: In spite of stress, which actually is resolving itself, I am down to somewhere between 20/40 and 20/100 depending on what the light is. The optometrist pegged me at 20/70 and gave me –1.50 diopters. This part of my life is probably the best part of my life—except maybe T'ai Chi. Bye.
31. T. N.: Some things are changing for me

vocationally. It is difficult to stay in a stressful work environment when your life is about relaxation.

32. N. N.: I am so excited with what is happening with my mother. She can now see the numbers on the kitchen timer—of course, with her glasses. But before, she used her glasses *and* her magnifying glass—and *still* she wasn't sure of numbers. Now she can also see the little arrow on her sewing machine. Thank you. (*Comment:* N. N. and her mother attended vision classes.)
33. B. T. (before attending classes): I was thinking about stress and eyesight, and I was thinking about the time when I realized I had cataracts, and I had blamed it on working in an office with two chain smokers and all the smoke drying out the lenses of my eyes. But I realized it was most the stressful job I had had in my whole entire life. I was *so tense* in that job. And then another time, when I was a student, I was far away from home, and I was homesick, and I almost went blind. And that was another stressful year of mine, and, God!, now when I put two plus two together, I keep thinking about stress, and my eyes *always* get worse when I am under stress. And all of the people in my retinitis pigmentosa group say their eyes get worse, too, when they are under stress.
34. O. H.: I want to share briefly a story with you. Today I picked up a book, and started to read the book, and realized I was not using my glasses! I was very excited by that! Things are moving!
35. B. U.: My clarity is coming back, after a lot of resistance. I notice my own willingness to relax, and vision does get clearer and more mobile every day. And, in fact, I have gotten over a hump of resistance. And I probably will encounter some more humps in the future. But it is truly very energizing and clarifying for my mind and emotions and vision to *give in* to the process of letting my clarity return.
36. K. I.: I went to the eye doctor, and I went through the whole exam, and I knew that my eyes had improved. He told me that with my (former) 20/40s I could now see 20/25. And my (former) 20/80s are definitely too strong for the computer, which I knew. So, it was really exciting to see how much my vision had improved!
37. M. K.: I have exciting news to tell you. I understand centralization! About two days ago, I started seeing a single point clearly. I tip my hat to you! Thank you very much.
38. D. N.: Just to give you an update. I am doing fine. I am reading in the sunshine without glasses a lot of the time. And, really, I am doing well with these +1.50s, although sometimes I have to get into a good light, because light has a lot to do with it, I discovered.
39. K. T.: I went to my optometrist this afternoon, and he said that the glasses he had prescribed for me to see 20/40, now I can see almost 20/20 through them. So, he is going to prescribe another pair of glasses for me. So I am really excited now—not that I wasn't excited before—but now I am really excited. I just want to tell you the good news. Thanks a lot.

40. K. N., again: I am so excited, I am really, every day, doing my vision habits—brush, breathe, and blink. Things I could not read before I can read, and it is very exciting.
41. T. R.: I am thinking that my life is pretty hectic right now, and I do not think I will be attending the remaining classes. I think I have the basic gist of it. I know I will be missing valuable information, but I feel like *right now I have to make some major lifestyle changes, such as relaxing and breathing.* I do have plans to go away for the next couple of weekends to make some money, which I really need, but I appreciate everything you have done. And, I do hope that through this gradual process things will begin to change for me. But, I see that it is really something very major. Like you always say, "It is not a trivial class." That's true. But I definitely have those *three things* down, and now I just need to apply them, and make changes in my life. So, thank you very much for your help, and I will be talking to you sometime in the future to let you know how things are going.
42. K. F.: I had your course about a month and a half ago. My vision has improved. I went to the DMV and passed. Now I can drive legally without glasses. I thought I would call you and say "Thank you" for your class. You have helped me make great improvements with my eyes.
43. B. H.: Just wanted to let you know my husband and I are moving . . . I wanted to thank you for everything, and I feel very fortunate to meet you and take your class. My vision continues to improve more and more every day. So, keep up the good work. Bye.
44. M. L.: I just wanted to tell you something really good is happening, because my eyes are getting so good, I can hardly believe it. My vision is improving a lot. I'm seeing a lot of things I could not see before. In the night, I can see my clock; I could not see it before. It was always blurry. I can see my television without my glasses, and a lot of really good things. I just wanted to let you know about my progress. I must be doing good vision habits.
45. L. M.: This vision is a lot of fun. It really works, and I am really psyched, and I want to thank you.
46. M. I.: Boy, I must have had 20/15 today over in the Marin Headlands. It was incredible. I could count the houses on the streets in the Sunset District of San Francisco. Actually, I was seeing from Tennessee Valley, which is farther than the Marin Headlands. Thanks for your good work.
47. B. T. (again, before attending classes): I have decided I would like to be your last, ninth student in your course beginning April 8. I just had a realization that I cannot afford *not* to take your class.
48. M. L.: I just thought I would call you and let you know that I have been having a lot of flashes. I mean, lots and lots and lots. I have just been noticing that I haven't been wearing my glasses for three weeks.
49. B. T. again: Reading on the trolley coming home last night, I had an intellectual appreciation that I would, could, will get better; that my progress is less

"iffy" now; it's more, like, definite. In my mind, it is definite. And last night I had a intellectual realization that it is definite. That I can do it. And then this morning I had the emotional realization. . . .

50. R. C.: I thought I would give you a progress report. I went to my eye doctor today, and I had a "micro" improvement, which I was thoroughly excited about, and certainly congratulated myself. Thanks a lot. I am very happy.

51. K. W.: I just wanted to let you know I had my first real flash. I saw clearly for a few seconds, and then I was staring at the thing I was looking at, and then it went away. But, it *did* happen. It was really magical! So, even though I have been really down on myself, and thinking that I was not doing well, something must be happening, right? Bye, and thanks.

52. F. G.: I just got a third reduction, which is getting pretty far down there. So, I am glad about that. Thanks, bye.

53. M. L.: I just went to my eye doctor last week, and he said that my naked eyes are 20/80, and that I do not need any more reduced glasses for up close.

54. G. I.: I am really *on* this thing. I am doing so much better, you would have been proud of me. I even went to a fair, and I went on one of those incredible rides that spins around backward and goes up and down at the same time. And I went by myself, and I had the courage to do that, and did OK. I want to keep consistent with this, and want to be able to make sure I practice correct reading and writing habits. The reading is going OK. (*Comment:* G. I. had serious difficulties reading before the vision class.)

55. M. U.: I had this great insight, or connection, in my own life. This thought came to me that I have to get focused in life, because I have been rather scattered. I have had a hard time looking for a job; I haven't really looked for a job. Just kind of been running from one interest to the next to the next. So, the word that came to me—about the way I was leading my life was—it is time to get more focused. Well, this seems to have something to do with vision, doesn't it?! What do you know? So, anyway, that seems like a good thing. Thanks very much.

56. M. C.: I want to thank you for the class. It is absolutely wonderful. I spent the entire day yesterday without my glasses on—even at work—which was a real milestone for me. I can't thank you enough for the class. It was really great. Thanks a lot.

57. K. N.: I just wanted to say that I love this class, and I am having such wonderful experiences. This has been such a happy day. Actually, it started yesterday on the way home from class.

58. K. N., again: I wanted to tell you I am seeing so wonderfully well. A couple of things have happened recently, and that is: I have been thinking about the woman who put reminder stickers all over her house, and how you said she improved fast. I keep thinking every day, "I am going to do that. I am going to put up reminder stickers." And I have a whole box of stickers, but I can't decide which one to use. But, because I have been thinking about it so much, I

think about where I am going to put them, so I am always thinking about centralizing and sketching and stuff. So, it's working even if I don't have stickers up! The other thing is I was putting make-up on yesterday, and I looked up, and I realized my eyes are together—seeing. Usually when I am up close at the mirror, one eye is down, and the other is up—and I am using only one eye, while the other is not seeing. So now they are coming together. I feel like I am holding my head straight. And my eyes are coming together! It is really fun! Even my boyfriend noticed it, when we are looking at each other, that one eye is not wandering off. I realize that a lot of this is staying conscious of my blinking, because the more I blink, the more it brings my eyes together somehow. I'm not sure why that works, but it does. And my yawning mechanism is just going "nuts"—it's great! Every time I get into one of these yawning spells, I realize it is when my eyes have been under some sort of stress. Like right after my computer class, all the way home I am yawning. It works! Anyway, I am very excited about life, and all of the things you helped us relearn. At a conference where I was just helping out, I met a lot of friends I had not seen for a long time, and it was really emotional for me to get up and introduce myself. I felt real powerful, just within myself; confident. I really attribute a big portion of that, of my excitement about life, and staying alive in each moment to the commitment I made when I started with your class. And I am really grateful. So, I think that is long enough. I hope your tape does not run out. Bye.

59. T. N., again: I just wanted to give you a little success story. I came into work today after having my work done with my chiropractor yesterday. He made some wonderful adjustments. He really helped loosen up my neck a lot. I was amazed at how tight some of the muscles had been for such a long time. At work I realized I could now see twice the distance as I could before with clarity, because when I first took my glasses off, I used to be able to see my computer screen at about 18 inches. And now, I can actually stretch out my arm to about a three-foot length, and I can now see the computer screen very clearly. Obviously, I have more improvement to go, but it is very impressive that after these months, and all the different things I have been doing, and with chiropractic, I have made a definite step forward. So, just wanted to let you know about that. Take care. Bye. (*Comment:* T. N. is now a Certified Natural Vision teacher.)

60. K. L.: Thank you so much for talking with me for so long after the class. It was a real beginning of my understanding. And now I can read the books and have a much better feeling for them. I am really excited about the centralizing principle, which I really got for the first time because of what you explained to another student. So now, when I look at the smallest thing, it becomes clear, and it's very, very nice. So, I just wanted to thank you for everything so much. Bye.

61. T. W.: I just wanted to pass on some good news. I just happened to be at the

DMV because I lost my driver's license. I requested a duplicate, and at the same time I asked if they could re-test my eyes because I had been taking a natural vision course. I took the test again, and I passed! So, I don't need corrective lenses. I wanted to thank you very, very much. Best wishes.

62. C. B.: I just laughed yesterday, because I went to have my renewal of my driver's license at the DMV, and they gave me an eye test. So, she asked me to read the lines; and so, I read the lines. And then she looked up at me and said, "Are you wearing contact lenses?" And I said, "No." She said, "Have you had any corrective surgery?" And I said, "No." And she was just in puzzlement. And I guess she looked up my old files, and I guess it said I needed glasses. And I just sort of smiled. And she said, "Well, you are supposed to be getting worse!" And I said, "No! I am getting better!" And, so it was just sort of a funny thing. I said, "Yeah, your eyes can improve. You do not have to go negative in the other direction." So, that was just sort of an interesting thing. My eyes are not quite 20/20 yet, but with all your support in fundamentals of natural vision, I have great faith that I will arrive at that point—20/20, if not better. And, like everything else, it's all associated with good mind-health and mind-spirit and general health. OK. Thanks, Tom. (*Comment:* C. B. is a medical doctor who teaches proper nutrition to his clients. He gave me a gift of a T-shirt which says, "Sketch, Breathe, and Blink—Oh, I See.")
63. H. T.: I just had a check-up with my eye doctor today, and my vision has improved once again. He was really amazed at how much my vision has improved. I am real excited about it. And the glaucoma test—he said that my pressure was like a teenager's. And I really attribute it to your class and all the good teaching I got. And my glasses keep getting lighter and lighter, and it's a wonderful feeling, so, I wanted to thank you very much for your good work. (*Comment:* H. T. integrates natural vision principles into the art classes she teaches to adults and children.)
64. S. T.: I have had a lot of vision improvement and a lot of "Wow's" lately, but I am calling because I wanted to get a bunch of your brochures, because there is a lot of interest in your classes at the Feldenkrais training I am attending. I will see you at the Review class.
65. D. B.: I am playing with this nose-feather, and it is pretty amazing the stuff that is coming up. I am seeing so much about how my vision is one more metaphor, one more way of how I live my life. This is, like, totally wonderful and I am so excited, and thank you.
66. S. I.: I was at a training yesterday with some people I have been working with for the last two years, and it was interesting what happened. I was relaxing and yawning, and the leader of the training apparently got very angry at me because I was yawning so much, and he accused me of not participating and being disrespectful, and, uh, I was not expecting that. So, I might want to have a talk with you about some of the social consequences of being relaxed. Maybe I am being an utter fanatic

about it, but it feels so good, I am having a hard time stopping! I ended up leaving this training. It just wasn't worth it for me to be there. Also, my right jaw has been popping very loudly, which is something that happened when I was 18 years old. It was pretty bad at that time. It was sort of like lock-jaw, and I would try to put food in my mouth, and my mouth would not open. It is not that bad, but it is sort of reminiscent of that, and it reminds me of what you said about going back through layers—that if there was an old injury or illness, a person might re-experience it in order to release it. So, I figure that is what is happening, but it's a little strange, 'cause I haven't been in that place for 10 or 15 years now. So, lots of interesting developments. And I am having fun! And I just wanted to call and check in and make use of your "staring hotline." Hope you are well. Bye. (*Comment:* S. I. identifies his own reversal.)

67. B. T.: I wanted to leave you this message of success. I had another reduction of my lenses. I am now using my original 20/80 correction lenses as my 20/40 lenses, which feels really good. And the other thing that is really significant is that I have noticed that my blur without any glasses is less. And when I noticed it, is when I just got my last 20/80 lenses. I just noticed that the blur without them is not that much worse than the blur with them. It was so neat to see that—that actually, I am really making progress. So, albeit it is slow, but I am really excited about that. This has been encouraging, and helps me to not wear my glasses more often. So, just wanted to let you know things are moving. Take care. Bye.

68. D. B., again: I just wanted to tell you I just had this amazing, wonderful—I can't remember what you called it—but it was just like a real, absolute miracle in my vision. It kind of subsided back now, but it was just phenomenal. It was like—just the clarity and the color and—I'm kind of rocking and reeling from it at this point. And it was just incredibly wonderful. I just wanted to share that with you, because I knew you would appreciate it. Bye. (*Comment:* This was a flash of better vision.)

69. S. H.: I went to the DMV this morning and managed to pass the darn vision test. And so, I will be in touch with you before the next time the DMV test comes up again four years from now *when I am 88.* Whooaahhh! Ah, gosh, Tom. I am sure your course helped me.

70. L. G.: I just wanted to give you the good news. I did the 3 B's all the way to the eye doctor's office yesterday, and with my previously reduced glasses I could see better than 20/20. That's exciting, isn't it!

71. S. H.: It is the middle of the night, but I just had to call and let you know that I really think that my amblyopia and strabismus are disappearing. And I am just very happy. I was just looking in the mirror at my eyes and they just seem so beautiful to me now. And when I turn my head in a direction that before my eyes would always go funny, so to speak, now they seem to go "in synch" in synchronicity with each other,

and they don't look strange. So, I just wanted to call and share the good news. (*Comment:* Before vision classes, S. H. could not drive a car because of very poor peripheral vision. Now she can.)

72. S. C., again: I am still having such wonderful improvement, and different things going on with my vision, and I am so excited about it!
73. S. I., again: I had another remarkable breakthrough today. At the gym, a very large gym in a large room, and I sketch the signs that are way against the far wall, and they are really teeny little signs, and I just sketch them because they are these brightly colored objects. And I noticed today that—um—I knew before that there were words on them, but they were just a total blur, just teeny little letters, and I had not even thought about the possibility of reading the words—it was enough that I could even see the signs. But, today I found myself reading the words! It was remarkable, I mean, there it was, "Unload all bars. Replace all weights." And, I never even considered the possibility of reading the signs, because the print just seemed so tiny; it's so far away! And there it was—I was reading it! It was just astounding! So, your program really does work. I guess you know that already. But, I just thought I would let you know of one more success story. Bye.
74. M. C.: I am about 20/40 now—with just my own eyes—and I have not worn glasses for a whole year! Cool! (*Comment:* M. C. is now a Natural Vision teacher.)
75. N. I.: My eyes are continuing to get better. I will probably be getting my third pair of reduced lenses within, I would say, the next month, which I am thrilled about, because that will probably be my last pair of glasses! Thanks a lot, Tom. Take care.
76. N. W.: I did have something of a special moment this month, where I had for the first time a flash of 3-D vision—without my glasses! I will be happy to share that at the next month's Review class.
77. T. L.: I very much enjoyed your Introductory Lecture last night. And my friend Sue, who thought the whole thing was hogwash before, was very pleased and was already, all the way home, talking about referring her neighbor's three-year-old boy, who has coke-bottle glasses, to me. (*Comment:* T. L. is a Natural Vision teacher and loves teaching children natural vision habits. Also, due to back pain, T. L. was unable to jog for many years before taking the vision classes. She now jogs again—pain-free.)
78. T. L., again: I have even—if it's possible—*more* enthusiasm. So, good!
79. F. N.: I had the most amazing thing happen this morning with my eyes when I was dancing. It kind of blew me away. All of a sudden my eyes began to centralize on their own completely. It's like the muscles had relaxed—*totally* relaxed. And, then I was dancing the whole time that way. I can't even do that blurry thing (diffusion) any more, because I *feel* it. And what was amazing, when I had to put on my glasses to drive home, I felt what the glasses do. They actually make me diffuse, because

they make my eyes lock up in a way that my eyes are pointing forward, instead of centralizing. And it creates this strain, when I want to just relax my eyes and centralize and everything—instead of the glasses, which tend to flatten them out and outward, if that makes any sense. But, it's amazing, and I am so excited, and I just wanted to tell you.

80. B. K.: I just have three things to say: Brush, Breathe, and Blink! And I will be at the next Review class.
81. L. C.: I will be attending your Staring Anonymous meeting (Review class) tomorrow night.
82. T. L., again: I went to the eye doctor on Monday because my eye was hurting me; my glasses were too strong. The right eye is now reduced to –1.00 DS from –1.50 DS the last time; of course, the left lense still has no correction. So that is very exciting.
83. A caller, but not my student: J. N: My mother healed herself with the Bates method, and she is now 85, and she did this Bates program at age 20, and she still does not wear glasses.
84. M. S.: Wanted to say that we both had really good success, and really appreciate your work. I have not used the reading glasses for any application for the last two weeks, and that includes the small print on the computer and all the fine print work that I have to do. And it is not perfect, but I certainly understand how to keep working toward that goal. I thank you very much. Bye.
85. S. I., again: I have not seen you in half a year or longer. I am still blinking and breathing, and what's the other one?—sketching! And my vision is actually excellent these days.
86. N. I., again: I went to the DMV today and I missed by one letter! So, I am disappointed, but I can tell I have come a really long way. And, I will be going back at some point, and trying again.
87. D. S.: I wanted to let you know I had my eyes re-tested today, and the eye doctor said there was a 5% improvement. (*Comment:* This was after only two classes.)
88. M. H.: Just a note to thank you for your course. It has allowed me to get the most out of my vision. Vision continues to improve and has affected my life for the better. I've given up a "Big Bucks" computer job which I had for 15 years. I will be looking for work more suitable to my body and the Earth. My good vision will see me through and I am confident I will find something in which I can work happily at. (*Comment:* M. H. now has a very successful San Francisco pet-sitting business.)
89. A. O.: I started wearing glasses for distance when I was fourteen years old. My vision was such that I would not cross the street if I did not have glasses on. By 1983, I was wearing bifocals and was having severe head and neck pains. I took Tom's class in 1984 and threw away my glasses and the severe head and neck pains were gone. I am sixty-four years old now and do not own a pair of glasses for either reading or distance. The Bates method really works.
90. L. N.: Thanks again for a really illuminating and life-changing course. It has affected my life in every direction.

HUNDREDS OF CASE HISTORIES NOW IN LITERATURE

There are hundreds of case histories of natural vision improvement in the references listed in the Bibliography. Several of these books are written by ophthalmologists, optometrists, and one medical doctor.

Most people who offer natural vision classes are private teachers.

"OUT OF THE NIGHT"— A VISION POEM

The poem on the next page was written by Adam Schwartz at the conclusion of the 1993 Natural Vision Teacher Training Program.

Notes

1 W. B. MacCracken, *Use Your Own Eyes* (Berkeley, California: Published by the author, 1937), p. ix.

2 Ibid., p. 227.

3 Ibid., pp. 232–36.

4 Harris Gruman, *New Ways to Better Sight* (New York: Hermitage House, 1950), p. 186.

5 Ibid., p. 187.

6 Janet Goodrich, *Natural Vision Improvement* (Berkeley, California: Celestial Arts, 1985), pp. 187–91.

7 Mary Dudderidge, "New Light Upon Our Eyes: An Investigation Which May Result in Normal Vision for All, Without Glasses," in *Scientific American* (January 12, 1918), p. 61.

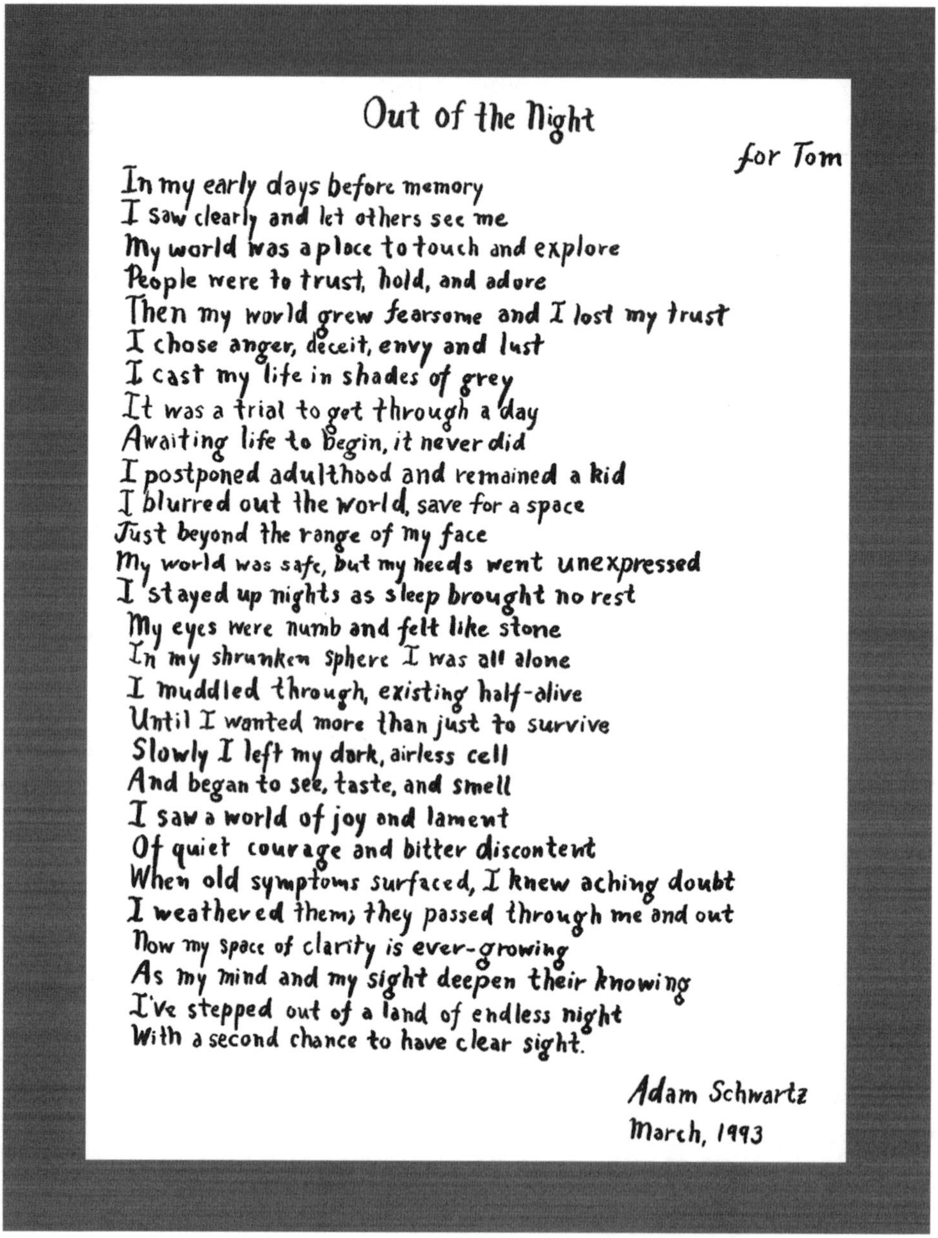

Out of the Night

for Tom

In my early days before memory
I saw clearly and let others see me
My world was a place to touch and explore
People were to trust, hold, and adore
Then my world grew fearsome and I lost my trust
I chose anger, deceit, envy and lust
I cast my life in shades of grey
It was a trial to get through a day
Awaiting life to begin, it never did
I postponed adulthood and remained a kid
I blurred out the world, save for a space
Just beyond the range of my face
My world was safe, but my needs went unexpressed
I stayed up nights as sleep brought no rest
My eyes were numb and felt like stone
In my shrunken sphere I was all alone
I muddled through, existing half-alive
Until I wanted more than just to survive
Slowly I left my dark, airless cell
And began to see, taste, and smell
I saw a world of joy and lament
Of quiet courage and bitter discontent
When old symptoms surfaced, I knew aching doubt
I weathered them; they passed through me and out
Now my space of clarity is ever-growing
As my mind and my sight deepen their knowing
I've stepped out of a land of endless night
With a second chance to have clear sight.

Adam Schwartz
March, 1993

Figure 29–1: "Out of the Night." Reprinted with permission from Adam Schwartz.

Chapter Thirty

Questions and Answers

HOW CAN I FIND A NATURAL VISION TEACHER?

The Natural Vision Center of San Francisco maintains a list of Natural Vision teachers around the world.

Send a self-addressed stamped envelope, including your name, address, and phone number, requesting the name of a Natural Vision teacher in your area, to:

Natural Vision Center of San Francisco
P.O. Box 16403
San Francisco, CA 94116 USA

HOW CAN I OBTAIN INFORMATION ABOUT BECOMING A CERTIFIED NATURAL VISION TEACHER?

See Appendix E, "Becoming a Natural Vision Teacher."

WHAT ARE THE LITTLE SPECKS I SEE FLOATING IN FRONT OF MY EYES SOMETIMES?

Bates has this to say in *Perfect Sight Without Glasses:*

A very common phenomenon of imperfect sight is the one known to medical science as *muscae volitantes* or *flying flies.* These floating specks are usually dark or black, but sometimes appear like white bubbles, and in rare cases may assume all the colors of the rainbow. They move somewhat rapidly, usually in curving lines, before the eyes, and always appear to be just beyond the point of centralization. If one tries to look at them directly, they seem to move a little farther away. Hence their name of *"flying flies."*

The literature of the subject is full of speculations as to the origin of these appearances. Some have attributed them to the presence of floating specks—dead cells, or the debris of cells—in the vitreous humor, the transparent substance that fills four-fifths of the eyeball behind the crystalline lens. [This is correct.] Similar specks on the surface of the cornea have also been held responsible for them. It has even been surmised that they might be caused by the passage of tears over the cornea. They are so common in myopia that they have been supposed to be one of the symptoms of this condition, although they occur also with other errors of refraction, as well as in eyes otherwise normal. They have been attributed to disturbances of the circulation, the digestion and the kidneys ...

A clergyman who was much annoyed by the continual appearance of floating specks before his eyes was told by his eye specialist that they were a symptom of kidney disease, and that in many cases of kidney trouble disease of the retina might be an early symptom. [Chinese healing philosophies connect the liver and kidneys to sight.] So at regular intervals he went to the specialist to have his eyes examined, and when at length the latter died, he looked around immediately for some one else to make the periodical examination. His family physician directed him to me.... the clergyman particularly wanted some one capable of making a thorough examination of the interior of his eyes and detecting at once any signs of kidney disease that might make their appearance. So he came to me, and at least four times a year for ten years he continued to come.

Each time I made a very careful examination of his eyes, taking as much time over it as possible, so that he would believe that it was careful; and each time he went away happy because I could find nothing wrong....

The specks are associated to a considerable extent with markedly imperfect eyesight, because persons whose eyesight is imperfect always strain to see; but persons whose eyesight is ordinarily normal may see them at times, because no eye has normal sight all the time. Most people can see muscae volitantes when they look at ... any uniformly bright surface....

Bates showed that when mental strain is present, these particles are seen more readily. Bates concluded, erroneously, that the floating specks are *solely* mental, and not physical.

Ophthalmologist Charles May writes in his book *Diseases of the Eye:*

> *Muscae Volitantes* is a term employed for the appearance of *spots* (motes) before the eyes, *without appreciable structural change* in the vitreous or other media. They are caused by the shadows cast upon the retina by the cells normally found in the vitreous, and are present in all eyes under certain circumstances, such as exposure to a uniform bright surface, or in looking through a microscope. They are found more frequently in *errors of refraction* (especially *myopia),* and the symptom may be aggravated temporarily during digestive derangements. They are *annoying* and sometimes alarm the person, but are of *no importance,* and do not affect the acuteness of vision. The [solution] consists in correcting errors of refraction, or in relieving the disturbance of digestion. They often persist until the person ceases to look for them and thus forgets their existence.[1]

Today, typical floating specks are considered to be remnants of the blood vessels which course the interior of the eye as the fetus develops.

Important: Some floating particles can be caused by blows to the head or eye diseases. Anyone with this concern should consult immediately with an ophthalmologist.

IS THE BATES METHOD A FORM OF MIND CONTROL OR HYPNOSIS?

No. The Bates method is an educational process of relearning the same natural, correct vision habits you had when you used to see clearly. Students are eliminating the strain they put on the visual system when they acquired blurred vision. There is no mind control or hypnosis involved in this educational program.

I FIND THERE ARE SOME PARALLELS BETWEEN THE BATES METHOD AND SPIRITUAL/METAPHYSICAL CONCEPTS. WHY DO YOU NOT MENTION OR TEACH THESE CONCEPTS IN YOUR CLASSES?

Eyesight improvement is not dependent upon understanding spiritual/metaphysical concepts. Also, some students in my group are not interested in my perceptions of spirituality and metaphysics. If a student is interested in such concepts, he may seek a teacher in that field.

One excellent New York Bates teacher offered her private students a very short optional metaphysical teaching at the end of each lesson during palming. (Natural vision students often palm for a few minutes at the end of each class.) Interestingly, more than 90% of her students elected to receive this optional teaching.

Notes

[1] Charles H. May, *Diseases of the Eye* (Baltimore, Maryland: William Wood and Company, 1943), pp. 264–65.

Chapter Thirty-One

Summary

An important scientific innovation rarely makes its way by gradually winning over and converting its opponents: it rarely happens that Saul becomes Paul. What does happen is that its opponents gradually die out and that the growing generation is familiarized with the idea from the beginning.

—Max Planck, *The Philosophy of Physics,* 1936

Because natural vision education is relatively unknown, I have attempted in this book to present and explain the work of Dr. William H. Bates as thoroughly, logically, and convincingly as I am able. I have presented both rational and empirical scientific facts to support Bates' discoveries about natural vision.

To summarize the key points of this book:

It is clear that compensating lenses are, at best, a crutch. At worst, they create more vision problems.

Bates' research proved that errors of refraction are functional problems—specifically, the extrinsic muscles contract chronically tight and change the shape of the eyeball to be long, short, or oval, creating nearsightedness, farsightedness, and astigmatism, respectively. Bates also showed that strabismus is caused by one or more recti muscles becoming chronically tight. Since Bates proved natural vision improvement is possible, regardless of age or parentage, the mechanism of how vision improves is only of academic interest.

Bates proved the two oblique muscles can accommodate the eye to see clearly up close. When these two muscles release their contractions, the eye sees clearly in the distance again.

Bates went further in his research to prove that functional vision problems are caused by mental strain. The entire basis of Bates' work on natural vision improvement is relaxation. The principles of movement and centralization are essential in order to achieve relaxation. The three principles of natural vision are not confined to the Bates method, but are universal in scope.

The specific habits of normal sight Bates described are the same habits (virtually) all people learn automatically and subconsciously in the first few years of life. Natural vision students are literally and simply relearning to see.

The sketching (or shifting) habit is simply

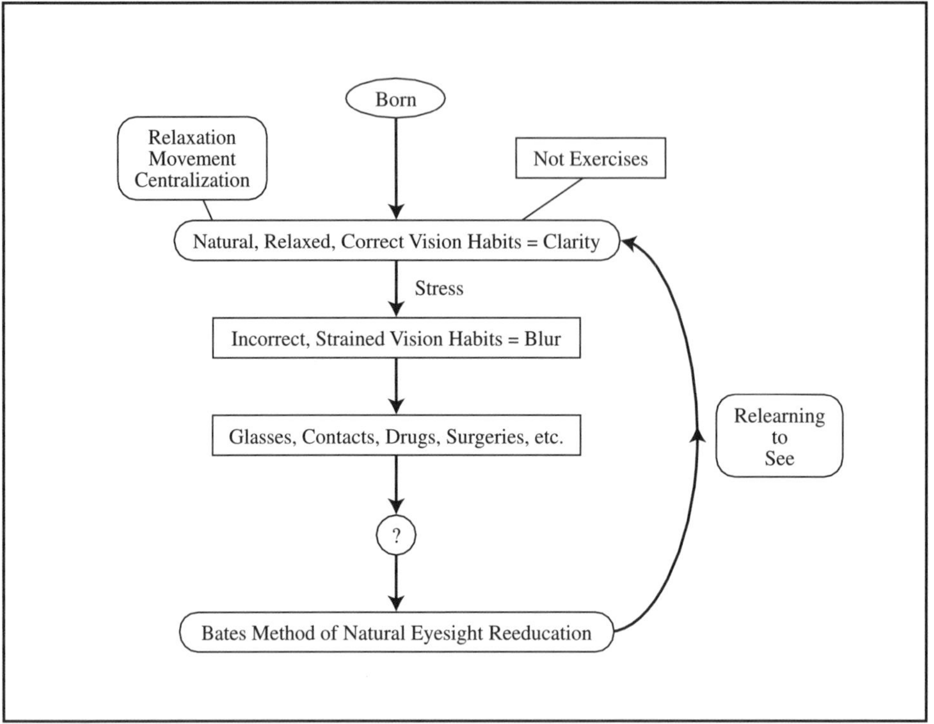

Figure 31–1: Born to See.

the combination of the principles of movement and centralization. Breathing correctly is, of course, natural and essential for normal health. The breathing habit is especially connected to the relaxation principle of natural vision. Blinking frequently is clearly an essential, normal vision habit.

Mary Dudderidge sums up her article on the Bates method in *Scientific American:*

> By means of this simple system of eye education Dr. Bates maintains that the organs of vision can be kept always in a normal condition. The savage presumably got this education from his daily life. He was obliged, as a condition of continued existence, to focus his eyes for accurate vision at all distances. If he didn't he was eliminated. We who are protected from all the dangers from which our savage forebears could protect themselves only by their good eyesight, and whose eyes are limited for a great part of the time to a narrow range of vision, quite [commonly] lose this power. Under similar conditions wild animals lose it also, becoming myopic in captivity, although they neither read nor write nor sew nor set type. The [solution] is not to close our schools and stop our printing presses and return to a primitive condition in which there was no astigmatism or short sight, but to practice the art of seeing perfectly....[1]

Modern right brain/left brain concepts provide a particularly valuable perspective on Bates' discoveries. We live in an extremely left-brain oriented, industrialized, literate society. Essentially, Bates discovered that normal vision is primarily a right-brain function. If the visual system is used in primarily a left-brain, strained manner, sight cannot be normal.

The personality of the individual appears to dictate what type of blurred vision a person will acquire if he forms strained vision habits. The re-integration of correct vision habits into the relatively "flat," left-brain activities of reading, computer work, and watching TV is especially important.

The overall health of an individual can have a large impact on the student's ability to relearn natural vision habits and principles. The epidemic of blurred vision in this society can be viewed as a subset of the many increasingly serious health problems. These problems appear to stem largely from our left-brain, rational approach to living, inappropriately applied to right-brain, empirical aspects of life. Massive, indiscriminate use of drugs and surgeries is one glaring example, and this has been particularly destructive. The *quality* of American life has lowered significantly in the last several decades. Improving vision naturally is one way of improving the quality of one's life.

ONE FINAL "NATURAL" VISION IMPROVEMENT STORY

> After the first Introductory Lecture I gave in San Francisco in 1983, I met a woman who was cooking in the yoga school's kitchen. She told me she used to wear glasses. During the stressful 1960s she left the US for Peru, where she lived with the natives in a peaceful, rural village. She woke up with the sunrise, planted, harvested, and ate natural food, drank crystal-clear, fresh mountain water, relaxed and enjoyed nature, and went to sleep at sunset.
>
> Noticing the natives did not use glasses, she began using her glasses less and less. She began seeing more and more *naturally—automatically and subconsciously.* At the end of her two-year visit, her vision had become clear. During her stay in Peru, she knew nothing about the Bates method or vision improvement concepts.

A person's vision is determined by that person's relationship with nature—regardless of any type of knowledge held by the person. Just as a person can "fall" out of proper vision habits without knowing consciously what she is doing, she can also "fall" back into the proper vision habits without conscious knowledge. This is what happened to this woman, and to several other people I have talked with. In each case, excessive stress was removed from their lives.

It was Bates' recognition of similar so-called "spontaneous remissions" of blurred sight which prompted him to discard orthodox "impossible to improve" theories of blurred vision, and allowed him to discover the truth of errors of refraction. Bates proved that natural vision principles and habits determine how well a person sees.

See *Plate 60: The Land of Sketch, Breathe, and Blink.*

One final reminder:

Sketch, Breathe, and Blink!

NOTES

1 Mary Dudderidge, "New Light Upon Our Eyes: An Investigation Which May Result in Normal Vision for All, Without Glasses," in *Scientific American* (January 12, 1918), p. 61.

APPENDIX A

Bibliography

VISION

Agarwal, J. *Yoga of Perfect Sight.* Pondicherry, India: Sri Aurobindo Ashram Press, 1979.

Agarwal, J., and Mrs. T. *Care of the Eyes.* Madras, India: Gnanodaya Press, 1978.

Agarwal, R. S. *Mind and Vision.* Pondicherry, India: Sri Aurobindo Ashram Press, 1935. Based on Bates' 1920 book *Perfect Sight Without Glasses.* An ophthalmologist teaching the Bates method.

American Optical. *The Human Eye.* Southbridge, Massachusetts: American Optical Corporation, 1972.

Banker, Deborah E. *Self-Help Vision Care.* Malibu, California: World Care, 1994. A holistic approach to improving vision naturally.

Bates, William H. *Perfect Sight Without Glasses.* New York: Central Fixation Publishing Co., 1920. Ophthalmologist who created an educational program for improving eyesight naturally. Difficult to find. (See following.)

——. *The Bates Method for Better Eyesight Without Glasses.* New York: Henry Holt & Co., 1940. Parts of Bates' 1920 *Perfect Sight Without Glasses* have been eliminated in this edition revised by Bates' wife Emily after his death.

——. *Better Eyesight.* New York: Central Fixation Co., July 1919-April 1930 (or later). A monthly magazine "Devoted to the Prevention of Imperfect Sight Without Glasses." Edited by Bates, these magazines contain a multitude of case histories of improved vision; articles contributed by other Natural Vision teachers, including at least one other ophthalmologist and several medical doctors. Difficult to find.

Benjamin, Harry. *Better Sight Without Glasses.* New York: Thorsons/HarperCollins, 1984.

Corbett, Margaret D. *Help Yourself to Better Sight.* North Hollywood, California: Wilshire Book Co., 1949. Corbett trained with Bates in 1930 to become a Natural Vision teacher. She trained many teachers on the West Coast.

——. *How to Improve Your Eyes.* Los Angeles: Willing Publishing Company, 1938.

——. *How to Improve Your Sight.* New York: Bonanza Books, 1953.

David, Thomas H. *Improve Your Vision with Television!* Los Angeles, California:

DeVorss & Co., 1951. This chiropractor studied with Bates in 1925, and then added vision improvement education to his chiropractic work. The booklet is brief, and is very difficult to find.

Downer, John. *Supersense: Perception in the Animal World.* New York: Henry Holt and Company, 1988.

Dudderidge, Mary. "New Light Upon Our Eyes: An Investigation Which May Result in Normal Vision for All, Without Glasses," in *Scientific American,* January 12, 1918.

Forrest, Elliot B. *Stress and Vision.* Santa Ana, California: Optometric Extension Program Foundation, 1988.

Frisby, John P. *Seeing: Illusion, Brain and Mind.* Oxford: Oxford University Press, 1979.

Gesell, Arnold, Francis L. Ilg, and Glenna E. Bullis. *Vision: Its Development in Infant and Child.* New York: Paul B. Hoeber, Inc., 1949. A classic.

Goodrich, Janet. *Natural Vision Improvement.* Berkeley, California: Celestial Arts, 1985. Book contains proof of natural vision improvement, verified by an optometrist, an ophthalmologist and a researcher. A modern Bates book with lots of good information.

Gottlieb, Raymond L. "Neuropsychology of Myopia," in *Journal of Optometric Vision Development,* Vol. 13, No. 1, March 1982, pp. 3–27. An optometrist who teaches natural vision improvement.

Gregg, James R., and Gordon G. Heath. *The Eye and Sight.* Boston: D. C. Heath and Company, 1964.

Gregory, R. L. *Eye and Brain: The Psychology of Seeing.* New York: McGraw-Hill Co., 1966.

——. *The Intelligent Eye.* New York: McGraw-Hill Co., 1970.

Grossinger, Richard. "Bates Method" in *Planet Medicine: Modalities.* Berkeley, California: North Atlantic Books, 1995. Natural vision student and publisher of North Atlantic Books.

Grow, Gerald. "Improving Eyesight: The Bates Method," in *The Holistic Health Handbook.* Edward Bauman, Armand Brint, Lorin Piper, and Pamela Amelia Wright, eds. Berkeley, California: And/Or Press, 1978.

Gruman, Harris. *New Ways to Better Sight.* New York: Hermitage House, 1950.

Hackett, Clara A., and Lawrence Galton. *Relax and See.* London: Faber and Faber, Limited, 1957. Difficult to find.

Hahn, Joan Elma. *Eyes and Seeing.* New York: Atheneum, 1981.

Hughes, Barbara. *Twelve Weeks To Better Vision.* New York: Pinnacle Books, Inc., 1981.

Huxley, Aldous. *The Art of Seeing.* New York: Harper & Brothers Publishers, 1942; republished by Berkeley, California: Creative Arts Book Co, 1982. Widely available and highly recommended. Huxley, author of *Brave New World,* published this book after taking lessons from Margaret Corbett and improving his vision. Huxley attempts to "correlate the methods of visual education with the findings of modern psychology and critical philosophy."

Kahn, Fritz. "The Eye," in *Man in Structure and Function, Vol. II.* New York: Alfred A. Knopf, 1943. Exceptional description of the eye and vision for the lay person.

Kavner, Richard S. *Your Child's Vision: A Par-*

ent's Guide to Seeing, Growing, and Developing. New York: Fireside/Simon & Schuster, 1985.

——, and Dusky, Lorraine. *Total Vision.* New York: A & W Publishers, Inc., 1978.

Kelley, Charles R. "Psychological Factors In Myopia" in *Journal of American Optometric Association,* 33(6): 833–837, 1967.

Kennebeck, Joseph J. *Why Eyeglasses are Harmful for Children and Young People.* New York: Vantage Press, 1969. An optometrist. Difficult to find.

Kessel, Richard G., and Randy H. Kardon. *Tissues and Organs: a text-atlas of scanning electron microscopy.* New York: W. H. Freeman and Company, 1979. Contains excellent high-magnification images of the eye.

Leviton, Richard. *Seven Steps to Better Vision: Easy, Practical and Natural Techniques That Will Improve Your Eyesight.* Brookline, Massachusetts: EastWest/Natural Health Books, 1992.

Liberman, Jacob. *Take Off Your Glasses and See.* New York: Crown Publishers, Inc., 1995. An optometrist who improved his eyesight naturally and eliminated his need for compensating lenses.

Life, The Editors of, and text by Richard Carington. *The Mammals.* New York: Time Incorporated, 1963.

MacCracken, W. B. *Normal Sight Without Glasses.* Berkeley, California: Published by the author, 1945. Difficult to find.

——. *Use Your Own Eyes.* Berkeley, California: Published by the author, 1937. A medical doctor who trained with Bates, and taught natural vision improvement in Berkeley. Excellent, but difficult to find.

MacFadyen, Ralph J. *See Without Glasses: The Correction of Eye Strain and the Science of Sight.* New York: Grosset & Dunlap Publishers, 1948. Difficult to find.

Markert, Christopher. *Seeing Well Again Without Your Glasses.* C. W. Daniel Co., 1981.

Mueller, Conrad G., and Mae Rudolph and the Editors of Time-Life Books. *Light and Vision.* New York: Time-Life Books, 1966. Excellent.

Murphy, Pat, ed. *The Eye.* San Francisco: The Exploratorium, 1985.

——. "In the Darkness," in *Exploring.* San Francisco: The Exploratorium, 1993.

Murphy, Wendy, and the Editors of Time-Life Books. *Touch, Taste, Smell, Sight and Hearing.* Alexandria, Virginia: Time-Life Books, Inc., 1982.

Peppard, Harold M. *Sight Without Glasses.* Garden City, New York: Garden City Books, 1940.

Peterson, Roger Tory, and the Editors of Life. *The Birds.* New York: Time, Inc., 1963.

Price, C. S. *The Improvement of Sight by Natural Methods.* London: Chapman & Hall Limited, 1934.

Rahn, Joan E. *Eyes and Seeing.* New York: R. R. Donnelley & Sons, Inc., 1981.

Raskin, Edith L. *Watchers, Pursuers and Masqueraders: Animals and Their Vision.* New York: McGraw-Hill Book Company, 1964.

Raskin, Ellen. *Nothing Ever Happens on My Block.* New York: Macmillan Publishing Co., 1966. For children.

Rodale, J. I. *The Natural Way to Better Eyesight.* New York: Pyramid Books, 1968.

Rosanes-Berrett, Marilyn B. *Do You Really Need Glasses?* Barrytown, New York: Pulse/Station Hill Press, 1990.

Rotte, Joanna, and Koji Yamamoto. *A Holistic Guide to Healing the Eyesight.* Japan Publications, 1986.

Samuels, Mike, and Samuels, Nancy. *Seeing With the Mind's Eye.* New York: Random House, 1975.

Schlossberg, Leon, and George D. Zuidema. *The Johns Hopkins Atlas of Human Functional Anatomy.* Baltimore: The Johns Hopkins University Press, 1972.

Scholl, Lisette. *Visionetics: The Holistic Way to Better Eyesight.* New York: Doubleday & Company, Inc., 1978.

Seiderman, Arthur S., and Steven E. Marcus. *20/20 Is Not Enough.* New York: Alfred A. Knopf, 1989.

Sinclair, Sandra. *How Animals See.* New York: Facts on File Publications, 1985. Filled with extraordinary color pictures and excellent descriptions of many different types of eyes. Difficult to find. Currently out of print.

Sutton-Vane, S. *The Story of the Eyes.* New York: The Viking Press, Inc., 1958. Difficult to find.

Tobe, John H. *Cataract, Glaucoma and Other Eye Disorders.* St. Catharines, Ontario: published by the author(?), 1973.

Wertenbaker, Lael, and the Editors of U.S. News Books. *The Eye: Window to the World.* Washington, D. C.: U.S. News Books, 1981. Excellent.

Windolph, Michael. *Do You Really Need Eyeglasses?* New York: Cornerstone Library, 1976. Difficult to find.

Yarbus, Alfred L. *Eye Movements and Vision.* New York: Plenum Press, 1967.

OTHER RECOMMENDED READING

Bauman, Edward, Armand Brint, Lorin Piper, and Pamela Amelia Wright, eds. *The Holistic Health Handbook.* Berkeley, California: And/Or Press, 1978.

——. *The Holistic Lifebook Handbook.* Berkeley, California: And/Or Press, 1981.

Becker, Robert O. *Cross Currents: The Perils of Electromagnetic Pollution, The Promise of Electromedicine.* Los Angeles: Jeremy P. Tarcher, Inc., 1990.

Bertherat, Therese, and Carol Bernstein. *The Body Has Its Reasons: Self-Awareness Through Conscious Movement.* Rochester, Vermont: Healing Arts Press, 1989.

Biermann, June, and Barbara Toohey. *The Woman's Holistic Headache Relief Book.* Los Angeles: J. P. Tarcher, Inc., 1979.

Brecher, Edward M., and Editors of Consumer Reports. *Licit and Illicit Drugs.* Boston: Little, Brown and Company, 1972.

Bricklin, Mark. *The Practical Encyclopedia of Natural Healing.* Emmaus, Pennsylvania: Rodale Press, 1976.

Carter-Scott, Chérie. *Negaholics: How to Overcome Negativity and Turn Your Life Around.* New York: Ballantine Books, 1989. Excellent.

——. *The New Species.* New York: Coleman Graphics, Inc., 1980.

Chopra, Deepak. *Quantum Healing.* New York: Bantam, 1989.

Coulter, Harris L. *Divided Legacy, A History of the Schism in Medical Thought, Vol. I: The Patterns Emerge: Hippocrates to Paracelsus.* Washington, DC: Weehawken Book Company, 1975.

——. *Divided Legacy, Vol. II: The Origins of Modern Western Medicine: J. B. Van Helmont to Claude Bernard.* Berkeley, California: North Atlantic Books, 1977.

——. *Divided Legacy, Vol. III: The Conflict Between Homeopathy and the American Medical Association: Science and Ethics in American Medicine 1800-1914.* Berkeley, California: North Atlantic Books, 1982.

——. *Divided Legacy, Vol. IV: Twentieth Century Medicine, The Bacteriological Era.* Berkeley, California: North Atlantic Books, 1994.

——. *Homeopathic Science and Modern Medicine: The Physics of Healing with Microdoses.* Berkeley, California: North Atlantic Books, 1981.

Crouch, Tammy, and Michael Madden. *Carpal Tunnel Syndrome and Overuse Injuries.* Berkeley, California: North Atlantic Books, 1992.

Dennison, Paul E. *Switching-On.* Ventura, California: Edu-Kinesthetics, Inc., 1981. Excellent.

——, and Gail E. Dennison. *Brain Gym.* Ventura, California: Edu-Kinesthetics, Inc., 1986. Many practical activities.

——, and Gail E. Hargrove. *Personalized Whole Brain Integration.* Ventura, California: Edu-Kinesthetics, Inc., 1985. Excellent.

——, and Gail Hargrove. *E-K for Kids.* Ventura, California: Edu-Kinesthetics, Inc., 1985. Many practical activities for children.

Diamond, John. *Your Body Doesn't Lie.* New York: Warner Books, 1979.

Dufty, William. *Sugar Blues.* New York: Warner Books, 1975. You may give up white sugar after reading this book.

Edwards, Betty. *Drawing on the Right Side of the Brain.* Los Angeles: Tarcher, Inc., 1979.

Elben. *Vaccination Condemned.* Los Angeles: Better Life Research, 1981.

Ferguson, Marilyn, ed. *Brain/Mind Bulletin.* Los Angeles: Interface Press. Periodical.

Gelb, Harold, and Paula M. Siegel. *Killing Pain Without Prescription.* New York: Harper & Row, 1980.

Glendinning, Chellis. *My Name is Chellis, & I'm in Recovery from Western Civilization.* Boston: Shambhala Publications, 1994.

Grossinger, Richard. *Planet Medicine: Modalities.* Berkeley, California: North Atlantic Books, 1995.

——. *Planet Medicine: Origins.* Berkeley, California: North Atlantic Books, 1995.

Hall, Dorothy. *Iridology. Personality and Health Analysis Through the Iris.* Melbourne, Australia: Nelson, 1980.

Harrison, John. *Love Your Disease: It's Keeping You Healthy.* Sydney: Angus & Robertson Publishers, 1984.

Hayfield, Robin. *Homeopathy for Common Ailments.* Berkeley, California: Frog, Ltd., and Homeopathic Educational Services, 1993.

Huggins, Hal A. *It's All In Your Head: The Link Between Mercury Amalgams and Illness.* Garden City Park, New York: Avery Publishing Group, Inc., 1993.

Hunter, Beatrice T. *Consumer Beware: Your Food and What's Being Done to It.* New York: Simon & Schuster, 1971.

Jensen, Bernard. *The Doctor-Patient Handbook.* Escondido, California: Bernard Jensen Enterprises, 1976. Excellent discussion about nutrition, iridology, detoxification, the healing crisis, and reversal processes.

——. *The Science and Practice of Iridology.* Escondido, California: Bernard Jensen, 1981.

——. *Tissue Cleansing through Bowel Management.* Escondido, California: Bernard Jensen, 1981.

Kime, Zane R. *Sunlight Could Save Your Life.* Penryn, California: World Health Publications, 1980.

Léboyér, Frederick. *The Art of Breathing.* Longmead, England: Element Books Ltd., 1985. Breathing for childbirth.

Liberman, Jacob. *Light: Medicine of the Future.* Santa Fe: Bear & Co., 1991. A must-read book; covers the impact of natural and artificial light on the mind, body, and emotions.

Lowen, Alexander. *Bioenergetics.* New York: Penguin Books, Inc., 1976.

Mendelsohn, Robert S. *Confessions of a Medical Heretic* (Chicago, Illinois: Contemporary Books, Inc., 1979). Uses a Church/Faith/Sacraments analogy for discussing the problems of modern medicine.

Miller, Neil. *Vaccines: Are They Really Safe and Effective?—A Parent's Guide to Childhood Shots.* Santa Fe, New Mexico: New Atlantean Press. 1993.

Ott, John N. *Health & Light.* New York: Simon & Schuster, 1973. A classic.

——. *Light, Radiation, and You: How to Stay Healthy.* New York: Simon & Schuster, 1982.

Panos, Maesimund B., and Jane Heimlich. *Homeopathic Medicine at Home.* New York: G. P. Putnam's Sons, 1980. Natural remedies for everyday ailments and minor injuries. My favorite "practical" homeopathy book.

Peck, M. Scott, *The Road Less Traveled.* New York: Simon and Schuster, 1978.

Pelletier, Kenneth R. *Holistic Medicine: From Stress to Optimum Health.* New York: Dell Publishing Co., Inc., 1979.

——. *Mind as Healer, Mind as Slayer: A Holistic Approach to Preventing Stress Disorders.* New York: Dell Publishing Co., Inc., 1977.

Pitchford, Paul. *Healing with Whole Foods.* Berkeley, California: North Atlantic Books, 1993.

Reubin, David, M.D. *Everything You Always Wanted to Know About Nutrition.* Boston: G. K. Hall & Co., 1979.

Ribot, T. *The Psychology of Attention.* Chicago: The Open Court Publishing Company, 1890. The Marcel Rodd Company, 1946 edition (New York) contains a foreword by Bates teacher Margaret D. Corbett.

Robertson, Laurel, Carol Flinders, and Bronwen Godfrey. *Laurel's Kitchen.* New York: Nilgiri Press, 1976.

Rosen, Marion, and Sue Brenner. *The Rosen Method of Movement.* Berkeley, California: North Atlantic Books, 1991.

Schmidt, Michael A., and Lendon H. Smith and Keith W. Sehnert. *Beyond Antibiotics: 50 (or so) Ways to Boost Immunity and Avoid Antibiotics.* Berkeley, California: North Atlantic Books, 1993.

Selby, Hans. *Stress Without Distress.* New York: Signet, 1975.

Smith, G. Kent. *Homeopathy: Medicine for Today's Living.* Glendale, California: (private printing?), 1978.

Turner, James S. *The Chemical Feast.* New York: The Colonial Press, 1970.

Ullman, Dana. *Homeopathy: Medicine for the 21st Century.* Berkeley, California: North Atlantic Books, 1988.

Vithoulkas, George. *A New Model for Health and Disease.* Berkeley, California: Health and Habitat and North Atlantic Books, 1991. Read this book!

——. *Homeopathy, Medicine of the New Man.* New York: Arco Publishing, Inc., 1979.

——. *The Science of Homeopathy.* New York: Grove Press, 1980. The single most important book I have read on health and healing.

Wigmore, Ann. *The Wheatgrass Book.* Wayne, New Jersey: Avery Publishing Group, Inc. 1985.

Wurtman, Richard J. "The Effects of Light on the Human Body," in *Scientific American,* July 1975, Vol. 233, No. 1, pp. 68–77. Excellent.

Zi, Nancy. *The Art of Breathing.* Glendale, California: Vivi Company, 1986.

APPENDIX B

Resources

HOLISTIC HEALTH

1. American College of Traditional Chinese Medicine, 455 Arkansas St., San Francisco, CA 94107. (415) 282–7600.
2. B. K. S. Iyengar Association of Northern California, 2404 27th Ave., San Francisco, CA 94116. (415) 753–0909. Yoga.
3. Feldenkrais Resources Center, 830 Bancroft Way, Berkeley, CA 94710. (510) 540–7600.
4. Hahnemann Medical Clinic, 828 San Pablo Ave., Albany, CA 94706. (510) 524–3117. Classical homeopathy.
5. Homeopathic Educational Services, 2124 Kittredge St., Berkeley, CA 94704. (510) 649–0294.
6. Mark E. Abramson, D.D.S., Inc., 35 Renato Ct., Redwood City, CA 94061. (415) 369–9227. Specializing in temporomandibular joint (TMJ), head, facial, neck, and oral alliance therapy for sleep apnea and snoring.
7. The MMS Institute, P. O. Box 30052, Santa Barbara, CA 93130. (805) 563–0789. Chérie Carter-Scott. Holistic Self-Esteem Workshops, plus more.
8. National Center for Homeopathy, 801 North Fairfax St., Suite 306, Alexandria, VA 22314. (703) 548–7790.
9. *Natural Health* magazine, 17 Station St., Box 1200, Brookline Village, MA 02147. (617) 232-1000.
10. Northern American Society of Teachers of Alexander Technique, P. O. Box 517, Urbana, IL 61801. (800) 473–0620.
11. San Leandro Chiropractic Center, Dr. Michael D. Pedigo, D.C., 144 Joaquin Ave., San Leandro, CA 95477. (510) 357–2343. A victorious plaintiff in the Wilk's chiropractic case against the AMA.
12. Severyn, Kristine, R.Ph., Ph.D., is founder and director of Ohio Parents for Vaccine Safety, 251 W. Ridgeway Dr., Dayton, OH 45459. As a registered pharmacist, Dr. Severyn has researched and published extensively on vaccine policy and has testified before state legislators in Ohio and Michigan, and in federal vaccine commissions in Washington, DC. For a free general information packet, call (513) 435–4750.

LIGHTING

1. GE Lighting, A Division of General Electric Company, 1975 Noble Rd., Nela Park, Cleveland, OH 44112. (800) 435–4448. The "C50" fluorescent tube made by General Electric Company is called "Chroma 50." Its spectral power distribution curve is shown in *Plate 26: Spectral Power Distribution Curves.*
2. OSRAM Sylvania, 18725 N. Union St., Westfield, IN 46074. (800) 255–5042. Design 50. Also manufactures blacklights.
3. Environmental Lighting Concepts, Inc., 3923 Coconut Palm Dr., Tampa, FL 33619. (800) 842–8848. Ott-Lite Tubes, Bulbs and Fixtures, and other products. Some ELC products provide mid- and near-UV light. The Ott-Lite Bulb, shown in *Figure 16–3: Lighting,* is an integral compact fluorescent rated at 5000K/CRI 84/10,000 hours/17 watts and uses an electronic ballast. *Maximum* UV-transmitting, neutral gray sunglasses. (Sunglasses sold in the US are required by federal regulations to block a certain minimum amount of UV light.)
4. Philips Lighting Company, 200 Franklin Square Dr., P. O. Box 6800, Somerset, NJ 08875. (908) 563–3000. Model 950. The "C50" fluorescent tube made by Philips Lighting Company is called "Colortone 50." Also manufactures blacklights.
5. Duro-Test Corporation, 185 Scoles Ave., Clifton, NJ 07012. (201) 472–1900. Vita-Lite, Vita-Lite Plus, Vita-Lite Supreme. In addition to the full spectrum of colors, these fluorescent lights provide mid- and near-UV light.
6. Real Goods, Ukiah, CA (800) 762–7325. Environmentally friendly products. Catalog with large section on lighting.
7. 3M Corporation, 3M Center, Saint Paul, MN 54144. (612) 733–1110. Lead-impregnated tape that can be wrapped around the cathodes of fluorescent tubes to block x-rays.

COSMOSIS

Cosmosis is a geological event that created a unique art form in a large rock over a billion years ago. It was discovered by Jim Quackenbush in 1975. In 1979, a Stanford University geologist stated that he had never seen minerals that had developed into "such artistic forms." Indeed, these artistic forms, samples of which are shown in *Plate 10: Cosmosis,* are unprecedented in art history. These artworks convey a pictorial story of Earth's history. The Cosmosis research was completed in 1994, resulting in an exhibit of 175 masterpieces. This exhibit is on tour in United States schools as a "hands-on" science, art, and history presentation.

The Cosmosis artwork project provides children with an opportunity to use their eyesight with many of the principles and artistic qualities of natural vision including: creativity, fine detail, colors, texture, and three-dimensionality. Cosmosis artworks have been used in Natural Vision classes for over a decade.

For more information, write to: Jim Quackenbush, Cosmosis, P. O. Box 721, Joshua Tree, CA 92252.

OTHER

1. Marine World Africa USA. Marine World Parkway, Vallejo, CA 94589. (707) 644–4000/(707) 643–6722. Endangered species education and more.
2. Monart School of the Arts, 1581 Roy Ave., Room 14, Berkeley, CA 94708. (510) 540–4877.

APPENDIX C

Biographical Sketch of William H. Bates, M.D.

• 1860
Born in Newark, New Jersey, on December 23, 1860, son of Charles and Amelia Bates.

• 1881
Graduated with a B.S. in Agriculture from Cornell University.

• 1885
Graduated from the College of Physicians and Surgeons, Columbia University. Initially directed his attention to all organs of the head. Practiced orthodox medicine for several years.

• 1886
Operated in many hospitals, including Manhattan Eye and Ear Hospital, Bellevue Hospital, Northwestern Dispensary, and Harlem Hospital.

• 1886–1896
Assistant surgeon at the New York Eye Infirmary, Northwestern Dispensary, and Harlem Hospital.

• 1886–1891
Instructor of ophthalmology at the New York Post-Graduate Medical School and Hospital. Successful and well-respected eye surgeon.

Taught medical students how to improve their nearsightedness.

Expelled from the faculty.

• 1886–1902
Research at the Pathology Laboratory of Dr. Pruden at the College of Physicians and Surgeons, Columbia University.

• May 16, 1886
Report on his discovery of the astringent and haemostatic properties of the aqueous extract of the suprarenal gland, later commercialized as adrenaline, published in the *New York Medical Journal*.

• 1903–1909
Licensed to practice medicine in Grand Forks, North Dakota.

• 1910
Elected president of the Grand Forks district Medical Society.

• 1910
Returned to New York City.

• 1912
Research at Physiological Laboratory of the College of Physicians and Surgeons. Assisted by Emily A. Lierman.

• 1919–1930
Published *Better Eyesight* monthly magazine.

• 1920
Published his book *Perfect Sight Without Glasses*.

• 1928
Married Emily Ackerman Lierman, his assistant and partner in experimental research on eyesight from 1911 to 1928.

• 1931
Died at age 70 at his residence in New York City on July 10, 1931, during a black flu epidemic.

The following letter was written by Emily A. Bates "To the Editor of *The New York Times*." The article is entitled "Carrying On Dr. Bates' Work," on July 18, 1931, p. 12:

> I wish to express my gratitude to R. R. A. for the fine tribute he paid my husband, William H. Bates, M.D., in his letter in *The New York Times* of July 16. What he said was true. I myself have had the honor and the privilege of assisting the doctor in his research work during a period of six years at the Physiological Laboratory of the College of Physicians and Surgeons in New York City, also working by his side for nine consecutive years at the clinic of the Harlem Hospital. I have also had the privilege of instructing students in his method of [reversing] imperfect sight without the use of glasses. I am now going on with the work, which he left for me to do, in an educational way. There is a Bates Academy in Johannesburg, South Africa, where students of Dr. Bates are doing his work, and we have representatives in Germany, England, and in various cities throughout the United States.
>
> Emily A. Bates. New York, July 16, 1931.

"July 16" in the first sentence is likely a typographical error because the date R. R. A.'s letter appeared in *The New York Times* was July 15.

Appendix D

Light Comparison Table

See the following two pages for the Light Comparison Table.

Light Comparison Table

ATTRIBUTES	SUNLIGHT	INCANDESCENT BULBS	"QUARTZ" HALOGEN BULBS
Mechanism	Nature	Glowing tungsten filament in glass bulb containing inert gas	
Sizes	N/A	Wide range; typically small	Small
Shapes	N/A	Many types	
CCT	Noontime: 4870-5000K	2500-2700K	3000K
CRI (1-100)[b]	100	90-95	95
Mid- and Near- UV	Yes	Negligible	
Initial Cost	Zero	Low	Medium
Initial Convenience	N/A	High	
Long-Term Cost	Zero	High	Medium
Long-Term Convenience	N/A	Low	Low, but better than regular incandescent
Efficiency (lumens/watt)	N/A	Very low	Medium
Bulb/Tube Lifetime (average hours)	N/A	750-1000	2000-2500
Ballast Required	N/A	No	
Flicker (cycles/second)	N/A	60	
Heat Output	N/A	High	
Point/Diffused	Point/Diffused	Point	
Contrast (shadows)	Excellent	High	
Glare	N/A	Possible	
Dimming	N/A	Yes[d]	
Start-up Tim	N/A	Instantaneous	
Design	N/A	Very Simple	Simple
Other		Violet-blue deficient	Bright, white light; spectrum is better than regular incandescent; some are pressurized.

[a] There is a wide range of other fluorescent tubes which fall between the standard cool-white and the newer full-spectrum versions.
[b] CRI comparisons are only valid when comparing light sources with the same CCT.
[c] One-piece (integral) CF models use either an electronic or magnetic, built-in ballast.
Two-piece (modular) CF models use a ballast contained in the screw-in base and a replaceable fluorescent tube. Modular CF model currently use only magnetic ballasts. The wattages of the tube and the ballast need to be added to get the total wattage of a modular CF.
[d] Halogen bulbs need to operate at full wattage periodically to provide maximum performance.
See Chapter 16, "Light," for more information regarding lighting.

HIGH-INTENSITY DISCHARGE (HID) BULBS	COMPACT FLUORESCENT (CF) TUBES	COOL-WHITE FLUORESCENT TUBES	FULL-SPECTRUM FLUORESCENT TUBES[a]
Highly pressurized gas "glows" due to mercury vapor/UV radiation	Phosphors (some special) "glow" due to mercury vapor/UV radiation	Phosphors "glow" due to mercury vapor/UV radiation	Special phosphors "glow" due to mercury vapor/UV radiation
Wide range	Small-medium; typically larger than incandescent	Short-long; Usually T-12	Short-long; common size is 4'; T-12, T-10; T-8
Various			
Mercury: 4000-5900K Sodium: 2100K Metal Halides: 3000-3800K	2700-5000K 2700-2800K typical	4100-4200K	5000-7500K 5000-5900K typical
Mercury/Sodium: 22-43 Metal Halide: 65-75	82-85; 82 typical	52-69; 62 typical	90-98
Negligible			Variable; some fixtures use a separate, replaceable UV lamp
High	High-Very High	Low	High-Very High
High		Low-Medium	
Low-Very Low	Low	Medium	Low
High		Low-Medium	High
Very high (Metal Halide)	High-Very High	Medium-High	Very High
20,000-24,000	9,000-20,000; 10,000 typical	6000-7500	20,000-33,000
Yes[c]			
60	Magnetic ballast: 60/Electronic ballast: 20,000-35,000		
Very High	Low		
Point	Diffused		
High	Low-Medium	Low	
Possible	No		
No	No (may be available in the future)	No	
Very slow	Medium-Fast (Ballast dependent)		
Complex	Medium complexity	Less complex than full-spectrum	Sophisticated, especially T-10 & T-8s
	Fit into most incandescent lamp fixtures; may need adapter.	Standard fluorescent	Excellent visible spectrum; some have mid- and near-UV.

APPENDIX E

Becoming a Natural Vision Teacher

The Natural Vision Center of San Francisco has been training Natural Vision teachers for over a decade.

The Teacher Trainee does not need to have clear vision to become a Natural Vision teacher. If you already have clarity, you will simply be teaching others the correct vision habits you already have—and the ones your students want to relearn.

Natural Vision teachers who teach children to improve their sight are especially needed.

For more information regarding the Natural Vision Center of San Francisco's Certified Teacher Training Program, please write to:

Natural Vision Center of San Francisco
P.O. Box 16403
San Francisco, CA 94116–0403
USA

or call:

(415) 665-2010

APPENDIX F

Eye Charts

DISTANCE EYE CHART

Assemble the Distance Eye Chart as indicated on the next page, and then place twenty feet away.

The numbers underneath each line refer to acuity at twenty feet. For example, "200" underneath the letter "S" indicates this is the 20/200 line; "70" underneath the letters "T-C-H" indicates this is the 20/70 line.

For more information on acuity and eye charts, refer to Chapter 3, "Understanding Lenses and Prescriptions."

To assemble the Distance Eye Chart, cut along the six dashed lines on the next three pages. Then, align the bottom edge of the first page, ab, with the top edge of the second page, a'b'. Tape them together. Similarly, align the bottom edge of the second page, cd, with the top edge of the third page, c'd'. Tape them together. The chart can then be pasted onto cardboard.

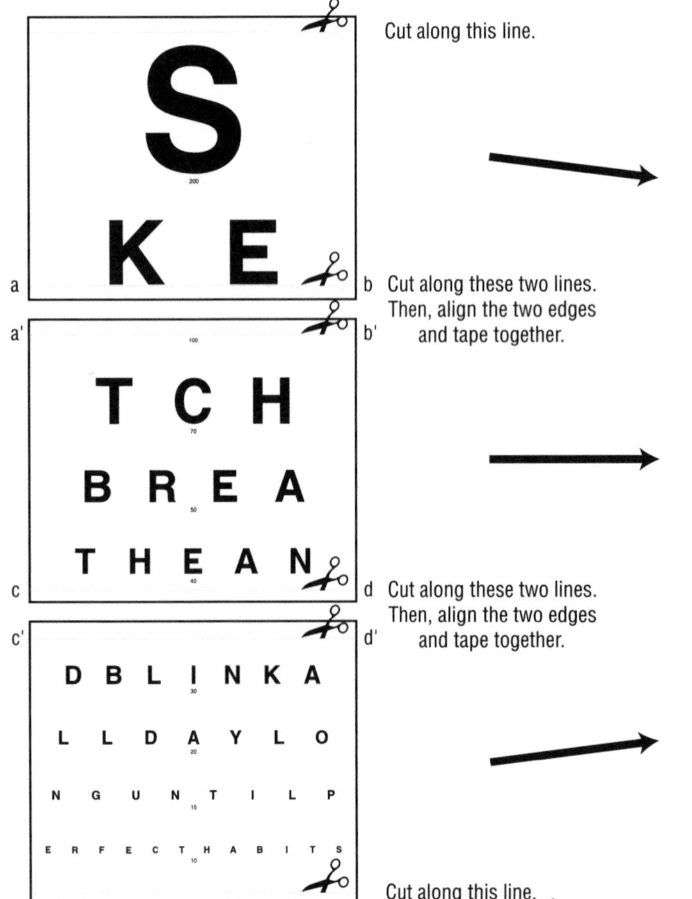

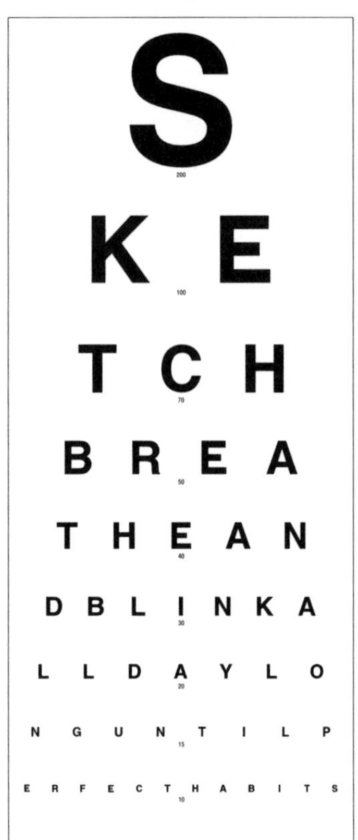

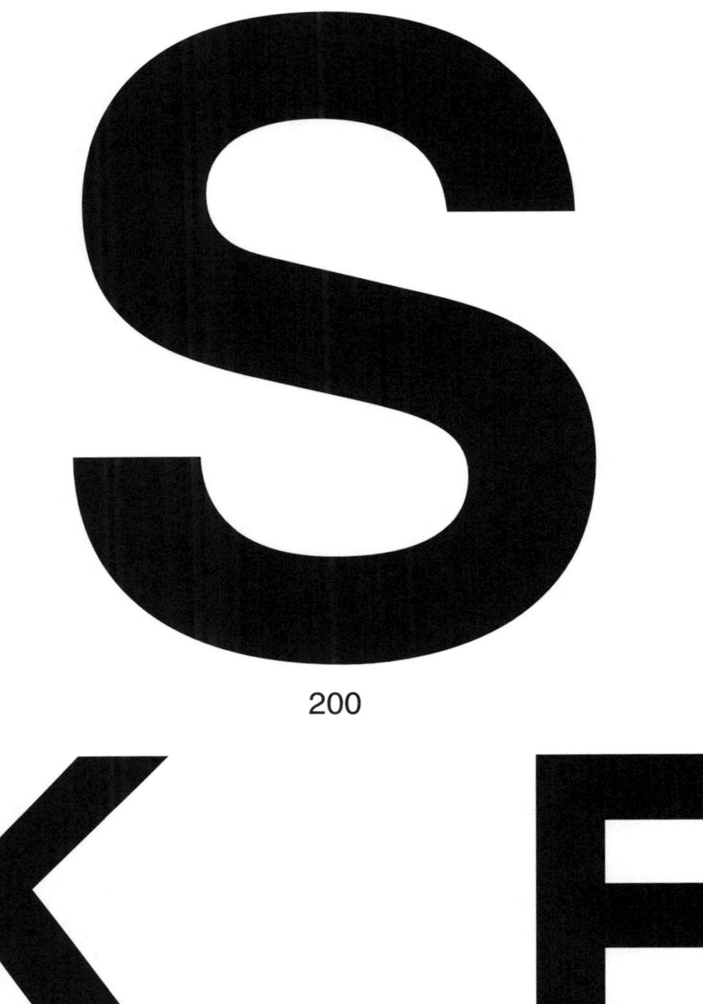
S
200
K E
a
b

a' b'

100

T C H

70

B R E A

50

T H E A N

40

c d

c' d'

D B L I N K A

30

L L D A Y L O

20

N G U N T I L P

15

E R F E C T H A B I T S

10

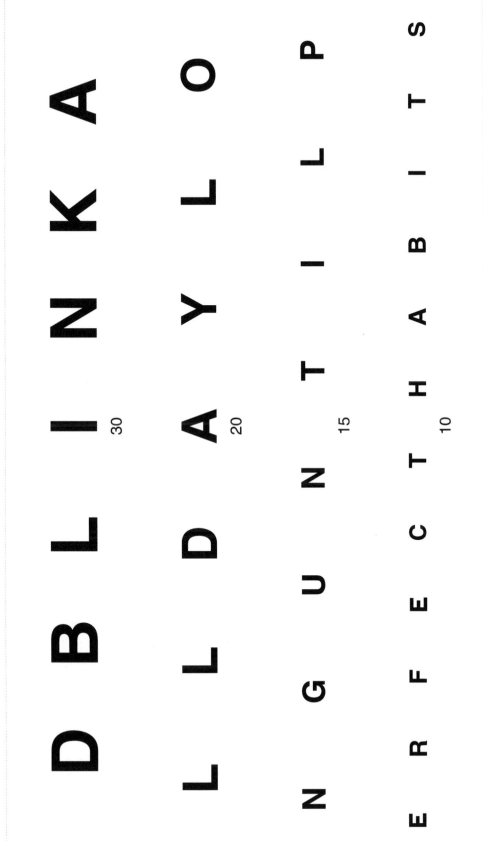

NEAR EYE CHART

Hold the Near Eye Chart (on the next page) fourteen inches away. The numbers underneath each line refer to acuity at a distance of fourteen inches. For example, "200" underneath the letter "S" indicates this is the 20/200 (equivalent) line; "70" underneath the letters "T-C-H" indicates this is the 20/70 line. The chart can be cut along the edges and pasted onto cardboard.

For more information on acuity and eye charts, refer to Chapter 3, "Understanding Lenses and Prescriptions." More small print can be found in *Figure 22–3, The Menace of Large Print: 7 and 6 point,* and *Figure 22–4, The Menace of Large Print: 5 to 1.5 point.*

S

200

K E

100

T C H

80

B R E A

70

T H E A N

50

D B L I N K A

40

L L D A Y L O

30

N G U N T I L P

25

E R F E C T H A B I T S

20

Appendix G

Additional Vision Stories

The following are additional fairy stories from the *Better Eyesight* magazines. The first story is located in Chapter 23, "Children and Schools."

From *Better Eyesight* magazine, February 1924:

> Editor's [Bates'] Note—We should read fairy stories for the benefit of our eyesight. It can be demonstrated that the imagination is a benefit to the vision and if fairy stories improve the imagination they will also improve the sight.
>
> THE BLACK FAIRY
>
> Zipp, bang, again and again, the cruel boys pasted the little boy with snowballs, calling: "Four eyes, four eyes," at him because he could not see well and wore glasses. The snow got down his neck, inside the collar of his little jacket, it stung the skin of his face, blurred his glasses and hurt him so that he cried in pain. He could not fight them, so he ran as fast as his little legs could travel. He stumbled and fell. It seemed to the little boy that he fell down a long, long way and kept on falling, falling so long that he could not remember how long it was. He closed his eyes, for only a moment it seemed, and then he stopped falling. When he opened his eyes and looked around him, he found himself lying on the grass, and the grass was soft and warm, like it is in fairy land. Above him the branches of the trees were moving from a light summer breeze. Around him were bright colored flowers, with the bees buzzing to and fro. Everywhere was the bright warm sunshine. He fell asleep for awhile and awoke feeling rested. On his breast lay a little puppy fox gazing kindly at his face. He touched it with his hand and gently smoothed the top of its head. Then another little fox puppy came out from the shadow of the grass, poked its nose close to the little boy's face and licked his cheek. Then two more came romping, toddling into view, all anxious to get close to the little boy and to be petted. But suddenly he lost all interest in the puppies, when the mother fox appeared with a tiny black fairy on her back. The puppies and the little boy crowded as close to her as they could. He petted the puppies while the mother fox looked on, happy and contented. A contented fox is not always, or often, seen. The mother fox said to the fairy, "Little Black Fairy, we found this boy all bruised and bloody. He is such a good lit-

tle boy and he is so gentle, kind and good that I wish someone would make him happy. That is why I asked you to come and see him."

And then the puppies began to all talk at once. They begged the fairy to be good to the little boy, the little boy whose heart was so full of love that he even loved baby foxes. The father fox called just then and all the foxes ran away quickly, so as not to keep him waiting. The little boy said to the black fairy:

"How beautiful you are. I like to look at you. Your eyes sparkle like the diamond in my mother's ring, when the sun shines on it, and your teeth are white like the pearl necklace my mother wears to parties; your lips are red like my sister's ruby ring; your ears are so like the fine sea shells at the seashore; your laugh sounds like the water bubbling over the pebbles in the brook, while your smile warms me inside my breast and makes me love you. Come closer to me little black fairy. Stay with me always and let me love you more than I have ever loved anybody else. When I look at you, the pain in my head leaves me, my eyes feel rested and cool, the light seems brighter. I can see everything clear, and the fog over the trees and flowers disappears."

After he spoke so nicely to the little black fairy, she giggled and laughed and blushed. She jerked her shoulders up and down, danced around on her toes, waved her hand to him, threw him many kisses and became so excited by her exertions she quite got out of breath. After she quieted down enough so she could speak she called to him:

"Oh, you dear little Foureyes, I love you for what you say. I love you so much that I want to help you as much as a fairy can help you. Let me improve your poor eyes, so that you will always have perfect sight without glasses. Love me enough and I will return your sight to normal. Never forget me. Please remember me so well that you will always see me, one tiniest part of me blacker than all the rest of me. See me on everything you look at, no matter how large or how small or how far away. Let me be your sweetheart fairy, the one little fairy you love best, and the world will be for you a heavenly place to live, with your eyes at rest with perfect sight as long as you are true to me, and never forget me."

And then she waved her hand to him and moved farther and farther away, until she appeared as small as a tiny black speck, the size of a period in the little boy's book. He remembered that he loved her, and did as she advised, and found that no matter how far away she was he was able to remember how she looked, one tiniest part of her blacker than all the rest. He loved her so much that he saw her better than everything else. The sight of her rested his eyes. And after she had disappeared from view he loved her so much better than the trees, the grass, the clouds, the flowers, that he believed he saw her better than anything else. And the better he imagined or remembered his little black fairy, or saw her in his heart better than all else, the more perfectly he saw the trees, the grass, the clouds and the flowers. He was true to his love, the little black fairy, and she was true to her promise to him that he would see perfectly without glasses as long as he remembered her perfectly. When he looked at a large tree she was a good-sized fairy. When he looked at a small blade of grass or a tiny flower, she was the tiniest little fairy that one could imagine.

His sight was good when he remembered how perfectly black she was; but, when she looked less black his sight was worse. He found that he had to remember his love perfectly, to be perfectly true to her in order to have perfect sight....

The next morning when his mother came into his room and wakened him with a kiss, he opened his eyes wide, with no dread of the bright sunlight which shone on his mother's face. He was all excited, laughing and talking eagerly, rapidly, of the good fortune that had come to him. Among other things he said:

"Oh, mother, I can see you without my glasses. I see the blue color of your eyes which I never saw before. The fog has gone from the pictures on the wall, I can look out the window and see the trees, the grass, the flowers, the people walking along the sidewalk, and there is father talking to a strange boy—oh no, he is the boy who lives next door. He is not a strange boy, but I see him so much clearer now without my glasses than I ever did before when I wore them. Aren't you glad? Please, I want to get dressed quickly, run down stairs and tell father all about it."

THE WHITE FAIRY

The teacher was tired. It was very warm, and through the open windows one heard in the distance the birds calling to each other. Her head was aching, her eyes throbbing with pain. She took off her glasses to rest her eyes and sat for a while with her eyes closed, and her head resting on her hands. And the students were tired, restless, anxious to get out in the bright sunshine and play on the cool green grass in the shade of the trees. Their eyes were continually looking out the windows.

George Smith saw her first, standing on the window sill waving her hands to the children, smiling such a beautiful smile of love with her tiny rosebud of a mouth. But it was her wonderful black eyes which smiled most. They sparkled and twinkled so merrily, they were so full of life and love and happiness. They were so cheery, so encouraging, so comforting, that all were intoxicated with delight. She was only a few inches tall, but every bit of her from the top of her head to her tiny feet was formed with a perfection of beauty rarely seen. And how graceful she was. She found her way somehow to the top of a vacant desk; and, after delighting the children for a few moments with the most wonderful, most delightful of fairy dances, sat herself down on the top of an inkstand—but she was not quiet a moment. Her feet and hands, her whole body seemed to swing from side to side, just like the pendulum of a clock swings; and, when you looked alternately from one eye to the other they seemed to swing also. This swing was very noticeable, and the strange thing about the swing was that it was so restful, and did the eyes of the children so much good. Those wearing glasses took them off and found that they could see the swinging eyes of the little white fairy as well as everything else quite perfectly. And the teacher noted that the fog over everything she formerly saw without glasses was gone, the pain in her eyes and head was gone. She saw everything clearly, so easily that she quite forgot that she had eyes....

Every time she read the Snellen Card it seemed to her that she read it more easily and better, and she found herself looking at the card every once in a while during the day. She acquired a certain amount of pleasure in looking at the card, and she found the students doing the same thing.

Standing twenty feet from the card, without her glasses, at the end of the month, she found that her vision with each eye was normal, and even a little better than the average normal vision. Furthermore her eyes, which formerly had bothered her more or less, although she wore glasses prescribed by a very prominent eye doctor, never gave her the relief that she now obtained without glasses, by reading the Snellen Card daily.

By teaching her students in the same way, she was very much pleased to note also that they were brighter and had better memories, and studied for longer periods without becoming tired or restless. Her attendance was better than it had ever been in any one month before.

One little boy told her that he no longer had headaches from studying his lessons, and that he could read what was written on the blackboard without half trying.

Other teachers became interested and they obtained the same beneficial results.

From *Better Eyesight* magazine, September 1924:

THE FAIRY SCHOOL

By George Guild

It was very hot. The school windows were wide open, but not a breath of air was stirring and the teacher and students were very uncomfortable from the heat. Freddie was only eight years old and he could not be blamed when his mind wandered from his work. In spite of all that he could do, his head would nod, his eyes would close and he would drop off to sleep. Then he heard the White Fairy talking to the children while she sat on the teacher's desk, waving her hands and dancing around to the amusement of the children. Her eyes were so bright and full of sympathy, kindness and love that not one of the boys or girls could keep their eyes from her face. She said:

"Now watch me as I swing from side to side. Please, all of you stand up, with your feet slightly apart, facing me, and move your whole body, your head and your eyes from side to side while I am moving.

"Now sit down, close your eyes, and cover them with the palms of your hands, resting your elbows on your desk. While you are doing this remember me standing up, smiling at you and loving you with all my heart." In five minutes she said: "Now open your eyes and watch me while I dance."

Freddie noticed how much more distinctly he could now see the face of the White Fairy.

Then all of a sudden the White Fairy stopped dancing. At first, the smiling eyes were very clear, but in a few seconds or so they began to blur and fade away. It was not long before he was unable to see her face or her tiny feet; they had become just a blur. He felt uncomfortable, and he must have looked uncomfortable because the White Fairy called out: "Freddie, swing your head from side to side." Freddie was only too glad to swing from side to side, and it was not long before he became able to see her tiny feet, her eyes and face just as clearly as before.

Then the White Fairy said: "Now, Freddie, close your eyes and remember me as well as you can. If you love me you will remember me."

And Freddie closed his eyes, and I am quite sure that he remembered the face of the White Fairy, because he loved her so much. After he had kept his eyes closed for a few minutes the White Fairy called out:

"Open your eyes and tell me what you see." And when Freddie opened his eyes the schoolroom was gone. It seemed as though he was in the woods; it seemed as though he was a fairy also and that all the other children were fairies, and he enjoyed being a fairy because when he imitated the look of love on the face of the White Fairy he thought of his mother and his father, his brothers and his sisters and other people that he could remember. He seemed to love all of them a great deal more than he had ever loved anybody in his life. The White Fairy invited him to dance with her. It was very strange to Freddie that he could dance for a long time without getting tired, and the more he danced the better did he feel. Then the White Fairy told him to stop dancing, and while he sat on the grass she walked around him, touching his head with the tips of her fingers until he fell asleep.

When he woke up the teacher was petting his head and loving him. At once he called out: "Oh, teacher, the White Fairy taught me to dance, how to see, and now I feel just like studying." When the teacher heard him say this she said:

"Freddie, I am curious. Show me what the White Fairy helped you to do." And so, before the whole school Freddie showed how the White Fairy taught him to swing, shift and palm, and how she showed him how staring and straining made his sight worse and that by moving his head and eyes from side to side his sight got better. Right away the children all did it, and after they had practiced with Freddie for a short time they were all very happy and told the teacher that they also felt a great deal better, and, like Freddie, they wanted to get to work because they felt just like studying.

From *Better Eyesight* magazine, June 1925:

THE SAND MAN

By George M. Guild

The little boy sat on the lap of his mother in a rocking chair. His name was Freddie. He had had a long day and was very, very tired. His mother rocked him back and forth, petted him with her cool hands and quieted him with her frequent kisses. He kept telling her: "Oh, mother, my eyes hurt, my head hurts, my arms hurt, my feet hurt, I am all hurt, and I am all tired out."

While she rocked him back and forth, a little old man came into the room with a bag of sand over his shoulder—the Sand Man. Freddie did not see him coming and Freddie's mother did not see him coming, but when he threw a little sand into their eyes they both became very sleepy. Freddie sat up and looked around, stretched his arms, and his big tortoise-shell glasses fell from his eyes onto the floor. Freddie jumped down to get his glasses, and then he saw the Sand Man pick them up from the floor and hold them behind his back where Freddie could not get them. Freddie was very indignant and scolded the Sand Man for taking his glasses, but the little old man smiled and said: "Do they help you to see?"

Freddie answered: "No, my eyes feel all right until I put them on in the morning, and then things are blurred, and my eyes begin to pain; but the Doctor said that if I did not wear them all the time, I would most surely go blind."

The Sand Man said to him: "Would you like to go with me and talk it over with the fairies? They don't like to see little boys wearing glasses."

So the little boy took the hand of the Sand Man and they ran, skipping and jumping around, out of the room, into the hall, down the stairs, out the front door, through the front gate, and then into the woods. There the moon was shining very brightly through the trees and lighted up a space where thousands of fairies were dancing, laughing, and joking and having a good time. Freddie was so glad to see the fairies, because in his heart he knew there were fairies, but all his uncles and aunts and cousins and grown people generally laughed at him and made fun of him for believing in fairies. When the fairies saw him coming, they all ran to him and climbed up on his shoulders and the top of his head, sat on his ears, tickled him under the chin, and made him laugh, and he had a good time from the very start.

The fairies had some difficulty in teaching him how to dance their way, but they finally got him to go through movements of various kinds. The one he liked best of all was to turn his head, eyes, and his whole body as far to the right and to the left as he possibly could without trying to see the things in front of him, which move in the opposite direction. He never heard fairies sing, but he heard them now and he liked the sound of their voices. He tried to sing with them, but he did so poorly and his voice was so harsh that he could not keep on singing. But the fairies encouraged him, and told him how to hold his lips and his tongue, and how to breathe, and very soon he was singing just as loud and just as musically as the rest of them. This was very strange, indeed, because he sang songs that he had never heard before, that is, consciously. Of course, when he was asleep, he would dream, perhaps, of the fairies singing, but when he woke up in the morning the dreams of the fairies, like all other dreams, were usually soon forgotten.

What surprised him most of all was the fact that his eyes did not bother him. He was no longer sleepy, no longer tired; every nerve in his body was just as happy as he was. There was no pain, only a feeling of delicious joyousness that no words could describe. Not only were his eyes comfortable, free from pain and fatigue, but he was able to see the fairies, the trees, the flowers, the birds, and the toadstools where the fairies sat to rest. It seemed to him that he could see through the trees, that he could see through the ground down into the other side of the Earth where China was. He felt as though he could see the Chinese fairies almost as well as he could see the fairies that surrounded him. His eyes never kept still, they were moving in all directions, and the more they moved the better they felt. When his eyes moved in one direction, it seemed as though his hands and feet moved in the other direction, but one could not catch the other. The movement of his eyes was all the time missing the movement of his toes. They seemed like two railroad trains on parallel tracks, which pass each other going in the opposite direction at full speed. He noticed that the fairies were moving in the same direction that his body was moving; the Sand Man, the trees, the grass, everything was moving with his body, opposite to the movement of his eyes. It seemed a very strange thing to him. The strangest thing about it was that for the first time in his life he felt his eyes were rested, although they were moving, and that for the first time in his life also, his body, and his nerves were at rest although they were, as he thought or imagined, constantly moving.

The next morning when his mother came to awaken him, she found him looking over toward the trees and smiling. Every once in a while he would laugh out loud, as loud as he could scream. His mother was worried and she said to him: "What is the trouble; why are you up so early? Why are you laughing, and why do you look over toward the trees?"

Then he told her what had happened to him on the previous night when the Sand Man took him over to see the fairies. She smiled indulgently, as mothers will, but the next question she asked him was the most important one of all: "Where are your glasses?"

Freddie looked up into the face of his mother, who leaned over and kissed him. He threw his arms around her and pressed his cheek against hers and said: "Mother, please forgive me. The Sand Man took them. The fairies told me how to see perfectly without glasses, so that I would have no pain and would never get tired. I want to get up early in the morning every morning and go over into the woods and play; play where the fairies played, where the fairies eliminated my poor sight."

From *Better Eyesight* magazine, December 1928:

PANSY LAND

By Emily C. Lierman

Once upon a time in a town near the Pacific Coast there lived a boy named George who suffered intensely from poor eyesight. One day he met a girl named Christine. The little boy had heard that Christine knew the great secret of good eyesight and begged her to tell him what he could do to improve his eyes. It did not take Christine long to teach George how to use his eyes right and keep from straining them. Christine soon found that George was not lonely like she was, for one day he brought Amy with him, the girl who made many children happy with her stories. She was beautiful to look at and had many friends. George and Amy were constant pals, and helped to make Christine happy. Amy's eyes also became wonderfully bright through Christine's guidance and help, and everyone in Pansy Land wanted to know how this came about.

One day these three friends of *Better Eyesight* took a trip to the land of pansies. Before they were allowed to enter the gate, they had to seek admission from the doorkeeper. They waited until he went to see whether or not the pansies had gone to bed, as it was near closing time. He soon came back to them and told them to enter, that the pansies still had their eyes open and would welcome them. They walked a great distance and found that with the exception of narrow paths, everything was covered with miles and miles of pansies. There were yellow pansies with eyes as blue as the skies, brown and tan pansies with rose-colored eyes, and others dressed in all the colors of the rainbow. All of them were swaying with the gentle breeze and they were most beautiful to see.

Suddenly, a jolly gnome appeared before them. They noticed that his eyes were shining brightly and that he had the kindliest face of anybody they had ever seen. George knew him right away. He said, "This is Horatio the Great. It is he who first discovered how to improve people's sight without glasses and help those who had pain and other troubles with their eyes." George also remarked that he had the biggest heart that anybody ever had, and was the best friend of poor children all over the world. Horatio the Great stood by listening to these kind remarks but was too modest to make any reply. He just listened.

After George got through talking, the kindly gnome invited them to sit in his parlor, which was made of the loveliest pink mushrooms imaginable. He told them to place their palms over their eyes and not to think of anything bad or wrong and then to make a wish. They wished that they could be two very little girls and a very little boy again.

All of a sudden, there was a rumbling sound like thunder, and George, Amy, and Christine became very much frightened. The good gnome knew what had happened. He said, "Take down your hands and let me see how badly you have been frightened, when there was nothing at all to be frightened about." He looked into their eyes and said, "Because you were frightened, you began to strain and your eyesight is now poor. You must be calm like I am, no matter how much trouble or worry you might have or how frightened you become. Don't you know that fear always affects good eyes and makes them poor?"

He then told them again to cover their eyes with the palms of their hands and he would tell them what caused their fright. He said, "You know I have many helpers in Pansy Land; some of them are my good gnomes. It was the good gnomes that you heard when they returned to their places on the roof of my palace. Don't be alarmed."

After this remark, there was no more fear and no more eyestrain. He then told them to remove their hands from their eyes. When they opened their eyes again he held in his hand a shining light, which was really a star on the end of a wand. With this he touched their eyelids and they were little children again.

When he touched the lonely little girl he said, "Now your name is Crystal, because you will always have crystal clear eyes. You will improve the sight of children and grown-ups all over the world in time to come. You are ordered to finish your work here on the West Coast of this great big world where many people want you. You must be strong in your mind and heart and know that when your enemies want to hurt you, the good gnome, Horatio the Great, will always be standing by you and will keep you from harm. You must never be afraid."

Amy and George stood by listening with their eyes wide open, but blinking all the time to be sure that they would not strain and displease Horatio the Great.

The good gnome then touched little Amy with the shining star and said, "You will do greater things than you have ever done, now that you have better eyesight and no longer need glasses. You will go to many boys and girls and you will take away all pain and sorrow from those who suffer with eye trouble. Sometimes you will go alone, but most of the time little Georgie will take you in his chariot so that you will not be weary in well-doing." This pleased little Georgie because he did not ever want to be separated from Amy, who had always made happiness and joy for him. Little Crystal knew in her heart how much they loved each other and this made her very happy.

The kindly gnome, Horatio the Great, then placed his wand with the shining star on the head of little George and said, "My book, which tells you how to take care of people's eyes, will help you to understand the work that you have to do. What you must enjoy is helping people with eyestrain. I give you my special blessing because of the good work you have already done. You will take Crystal and Amy to your beautiful home in Marston Hills."

This made Georgie very happy. His beautiful home has a frog pond in a lovely garden. In the pond lives one large frog. He has many friends who live near him all the time. Their names are Climbing Rose, American Beauty, Geranium, Calla Lily, Honey Suckle, and many others that would take much time to name.

This kindly frog is never thirsty and is ever ready to share with you the sparkling water that flows from his mouth. Even the frog has his work to do. In the pond directly under the throne on which the frog sits during the day, there lives a family by the name of Goldfish. Not so long ago the family increased in great numbers. They are lively and hungry all the time, and Amy and George always feed them. All of the goldfish have perfect eyesight. The frog will tell you that at no time is eyestrain allowed in his kingdom. He has for his kindly assistant Mary, who looks after things not only in the garden, but in the house that George built.

Horatio the Great led the procession to a little woodland which belonged to the pansies. Little Crystal noticed that a beautiful palm had been crushed on one side and many leaves were scattered on the grassy carpet. The two little girls and the little boy closed their eyes while the gnome told them the story of the crushed palm, and what had happened on that day. He told how the Queen of the Fairies had been honored by all the fairies of Pansy Land. No disorder is ever allowed, because it causes much work and strain to those who are the care-takers, but on this special occasion when the Queen of the Fairies that live all over the world had been given a reception, he made excuses for the fairies because of the disorder of the place.

From there he led them away to the center of the pansy bed that had the most colors. He told them to palm again and remember the color of any pansy they saw. While their eyes were closed and covered, the good gnome passed his wand with the shining star over the heads of the pansies. When Crystal, Amy and Georgie opened their eyes, lo and behold, there was a beautiful fairy on the top of every pansy, right before their eyes. What a beautiful sight it was and how happy these children were. The sun never shone more brightly; never in their lives did they smell more wonderful perfume. Immediately there was a beautiful fairy dance and the more the children blinked, the more wonderful the fairies danced.

All good things must come to an end, for a little time at least, and soon the kindly gnome remarked that it was bed time for the fairies and the pansies. Horatio the Great, with his kindly manner, led the way to the gate and gently bowed before the two little girls and the little boy, who honored him with their smiles and good wishes and said good bye for a while.

Georgie remembered what he had promised the gnome, and placing little Amy and Crystal in his chariot, drove on to his home in the hills to the frog pond and the flowers.

Because of their happiness, the good gnome did not wish to change them into grown-ups again, so they will always be children and live happily ever after.

Index

P